Frontiers in Nanobiotechnology

(Volume 1)

Advances in Biosensing Technology for Medical Diagnosis

Edited by

Han-Sheng Chuang
*Department of Biomedical Engineering,
National Cheng Kung University,
Tainan,
Taiwan*

&

Yi-Ping Ho
*Department of Biomedical Engineering,
The Chinese University of Hong Kong,
Shatin,
Hong Kong,
China, SAR*

Frontiers in Nanobiotechnology

Volume # 1

Advances in Biosensing Technology for Medical Diagnosis

Editors: Han-Sheng Chuang and Yi-Ping Ho

ISBN (Online): 978-981-14-6480-5

ISBN (Print): 978-981-14-6476-8

ISBN (Paperback): 978-981-14-6478-2

need for a court order if at any point you breach any terms of this License Agreement. In no event will any delay or failure by Bentham Science Publishers in enforcing your compliance with this License Agreement constitute a waiver of any of its rights.

3. You acknowledge that you have read this License Agreement, and agree to be bound by its terms and conditions. To the extent that any other terms and conditions presented on any website of Bentham Science Publishers conflict with, or are inconsistent with, the terms and conditions set out in this License Agreement, you acknowledge that the terms and conditions set out in this License Agreement shall prevail.

Bentham Science Publishers Pte. Ltd.
80 Robinson Road #02-00
Singapore 068898
Singapore
Email: subscriptions@benthamscience.net

BENTHAM
SCIENCE

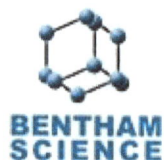

CONTENTS

PREFACE

Medical diagnosis is set to discover the cause of a person's symptoms and to find the right treatment. An accurate medical diagnosis made in a timely manner is, therefore, the key to effective medical interventions and the subsequent survivorship. The existing clinical measures, usually involving invasive procedures, expensive and tedious operations, long turnaround time, or sometimes labor-intensive steps, may delay the clinical decisions. Biosensing technology is flourishing rapidly in recent years because of the advancement of micro/nano-fabrications. Despite the booming in all sorts of modern biosensors, most clinicians still prefer conventional medical instruments in diagnosis or making their therapeutic decisions. The barriers preventing the clinical communities from embracing new diagnostic technologies may be attributed to different levels of issues, including reproducible clinical validation, regulatory hurdles, compensations for the coverage of a new diagnostic procedure, and ethical concerns. To disseminate the cutting-edge diagnostic tools into routine clinical practice, the research and healthcare communities shall join the efforts to maximize the potential of recent biosensing advances. As a headway to broaden the readers' horizon and to guide the readers in tailoring up-to-date biosensing techniques for specific embodiments, this book is aimed to bridge the gap between the scientific and clinical communities by providing valuable insights on the working principle of advanced biosensing technologies, and the scientific/clinical validations in establishing the analytical measures, especially, in medical applications. The inclusion of adequate background on the advancement in biosensing is expected to clear the hesitations of healthcare providers for adopting new diagnostic methods, encouraging the policy makers to reshape the regulations and compensations for diagnostic research and development, educating the next generation scientists to continue the efforts, as well as exposing the general audience to the latest development in relevant fields.

To this end, this book is organized in three parts, including part I: fundamentals of biosensors, part II: state-of-the-art biosensing technology, and part III: clinical practice with medical diagnostics. The opening chapter in part I describes the essentials of biosensors in medical diagnosis and how to evaluate the performance of a biosensor. In chapter 2, the micro-/nan--scale fabrication techniques are introduced to lay the foundation for subsequent realizations of biosensors in the following chapters. In part II, biosensors that cover five representative technological domains, including electrochemistry, electrical engineering, biochemistry, optical engineering, and fluid mechanics, are respectively discussed in chapters 3 through 7. In the last part, biosensors applied for different clinical purposes are specifically discussed in chapters 8 through 12 to highlight the potential use of biosensors in the clinical setting in the foreseeable future.

The editors are sincerely grateful to all the authors for their efforts in preparing the excellent and up-to-date chapters contained in the book. On behalf of these world-renowned experts in the field, the editors expect that this book will give the readers: (a) the state-of-the-art biosensing technologies developed in broad fields, (b) specific examples of novel biosensors used in medical diagnosis, and (c) step-by-step guidance of micro- and nano-fabrications in current biosensors. We hope readers who are interested in learning advances in biosensing technology may find this book not only containing plenty of scientific merits in this emerging field but also as informative as a tool book in their daily life.

Han-Sheng Chuang
National Cheng Kung University
Tainan
Taiwan

&

Yi-Ping Ho
The Chinese University of Hong Kong
Shatin
Hong Kong
China, SAR

List of Contributors

An-Chi Wei	Graduate Institute of Biomedical Electronics and Bioinformatics, National Taiwan University, Taipei, Taiwan
Birgitta Ruth Knudsen	Department of Molecular Biology and Genetics, Aarhus University, Denmark
Ching-Hua Lu	Department of Neurology, China Medical University Hospital, Taiwan School of Medicine, China Medical University, Taiwan
Changchun Liu	Mechanical Engineering and Applied Science, School of Engineering and Applied Sciences, University of Pennsylvania, Philadelphia, PA, USA UCONN Health, University of Connecticut, USA
Dean Chou	Department of Mechanical Engineering, National Central University, Taoyuan, Taiwan
Donghyun Kim	School of Electrical and Electronic Engineering,, Yonsei University, 50 Yonsei-ro, Seodaemun-gu, Seoul, Republic of Korea, South Korea
Di-Hua Luo	Department of Psychology, College of Science, National Taiwan University, Taipei, Taiwan
Eunseop Yeom	School of Mechanical Engineering, Pusan National University, Busan, South Korea
Hao-Hsiang Chang	Department of Family Medicine, National Taiwan University Hospital, Taipei, Taiwan
Huan Hu	ZJUI Institute, Zhejiang University, Haining, Zhejiang Province, 314400, China
Huong T. Vu	Department of Biomedical Engineering, The University of Texas at Austin, USA
Hsien-Chang Chang	Department of Biomedical Engineering, National Cheng Kung University, Tainan, 70101, Taiwan
Hsin-Chih Yeh	Department of Biomedical Engineering, The University of Texas at Austin, USA Department of Biomedical Engineering and Texas Materials Institutes, The University of Texasat Austin, USA
Jinzhao Song	Mechanical Engineering and Applied Science, School of Engineering and Applied Sciences, University of Pennsylvania, Philadelphia, PA, USA
Jacky Fong-Chuen Loo	Department of Biomedical Engineering, The Chinese University of Hong Kong, Hong Kong, SAR Department of Neuroscience and Biomedical Engineering, Aalto University School of Science, Aalto, Finland
Kamilla Vandsø Petersen	Department of Molecular Biology and Genetics, Aarhus University, Denmark
Ko-Hong Lin	Graduate Institute of Biomedical Electronics and Bioinformatics, National Taiwan University, Taipei, Taiwan
Lærke Bay Marcussen	Department of Biomedicine, Aarhus University, Denmark Department of Molecular Biology and Genetics, Aarhus University, Denmark

Lei Li	CAS Key Laboratory of Cryogenics, Technical Institute of Physics and Chemistry, Chinese Academy of Science, Beijing 100190, China
Lester U. Vinzons	Graduate Institute of Biomedical Engineering, National Chung Hsing University, Taichung, Taiwan
Michael G. Mauk	Mechanical Engineering and Applied Science, School of Engineering and Applied Sciences, University of Pennsylvania, Philadelphia, PA, USA
Marianne Smedegaard Hede	VPCIR.COM, Denmark
Neil Adrian P. Ondevilla	Department of Biomedical Engineering, National Cheng Kung University, Tainan, 70101, Taiwan
Po-Yen Chen	Department of Mechanical Engineering, National Central University, Taoyuan, Taiwan
Ru-Yi Youh	Department of Mechanical Engineering, National Central University, Taoyuan, Taiwan
Seongmin Im	School of Electrical and Electronic Engineering,, Yonsei University, 50 Yonsei-ro, Seodaemun-gu, Seoul, Republic of Korea, South Korea
Soonwoo Hong	Department of Biomedical Engineering, The University of Texas at Austin, USA
Shu-Ping Lin	Graduate Institute of Biomedical Engineering, National Chung Hsing University, Taichung, Taiwan Research Center for Sustainable Energy and Nanotechnolog, National Chung Hsing University, Taichung, Taiwan
Tien-Chun Tsai	Department of Biomedical Engineering, National Cheng Kung University, Tainan, 70101, Taiwan
Tza-Huei Wang	Department of Biomedical Engineering, Johns Hopkins University, Baltimore, Maryland, USA Department of Mechanical Engineering, Johns Hopkins University, Baltimore, Maryland, USA
Wonju Lee	Korea Electrotechnology Research Institute, 111 Hanggaul-ro, Ansan, Gyeonggi-do, Republic of Korea, South Korea
Wei-Min Liu	Department of Chemistr, Fu Jen Catholic University, New Taipei City, Taiwan
Wen-Wei Tseng	Graduate Institute of Biomedical Electronics and Bioinformatics, National Taiwan University, Taipei, Taiwan
Xianbo Qiu	College of Information Science and Technology, Beijing University of Chemical Technology, Beijing, China
Yu-De Lin	Graduate Institute of Biomedical Electronics and Bioinformatics, National Taiwan University, Taipei, Taiwan
Yi-Chia Wei	Department of Neurology, Keelung Chang Gung Memorial Hospital, and Chang Gung University College of Medicine, Keelung, Taiwan
Yi-Ping Ho	Department of Biomedical Engineering, The Chinese University of Hong Kong, Hong Kong, SAR Centre for Novel Biomaterials, The Chinese University of Hong Kong, Hong Kong, SAR

Yen-Cheng Chao Department of Chemistr, Fu Jen Catholic University, New Taipei City, Taiwan

Yi Zhang School of Mechanical and Aerospace Engineering, Nanyang Technological University, Singapore

Yu-Ling Chang Department of Psychology, College of Science, National Taiwan University, Taipei, Taiwan

Zih-Hua Chen Graduate Institute of Biomedical Electronics and Bioinformatics, National Taiwan University, Taipei, Taiwan

CHAPTER 1

Essentials of Biosensors

Jacky Fong-Chuen Loo[1,2,*], **Tza-Huei Wang**[3,4] and **Yi-Ping Ho**[1,5]

[1] *Department of Biomedical Engineering, The Chinese University of Hong Kong, Hong Kong, SAR*

[2] *Department of Neuroscience and Biomedical Engineering, Aalto University School of Science, Aalto, Finland*

[3] *Department of Biomedical Engineering, Johns Hopkins University, Baltimore, Maryland, USA*

[4] *Department of Mechanical Engineering, Johns Hopkins University, Baltimore, Maryland, USA*

[5] *Centre for Novel Biomaterials, The Chinese University of Hong Kong, Hong Kong, SAR*

Abstract: The primary objective of medical diagnosis is to precisely detect the disease onset in a timely manner for effective treatments. The rising demand in medical diagnosis, given the rapidly aging populations, increasing population mobility and complex healthcare needs, has called for support of effective diagnostic approaches, where biosensors have provided well-suited solutions. To this end, biosensors are typically examined by the yardstick of specificity, sensitivity, dynamic range, and reliability or robustness. The advancements in biomarker discoveries and signal transduction schemes have led to biosensors of improved performances; however, challenges remain particularly for translating the biosensors into clinical uses. This chapter is therefore aimed to prepare the audience with essentials of biosensors and roadblocks associated with clinical translations. Comprehension of these prerequisites is expected to accelerate the development of biosensors from lab bench to bed.

Keywords: Molecular biosensing, Medical diagnosis, Point-of-care, Signal transduction.

INTRODUCTION

The ultimate goal in medical diagnosis is to pinpoint the onset of diseases precisely for timely and proper treatments. The demand has continued to escalate given the rapidly aging populations, increasing population mobility and complex healthcare needs. Detection of clinically relevant target biomarkers has long been a way for accurate medical diagnosis. Clinicians have been using an optical mic-

* **Corresponding author Jacky Fong-Chuen Loo:** Department of Biomedical Engineering, The Chinese University of Hong Kong, Hong Kong, SAR & Department of Neuroscience and Biomedical Engineering, Aalto University School of Science, Aalto, Finland; E-mail: jacky.loo@aalto.fi

Han-Sheng Chuang & Yi-Ping Ho (Eds.)

roscope to detect *Mycobacterium tuberculosis*, the bacilli responsible for tuberculosis, from samples of the patients as early as in the late 19th century [1]. Radioimmunoassay, a conventional biochemical assay relying on the interaction between the antigen and the antibody, has been developed in the 1950s [2]. These two tests utilize cell staining techniques, radioactive materials processing and operation of scintillation counters. However, in order to obtain reliable results for appropriate downstream treatment, these traditional detection methods required a centralized laboratory and well-trained technicians to handle a series of laboratory processes, including sample pre-processing, preparation of reagents, performing assays, operating equipment, and interpretation of obtained results. Take the COVID-19 pandemic in 2020 as an example, hospitals and centralized laboratories have been overloaded worldwide. Biosensors suit the so-called point-of-care (POC) setting may help to delay the outbreak by enabling self-diagnosis of viral infection or immunity without the needs of advanced equipment or trained staff [3].

Defined as "a device that uses specific biochemical reactions mediated by isolated enzymes, immunosystems, tissues, organelles or whole cells to detect chemical compounds usually by electrical, thermal or optical signals" by the International Union of Pure and Applied Chemistry (IUPAC), biosensors have become a natural choice for the applications in medical diagnostics, since the first invention of glucose biosensors based on electrochemical sensing in the 1970s [4]. The development has further fueled by the advanced engineering and biotechnological approaches starting from the 1980s [5, 6]. The earliest biosensors are mostly based on catalytic systems, integrating enzymes, cellular organelles, or even whole microorganisms with transducers that convert a biological response into a digital electronic signal [7]. Later advancements in the discovery of new biomarkers and exploration of novel biosensing mechanisms have led to the booming interests of molecular diagnosis based on the detection of small molecules or nucleic acids, setting the foundation of the POC diagnosis. In addition to solving the traditional medical diagnosis, the recent development on advanced technologies, such as microelectromechanical systems (MEMS), nanophotonics, or methodologies, such as CRISPR/Cas9 system for both genetic biomarker recognition and signal amplification, can be quickly adopted in the development of novel biosensors that continuously improve its performance and accuracy for medical diagnosis [8].

Based on the definition of IUPAC, a biosensor shall comprise the following three parts: a bioreceptor, a transducer and a signal readout unit, as illustrated in the schematics of Fig. (1). Bioreceptors can be regarded as recognition elements, such as antibodies, aptamers, or nucleic acid probes, that bind to the target analytes specifically [9, 10]. Binding affinity and reaction kinetics between the recognition element and the target jointly determine the sensitivity and dynamic range for the "sensing" of targeted biomolecules, while the stability under different conditions or prolonged storage determines the reliability of biosensing. Interpretation of the acquired data perhaps remains challenging in POC diagnosis. Optical and electrochemical are the two most commonly employed approaches to transduce the "sensed" events into detectable signals. Absorbance, fluorescence and luminescence sensing mechanisms are commonly used in the optical-based sensors, while potentiometric and amperometric sensing mechanisms are commonly used in the electrochemical-based sensors for signal readout [11]. For optical transducers, quantification of the detectable "photons" to signify the presence of targeted analyst is achieved with optoelectronic components such as photodiodes, photomultipliers and charge-coupled devices, which convert the detectable "photons" into electronic signal readout for downstream computation and display. For electrochemical based transducers, electrodes coated with enzymes are often applied to detect the oxidation of the targeted analyte, such as glucose, upon catalysis by an oxidoreductase enzyme, *i.e.* glucose oxidase [12]. The electrons liberated during this redox reaction are shuttled to the electrode through artificial electron acceptors or mediators, *i.e.* ferrocene, where the current generated and detected by a potentiostat is directly related to the concentration of targeted analytes.

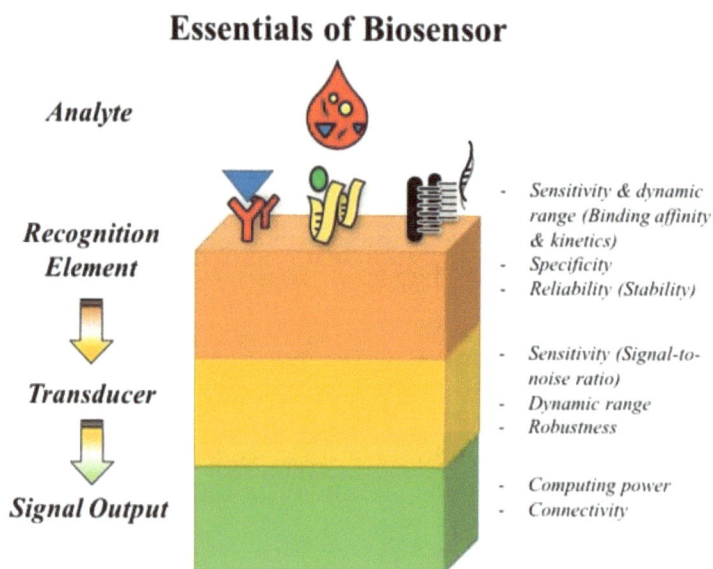

Fig. (1). Schematics of a biosensor. The recognition elements (*i.e.* antibodies, aptamers, and nucleic acid probes) are essential for the specific capture of the corresponding target analytes. The interaction between the recognition element and the target analyte is registered by a detector and subsequently transduced into a signal output in the form of for example fluorescence or electricity. The associated assessment criteria are listed on the right.

Targeting POC diagnostics, biosensors are typically examined by at least the following yardsticks: specificity, sensitivity, dynamic range, and reliability or robustness. These performance factors may be interlinked and shall be considered based upon the needs. Among these, specificity and sensitivity are equally important in most cases. Take the matrix of specificity and sensitivity as illustrated in Fig. **(2)** for example, high specificity and sensitivity is the best scenario. For screening of viral infection, such as the Zika virus, by detecting the viral RNA in urine, where the viral nucleic acids may be presented as low as a few copies, the diagnostic strategy would opt for high sensitivity [13]. For sensing of blood glucose and sodium, which lies in a concentration range of millimolar, high sensitivity is unnecessary, but sufficiently high specificity is critical [14]. In this chapter, we intend to give the audience a brief introduction to the essential elements of a biosensor and the evaluators for the development of a reliable biosensor particularly in the POC setting in medical diagnosis.

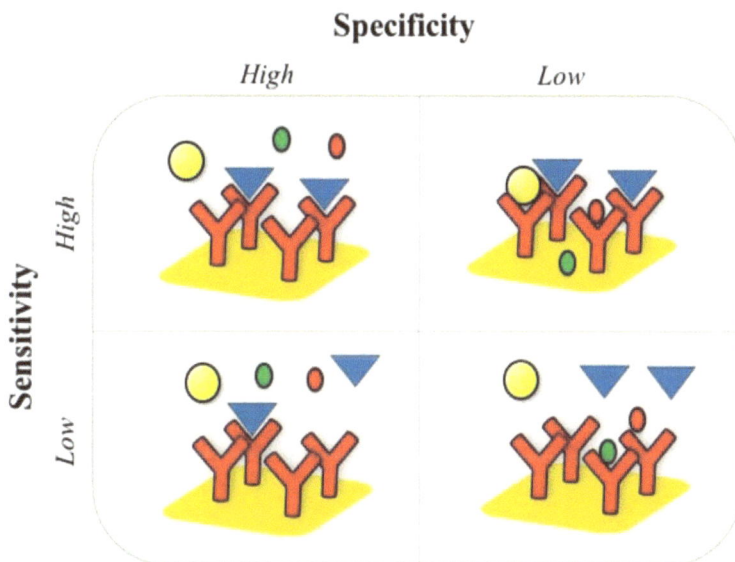

Fig. (2). The matrix of sensitivity and specificity in biosensing. Possible scenarios are exemplified by the interaction between the antibody (red y-shape) and the target analyte (blue triangle). (Top left) High sensitivity and specificity: specific interaction between the two entities with high sensitivity; (Top right) High sensitivity but low specificity: non-specific interaction although the detection sensitivity is sufficiently high; (Bottom left) High specificity but low sensitivity: incapable of detecting target analytes of low concentration; (Bottom right) Low sensitivity and specificity: non-target molecules are detected.

SPECIFICITY

In the clinical setting, specificity may be broadly referred to as the specificity of both disease confirmation and biosensing of targeted biomarkers. Specificity in disease confirmation is often optimized by screening biomarkers with high clinical relevance to a particular disease, such as neurodegenerative disorders and infectious diseases. For example, 2N4R tau protein and Aβ oligomers are currently recognized as specific biomarkers for the diagnosis of Alzheimer's disease, whereas C-reactive protein, Interleukin 6 (IL-6) and microRNA-16 are biomarkers associated with sepsis [15, 16].

The specificity of biosensing hinges heavily on the recognition element, as hinted by the configuration in Fig. (1). "Specific" interaction has implied not only a high binding affinity between the recognition element and target analyte but also a low binding affinity between the recognition element to non-targets. Non-specific binding to non-targeted analytes resulted in the so-called false positive signals, which may lead to unnecessary treatments and a waste of clinical resources. For nucleic acids, the detection relies on the Watson-Crick base pairing. The nucleic acid probes may be designed to identify complementary strand or discriminate one-base-mismatched sequence in the targets [17]. For the case of protein markers, antibody fragments, synthetic receptors, and aptamers have been developed to specifically bind to the targeted proteins. Antibody fragments, relying on specific binding between the variable fragment (Fv) region and the target antigen, do not have the fragment crystallizable region (Fc region) to bind with non-targets [18]. Synthetic receptors and molecularly imprinted polymers, which is molded into a shape with cavities complementary to the target analyte for high affinity binding, are produced with the aid of computational chemistry and molecular imprinting for rational design of specific molecular recognition [19, 20]. Aptamer, on the other hand, typically requires an artificial selection process, *i.e.* systematic evolution of ligands by exponential enrichment (SELEX) method. Negative selection is also necessary for SELEX to rule out the aptamer sequences with possible binding to non-targets [21, 22]. Compared to antibody development, which requires multiple screening after an antibody with high binding affinity is raised, the aptamer SELEX process can tune its specificity to the target during the selection cycles. In addition, aptamer can be easily linked with ribozyme which acts as an on/off switch, as shown in Fig. (**3A**), upon binding to the target analyte, theophylline. Afterwards, the activated ribozyme triggers the downstream signal amplification process for visible signal readout Fig. (**3B**) [23].

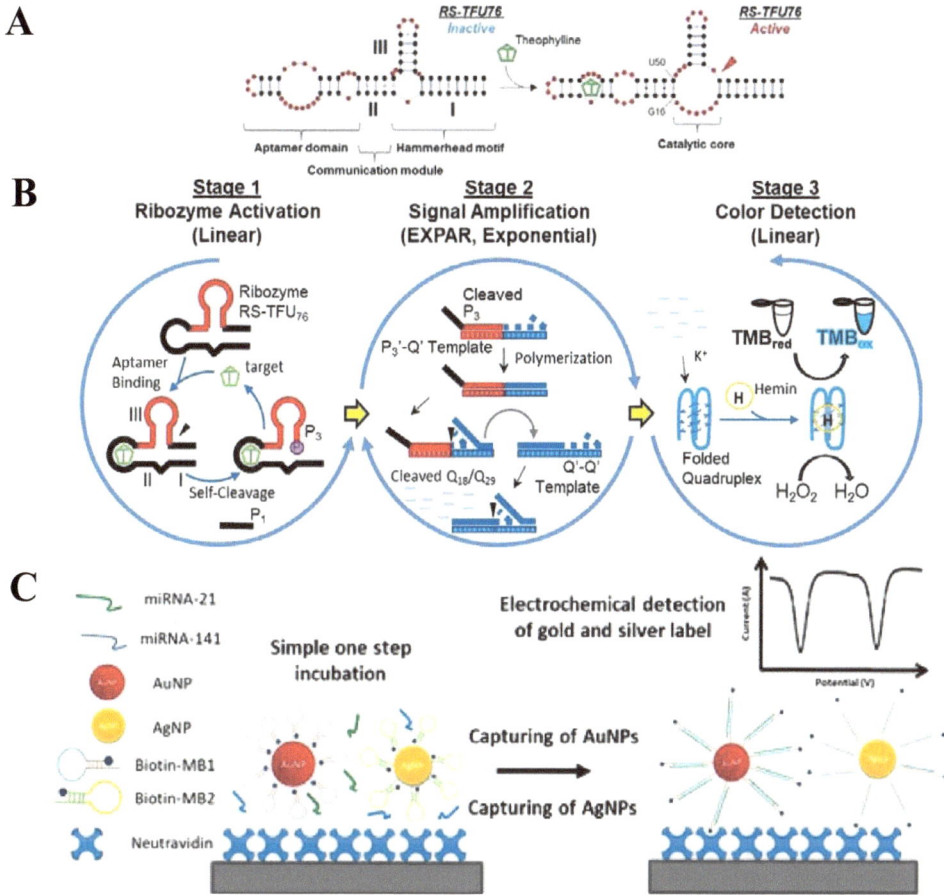

Fig. (3). Various approaches to achieve high specificity of biosensing. **A.** Sequence and conformational change of modified theophylline ribozyme (RS-TFU76) with an aptamer-binding domain (left, stem II), a communication module (middle, stem II), and a hammerhead ribozyme motif (right, stems I and III) from inactive to active after adhesion of theophylline (T) to the putative binding site and activates RS-TFU76 (right). **B.** The schematic diagram showing the whole ligand-induced ribozyme targeting and sensing system. After theophylline target (T) binds to the aptamer domain linked to a cis-acting hammerhead ribozyme (RS-TFU76) and causes the conformational change to the "ON" state and subsequent self-cleavage that forms two products, P1 and P3 in stage 1, downstream EXPAR amplification is triggered by the cleaved kinase-treated ribozyme (P3) and from the given templates produces ssDNA guanine quadruplex precursors (Q) in stage 2. Peroxidase activity is generated from ssDNA Q folding with hemin (H) to oxidize 3,3',5,5'-tetramethylbenzidine substrate from clear (TMBred) to blue state (TMBox) for visualization. **C.** The schematics showing the assay design of the electrochemical biosensor for the multiplexed detection of miRNAs with neutravidin-coated biosensing surface based on a simple one-pot assay approach where simultaneous detection of miRNAs by specific hybridization between the target miRNA and biotin-MB1-AuNP or miRNA-141/biotin-MB2-AgNP onto the neutravidin electrode followed by SSWV. The binding results in the increase in the different peak currents corresponding to AuNPs and AgNPs, which allows different signal responses from respective miRNAs to be differentiated due to the intrinsic electrochemical signature of the nanolabels. Reprinted with permission from references [23, 31].

Clinically speaking, the test specificity also concerns with the validity of targeted biomarkers among other interferential substances in the clinical samples, such as blood pigment. Take a commercially available coronavirus rapid paper-strip POC test for example, the test is based on detecting antibodies against SARS-CoV-2 for the evaluation of immunity. However, a positive signal may be acquired in the presence of SARS-CoV-2 binding antibodies, which do not provide a long-term immunity, in patients recovered from the viral infection [24]. The false positive may mislead the individual into believing that they have already been infected and developed an immunity. Apart from the detection of SARS-CoV-2 viral genome, surface protein antigens and specific antibodies, the discovery of appropriate biomarkers related to its infection is also challenging. Cytokine storm, an immune indicator of severity, is usually found in patients infected with SARS but not SARS-CoV-2 [25]. To identify highly specific human biomarkers related to SARS-CoV-2 infection, the mechanism of its infection and recovery needs further investigation.

Several optimization approaches can be adopted to enhance sensing specificity. Optimization of the reaction conditions, such as the amount of recognition elements coated on the sensing surface, pH values and ionic conditions may enhance the binding affinity between the recognition element and the target analyte, as well as reduce the background noise generated by nonspecific bindings [26, 27]. Recognition by, for example, dual- or multiple-antibodies targeting different epitopes of the same target, generating a sandwich-like 'Antibody 1-Antigen-Antibody 2' complex, functions as an AND gate. The specificity is enhanced by the signal generated from the event dual-recognized by two antibodies, such as the demonstration of whole bacteria detection [28]. Aptamer split, similar to the concept of dual antibodies, has also been used to further increase the detection specificity [29]. Additionally, the removal of the non-specific binding by charge-charge interaction is another strategy to reduce the background noise for increased specificity. Alternative recognition elements, such as peptide nucleic acid, remove the negative surface charge of nucleic acid backbone, and neutravidin minimizes the surface charge in neutral pH value in place of streptavidin during sensing [30, 31]. Fig. (**3C**) shows an example on the use of a neutravidin-coated surface to capture biotinylated probe-nanoparticl--microRNA complex specifically. In this configuration, there is a low chance of nonspecific charge-charge interaction between nanoparticles or microRNA and the neutravidin-coated surface. Coating of proper blockers, such as PEG, reduces hydrophobic interaction and adsorption of nonspecific protein or nucleic acid on the bare sensing surface [32].

SENSITIVITY

Sensitivity, or the limit of detection (LOD), is referred to the minimal amount of analyte that can be detected by a biosensor. The development of biosensors has been pushing the detection limit, making the early diagnostics possible by detecting extremely low amounts of the analyte. The state-of-art is already capable of analyzing single cells or even single molecules, which allows not only sensitive disease diagnosis but also further understanding of the disease progression [33]. As illustrated in Fig. (1), sensitivity of a biosensor is determined by the binding of the recognition element and the target analyte in concert with the efficiency of signal transduction. Binding of the recognition element and the target analyte is preferred in a fast kinetic and high affinity. High sensitivity in a POC test is highly desirable, so that early identification of the disease onset and accurate frequent monitoring of the disease status may become possible during regular checkup. In the COVID-19 pandemic, the sensitive viral RNA detection with a detection limit below 10^5 copies/swab would have provided effective screening of SARS-CoV-2 infection at an early stage, when the transmission rate is high in the absence of commonly developed symptoms such as fever and coughing [34, 35]. Tests of high sensitivity would also help the SARS-CoV-2 surveillance and pandemic control by pinpointing the asymptomatic patients.

Take the nucleic acids based biosensors for example, strategies such as increasing the bound events, as shown in Fig. (4A) [36], are often used "amplify" the signal. For the recognition of antibodies, the affinity of rabbit polyclonal antibodies is usually 10-1000 times higher than that of a mouse monoclonal because of the high efficiency of affinity optimization during antibody production in the rabbit immune system [37]. The drawback of this polyclonal feature, *i.e.*, multiple epitope targeting, in rabbit antibody is further tackled by the development of monoclonal antibodies with hybridoma technique [38]. On the other hand, avidin has been used to capture biotinylated molecules with a high affinity, with a K_d as low as 10^{-14} M between streptavidin and biotin. Also, their tight interaction is not easily affected by temperature, pH values, or osmotic pressure change, which makes it useful in the sensitive detection of biomolecules with biotin tagged in the robust screening of clinical samples.

Besides the choice of recognition elements, enzyme is widely used as a biological catalyst that increases the rate of biochemical reaction of signal generation to amplify the signal. Enzyme-linked immunosorbent assay (ELISA), an assay conjugating enzymes with recognition elements, was the first demonstrated technique to increase sensitivity in place of radioimmunoassay (RIA) in the 1950s [39, 40]. Horseradish peroxidase is widely used for colorimetric or chemil-uminescent detection *via* the ability of HRP of converting a substrate, such as

3,3',5,5'-Tetramethylbenzidine (TMB), into a colored product or emission of light [41, 42]. Apart from acting on the signal generation molecules, other enzymes have been employed to act on the target analyte during biosensing. Fig. (4B-C) shows two examples of signal amplification. RNA-cleaving DNAzymes have been developed for diagnostic POC tests that recognize bacterial pathogens, such as *Escherichia coli* [43]. RNase H has been used in repeated cycles of digesting the RNA probe in the DNA-RNA hybrid for sensitive microRNA detection, which could reveal the hidden disease for early diagnosis, as shown in Fig. (4B) [15, 44].

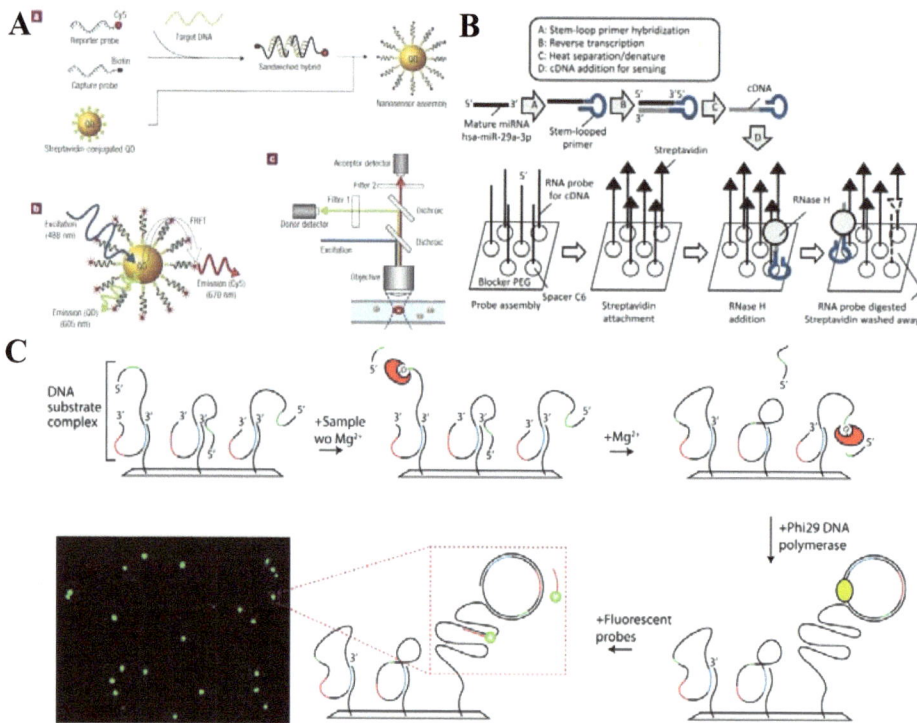

Fig. (4). Various methods of signal amplification to increase sensitivity of biosensing. **A.** The schematic diagram showing the formation of a nanosensor assembly with fluorescence emission caused by FRET between Cy5 acceptors and a QD donor in the presence of targets. **B.** The schematic diagram showing the design and workflow for microRNA sensing with the MicroRNA-RNase-SPR assay, which relies on a repeated cycle of RNA probe digestion by RNase H after mature microRNA-converted cDNA (top A to D) bound on the probe to form hybridized RNA-cDNA in the gold SPR surface (bottom). It resulted in the change of the SPR signal to be measured. **C.** Schematic illustration of the mycobacteria biosensing system using DNA substrate complex containing scissile DNA oligonucleotide hybridized to the immobilized DNA primer captures mycobacterial TOP1A. Signal sensitivity is enhanced with rolling circle amplification (RCA) to amplify the scissile DNA circle formed by the ligation step of the mycobacterial TOP1A catalytic cycle. Reprinted with permission from references [36, 44, 48].

Moreover, enzymes, including polymerase and ligase, have been used in the nucleic acid amplification on the target nucleic acid or reporter, such as aptamers that correlate to the concentration of the target analyte. For example, Fig. (**4C**) shows the rolling circle amplification (RCA), an isothermal amplification technique. On the other hand, fluorescence labels using chemical dyes have been popular in the last two decades. Intercalating dyes, molecular beacons (MB), and TaqMan probes are employed to label the target nucleic acid molecule, while fluorescein-based probes that bind to ions, such as Cl⁻, have been coupled with Förster resonance energy transfer (FRET) to detect the presence and quantitation of these molecules [45]. Fluorescence protein, such as green fluorescence protein (GFP), are also used in cell-based biosensors because of the genetically encoded fluorescent. Split GFP fusion with surface receptors has been used to detect target molecules, where the interaction between the target and the receptor causes the split GFPs to form a functional GFP and give out fluorescence. Upconverting nanoparticles (UCNPs), on the other hand, rely on the use of non-photobleaching and non-harmful infrared spectrum, and could overcome both the limitation in photo-bleaching and background noise from excitation in the visible spectrum [46]. The increase in signal intensity, together with the decrease in noise, eventually boosts the signal-to-noise ratio for sensitivity biosensing. In addition, the use of the infrared spectrum increases the depth of excitation light to be passed, which is feasible for *in vivo* high-contrast imaging [47].

On the other hand, the sensitivity of biosensor is also determined by the signal-to-noise ratio during signal acquisition, where the noise could be the system noise such as background fluorescence. Although there are many labeling techniques available, the background fluorescence, procedures and time needed for labeling usually hinder their practical use in biosensing. In this regard, surface plasmon resonance (SPR) has been developed as a label-free, highly sensitive sensing method [49]. Three interrogations, *i.e.* angular, wavelength and phase interrogations, have been investigated for the SPR measurement. Among these, phase measurement has shown with a superior detection sensitivity. It achieves the ultra-low detection limit, compared to conventional biochemical reactions using enzymes for signal amplification [50]. With the use of molecular imprinted film, such as amoxicillin-imprinted p(HEMAGA) film for amoxicillin detection, sensitive detection of the target as low as in pg/mL level can be achieved since the SPR sensing surface is well covered by the film to maximize its ability on target recognition [51, 52]. Coupling enzymatic reactions with SPR can also further increase its sensitivity [44, 53]. Besides, SPR imaging further extends its capacity for simultaneous multiplex detection to increase the throughput without compromising its sensing sensitivity [54 - 56]. It is particularly useful when more than one analyst is required for measurement and result interpretation, such as olfactory sensing [57]. SPR imaging on real-time multiple targets tracking can be performed after the multiple recognition elements are printed in an array format on the SPR sensing surface [58]. SPR image scanning using a mechanical stage usually creates vibration that affects the signal detection, where the use of MEMS system, such as digital micromirror devices, could stabilize the whole sensor for stable optical measurement [59, 60]. The SPR image resolution could be further enhanced by phase measurement or nanomaterials, such as random nanodot arrays and gold nanoparticle arrays [61 - 63]. Unfortunately, these sensitive sensing devices are usually not portable to meet the POC need. In light of this, there are increasing research and development of the fiber-SPR sensing method, by integrating all the optical sensing in a gold-coated fiber, optical paths with fiber and junctions to connect all the components, from a light source to the spectrometer [64]. It could tackle not only the portable issue but also the instability issue for robust biosensing with conventional SPR method [65 - 67]. Apart from this, the use of nanoparticles, such as gold nanorods (AuNRs) that generate localized SPR (LSPR), can achieve high sensitive sensing for visible discrimination in a test-tube format [68 - 71]. For example, cortisol, a stress biomarker that causes mental disorders, can be quantified simply by adding single drop of saliva supernatant to the aptamer-coated nanoparticles, which has been immobilized on sensing surface, without further reagent addition or washing [72].

Concentration or localization of the target analyte is another approach to enhance sensitivity. In conventional test-tube based assays, magnetic micro-beads conjugated with recognition elements isolate the target analyte from the sample mixture, and the magnetic action assembles the microbead-analyte complexes into a tiny region [73, 74]. The alternative, created by the advancement in micro-fluidics, utilizes micro-chambers in a microfluidic to gather target molecules in a micro- or nano-scale localized zone. This also helps in the downstream capture by recognition elements and hence the sensitivity. Droplet encapsulation not only concentrates the biochemical reaction in a pico-liter droplet to increase the chance of interaction between molecules but also enables digital analysis, such as digital polymerase chain reaction (dPCR) [75]. Rapid pathogen-specific phenotypic antibiotic susceptibility testing with a high sensitivity using digital loop-mediated amplification (dLAMP) has also been developed [76]. On the other hand, optical trapping is a non-contact based concentration and defined localization of the target analyte with a laser beam or plasmonic waveguide [77, 78]. The detection can be enhanced for single-cell analysis when assisted with micro-chambers, and its ability is demonstrated in the analysis of DNA [79] and protein [80, 81]. Thermal gradient trapping is similar to optical trapping with the additional benefit of sample heating to accelerate biochemical reactions, such as DNA amplification [82, 83].

DYNAMIC RANGE

In human bodies, the physiological range of biomolecules is usually as narrow as within two orders of magnitude. Most of the conventional biochemical assays, such as ELISA, could cover the range effectively. The integrated printed biosensor was reported to have a linear response between 0 and 5 mM glucose, suitable for glucose monitoring in interstitial fluid [84]. Although the dynamic range is relatively small, the sensitivity is high and accurate enough to measure the fasting blood glucose level. On the other hand, the high dynamic range provides the addition benefit of robustness in disease screening and in-depth understanding of the pathological development of diseases, since target biomarkers show a high dynamic range in different stages. For example, the dynamic in cytokine IL-2 secretion is correlated with the pathophysiological roles in the immune system, and the high dynamic range detection support the analysis of its secretion profile for a comprehensive understanding of the role of IL-2 during a disease [81]. Also, dynamics in a single red blood cell (RBC) triggered by an environmental stimulation, such as photo-induced oxidation of the RBC, can be monitored over time [85, 86].

A POC test with a higher dynamic range could extend the biosensing ability from detecting target biomarkers in a particular type to multiple types of specimen, since the concentration of target biomarkers may vary in different body fluids. For example, the viral RNA concentration of SAR-CoV-2 is ranged from 10^3 to 10^6 copy/mL in the respiratory tract specimens such as saliva and sputum, and from 10^2 to 10^4 copy/mL in human plasma sample [35, 87]. A POC test covering the said ranges would be versatile for different samples, provide additional safeguard on multiple screening of different samples from the same individual to validate their immunity, and facilitate the quantitative study of viral infection pathways and their migration inside human body by helping in the understanding of the mechanism of infection.

Various methods have been used to increase the dynamic range. A combination of several aptamers with various affinities to the target analyst was employed to detect different concentration ranges of the target [88]. The dynamic response range, adjustable by changing the environmental pH value in accordance to the isoelectric point of the target protein enables a high dynamic range of target *Plasmodium falciparum* lactate dehydrogenase detection from 100 pM to 10 nM [89]. In addition, duplexed aptamers, the hybridization between an aptamer and an aptamer-complementary element, *i.e.* a DNA oligonucleotide, was demonstrated as a ligand-responsive construct with a tunable dynamic range through base mutations on the bound DNA and screening by aptamer-complementary element scanning [90]. It was demonstrated with adenosine triphosphate (ATP) sensing with two orders of magnitude in aptamer-based electrochemical sensors [91]. Reducing the background noise to boost the detection limit, such as the use of nanomaterials UCNP@PDA@AP, supported a high linear dynamic range on cytochrome c sensing, from 50 nM to 10 µM [92]. Moreover, signal amplification with enzymes by increasing the detection limit without affecting the maximum detectable concentration helps increase the dynamic range in biosensing. For instance, immunosignal hybridization chain reaction by combining antibody-antigen interactions with hybridization chain reaction technology, has provided a broader dynamic range than the enzyme-based chemiluminescent detection method [93, 94]. The use of platinum nanocatalyst amplification on lateral-flow devices provided a broad linear dynamic range across four orders of magnitude from 1 to 10000 pg/mL on HIV diagnosis [95]. For the optical transducer for signal acquisition, the requirements for both high sensitivity and a broad dynamic range suggests that the interferometric sensor is the most fit compared to the absorbance and fluorescence measurement. SPR coupled with a continuous white light source in place of a single-wavelength laser could provide a wider coverage range of the measurable concentration, but the sensitivity will be sacrificed when using white light [96]. In this regard, the implementation of phase measurement, instead of intensity, could tackle the detection sensitivity, without compromising the dynamic range [97, 98]. This was demonstrated with a wide dynamic range for monitoring cytochrome-c leakage from 80 pM to 80 nM during cancer cell death for anti-cancer drug screening [50]. The wider coverage range of measurable concentration of the SPR method was investigated and in some recent works, such as the use of erythrocyte membrane (EM)-blanketed gold nanoparticle provide a sensitive and wide range, from 0.001–5.000 mg/mL, detection of fibrinogen in blood sample [99].

RELIABILITY AND ROBUSTNESS

Reliability and robustness of biosensors produce consistent quantitative results at the POC, which are essential to clinical decision making as valid clinical data. Fig. (5A) shows an example of an integrated biosensor platform, by merging the technical advances in printed electronics, sensing probe, and readout display for electrochemical sensing on the glucose level [84]. This portable platform in a card format supports the in-field applications, without the technical support of experts and clinical facilities. Regarding protein and nucleic acid-based biosensing, stability of recognition elements and molecular reactions are some of the key factors to generate reproducible results, but, unfortunately, the biological elements and reagents have a finite shelf life. In order to overcome this limitation, stability of the reagents is enhanced by, for example, a polymer coating and the addition of lyophilization and sugar stabilizers to reagents extend their lifetime from days to years [100]. Among various types of recognition elements, aptamers show many benefits over antibodies. The popularity of aptamer-based assays is growing among diagnostic applications, especially paper-based biosensors. Resistant to heat, aptamers can be stored in room temperature for months without losing its binding ability to the target [101]. An aptamer could also replace enzymes to convert immunoassay substrate TMB to color products in the immunoassay [23, 102]. Nevertheless, there are drawbacks of using enzymes in biological reactions to increase the signal, for instance, inconsistent reaction rates in different logs and reduction in activity over time, which hinders its practical use in stable biosensing. Enzyme-free signal generation is therefore desirable. Hybridization chain reaction is one of the enzyme-free methods for DNA amplification [93, 103]. Native DNA and even artificial DNA, *e.g.* locked nucleic acid (LNA) commonly used because of its resistance to nuclease, can be amplified using this method [104].

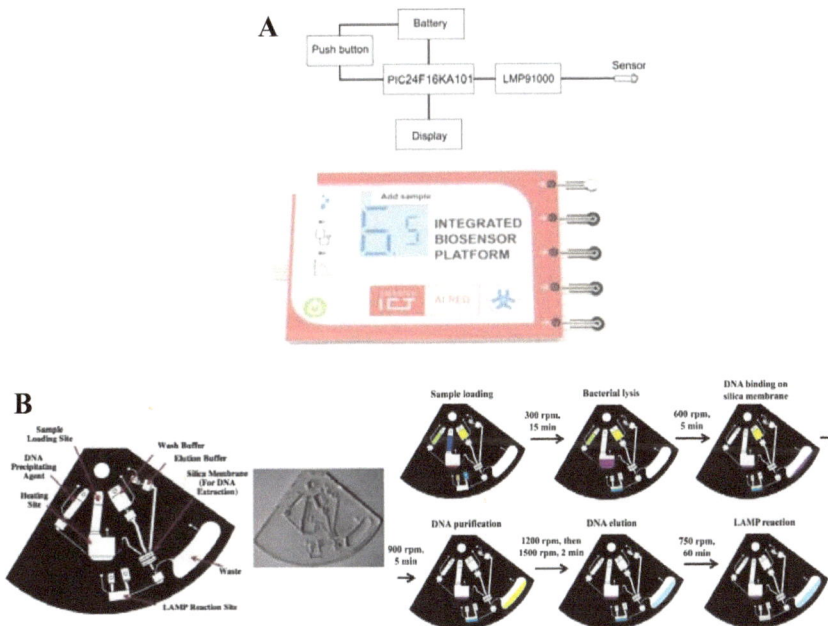

Fig. (5). Examples of portable biosensors demonstrated with high stability and robustness. **A.** schematic representation of the (Upper) hybrid printed circuit design and (Lower) printed integrated system, containing the printed circuitry and battery for micro-controller programming, actuation, communication and actuation, a potentiostat chip, and display for sensing. **B.** Schematic diagram of a self-contained microfluidic disc (one-quarter of a full disc area) to perform sample-to-answer nucleic acid-based molecular diagnosis of specific target bacteria from clinical samples, such as blood and sputum. The operation flow of microfluidic disc in the right panel shows the fluid movement sequentially at each step, controlled by a spinning force and valves to perform sample lysis, DNA extraction, and isothermal DNA amplification (real-time loop-mediated isothermal amplification (RT-LAMP)) automatically. Reprinted with permission from references [84, 114].

The use of nanomaterials is also on the rise. In conventional fluorescence labeling, the signal output is unstable because the chemical dyes or fluorescence proteins are easily degraded by enzymes or quenched by a high-power laser input, but nanomaterials show no such limitations [36]. Fluorescence-based nanoparticles (NPs), such as gold nanorod (AuNR), quantum dot (QD), are promising alternatives [105, 106]. Conductive nanomaterials, such as graphene, could enhance electrochemical sensing stability to be more reliable in low concentration biomolecules detection by simply coating on the current sensing electrodes [107]. Graphene oxide, carbon nanotube and carbon nanosphere have been evaluated with a peroxidase-like activity, which can be applied in immunoassays in place of the unstable peroxidase [108 - 110].

Sample actuation is another issue in robustness of biosensors. Considering the tedious and laborious operation of sample handling and processing, modern clinical equipment in centralized laboratories in hospitals are designed in an automated action. The only procedure is to insert the sample into sample racks and assay cassettes containing the reagent for the assay into the machine and to read the result generated. To construct a miniaturized biosensor, the use of microfluidics and a MEMS device, could benefit the automatic sample actuation, instead of using traditional pipette robots. More importantly, sample-to-answer can be achieved with lab-on-a-chip, designed to complete all the actions, *e.g.* cell isolation and enrichment of target biomolecules, in a robust, sensitive and automated manner [111]. The use of microfluidics facilitates the accurate temperature control, such as thermocycling, of a limited volume of fluid in a portable and lightweight processing device, regardless of the large specific heat capacity of water. Yet, the network of external pump connections is not robust when translated into POC use. Lab-on-a-disc (LOAD) therefore provides robustness in operation because of its fully automation of liquid handling [112, 113]. In addition, the high throughput, highly parallel and quantitative analysis are enabled to support simultaneous multi-dimensional analysis, such as multiple single-cell analysis in a sample. Multiple disease diagnosis for sample-to-answer on molecular diagnosis of bacterial infection can be performed in a disc, as shown in Fig. **(5B)**, where fluidic actuation is simply controlled with the centrifugal force only in a sequential order [114, 115]. Further combination of the advantages of label-free multiplexed SPR detection and LOAD achieve completely automated sensitive immunoassays [116]. While conventional microfluidics handle liquids continuously in microchannels, the digital microfluidic is a new type of microfluidics that manipulate fluids in discrete volumes in the form of droplets, with couplings with magnetic actuation or electrowetting-on-dielectrics (EWOD) actuation with demonstration of their potential for POC test in remote settings [117,118]. An additional benefit of digital microfluidics is that the formed droplets act as tiny micro-reactors to localize the reactant, thus increasing the sensitivity of diagnostic platforms.

Advancement of fabrication techniques, such as printing, engraving and molding, are useful in facilitating the production of biosensors and accelerating the turnaround time in development cycles. It also provides an ease of customization and supports just-in-time on-site manufacture. Integrating microfluidic biosensor development has a long history in the healthcare industry. One typical example is lateral-flow immunoassay, a biochemical test integrating recognition elements and transducers in a paper-strip format, commercially available worldwide as lateral flow dipstick for POC use, such as rapid HIV tests and rapid bacteria detection [43, 119]. Recent development shows that signal amplification, *e.g.* isothermal DNA amplification loop-mediated amplification (LAMP), can be accomplished in this paper-based sensor, besides protein-based immunoassays [120]. Furthermore, the evolution of affinity sensors from conventional lateral-flow paper test strips to wearable or implantable devices with soft and flexible materials, such as plastic membrane and polymers, have worked successfully in POC multifarious polymer designs that provide the base materials for sensor designs [121, 122]. Recent progress in 2D and 3D printed microfluidics biosensor has reduced the difficulties in prototyping and research development, where cycles of prototyping and optimization has been sped up [123 - 126].

To date, technological advancement has enabled comprehensive data analysis with high computational power. Limit of quantification (LOQ), defined as signal detection above the mean of the blank measures plus a $10\times$ standard deviation generally, could evaluate whether the low-level signal output is valid in not only qualitatively, *i.e.* yes/no determination but quantitatively and reliable with a low chance of false negative signal. One major technical breakthrough in biosensor development is the image analysis technique of parallel processing of multiple optical images and effective identification of target markers in the images automatically. Machine learning, one of the categories in narrow artificial intelligence, provides more accurate image analysis, especially those based on images and large dataset, to outperform that with manual operation for disease diagnosis [127]. Machine learning is well-known for its effective and automatic cellular image analysis and therefore has a high potential to replace labor- and skill-intensive image analysis [128]. Yet, the data-processing speed becomes a key factor when handling a large sum of data, especially arrays of dataset, and only a desktop computer is capable of handling such tasks. Cloud computing may be incorporated in portable biosensors for in-field operation, unlike traditional biosensors that are linked to a personal computer. Connected to a cloud network for further analysis, cloud computing further reduces the size, electricity, and hardware requirement for data processing of biosensors, especially image-based ones [129]. As a result, cloud-based or smartphone technologies are coupled with computing algorithms for high throughput and automated quantitative analysis with a short turnaround time. Biosensors that are connected to mobile phones for data processing and signal readout have been used for rapid bacteria detection [130 - 132]. By leveraging machine learning algorithms and advanced optical transducers in a compact biosensor, accurate optical-based biosensing with intelligent analysis for POC use can be realized. In fact, the same advances in digital technology that are boosting the fortunes of next-generation diagnosis are also extending the lifespan of an image-based biosensor used in the current diagnosis.

CONCLUDING REMARKS

No doubt, the development of a reliable and user-friendly POC biosensor is a formidable task, which will benefit not only to the clinicians but also the public community, addressing the rapidly growing demand on frequent health check-ups, long-term continuous screening of disease biomarkers in an individual. Many technical challenges await innovative solutions, particularly considering the translation into clinical uses for medical applications, such as personalized medicine. Furthermore, clinical evaluation of the diagnostic applicability holds the key to validate a biosensor for clinical requirements. Currently, the duration from evaluation to authority approval by, for example, The Food and Drug Administration (FDA) of United States may take years. While technical innovations may improve the performance factors, revised measures shall also be included to shorten the overall idea-to-market time, to address the increasing demand in healthcare. Overall, the applications of biosensors are obvious and the perspective is optimistic. However, cautions are required for considering the performance factors for different diagnostic applications. For example, an ideal biosensor suited for POC diagnostics shall bear the essentials of cost, speed, portability and device robustness in mind. The ultimate aspiration, as a biosensor engineer, is to witness a shift in current medical intervention from reactive care to predictive or preventive care in future.

CONSENT FOR PUBLICATION

Not applicable.

CONFLICT OF INTEREST

The authors confirm that this chapter contents have no conflict of interest.

ACKNOWLEDGEMENTS

The authors would like to acknowledge the support of the Startup Fund provided by the Chinese University of Hong Kong, the Endowment Fund Research Grant provided by the United College in the Chinese University of Hong Kong (#CA11278), and the General Research Fund provided by the Research Grants Council of the Hong Kong Special Administrative Region (Project No. CUHK 14201317). The authors would also like to acknowledge the support of the Innovative Technology Fund (ITS/061/18, GHX/004/18SZ) and the Area of Excellence scheme funding (AoE/P-0/12) provided by the Hong Kong Special Administrative Region.

REFERENCES

[1] Julián E, Roldán M, Sánchez-Chardi A, Astola O, Agustí G, Luquin M. Microscopic cords, a virulence-related characteristic of Mycobacterium tuberculosis, are also present in nonpathogenic mycobacteria. J Bacteriol 2010; 192(7): 1751-60.
[http://dx.doi.org/10.1128/JB.01485-09] [PMID: 20097851]

[2] Berson SA, Yalow RS, Bauman A, Rothschild MA, Newerly K. Insulin-I131 metabolism in human subjects: demonstration of insulin binding globulin in the circulation of insulin treated subjects. J Clin Invest 1956; 35(2): 170-90.
[http://dx.doi.org/10.1172/JCI103262] [PMID: 13286336]

[3] Udugama B, Kadhiresan P, Kozlowski HN, *et al.* Diagnosing COVID-19: The Disease and Tools for Detection. ACS Nano 2020; 14(4): 3822-35.
[http://dx.doi.org/10.1021/acsnano.0c02624] [PMID: 32223179]

[4] McNaught AD, Wilkinson A. Compendium of Chemical Terminology. 2nd ed., Blackwell Scientific Publication 2019.

[5] Williams DL, Doig AR Jr, Korosi A. Electrochemical-enzymatic analysis of blood glucose and lactate. Anal Chem 1970; 42(1): 118-21.
[http://dx.doi.org/10.1021/ac60283a032] [PMID: 5409504]

[6] Wang J. Glucose Biosensors: 40 Years of Advances and Challenges. Electroanalysis 2001; 13: 983-8.
[http://dx.doi.org/10.1002/1521-4109(200108)13:12<983::AID-ELAN983>3.0.CO;2-#]

[7] Turner APF. Biosensors: sense and sensibility. Chem Soc Rev 2013; 42(8): 3184-96.
[http://dx.doi.org/10.1039/c3cs35528d] [PMID: 23420144]

[8] Pardee K, Green AA, Takahashi MK, *et al.* Rapid, Low-Cost Detection of Zika Virus Using Programmable Biomolecular Components. Cell 2016; 165(5): 1255-66.
[http://dx.doi.org/10.1016/j.cell.2016.04.059] [PMID: 27160350]

[9] Ellington AD, Szostak JW. *In vitro* selection of RNA molecules that bind specific ligands. Nature 1990; 346(6287): 818-22.
[http://dx.doi.org/10.1038/346818a0] [PMID: 1697402]

[10] Tyagi S, Kramer FR. Molecular beacons: probes that fluoresce upon hybridization. Nat Biotechnol 1996; 14(3): 303-8.
[http://dx.doi.org/10.1038/nbt0396-303] [PMID: 9630890]

[11] Maduraiveeran G, Sasidharan M, Ganesan V. Electrochemical sensor and biosensor platforms based on advanced nanomaterials for biological and biomedical applications. Biosens Bioelectron 2018; 103: 113-29.
[http://dx.doi.org/10.1016/j.bios.2017.12.031] [PMID: 29289816]

[12]   Turner APF. Tech.Sight. Biochemistry. Biosensors--sense and sensitivity. Science 2000; 290(5495): 1315-7.
[http://dx.doi.org/10.1126/science.290.5495.1315] [PMID: 11185408]

[13]   Li L, He JA, Wang W, *et al.* Development of a direct reverse-transcription quantitative PCR (dirRT-qPCR) assay for clinical Zika diagnosis. Int J Infect Dis 2019; 85: 167-74.
[http://dx.doi.org/10.1016/j.ijid.2019.06.007] [PMID: 31202908]

[14]   Yamada K, Henares TG, Suzuki K, Citterio D. Paper-based inkjet-printed microfluidic analytical devices. Angew Chem Int Ed Engl 2015; 54(18): 5294-310.
[http://dx.doi.org/10.1002/anie.201411508] [PMID: 25864471]

[15]   Dong H, Lei J, Ding L, Wen Y, Ju H, Zhang X. MicroRNA: function, detection, and bioanalysis. Chem Rev 2013; 113(8): 6207-33.
[http://dx.doi.org/10.1021/cr300362f] [PMID: 23697835]

[16]   Fabri-Faja N, Calvo-Lozano O, Dey P, *et al.* Early sepsis diagnosis *via* protein and miRNA biomarkers using a novel point-of-care photonic biosensor. Anal Chim Acta 2019; 1077: 232-42.
[http://dx.doi.org/10.1016/j.aca.2019.05.038] [PMID: 31307714]

[17]   Tyagi S, Bratu DP, Kramer FR. Multicolor molecular beacons for allele discrimination. Nat Biotechnol 1998; 16(1): 49-53.
[http://dx.doi.org/10.1038/nbt0198-49] [PMID: 9447593]

[18]   Nelson AL, Reichert JM. Development trends for therapeutic antibody fragments. Nat Biotechnol 2009; 27(4): 331-7.
[http://dx.doi.org/10.1038/nbt0409-331] [PMID: 19352366]

[19]   Smolinska-Kempisty K, Ahmad OS, Guerreiro A, Karim K, Piletska E, Piletsky S. New potentiometric sensor based on molecularly imprinted nanoparticles for cocaine detection. Biosens Bioelectron 2017; 96: 49-54.
[http://dx.doi.org/10.1016/j.bios.2017.04.034] [PMID: 28472729]

[20]   Canfarotta F, Poma A, Guerreiro A, Piletsky S. Solid-phase synthesis of molecularly imprinted nanoparticles. Nat Protoc 2016; 11(3): 443-55.
[http://dx.doi.org/10.1038/nprot.2016.030] [PMID: 26866789]

[21]   Guo KT, Schäfer R, Paul A, Ziemer G, Wendel HP. Aptamer-based strategies for stem cell research. Mini Rev Med Chem 2007; 7(7): 701-5.
[http://dx.doi.org/10.2174/138955707781024481] [PMID: 17627582]

[22]   Tang Z, Parekh P, Turner P, Moyer RW, Tan W. Generating aptamers for recognition of virus-infected cells. Clin Chem 2009; 55(4): 813-22.
[http://dx.doi.org/10.1373/clinchem.2008.113514] [PMID: 19246617]

[23]   Liao AM, Pan W, Benson JC, Wong AD, Rose BJ, Caltagirone GT. A Simple Colorimetric System for Detecting Target Antigens by a Three-Stage Signal Transformation-Amplification Strategy. Biochemistry 2018; 57(34): 5117-26.
[http://dx.doi.org/10.1021/acs.biochem.8b00523] [PMID: 30064210]

[24]   Pelegrin M, Naranjo-Gomez M, Piechaczyk M. Antiviral Monoclonal Antibodies: Can They Be More Than Simple Neutralizing Agents? Trends Microbiol 2015; 23(10): 653-65.
[http://dx.doi.org/10.1016/j.tim.2015.07.005] [PMID: 26433697]

[25]   Thevarajan I, Nguyen THO, Koutsakos M, *et al.* Breadth of concomitant immune responses prior to patient recovery: a case report of non-severe COVID-19. Nat Med 2020; 26(4): 453-5.
[http://dx.doi.org/10.1038/s41591-020-0819-2] [PMID: 32284614]

[26]   Lequin RM. Enzyme immunoassay (EIA)/enzyme-linked immunosorbent assay (ELISA). Clin Chem 2005; 51(12): 2415-8.
[http://dx.doi.org/10.1373/clinchem.2005.051532] [PMID: 16179424]

[27] Mousavi SF, Fatemi S, Siadat SD, *et al.* Development and Optimization of a Homemade ELISA Kit for Detection of Antibodies Against Haemophilus influenzae Type b. Jundishapur J Microbiol 2016; 9(5): e30629-9.
[http://dx.doi.org/10.5812/jjm.30629] [PMID: 27540453]

[28] Templier V, Roux A, Roupioz Y, Livache T. Ligands for label-free detection of whole bacteria on biosensors: A review. Trends Analyt Chem 2016; 79: 71-9.
[http://dx.doi.org/10.1016/j.trac.2015.10.015]

[29] Melaine F, Coilhac C, Roupioz Y, Buhot A. A nanoparticle-based thermo-dynamic aptasensor for small molecule detection. Nanoscale 2016; 8(38): 16947-54.
[http://dx.doi.org/10.1039/C6NR04868D] [PMID: 27714066]

[30] Gupta A, Mishra A, Puri N. Peptide nucleic acids: Advanced tools for biomedical applications. J Biotechnol 2017; 259: 148-59.
[http://dx.doi.org/10.1016/j.jbiotec.2017.07.026] [PMID: 28764969]

[31] Azzouzi S, Fredj Z, Turner APF, Ali MB, Mak WC. Generic Neutravidin Biosensor for Simultaneous Multiplex Detection of MicroRNAs *via* Electrochemically Encoded Responsive Nanolabels. ACS Sens 2019; 4(2): 326-34.
[http://dx.doi.org/10.1021/acssensors.8b00942] [PMID: 30730699]

[32] Knowles DB, LaCroix AS, Deines NF, Shkel I, Record MT Jr. Separation of preferential interaction and excluded volume effects on DNA duplex and hairpin stability. Proc Natl Acad Sci USA 2011; 108(31): 12699-704.
[http://dx.doi.org/10.1073/pnas.1103382108] [PMID: 21742980]

[33] Loo JF, Ho HP, Kong SK, Wang T, Ho Y. Technological Advances in Multiscale Analysis of Single Cells in Biomedicine. Advanced Biosystems 2019; 1900138
[http://dx.doi.org/10.1002/adbi.201900138]

[34] Wölfel R, Corman VM, Guggemos W, *et al.* Virological assessment of hospitalized patients with COVID-2019. Nature 2020; 581(7809): 465-9.
[http://dx.doi.org/10.1038/s41586-020-2196-x] [PMID: 32235945]

[35] To KK-W, Tsang OT-Y, Leung W-S, *et al.* Temporal profiles of viral load in posterior oropharyngeal saliva samples and serum antibody responses during infection by SARS-CoV-2: an observational cohort study. Lancet Infect Dis 2020; 20(5): 565-74.
[http://dx.doi.org/10.1016/S1473-3099(20)30196-1] [PMID: 32213337]

[36] Zhang C-Y, Yeh H-C, Kuroki MT, Wang T-H. Single-quantum-dot-based DNA nanosensor. Nat Mater 2005; 4(11): 826-31.
[http://dx.doi.org/10.1038/nmat1508] [PMID: 16379073]

[37] Rossi S, Laurino L, Furlanetto A, *et al.* Rabbit monoclonal antibodies: a comparative study between a novel category of immunoreagents and the corresponding mouse monoclonal antibodies. Am J Clin Pathol 2005; 124(2): 295-302.
[http://dx.doi.org/10.1309/NR8HN08GDPVEMU08] [PMID: 16040303]

[38] Spieker-Polet H, Sethupathi P, Yam PC, Knight KL. Rabbit monoclonal antibodies: generating a fusion partner to produce rabbit-rabbit hybridomas. Proc Natl Acad Sci USA 1995; 92(20): 9348-52.
[http://dx.doi.org/10.1073/pnas.92.20.9348] [PMID: 7568130]

[39] Engvall E, Perlmann P. Enzyme-linked immunosorbent assay (ELISA). Quantitative assay of immunoglobulin G. Immunochemistry 1971; 8(9): 871-4.
[http://dx.doi.org/10.1016/0019-2791(71)90454-X] [PMID: 5135623]

[40] Engvall E, Perlmann P. Enzyme-Linked Immunosorbent Assay, Elisa : III. Quantitation of Specific Antibodies by Anti-Immunoglobulin in Antigen-Coated Tubes. J Immunol 1972.

[41] Bos ES, van der Doelen AA, van Rooy N, Schuurs AH. 3,3',5,5' - Tetramethylbenzidine as an Ames test negative chromogen for horse-radish peroxidase in enzyme-immunoassay. J Immunoassay 1981;

2(3-4): 187-204.
[http://dx.doi.org/10.1080/15321818108056977] [PMID: 7047570]

[42]   Harpaz D, Eltzov E, Ng TSE, Marks RS, Tok AIY. Enhanced Colorimetric Signal for Accurate Signal Detection in Paper-Based Biosensors. Diagnostics (Basel) 2020; 10(1)E28
[http://dx.doi.org/10.3390/diagnostics10010028] [PMID: 31936174]

[43]   Ali MM, Brown CL, Jahanshahi-Anbuhi S, *et al.* A Printed Multicomponent Paper Sensor for Bacterial Detection. Sci Rep 2017; 7(1): 12335.
[http://dx.doi.org/10.1038/s41598-017-12549-3] [PMID: 28951563]

[44]   Loo JFC, Wang SS, Peng F, *et al.* A non-PCR SPR platform using RNase H to detect MicroRNA 29a-3p from throat swabs of human subjects with influenza A virus H1N1 infection. Analyst (Lond) 2015; 140(13): 4566-75.
[http://dx.doi.org/10.1039/C5AN00679A] [PMID: 26000345]

[45]   Algar WR, Hildebrandt N, Vogel SS, Medintz IL. FRET as a biomolecular research tool - understanding its potential while avoiding pitfalls. Nat Methods 2019; 16(9): 815-29.
[http://dx.doi.org/10.1038/s41592-019-0530-8] [PMID: 31471616]

[46]   Loo JF-C, Chien Y-H, Yin F, Kong S-K, Ho H-P, Yong K-T. Upconversion and downconversion nanoparticles for biophotonics and nanomedicine. Coord Chem Rev 2019; 400213042
[http://dx.doi.org/10.1016/j.ccr.2019.213042]

[47]   Park YI, Lee KT, Suh YD, Hyeon T. Upconverting nanoparticles: a versatile platform for wide-field two-photon microscopy and multi-modal *in vivo* imaging. Chem Soc Rev 2015; 44(6): 1302-17.
[http://dx.doi.org/10.1039/C4CS00173G] [PMID: 25042637]

[48]   Franch O, Han X, Marcussen LB, *et al.* A new DNA sensor system for specific and quantitative detection of mycobacteria. Nanoscale 2019; 11(2): 587-97.
[http://dx.doi.org/10.1039/C8NR07850E] [PMID: 30556557]

[49]   Liedberg B, Nylander C, Lunström I. Surface plasmon resonance for gas detection and biosensing. Sens Actuators 1983; 4: 299-304.
[http://dx.doi.org/10.1016/0250-6874(83)85036-7]

[50]   Loo F-C, Ng S-P, Wu C-ML, Kong SK. An aptasensor using DNA aptamer and white light common-path SPR spectral interferometry to detect cytochrome-c for anti-cancer drug screening. Sens Actuators B Chem 2014; 198
[http://dx.doi.org/10.1016/j.snb.2014.03.077]

[51]   Yola ML, Eren T, Atar N. Molecular imprinted nanosensor based on surface plasmon resonance: Application to the sensitive determination of amoxicillin. Sens Actuators B Chem 2014; 195: 28-35.
[http://dx.doi.org/10.1016/j.snb.2014.01.011]

[52]   Atar N, Eren T, Yola ML. A molecular imprinted SPR biosensor for sensitive determination of citrinin in red yeast rice. Food Chem 2015; 184: 7-11.
[http://dx.doi.org/10.1016/j.foodchem.2015.03.065] [PMID: 25872420]

[53]   Loo JF-C, Yang C, Tsang HL, *et al.* An Aptamer Bio-barCode (ABC) assay using SPR, RNase H, and probes with RNA and gold-nanorods for anti-cancer drug screening. Analyst (Lond) 2017; 142(19): 3579-87.
[http://dx.doi.org/10.1039/C7AN01026E] [PMID: 28852760]

[54]   Wang D, Loo JFC, Chen J, *et al.* Recent Advances in Surface Plasmon Resonance Imaging Sensors. Sensors (Basel) 2019; 19(6): 1266.
[http://dx.doi.org/10.3390/s19061266] [PMID: 30871157]

[55]   Ho HP, Loo FC, Wu SY, Gu D, Yong K-T, Kong SK. MicroRNA Biosensing with Two-Dimensional Surface Plasmon Resonance Imaging. 2017.
[http://dx.doi.org/10.1007/978-1-4939-6848-0_8]

[56]   Shao Y, Li Y, Gu D, *et al.* Wavelength-multiplexing phase-sensitive surface plasmon imaging sensor.

Opt Lett 2013; 38(9): 1370-2.
[http://dx.doi.org/10.1364/OL.38.001370] [PMID: 23632487]

[57]   Hurot C, Brenet S, Buhot A, *et al.* Highly sensitive olfactory biosensors for the detection of volatile organic compounds by surface plasmon resonance imaging. Biosens Bioelectron 2019; 123: 230-6.
[http://dx.doi.org/10.1016/j.bios.2018.08.072] [PMID: 30201334]

[58]   Dey P, Fabri-Faja N, Calvo-Lozano O, *et al.* Label-free Bacteria Quantification in Blood Plasma by a Bioprinted Microarray Based Interferometric Point-of-Care Device. ACS Sens 2019; 4(1): 52-60.
[http://dx.doi.org/10.1021/acssensors.8b00789] [PMID: 30525470]

[59]   Wang D, Loo F-C, Cong H, *et al.* Real-time multi-channel SPR sensing based on DMD-enabled angular interrogation. Opt Express 2018; 26(19): 24627-36.
[http://dx.doi.org/10.1364/OE.26.024627] [PMID: 30469576]

[60]   Wang D, Loo JF. Development of a sensitive DMD-based 2D SPR sensor array using single-point detection strategy for multiple aptamer screening. Sens Actuators B Chem 2020; 305127240
[http://dx.doi.org/10.1016/j.snb.2019.127240]

[61]   Halpern AR, Chen Y, Corn RM, Kim D. Surface plasmon resonance phase imaging measurements of patterned monolayers and DNA adsorption onto microarrays. Anal Chem 2011; 83(7): 2801-6.
[http://dx.doi.org/10.1021/ac200157p] [PMID: 21355546]

[62]   Belushkin A, Yesilkoy F, Altug H. Nanoparticle-Enhanced Plasmonic Biosensor for Digital Biomarker Detection in a Microarray. ACS Nano 2018; 12(5): 4453-61.
[http://dx.doi.org/10.1021/acsnano.8b00519] [PMID: 29715005]

[63]   Kang K, Kim D. Effective optical properties of nanoparticle-mediated surface plasmon resonance sensors. Opt Express 2019; 27(3): 3091-100.
[http://dx.doi.org/10.1364/OE.27.003091] [PMID: 30732335]

[64]   Yin M, Gu B, An Q-F, Yang C, Guan YL, Yong K-T. Recent development of fiber-optic chemical sensors and biosensors: Mechanisms, materials, micro/nano-fabrications and applications. Coord Chem Rev 2018; 376: 348-92.
[http://dx.doi.org/10.1016/j.ccr.2018.08.001]

[65]   Lu J, Van Stappen T, Spasic D, *et al.* Fiber optic-SPR platform for fast and sensitive infliximab detection in serum of inflammatory bowel disease patients. Biosens Bioelectron 2016; 79: 173-9.
[http://dx.doi.org/10.1016/j.bios.2015.11.087] [PMID: 26706938]

[66]   Wang W, Mai Z, Chen Y, *et al.* A label-free fiber optic SPR biosensor for specific detection of C-reactive protein. Sci Rep 2017; 7(1): 16904.
[http://dx.doi.org/10.1038/s41598-017-17276-3] [PMID: 29203814]

[67]   Arghir I, Delport F, Spasic D, Lammertyn J. Smart design of fiber optic surfaces for improved plasmonic biosensing. N Biotechnol 2015; 32(5): 473-84.
[http://dx.doi.org/10.1016/j.nbt.2015.03.012] [PMID: 25858811]

[68]   Mayer KM, Lee S, Liao H, *et al.* A label-free immunoassay based upon localized surface plasmon resonance of gold nanorods. ACS Nano 2008; 2(4): 687-92.
[http://dx.doi.org/10.1021/nn7003734] [PMID: 19206599]

[69]   Mayer KM, Hafner JH. Localized surface plasmon resonance sensors. Chem Rev 2011; 111(6): 3828-57.
[http://dx.doi.org/10.1021/cr100313v] [PMID: 21648956]

[70]   Vilela D, González MC, Escarpa A. Sensing colorimetric approaches based on gold and silver nanoparticles aggregation: chemical creativity behind the assay. A review. Anal Chim Acta 2012; 751: 24-43.
[http://dx.doi.org/10.1016/j.aca.2012.08.043] [PMID: 23084049]

[71]   Loo JF, Lau P-M, Kong S-K, Ho H-P. An Assay Using Localized Surface Plasmon Resonance and Gold Nanorods Functionalized with Aptamers to Sense the Cytochrome-c Released from Apoptotic

Cancer Cells for Anti-Cancer Drug Effect Determination. Micromachines (Basel) 2017; 8(11): 338.
[http://dx.doi.org/10.3390/mi8110338] [PMID: 30400530]

[72]   Jo S, Lee W, Park J, Kim W, Kim W, Lee G, *et al.* Localized surface plasmon resonance aptasensor
       for the highly sensitive direct detection of cortisol in human saliva. Sens Actuators B Chem 2020;
       304127424
       [http://dx.doi.org/10.1016/j.snb.2019.127424]

[73]   Vinayaka AC, Ngo TA, Kant K, *et al.* Rapid detection of Salmonella enterica in food samples by a
       novel approach with combination of sample concentration and direct PCR. Biosens Bioelectron 2019;
       129: 224-30.
       [http://dx.doi.org/10.1016/j.bios.2018.09.078] [PMID: 30318404]

[74]   Zhao Q, Li X-F, Le XC. Aptamer capturing of enzymes on magnetic beads to enhance assay
       specificity and sensitivity. Anal Chem 2011; 83(24): 9234-6.
       [http://dx.doi.org/10.1021/ac203063z] [PMID: 22098163]

[75]   Mak WC, Cheung KY, Trau D. Diffusion Controlled and Temperature Stable Microcapsule Reaction
       Compartments for High-Throughput Microcapsule-PCR. Adv Funct Mater 2008; 18: 2930-7.
       [http://dx.doi.org/10.1002/adfm.200800388]

[76]   Schoepp NG, Schlappi TS, Curtis MS, *et al.* Rapid pathogen-specific phenotypic antibiotic
       susceptibility testing using digital LAMP quantification in clinical samples. Sci Transl Med 2017;
       9(410)eaal3693
       [http://dx.doi.org/10.1126/scitranslmed.aal3693] [PMID: 28978750]

[77]   Ashkin A, Dziedzic JM. Optical trapping and manipulation of viruses and bacteria. Science 1987;
       235(4795): 1517-20.
       [http://dx.doi.org/10.1126/science.3547653] [PMID: 3547653]

[78]   Maragò OM, Jones PH, Gucciardi PG, Volpe G, Ferrari AC. Optical trapping and manipulation of
       nanostructures. Nat Nanotechnol 2013; 8(11): 807-19.
       [http://dx.doi.org/10.1038/nnano.2013.208] [PMID: 24202536]

[79]   Cong H, Loo F-C, Chen J, Wang Y, Kong S-K, Ho H-P. Target trapping and*in situ* single-cell genetic
       marker detection with a focused optical beam. Biosens Bioelectron 2019; 133: 236-42.
       [http://dx.doi.org/10.1016/j.bios.2019.02.009] [PMID: 30953882]

[80]   Lin S, Crozier KB. Trapping-assisted sensing of particles and proteins using on-chip optical
       microcavities. ACS Nano 2013; 7(2): 1725-30.
       [http://dx.doi.org/10.1021/nn305826j] [PMID: 23311448]

[81]   Li X, Soler M, Szydzik C, *et al.* Label-Free Optofluidic Nanobiosensor Enables Real-Time Analysis of
       Single-Cell Cytokine Secretion. Small 2018; 14(26)e1800698
       [http://dx.doi.org/10.1002/smll.201800698] [PMID: 29806234]

[82]   Chen J, Cong H, Loo FC, *et al.* Thermal gradient induced tweezers for the manipulation of particles
       and cells. Sci Rep 2016; 6: 35814.
       [http://dx.doi.org/10.1038/srep35814] [PMID: 27853191]

[83]   Chen J, Loo JF, Wang D, Zhang Y, Kong S, Ho H. Thermal Optofluidics: Principles and Applications.
       Adv Opt Mater 2019; 1900829
       [http://dx.doi.org/10.1002/adom.201900829]

[84]   Beni V, Nilsson D, Arven P, Norberg P, Gustafsson G, Turner APF. Printed Electrochemical
       Instruments for Biosensors. ECS J Solid State Sci Technol 2015; 4: S3001-5.
       [http://dx.doi.org/10.1149/2.0011510jss]

[85]   Ramser K, Enger J, Goksör M, Hanstorp D, Logg K, Käll M. A microfluidic system enabling Raman
       measurements of the oxygenation cycle in single optically trapped red blood cells. Lab Chip 2005;
       5(4): 431-6.
       [http://dx.doi.org/10.1039/B416749J] [PMID: 15791341]

[86] Ramser K, Logg K, Goksör M, Enger J, Käll M, Hanstorp D. Resonance Raman spectroscopy of optically trapped functional erythrocytes. J Biomed Opt 2004; 9(3): 593-600.
[http://dx.doi.org/10.1117/1.1689336] [PMID: 15189098]

[87] Chan JF-W, Yip CC-Y, To KK-W, *et al.* Improved Molecular Diagnosis of COVID-19 by the Novel, Highly Sensitive and Specific COVID-19-RdRp/Hel Real-Time Reverse Transcription-PCR Assay Validated *In Vitro* and with Clinical Specimens. J Clin Microbiol 2020; 58(5): e00310-20.
[http://dx.doi.org/10.1128/JCM.00310-20] [PMID: 32132196]

[88] Drabovich AP, Okhonin V, Berezovski M, Krylov SN. Smart aptamers facilitate multi-probe affinity analysis of proteins with ultra-wide dynamic range of measured concentrations. J Am Chem Soc 2007; 129(23): 7260-1.
[http://dx.doi.org/10.1021/ja072269p] [PMID: 17503828]

[89] Figueroa-Miranda G, Feng L, Shiu SC-C, Dirkzwager RM, Cheung Y-W, Tanner JA, *et al.* Aptamer-based electrochemical biosensor for highly sensitive and selective malaria detection with adjustable dynamic response range and reusability. Sens Actuators B Chem 2018; 255: 235-43.
[http://dx.doi.org/10.1016/j.snb.2017.07.117]

[90] Munzar JD, Ng A, Juncker D. Comprehensive profiling of the ligand binding landscapes of duplexed aptamer families reveals widespread induced fit. Nat Commun 2018; 9(1): 343.
[http://dx.doi.org/10.1038/s41467-017-02556-3] [PMID: 29367662]

[91] Wei B, Zhang J, Ou X, Lou X, Xia F, Vallée-Bélisle A. Engineering Biosensors with Dual Programmable Dynamic Ranges. Anal Chem 2018; 90(3): 1506-10.
[http://dx.doi.org/10.1021/acs.analchem.7b04852] [PMID: 29300471]

[92] Ma L, Liu F, Lei Z, Wang Z. A novel upconversion@polydopamine core@shell nanoparticle based aptameric biosensor for biosensing and imaging of cytochrome c inside living cells. Biosens Bioelectron 2017; 87: 638-45.
[http://dx.doi.org/10.1016/j.bios.2016.09.017] [PMID: 27619527]

[93] Lin R, Feng Q, Li P, *et al.* A hybridization-chain-reaction-based method for amplifying immunosignals. Nat Methods 2018; 15(4): 275-8.
[http://dx.doi.org/10.1038/nmeth.4611] [PMID: 29481551]

[94] Dirks RM, Pierce NA. Triggered amplification by hybridization chain reaction. Proc Natl Acad Sci USA 2004; 101(43): 15275-8.
[http://dx.doi.org/10.1073/pnas.0407024101] [PMID: 15492210]

[95] Loynachan CN, Thomas MR, Gray ER, *et al.* Platinum Nanocatalyst Amplification: Redefining the Gold Standard for Lateral Flow Immunoassays with Ultrabroad Dynamic Range. ACS Nano 2018; 12(1): 279-88.
[http://dx.doi.org/10.1021/acsnano.7b06229] [PMID: 29215864]

[96] Ho HP, Wu SY, Yang M, Cheung AC. Application of white light-emitting diode to surface plasmon resonance sensors. Sens Actuators B Chem 2001; 80: 89-94.
[http://dx.doi.org/10.1016/S0925-4005(01)00881-4]

[97] Ng SP, Wu CM, Wu SY, Ho HP, Kong SK. Differential spectral phase interferometry for wide dynamic range surface plasmon resonance biosensing. Biosens Bioelectron 2010; 26(4): 1593-8.
[http://dx.doi.org/10.1016/j.bios.2010.07.128] [PMID: 20800466]

[98] Ng SP, Loo FC, Wu SY, Kong SK, Wu CML, Ho HP. Common-path spectral interferometry with temporal carrier for highly sensitive surface plasmon resonance sensing. Opt Express 2013; 21(17): 20268-73.
[http://dx.doi.org/10.1364/OE.21.020268] [PMID: 24105572]

[99] Jo S, Kim I, Lee W, *et al.* Highly sensitive and wide-range nanoplasmonic detection of fibrinogen using erythrocyte membrane-blanketed nanoparticles. Biosens Bioelectron 2019; 135: 216-23.
[http://dx.doi.org/10.1016/j.bios.2019.04.030] [PMID: 31026776]

[100] Liu M, Hui CY, Zhang Q, *et al.* Target-Induced and Equipment-Free DNA Amplification with a Simple Paper Device. Angew Chem Int Ed Engl 2016; 55(8): 2709-13.
[http://dx.doi.org/10.1002/anie.201509389] [PMID: 26748431]

[101] Carrasquilla C, Little JRL, Li Y, Brennan JD. Patterned paper sensors printed with long-chain DNA aptamers. Chemistry 2015; 21(20): 7369-73.
[http://dx.doi.org/10.1002/chem.201500949] [PMID: 25820300]

[102] Cheng X, Liu X, Bing T, Cao Z, Shangguan D. General peroxidase activity of G-quadruplex-hemin complexes and its application in ligand screening. Biochemistry 2009; 48(33): 7817-23.
[http://dx.doi.org/10.1021/bi9006786] [PMID: 19618960]

[103] Dirks RM, Pierce NA. Triggered amplification by hybridization chain reaction nd:4

[104] Komiya K, Komori M, Noda C, Kobayashi S, Yoshimura T, Yamamura M. Leak-free million-fold DNA amplification with locked nucleic acid and targeted hybridization in one pot. Org Biomol Chem 2019; 17(23): 5708-13.
[http://dx.doi.org/10.1039/C9OB00521H] [PMID: 30964494]

[105] Xu G, Zeng S, Zhang B, Swihart MT, Yong KT, Prasad PN. New Generation Cadmium-Free Quantum Dots for Biophotonics and Nanomedicine. Chem Rev 2016; 116(19): 12234-327.
[http://dx.doi.org/10.1021/acs.chemrev.6b00290] [PMID: 27657177]

[106] Wongkaew N, Simsek M, Griesche C, Baeumner AJ. Functional Nanomaterials and Nanostructures Enhancing Electrochemical Biosensors and Lab-on-a-Chip Performances: Recent Progress, Applications, and Future Perspective. Chem Rev 2019; 119(1): 120-94.
[http://dx.doi.org/10.1021/acs.chemrev.8b00172] [PMID: 30247026]

[107] Kovalska E, Lesongeur P, Hogan BT, Baldycheva A. Multi-layer graphene as a selective detector for future lung cancer biosensing platforms. Nanoscale 2019; 11(5): 2476-83.
[http://dx.doi.org/10.1039/C8NR08405J] [PMID: 30672548]

[108] Song Y, Qu K, Zhao C, Ren J, Qu X. Graphene oxide: intrinsic peroxidase catalytic activity and its application to glucose detection. Adv Mater 2010; 22(19): 2206-10.
[http://dx.doi.org/10.1002/adma.200903783] [PMID: 20564257]

[109] Wang H, Li P, Yu D, *et al.* Unraveling the Enzymatic Activity of Oxygenated Carbon Nanotubes and Their Application in the Treatment of Bacterial Infections. Nano Lett 2018; 18(6): 3344-51.
[http://dx.doi.org/10.1021/acs.nanolett.7b05095] [PMID: 29763562]

[110] Fan K, Xi J, Fan L, *et al. In vivo* guiding nitrogen-doped carbon nanozyme for tumor catalytic therapy. Nat Commun 2018; 9(1): 1440.
[http://dx.doi.org/10.1038/s41467-018-03903-8] [PMID: 29650959]

[111] Nasseri B, Soleimani N, Rabiee N, Kalbasi A, Karimi M, Hamblin MR. Point-of-care microfluidic devices for pathogen detection. Biosens Bioelectron 2018; 117: 112-28.
[http://dx.doi.org/10.1016/j.bios.2018.05.050] [PMID: 29890393]

[112] Strohmeier O, Keller M, Schwemmer F, *et al.* Centrifugal microfluidic platforms: advanced unit operations and applications. Chem Soc Rev 2015; 44(17): 6187-229.
[http://dx.doi.org/10.1039/C4CS00371C] [PMID: 26035697]

[113] Kong LX, Perebikovsky A, Moebius J, Kulinsky L, Madou M. Lab-on-a-CD: A Fully Integrated Molecular Diagnostic System. J Lab Autom 2016; 21(3): 323-55.
[http://dx.doi.org/10.1177/2211068215588456] [PMID: 26082453]

[114] Loo JFC, Kwok HC, Leung CCH, *et al.* Sample-to-answer on molecular diagnosis of bacterial infection using integrated lab-on-a-disc. Biosens Bioelectron 2017; 93: 212-9.
[http://dx.doi.org/10.1016/j.bios.2016.09.001] [PMID: 27660018]

[115] Yan H, Zhu Y, Zhang Y, *et al.* Multiplex detection of bacteria on an integrated centrifugal disk using bead-beating lysis and loop-mediated amplification. Sci Rep 2017; 7(1): 1460.

[http://dx.doi.org/10.1038/s41598-017-01415-x] [PMID: 28469259]

[116] Miyazaki CM, Kinahan DJ, Mishra R, *et al.* Label-free, spatially multiplexed SPR detection of immunoassays on a highly integrated centrifugal Lab-on-a-Disc platform. Biosens Bioelectron 2018; 119: 86-93.
[http://dx.doi.org/10.1016/j.bios.2018.07.056] [PMID: 30103158]

[117] Ng AHC, Fobel R, Fobel C, *et al.* A digital microfluidic system for serological immunoassays in remote settings. Sci Transl Med 2018; 10(438): 1-13.
[http://dx.doi.org/10.1126/scitranslmed.aar6076] [PMID: 29695457]

[118] Peng C, Zhang Z, Kim C-J, Ju YS. EWOD (electrowetting on dielectric) digital microfluidics powered by finger actuation. Lab Chip 2014; 14(6): 1117-22.
[http://dx.doi.org/10.1039/c3lc51223a] [PMID: 24452784]

[119] Mak WC, Beni V, Turner APF. Lateral-flow technology: From visual to instrumental. Trends Analyt Chem 2016; 79: 297-305.
[http://dx.doi.org/10.1016/j.trac.2015.10.017]

[120] Nurul Najian AB, Engku Nur Syafirah EAR, Ismail N, Mohamed M, Yean CY. Development of multiplex loop mediated isothermal amplification (m-LAMP) label-based gold nanoparticles lateral flow dipstick biosensor for detection of pathogenic Leptospira. Anal Chim Acta 2016; 903: 142-8.
[http://dx.doi.org/10.1016/j.aca.2015.11.015] [PMID: 26709307]

[121] Meng L, Turner APF, Mak WC. Soft and flexible material-based affinity sensors. Biotechnol Adv 2020; 39107398
[http://dx.doi.org/10.1016/j.biotechadv.2019.05.004] [PMID: 31071431]

[122] Kim J, Campbell AS, de Ávila BE-F, Wang J. Wearable biosensors for healthcare monitoring. Nat Biotechnol 2019; 37(4): 389-406.
[http://dx.doi.org/10.1038/s41587-019-0045-y] [PMID: 30804534]

[123] Loo JFC, Ho AHP, Turner APF, Mak WC. Integrated Printed Microfluidic Biosensors. Trends Biotechnol 2019; 37(10): 1104-20.
[http://dx.doi.org/10.1016/j.tibtech.2019.03.009] [PMID: 30992149]

[124] Au AK, Huynh W, Horowitz LF, Folch A. 3D-Printed Microfluidics. Angew Chem Int Ed Engl 2016; 55(12): 3862-81.
[http://dx.doi.org/10.1002/anie.201504382] [PMID: 26854878]

[125] Ho CMB, Ng SH, Li KHH, Yoon YJ. 3D printed microfluidics for biological applications. Lab Chip 2015; 15(18): 3627-37.
[http://dx.doi.org/10.1039/C5LC00685F] [PMID: 26237523]

[126] Dirkzwager RM, Liang S, Tanner JA. Development of Aptamer-Based Point-of-Care Diagnostic Devices for Malaria Using Three-Dimensional Printing Rapid Prototyping. ACS Sens 2016; 1: 420-6.
[http://dx.doi.org/10.1021/acssensors.5b00175]

[127] Ardila D, Kiraly AP, Bharadwaj S, *et al.* End-to-end lung cancer screening with three-dimensional deep learning on low-dose chest computed tomography. Nat Med 2019; 25(6): 954-61.
[http://dx.doi.org/10.1038/s41591-019-0447-x] [PMID: 31110349]

[128] Moen E, Bannon D, Kudo T, Graf W, Covert M, Van Valen D. Deep learning for cellular image analysis. Nat Methods 2019; 16(12): 1233-46.
[http://dx.doi.org/10.1038/s41592-019-0403-1] [PMID: 31133758]

[129] Zhang YS, Busignani F, Ribas J, *et al.* Google Glass-Directed Monitoring and Control of Microfluidic Biosensors and Actuators. Sci Rep 2016; 6: 22237.
[http://dx.doi.org/10.1038/srep22237] [PMID: 26928456]

[130] Gahlaut SK, Kalyani N, Sharan C, Mishra P, Singh JP. Smartphone based dual mode *in situ* detection of viability of bacteria using Ag nanorods array. Biosens Bioelectron 2019; 126: 478-84.
[http://dx.doi.org/10.1016/j.bios.2018.11.025] [PMID: 30472445]

[131] Hu J, Cui X, Gong Y, *et al.* Portable microfluidic and smartphone-based devices for monitoring of cardiovascular diseases at the point of care. Biotechnol Adv 2016; 34(3): 305-20.
[http://dx.doi.org/10.1016/j.biotechadv.2016.02.008] [PMID: 26898179]

[132] Yang J. Blood glucose monitoring with smartphone as glucometer. Electrophoresis 2019; 40: 1144-47.
[http://dx.doi.org/10.1002/elps.201800295] [PMID: 30136730]

CHAPTER 2

Micro/nanofabrication of IVD/POCT Biosensors

Huan Hu[1,*] and Lei Li[2]

[1] *ZJUI Institute, Zhejiang University, Haining, Zhejiang Province, 314400, China*

[2] *CAS Key Laboratory of Cryogenics, Technical Institute of Physics and Chemistry, Chinese Academy of Sciences, Beijing, 100190, China*

Abstract: Point-of-care technologies (POCT), defined as "the testing performed near or at the site of a patient with the result leading to a possible change in the care of the patient" by ISO 22870:2006, are transforming the healthcare system. With the growing global aging population, healthcare cost is becoming a huge burden for human society. IVD/POCT sensors can play an important role in alleviating this urgent social issue. First, they provide medical test and even therapy near the patient, saving the time and cost for commuting to hospitals. Second, with more frequent and even continuously test, more precise and even earlier diagnosis can be achieved, which further reduces the required treatment and gives doctors more information to determine more appropriate therapies. POCT sensors demand miniaturized devices and cheaper equipment. Micro/nanofabrication uses mass-production manufacturing methods to produce miniaturized sensors, which later can be packaged and fitted into a small equipment [1]. In this chapter, we will introduce the main microfabrication and nanofabrication techniques for POCT sensors.

Keywords: Etching, IVD/POCT biosensors, Microfabrication, Micro-Electro-Mechanical Systems (MEMS), Nanofabrication.

INTRODUCTION TO IVD/POCT BIOSENSORS

Point-of-care technologies (POCTs), defined as "the testing performed near or at the site of a patient with the result leading to a possible change in the care of the patient" in ISO 22870:2006, are transforming the healthcare system. With a global elderly population that is growing rapidly, healthcare cost is becoming a substantial burden for the society. *In vitro* diagnostic (IVD) or POCT sensors can play an important role in addressing this urgent social issue. First, these sensors enable medical tests and even therapy to be performed near the patient, saving the time and cost of commuting to hospitals. Second, with more frequent and conti-

---

[*] **Corresponding author Huan Hu:** ZJUI Institute, Zhejiang University, Haining, Zhejiang Province 314400, China; E-mail: huanhu@intl.zjn.edu.cn

Han-Sheng Chuang & Yi-Ping Ho (Eds.)

nuous testing, more precise and earlier diagnosis can be achieved, which reduces the required treatment further and provides doctors additional information to decide the appropriate therapies.

POCT sensors require miniaturized devices and cheaper equipment. Micro/nanofabrication uses mass-production manufacturing methods to produce miniaturized sensors, which can be subsequently packaged in small-size equipment [1]. In this chapter, we introduce the main microfabrication and nanofabrication techniques for POCT sensors.

MICROFABRICATION

Conventional thin-film Processing from Semiconductor Manufacturing

This technology originates from semiconductor manufacturing. Fig. (**1**) shows an overview of the manufacturing process used in the microelectronic industry. It mainly consists of thin-film formation, lithography, etching, dicing, and packaging. The fabrication process starts with a thin-film formation process, such as oxidation and thin-film deposition. This is followed by a lithography step, which involves using a photomask to expose a photoresist to ultraviolet (UV) light selectively. The exposed photoresist is then dissolved in the development stage, and the photoresist layer is patterned. Subsequently, an etching step is employed to etch the thin film underneath the remaining photoresist. Subsequently, the patterns are transferred from the photomasks to the thin films. These steps are normally iterated several times for producing microelectronic circuits. Finally, the substrate, normally a wafer, is diced into several small pieces named "dies," and these dies are then packaged into each individual component by attaching them to a package. Inside the package, an electrical connection is established through wire bonding, and the dies are encapsulated with epoxies.

Thin Film Formation

Thin films with different functions are required for different applications. Biosensors normally require metal materials for electrodes, semiconductor materials for sensing materials, and dielectric materials for electrical insulation.

Thin-film formation in microfabrication generally consists of oxidation, diffusion, implantation, and thin-film deposition. Oxidation involves growing an oxide layer from the substrate materials. For example, silicon oxide is grown from a silicon substrate at high temperatures in a furnace. The thin film is usually the oxide of the substrates. Diffusion and implantation are generally used for doping semiconductor materials with different elements. For example, phosphorous ions are doped into silicon to obtain n-type silicon, and boron ions are doped into silicon to obtain p-type silicon.

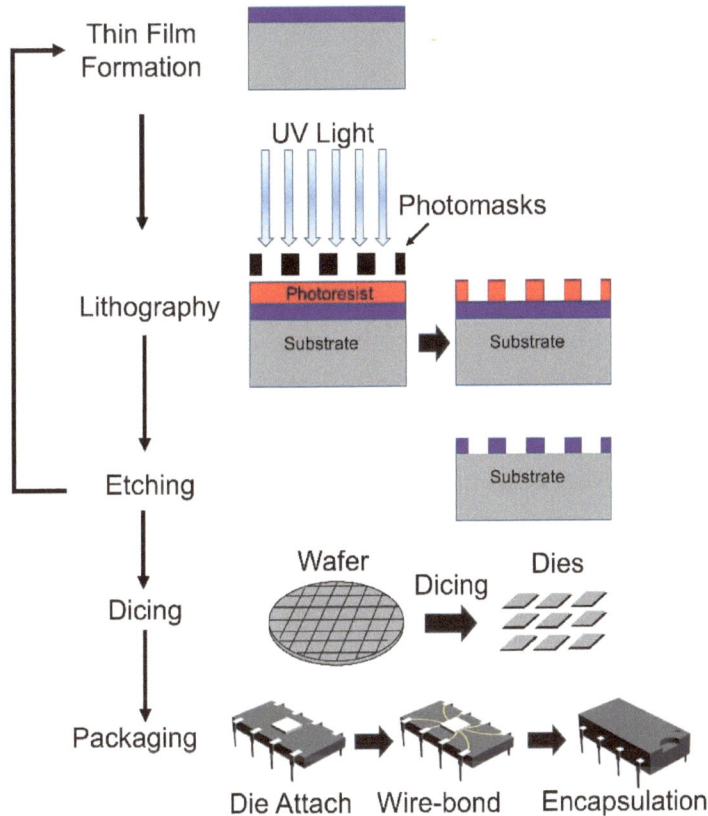

Fig. (1). Schematic illustrating the basic fabrication process of integrated circuits.

Thin-film deposition involves preparing a thin film on top of the substrate. The deposited materials are usually different from the substrate material. Several mechanisms exist for thin-film deposition. Generally, the deposition processes can be categorized into two types: physical and chemical processes, as shown in Fig. (**2a**).

In physical deposition methods, an electron beam evaporator uses a high-energy electron beam emitted from a tungsten filament under a high-vacuum condition to bombard the source materials, knocking the atoms off the substrate and converting them into the gaseous phase, which will precipitate on the substrate and turn into a solid form. A thermal evaporator uses electrical resistors to heat a metal boat that carries the pellets of target materials into vapor, which then travel directly to the target substrate in a vacuum and condense back into solid form.

Another type of physical method is sputtering deposition. In sputtering, inertial gas ions such as argon are bombarded on the target source, displacing atoms or ions, which are then deposited on the substrate. Different methods of generating gas ions exist, such as using direct current (DC) signals or radio frequency (RF) signals.

Some differences exist between evaporation and sputtering. First, evaporation normally occurs under a high-vacuum condition, and the mean free path of the atom is thus longer; this indicates that the atoms travel almost linearly at an angle. When the substrate has some microstructures, the deposited films will exhibit non-uniform coverage, as shown in the left figure of Fig. (**2b**). In contrast, in sputtering, the vacuum is not as high as that in evaporation; therefore, the atoms are likely to collide with other atoms, causing scattering before they reach the substrate. Hence, the coverage is more uniform as shown in the right figure of Fig. (**2b**). In some cases, such as filling a cavity for creating a photonic waveguide, uniform coating is preferred, whereas in other cases, such as metal lift-off processes, non-uniform coating is preferred.

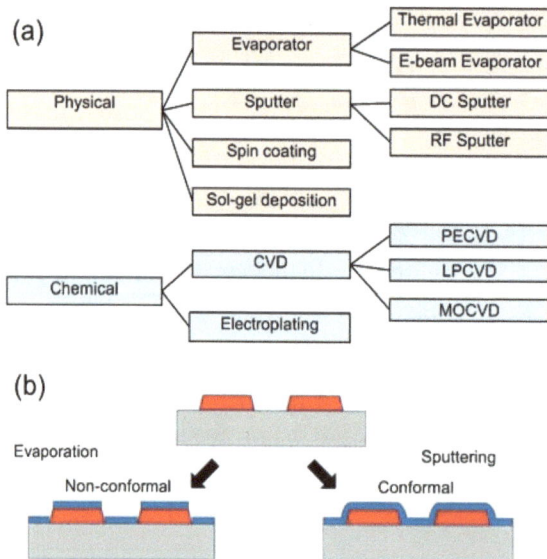

Fig. (2). (**a**) Thin-film deposition techniques; (**b**) two different thin-film coverage profiles.

Spin coating uses centrifugal forces along with the surface tension and viscosity of the solutions to spread a film into a uniform thickness. During the spinning process, the solvent also evaporates, thus increasing the viscosity of the film. After spinning, a baking process is normally used to remove the remaining solvent and cure the thin film. The photoresist layer and polyimides are generally prepared *via* spin coating.

Sol-gel deposition is typically used to form various oxides by sintering a deposited sol gel layer containing a precursor, such as the spin-on glasses and lead zirconate titanate (PZT) used for piezoelectric resonator biosensors.

Chemical vapor deposition (CVD) is a major chemical method for depositing thin films. In CVD, source gases are supplied into a chamber. Subsequently, they undergo chemical reactions on the substrates, which are usually heated to high temperatures. Some materials cannot adequately withstand high temperatures; therefore, plasma-enhanced CVD (PECVD) technology is generally used. PECVD uses RF voltages to excite plasma in reactive gases; therefore, chemical reactions can occur at a lower temperature. Low-pressure CVD (LPCVD) can produce thin films with excellent uniformity, but it requires high temperatures, and its deposition rate is slow. LPCVD is primarily used for polysilicon, oxides, phosphosilicate glass (PSG), and silicon nitride. Metal organic CVD (MOCVD) produces single-crystal or polycrystalline thin films in a moderate-pressure environment instead of a vacuum environment. III–V materials, such as aluminum nitride (AlN) and gallium arsenide (GaAs) are typically prepared *via* MOCVD.

Another chemical method for preparing thin films is electroplating [2]. Thick metal layers, such as copper exceeding one micrometer, are generally prepared using this method. For example, copper used in through-silicon vias (TSV) is prepared through electroplating. Copper thus prepared is used for filling the TSVs to establish electrical connections between chips. Electroplating can be used to fill predefined nanotemplates to produce nanowires useful for sensing gases, such as H_2S [3].

Etching

Three main types of etching methods exist based on the etching profiles. The first type is isotropic etching, in which the etchant etches the substrate at the same etching rate in all directions. Consequently, there will be an undercut region under the etch mask shown in Fig. (**3a**). Typical chemical etching systems such as HNO_3 and HNA (Hydrofluoric, Nitric, Acetic) systems belong to the category of isotropic etching. Sometimes, dry etching methods, such as reactive-ion etching, are also isotropic if the ions are not significantly accelerated to damage the structure physically, and only chemical etching occurs.

The second type of etching method is anisotropic etching, wherein the etchants favor substrate etching in certain directions. For example, potassium hydroxide (KOH) is a common etchant for silicon etching. It etches (100) single-crystal silicon much faster in the (100) direction but very slowly in the (111) crystal direction; therefore, the etching profile will exhibit anisotropy as shown in Fig. (**3b**).

Recently, a new type of etching method known as metal-assisted chemical etching (MacEtch) has been proposed [4, 5]. As shown in Fig. (**3c**), it uses metal catalysts, such as Au, Ag, and Pt, to induce the chemical etching of substrates, such as silicon, germanium, and III–V materials. The etching profile can be vertical and have very smooth sidewalls. It is useful for fabricating high-aspect-ratio structures. In addition, MacEtch can function under room-temperature and ambient conditions. Compared with the Bosch process, MacEtch is considerably less expensive and does not require sophisticated equipment.

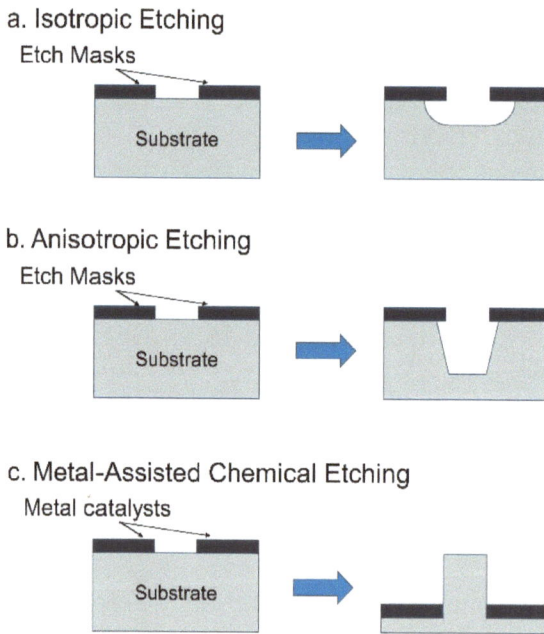

a. Isotropic Etching

b. Anisotropic Etching

c. Metal-Assisted Chemical Etching

Fig. (3). Three major etching techniques categorized based on the etching profiles. (**a**) isotropic etching wherein etching rates are equal in all directions; (**b**) anisotropic etching wherein etching rates are faster in one direction than in other directions; (**c**) metal-assisted chemical etching where etching only occurs in one direction.

Micro-electro-mechanical Systems (MEMS) Processing

MEMS such as micropumps or microresonators have moving components. Therefore, suspended structures are crucial components for MEMS. Suspended microstructures can be manufactured using two methods, as shown in Fig. (**4**).

The first method is to deposit the structure layer atop a sacrificial layer. Then, the sacrificial layer is selectively etched to release the structure layer to produce a suspended structure, as shown in Fig. (**4a**). A typical biosensor, such as a mechanical resonator, that employs a frequency shift to measure cell mass is also shown in Fig. (**4a**). Such a sensor uses this process to release the suspended beams [6]. The second type of method uses isotropic etching to achieve an undercut region that releases the structures, as shown in Fig. (**4b**). A typical CMOS-MEMS gyroscope is fabricated by using this method, as shown in Fig. (**4b**) [7].

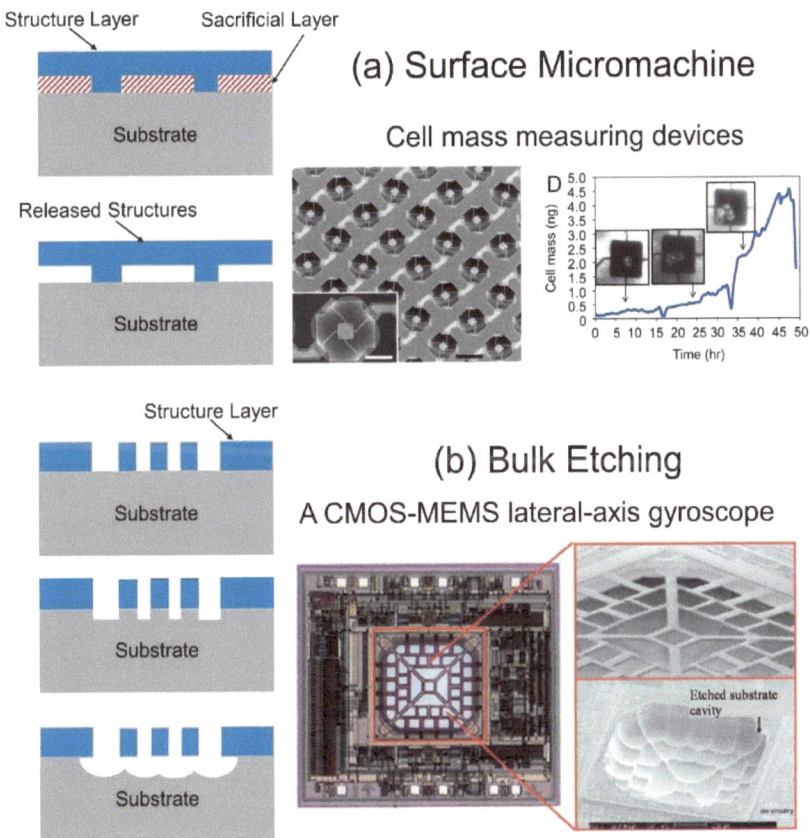

Fig. (**4**). Two types of methods for fabricating suspended structures for MEMS devices. (**a**) Sacrificial layer release; (**b**) front-side release using isotropic etching to achieve undercut region to release the structures.

Soft Lithography

Soft lithography, developed by the research group of Prof. Whitesides at Harvard University [8], refers to a set of methods that involve using a patterned elastomer as the mask, stamp, or mold to fabricate patterns. As a soft elastomeric material is used, this method is called "soft lithography." Several techniques can be categorized as soft lithography. Due to length limitations of this book chapter, we only introduce the most popular techniques, *i.e.*, molding and microcontact printing. The most common material used in soft lithography is polydimethylsiloxane (PDMS). In this process, the matrix agent and the curing agent are first mixed at a certain volume ratio, usually 10:1, and then baked at either room temperature for roughly 24 h or at elevated temperatures for shorter durations.

Soft lithography has several distinctive advantages that render it appealing for biosensor applications. First, it is considerably less expensive than traditional lithography is because the patterns can be repeatedly replicated from a mold. Second, it uses a self-assembly of biomolecules and can print biomolecules with micrometer to nanometer scale resolution [9].

As shown in Fig. (**5a**), the mold is usually prepared *via* the direct lithography of thick photoresists such as SU-8 or using prefabricated silicon. Silane is usually applied on top of the mold for facilitating the detachment of PDMS. Then, PDMS is poured on the mold and cured. Finally, the PDMS is detached from the mold and bonded to a glass substrate to form a sealed microchannel. This simple process enables various functions such as mixing [10], separation [11, 12], isolation [13], and capture [14]. These functions are crucial for realizing rapid and accurate biosensing. In addition, soft lithography can enable some unique devices. For example, Fig. (**5c**) shows a biosensor produced using a microfluidic droplet generator to detect single bacteria rapidly [15]. These kinds of droplets can enable cell encapsulation, cell culture [16], analysis such as digital PCR tests [17], which are particularly promising for drug screening, and the detection of pathogens with small concentration [18].

Microchannels fabricated *via* soft lithography can also be used to pattern biological molecules, such as immunoglobulins. This enables the preparation of simultaneous and highly localized immunoassays for the detection of different immunoglobulins [19].

In addition to microchannels, micropillars or microneedles of PDMS can be fabricated *via* the molding process and they have promising applications in measuring cellular forces [20]. The surface of a PDMS micropillar or microneedle is functionalized to allow cell culture and the force exerted by the cell on the PDMS micropillar causes bending, which can be observed under an optical microscope to derive the force based on the deflection of the pillars or needles [21].

As shown in Fig. (**5b**), soft lithography can enable the contact printing of biomolecules, which enables controlling cell shapes [22], bacteria assembly [23], and studying cell homeostasis [24]. Fig. (**5d**) shows a HeLa cell constrained by micrometer-scale strip patterns of fibronectin prepared *via* microcontact printing [24].

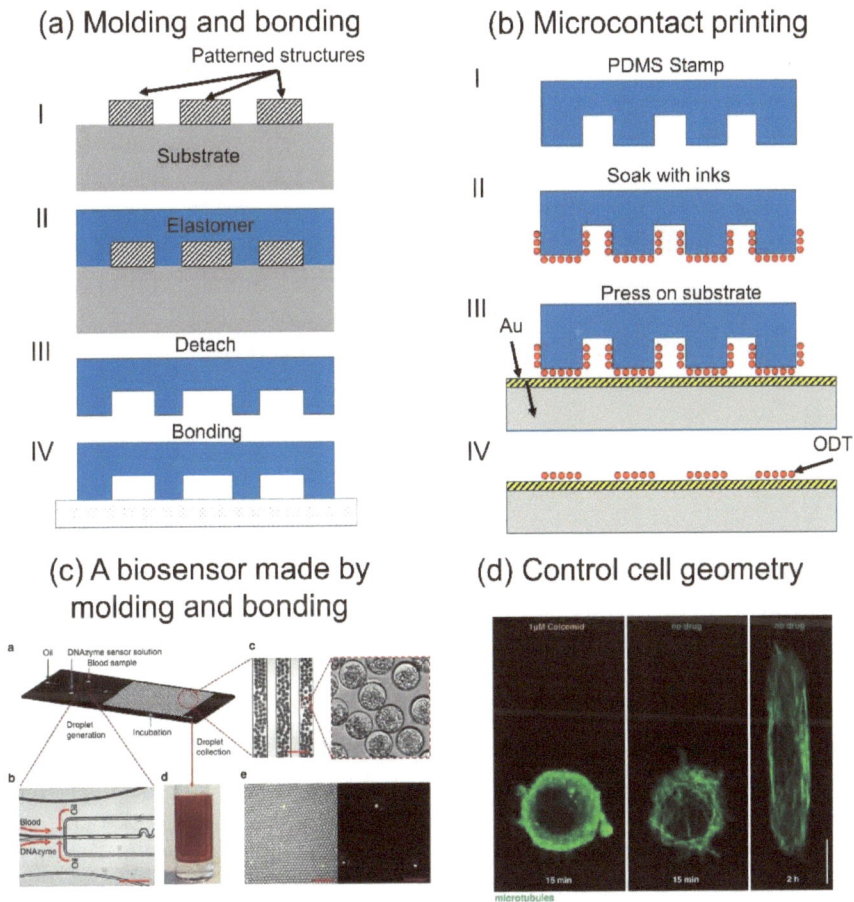

Fig. (**5**). Basic principle of soft lithography and its two major contributions to biosensors. (**a**) Schematic illustrating the major steps of molding; (**b**) schematic illustrating the major steps of producing a PDMS stamp and print molecules; (**c**) microfluidic droplet generator fabricated *via* molding and bonding process [15]; (**d**) micropatterned fibronectin lines prepared *via* microcontact printing to limit the extension of HeLa cells to fixed width [24].

Nanofabrication Techniques for IVD/POCT Sensors

The major difference between nanofabrication and microfabrication is the lithography technique used. Microfabrication uses conventional UV lithography and produces structures with dimensions as small as approximately one micron. Nanofabrication uses nanolithography to define patterns below one micron down to several nanometers. After the pattern is generated (on a resist layer in most cases), the procedures for transferring the pattern onto other materials such as etching and lift-off process are the same for both microfabrication and nanofabrication. Nanofabrication offers higher sensitivity, smaller volume, less energy consumption, and better portability to IVD/POCT sensors.

Nanolithography approaches can generally be categorized into two types: top-down and bottom-up approaches. However, as emerging nanofabrication technologies are being increasingly developed, they cannot be easily fitted into this simple classification. Therefore, a third category termed "unconventional" is established herein to include miscellaneous technologies for IVD/POCT sensors. Several nanofabrication technologies exist and covering them comprehensively is beyond the scope of this chapter. We focus on the nanofabrication technologies that have been used or have the potential to be used for producing POCT biosensors.

Top-down Nanofabrication

Top-down approaches mainly originate from semiconductor manufacturing, wherein lithography is used to nanopattern a resist, and the resist pattern is transferred to the substrate materials *via* etching. The final structure is achieved by selectively removing materials from the initial structure. Several types of top-down approaches exist.

The first type of top-down nanolithography approach is using beams, such as electron beams, light beams, X-rays, and ion beams, to expose the resist for producing nanostructures, as illustrated in Fig. (**6**). Such beam-based technologies include deep ultraviolet lithography (DUV), extreme ultraviolet lithography (EUV), electron beam lithography (EBL), ion beam lithography (IBL), and focused ion beam milling (FIB).

DUV [25] and EUV [26] are optical lithography techniques. They are the main technologies used in semiconductor manufacturing owing to the advantage of mass production. DUV and EUV use photon energy to induce the photochemical reaction of the resist to achieve nanopatterning. However, these techniques can only duplicate patterns predefined in a photomask and cannot produce arbitrary patterns. Recently, laser technology has also been used to write hundreds of nanometers of patterns directly.

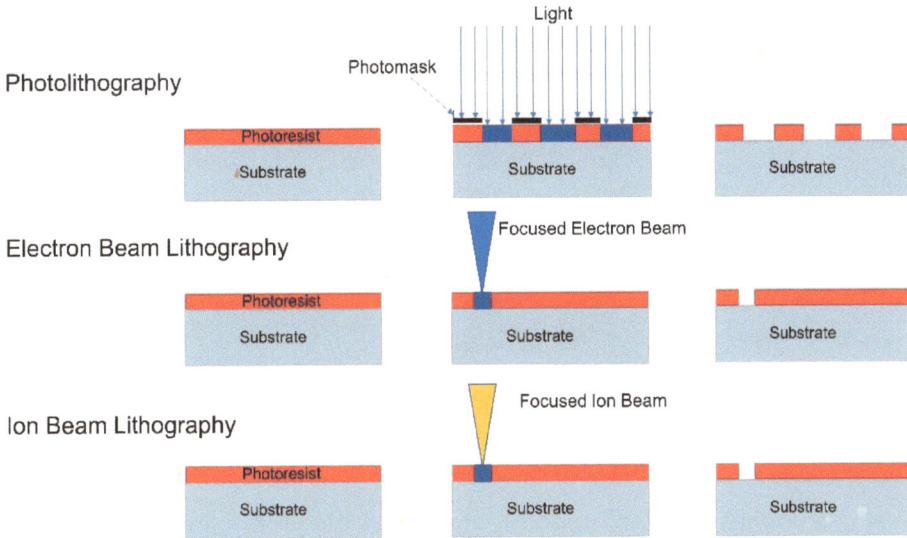

Fig. (6). Nanolithography using photons, electrons, and ions. (**a**) Photolithography requires a photomask; (**b**) electron beam lithography uses a controlled electron beam to expose the resist directly in the desired patterns and does not need a mask; (**c**) electron beam lithography uses a controlled focused ion beam to bombard the resist to generate low-voltage secondary electrons, which expose the resist in a predefined route.

Electron beam lithography (EBL) uses a focused electron beam instead of photons to induce the photochemical reaction of the resist in the desired region and achieve nanolithography. The feature size achieved *via* EBL is affected by the size of the focused electron beam spot, beam energy, resist, and substrate. The proximity effect occurs around a feature size of 10 nm, which prevents the size from decreasing further [27]. EBL has been used for fabricating nanoelec-tromechanical systems (NEMS) including sensors and actuators [28].

Ion beam lithography (IBL) uses a focused ion beam to perform nanolithography. When a focused ion beam hits the resist, secondary electrons are produced, and they induce the photochemical reaction of the photoresist. Focused gallium ions can conventionally provide a resolution of 50 nm. Recently, helium ion beams providing sub-5-nm resolution of fabrication have emerged [29, 30].

Fig. (**7**) shows a nanoplasmonic sensor with nanostructures defined *via* EBL. The sensor allows improved analyte detection because the analysts can be transported through the suspended nanohole [31].

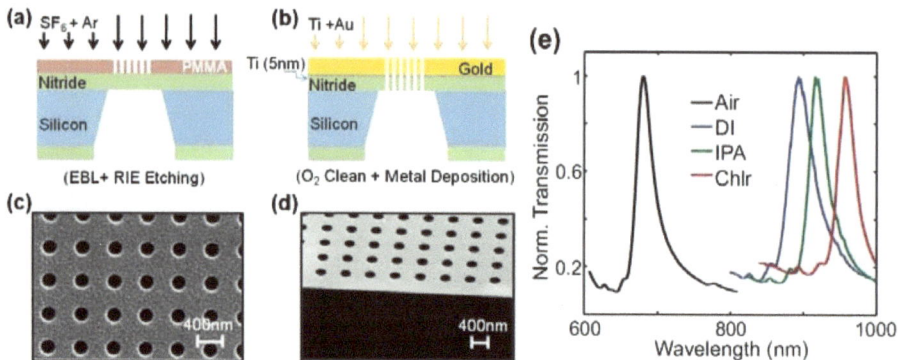

Fig. (7). Typical process flow of fabricating nanoplasmonic sensor using EBL combined with microfabrication.

The second type of top-down nanolithography approach is scanning-probe-based technology, in which a nanoscale tip interacts with substrates to form nanometer-scale patterns [32]. This type of approach can be categorized into material removal type, material transition type, and material addition type [33], as shown in Fig. (**8**). Each type can utilize different physical mechanisms such as thermal additives [34], thermal-chemical [35], mechanical [36], electrical [37], and electrochemical [38] reactions, and diffusion [39] to produce nanostructures. These mechanisms can be readily combined with the conventional microfabrication technology to produce nanodevices, as nanodevices typically require micropads for establishing electrical connections or micro-anchors for mechanical support

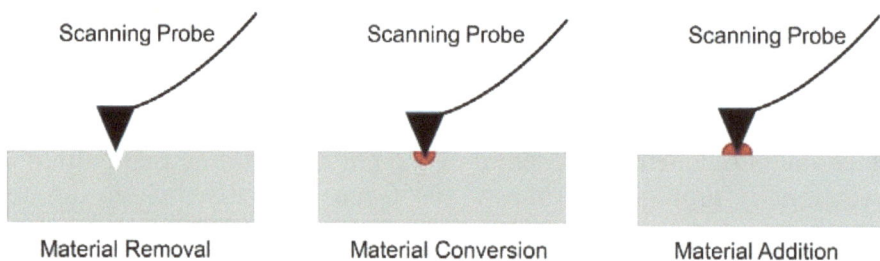

Fig. (8). Three major types of scanning-probe-based nanofabrication technologies: material removal, material conversion, and material addition.

Fig. (**9**) shows a representative methodology of combining scanning-probe-based nanofabrication with conventional microfabrication [40]. The process starts with a silicon-on-insulator (SOI) substrate. Aluminum micropads are first fabricated *via* conventional microfabrication, as shown in Fig. (**9a**). Then, polystyrene nanowires are deposited between two microfabricated aluminum pads using scanning-probe-based nanolithography (Fig. **9b**). After a step of silicon etching, the nanopatterns of the polymer nanowires and the micropatterns of the aluminum micropads are both transferred to the top silicon of the SOI substrate (Fig. **9c**). Subsequently, acetone and oxygen plasma etching are used to clean the remaining polymer nanowires (Fig. **9d**). Finally, the buried oxide layer is etched to release the nanobeam structure, and a suspended mechanical nanoresonator is thus obtained (Fig. **9e**). Fig. (**9f**) shows a scanning electron microscope (SEM) image of the resonator fabricated *via* this methodology and Fig. (**9g**) shows the measured resonance frequency of the resonator.

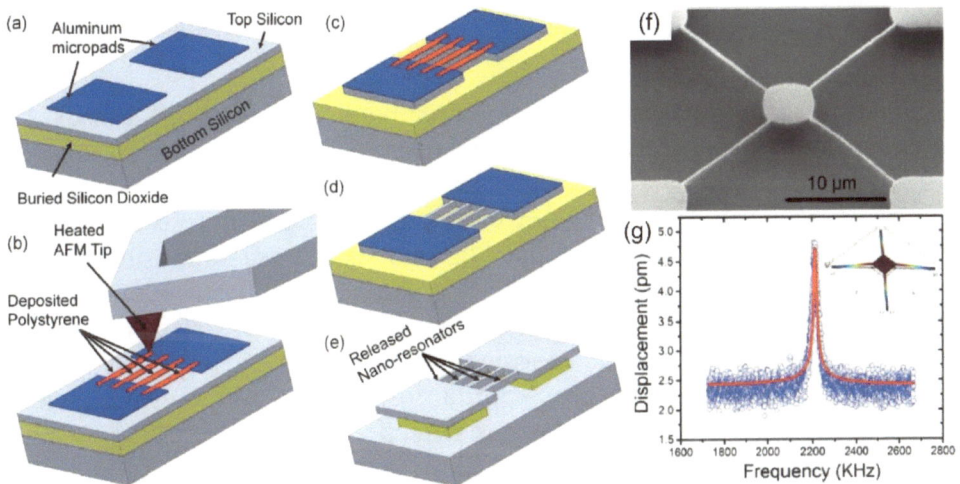

Fig. (9). Representative methodology of combining scanning-probe-based nanolithography with conventional microfabrication to fabricate nanomechanical resonators (reprinted with permission from [40]; copyright 2007 American Chemical Society).

The third type of top-down nanolithography approach is nanoimprint lithography (NIL), which involves replicating nanopatterns predefined in a master mold into samples [41]. It is a very important nanofabrication technology because it enables large-area and low-cost manufacturing of nanostructures and nanodevices, and is thus promising for the commercialization of IVD/POCT biosensors. Primarily two types of NIL exist—which are thermal-based curing and UV-light-based curing. These are illustrated in Fig. (**10**).

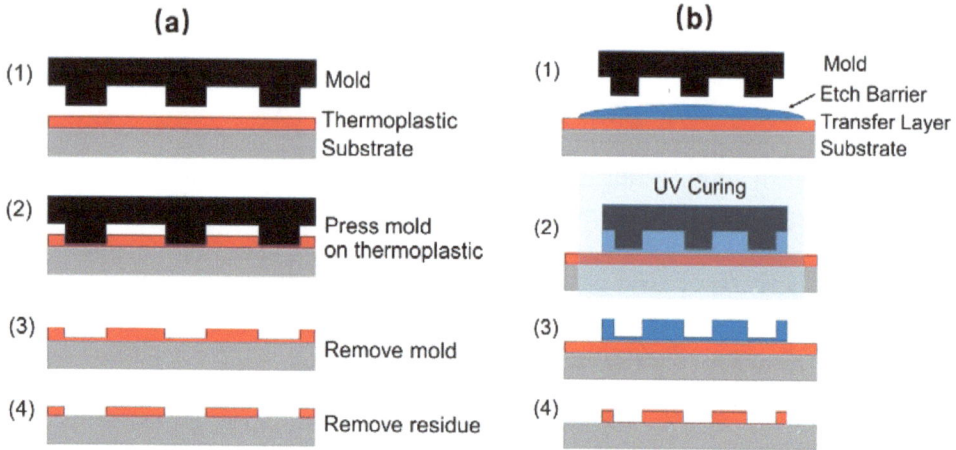

Fig. (10). Schematics of two major types of NIL. (**a**) Thermal-based curing; (**b**) UV-light-based curing.

NIL is very efficient in fabricating large-area nanostructures [42]. For example, photonic crystal sensors are mass-produced using NIL for detecting biomolecules. Fig. (**11**) shows a photonic crystal sensor fabricated *via* NIL. It can detect the presence of 65-nm-long and 30-nm-wide single gold nanorods (AuNRs) *via* resonance frequency shift and even provide an image by reading results across the sensor pixel-by-pixel [43]. Each pixel is a square of 500 nm × 500 nm. This technology is called photonic crystal-enhanced microscopy (PCEM), and it can provide information such as the adhesion between cells and substrate [44]. This type of photonic crystal sensor mass-produced *via* NIL can be further combined with smartphones to achieve point-of-care detection with low cost [45].

The fourth type of top-down nanolithography approach is laser interference lithography (LIL), which is also called holographic lithography. In LIL, a substrate with a photoresist film is arranged perpendicular to a mirror. The lasers incident on the mirror and reflected from the mirror form interference patterns on the photoresist and generate two-dimensional (2D) regular patterns of bright and dark spots, which further expose the photoresist and produce periodic nanopatterns. Fig. (**12a**) shows the classic Lloyd's interferometer setup. Fig. (**12b**) shows an actively stabilized setup to provide fast-configurable and stable fabrication results for LIL [46].

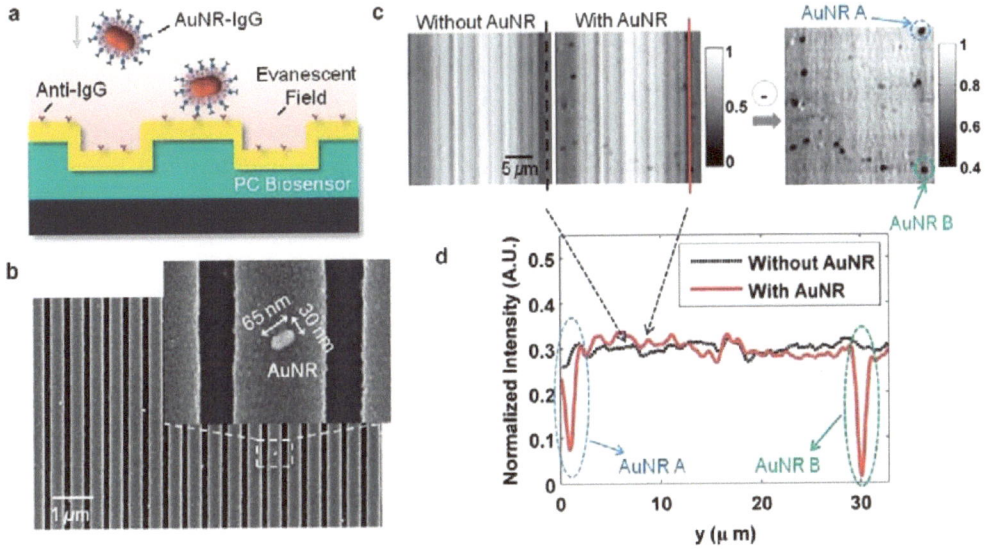

Fig. (11). (**a**) Schematic illustrating the attachment of AuNRs to the photonic crystal sensor surface; (**b**) SEM images of photonic crystal sensor surface with AuNR attached; (**c**) PCEM image of the sensor surface with and without AuNRs; (**d**) two representative cross-section lines of the normalized intensity images with/without two AuNRs on the photonic crystal sensor surface.

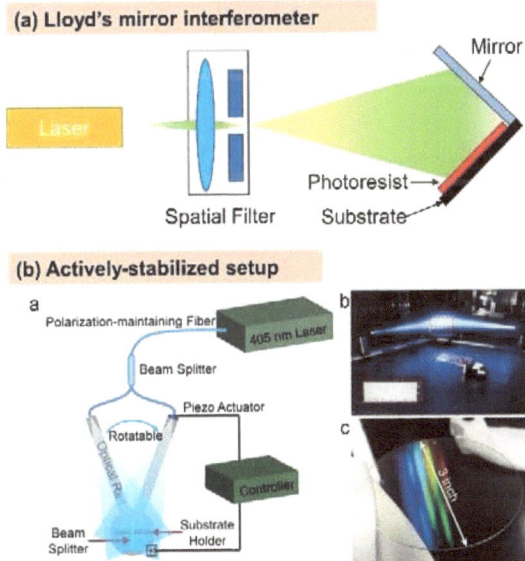

Fig. (12). Two setups for LIL. (**a**) Lloyd's mirror interferometer; (**b**) actively stabilized setup for producing gratings in a 3-inch wafer.

Although the design flexibility of LIL is limited to a certain degree and cannot match the design flexibility offered by a direct writing technology such as EBL, pattern types generated *via* LIL such as hole arrays and pillar arrays are still sufficient for several applications in optical biosensors such as plasmonic biosensors [47], surface-enhanced Raman spectroscopy (SERS) [48], and photonic crystals sensors [49, 50]. An LIL-made array of plasmonic nanoholes can detect the attachment of proteins [51]. Fig. (**13**) shows a metal–insulator–metal (MIM) device fabricated *via* LIL, which can enhance the up-conversion luminescence over 1000-fold and can potentially be used in medical applications such as photothermal therapy [52].

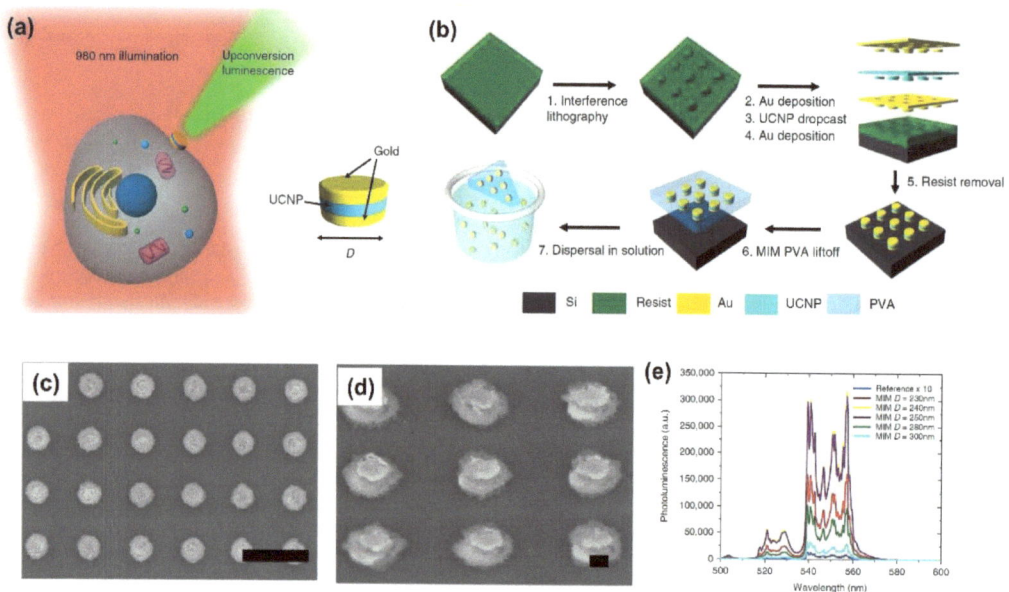

Fig. (13). Use of LIL to produce MIM devices for enhancing up-conversion luminescence [52]. (**a**) Schematic illustrating that MIM can be attached to cells for phototherapy; (**b**) fabrication process of MIM devices using LIL; (**c**) a top-view SEM image of an array of MIM devices; (**d**) a tilted-view SEM image of an array of MIM devices showing the three layers; (**e**) measured results showing different enhancements of photoluminescence for MIM devices with different geometries.

SUBSTRTE MATERIALS FOR BIOSENSORS

Conventional substrate materials for constructing biosensors include borosilicate glass [53, 54], metallic glass [55], single-crystal silicon [56], porous silicon [57], polyimide [58], polycarbonate [59], elastomers [60], and textiles [61], as shown in Fig. (**14**). In this section, we introduce two representative substrate materials—quartz and paper—and describe their applications in POCT biosensors.

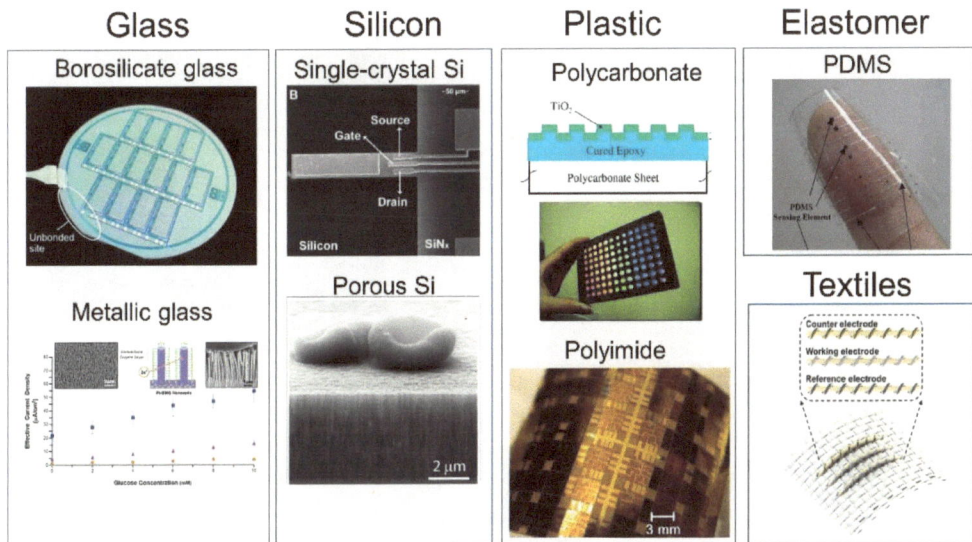

Fig. (14). Substrate materials for POCT biosensors including glass, silicon, plastic, elastomer, and textiles.

Quartz

Resonators made of quartz crystals usually have a very high Q factor, defined as the ratio of energy stored divided by energy dissipated. Generally, the higher the Q factor, the better is the sensing resolution of the biosensor. Quartz crystal microbalances (QCM) resonate with a certain frequency, which changes when there are biological targets binding to or biological events occurring on the sensing surface. As shown in Fig. (**15**), QCM has been used to monitor the transformation of supported bilipid layers in real time [62]. QCM has been demonstrated to detect a single virion on its surface with >90% confidence, and 10 virions with >99% confidence. In a serum, it can reliably detect 10 virions with >90% confidence and 100 virions with >99% confidence [63]. DNA is also successfully sensed by QCM [64].

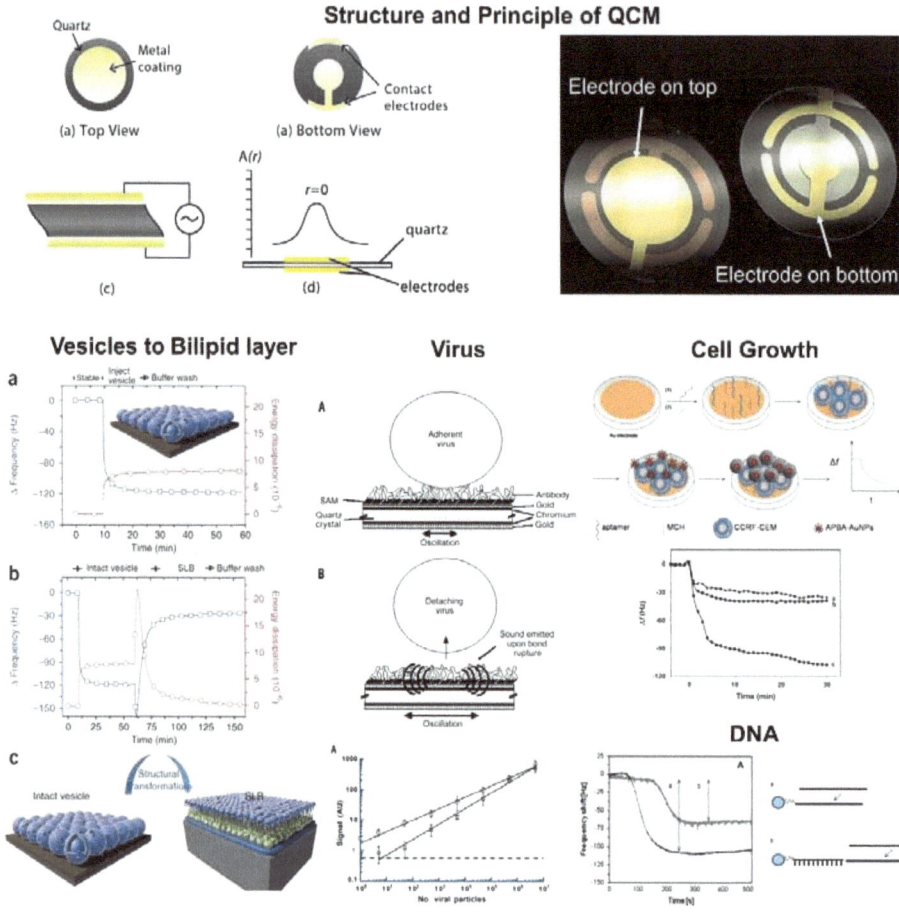

Fig. (15). (**a**) Structure and principle of QCM. (**b**) Applications of QCM in liquid layer, virus, cell, and DNA sensing.

Papers

Since the development of the paper microfluidic chip by the group of Prof. Whitesides at Harvard University in 2007 [65], microfluidic-paper-based analytical devices (μPADs) have been rapidly developed. This type of biosensor is generally based on chromatography or filter papers with hydrophobic or hydrophilic processing of the desired regions to create fluidic channel networks, as shown in Fig. (**16**). The hydrophilic region is used as a microfluidic analysis channel, and the liquid follows the hydrophilic wicking matrices owing to capillary forces, to achieve the loading of samples and reagents and the subsequent reaction and detection. Compared with the commercial POCT test strips, such as blood glucose test strips, μPAD can provide high-throughput parallel analysis with multiple channels and multiple indicators. Compared with silicon, glass, and PDMS, paper-based fabrication is inexpensive, rapid, user-friendly, and easy to operate.

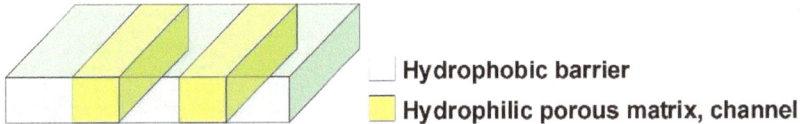

Hydrophobic barrier

Hydrophilic porous matrix, channel

Fig. (16). Schematic of the fluid channel and the hydrophobic barrier of a μPAD. The channel consists of a porous matrix of hydrophilic cellulose fibers and the sides of the channel are bounded by hydrophobic barriers because the hydrophilic solution cannot penetrate the hydrophobic barrier.

Fabrication of the 2D and 3D μPADs

The first reported method in this regard used photolithography and conventional photoresists to construct the hydrophobic barriers [65]. Briefly, the entire sheet of paper is soaked in a photoresist and then exposed to UV light through a mask with the designed pattern. Then, the unexposed photoresist is washed away, and the remaining photoresist is used as the hydrophobic barriers (Fig **17A**). Through this method, traditional photolithography, which is performed on a silicon wafer, can be extended to paper. Subsequently, various unique techniques have been developed for paper materials, such as paper cutting [66, 67], hydrophobic polymer plotting [68], wax printing [69], wax screen-printing [70], inkjet printing [71, 72], plasma treatment [73], flexographic printing [74], and laser treatment [75]. Among these methods, paper cutting is the simplest, involving only a single-step operation to cut the paper by blade or laser according to the pattern. Inkjet printing technology is based on "inkjet etching." A filter paper is soaked in a polystyrene solution and then etched with the toluene droplets ejected from an inkjet printer (Fig. **17B**). The wax screen-printing method first prints wax as the desired pattern on the paper, and then heats the paper to melt the wax penetration into the paper (Fig. **17C**). In addition to wax, polymers can be used in the screen-printing process.

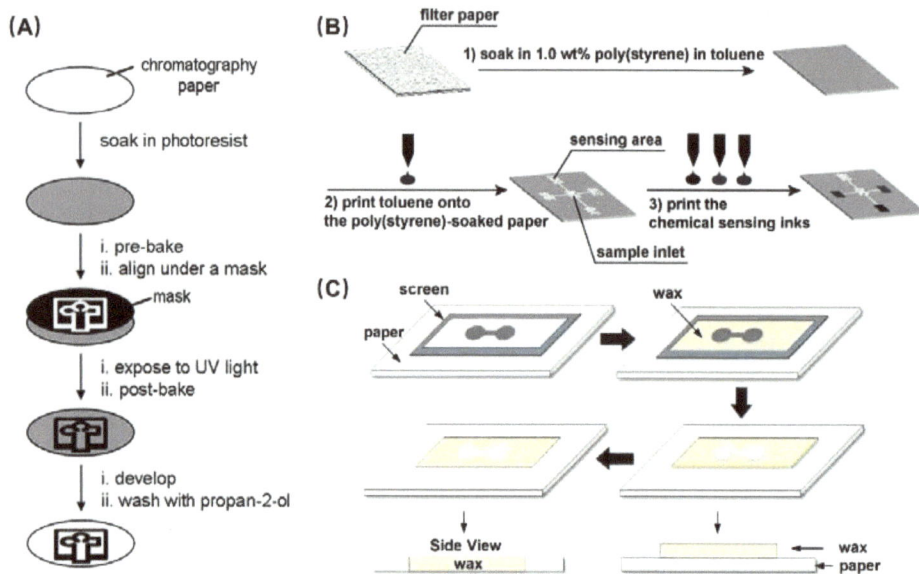

Fig. (17). Schematic diagrams for the fabrication of 2D μPAD. (**A**) Photolithography [65], (**B**) inkjet printing [71], and (**C**) wax screen-printing.

A three-dimensional (3D) μPAD can be fabricated by stacking alternating layers of patterned paper and using a water-impermeable double-sided adhesive tape with patterned holes in between papers [76]. The double-sided adhesive tape can separate the channels in the adjacent layers and the holes provide connections between channels in different layers (Fig. **18A**). Therefore, multiple analytes can be integrated on a single 3D μPAD [77]. In addition to the aforementioned stacking-layers method, a 3D μPAD can be fabricated using a digital light processing (DLP) printer [78] or even directly printed using a desktop 3D printer [79]. In the DLP printing method, liquid resin is printed on both sides of the paper *via* photopolymerization and is cured through exposure to light to form hydrophobic barriers. The 3D printed method first prints the polymer substrate and then fabricates the recyclable hydrophilic channels (Fig. **18B**).

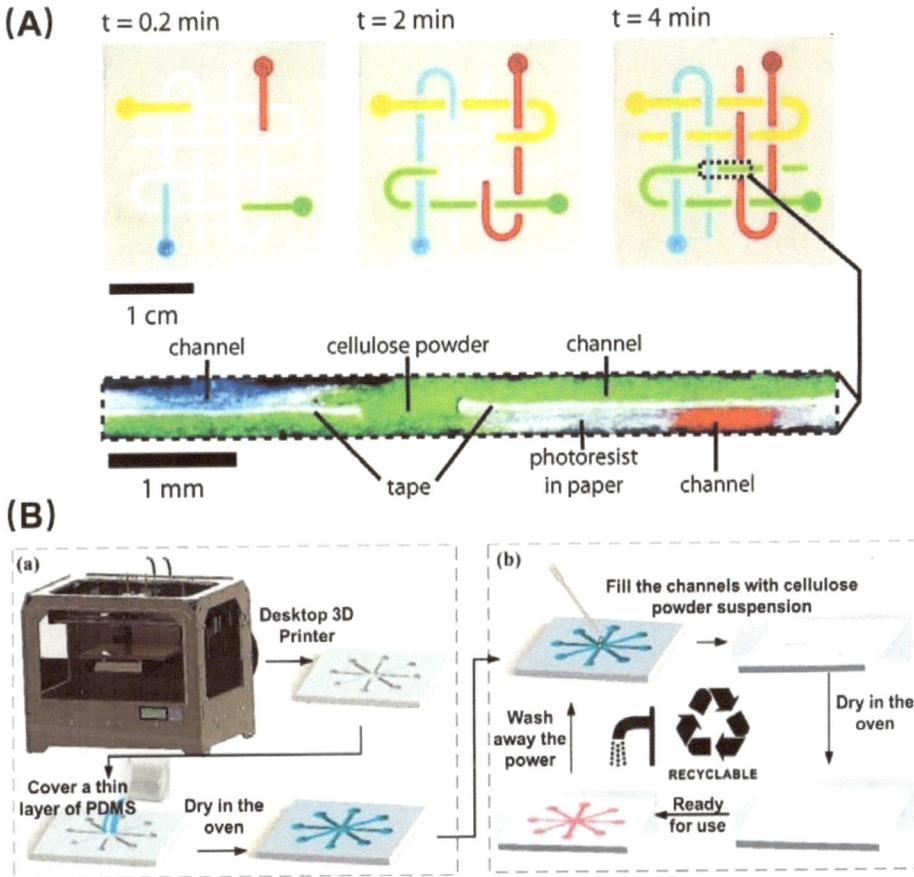

(A) t = 0.2 min   t = 2 min   t = 4 min

1 cm

channel   cellulose powder   channel

1 mm   tape   photoresist in paper   channel

(B)

(a)   Desktop 3D Printer

Cover a thin layer of PDMS   Dry in the oven

(b)   Fill the channels with cellulose powder suspension

Wash away the power   RECYCLABLE   Dry in the oven

Ready for use

Fig. (18). (A) 3D μPAD made from two layers of patterned paper and one layer of double-sided adhesive tape. Four channels cross each other without their contents becoming mixed [77]. (B) Schematic of the 3D printing method for the fabrication of the 3D μPAD [79].

OUTLOOK

Incorporation of Nanomaterials for Improved Sensing

One of the critical challenges of POCT biosensors is to detect small concentrations of targets [80]. Nanomaterials are capable of improving the performance of biosensors in terms of sensitivity and detection limit, due to their large surface/volume ratio and the various benefits resulting from their small dimensions. In addition, several nanomaterials can be synthesized in large amounts using cost-effective methods. Fig. (**19**) shows the commonly used nanomaterials categorized into three types: 0D, 1D, and 2D.

Among 0D nanomaterials, Au nanoparticles (AuNPs) are the most widely used, due to their good biocompatibility, simple production, and mature surface modifications [81]. AuNPs exhibit the surface plasmon resonance (SPR) effect upon irradiation with light of certain frequencies. Once the size of the AuNPs is less than the wavelength of the light, oscillating electrons cannot propagate along the surface but remain inside the NPs, thus creating plasmons in resonance with the incident light. The resonance frequency is dependent on the size, shape, and dielectric constant of the AuNPs [82]. The detection of certain analytes can cause a change in the oscillation frequency, manifested by a change in color observable by the naked eye, which provides the sensing capability. A representative type of biosensor is a colorimetric biosensor utilizing AuNPs [83]. Fig (**19A3**) shows the direct sensing of Hg^+ ions in human urine based on color change [84], which represents a useful POCT application.

Quantum dots (QDs) and AuNPs, which are luminescent semiconducting nanocrystals, are the most popular materials used for biosensing. The bandgap of QDs is highly dependent on their sizes. The emission spectrum will change upon biomolecular absorption. Moreover, QDs have become alternatives for organic fluorophores due to their photochemical stability, high quantum yield, and brightness [85]. Fig. (**19A4**) illustrates a mechanism for detecting food pathogens, such as bacteria, based on the change in emission spectrum. Pathogens such as *E. coli* [86], *Campylobacter jejuni* [87], *Salmonella* [88], and *Listeria monocytogenes* [89] have been detected using this method.

Examples of 1D nanomaterials include nanowires [90, 91], nanotubes [92], nanorods [93], and nanospikes [94, 95]. Fig. (**19B1 - B2**) lists the most widely used nanowires and nanotubes. Carbon nanotubes can be employed to detect changes in surface charge due to biochemical reactions, by being connecting to electrodes for current–voltage measurement, as shown in Fig. (**19B3**). Nanowires can be directly incorporated into a field-effect transistor (FET) for detecting small nucleic acid oligomers [96], and are used together with other fibers for wearable sensor applications, as shown in Fig. (**19B4**) [97].

Examples of 2D materials include graphene, black phosphorous, and MoS_2. Fig. (**19C1 - C3**) show illustrations of monolayer graphene, black phosphorus, and MoS_2. Fig. (**19C4**) shows direct DNA detection below the ppb level using MoS_2 electrochemical sensors [98]. Fig. (**19C5**) shows highly efficient graphene-based fluorescence resonance energy transfer (FRET) biosensors developed for DNA sensing. When the receptor DNA is absorbed on the surface of graphene oxide, the fluorescence is quenched. After hybridization with the analyte DNA, the dye is released and the fluorescence is re-established [80].

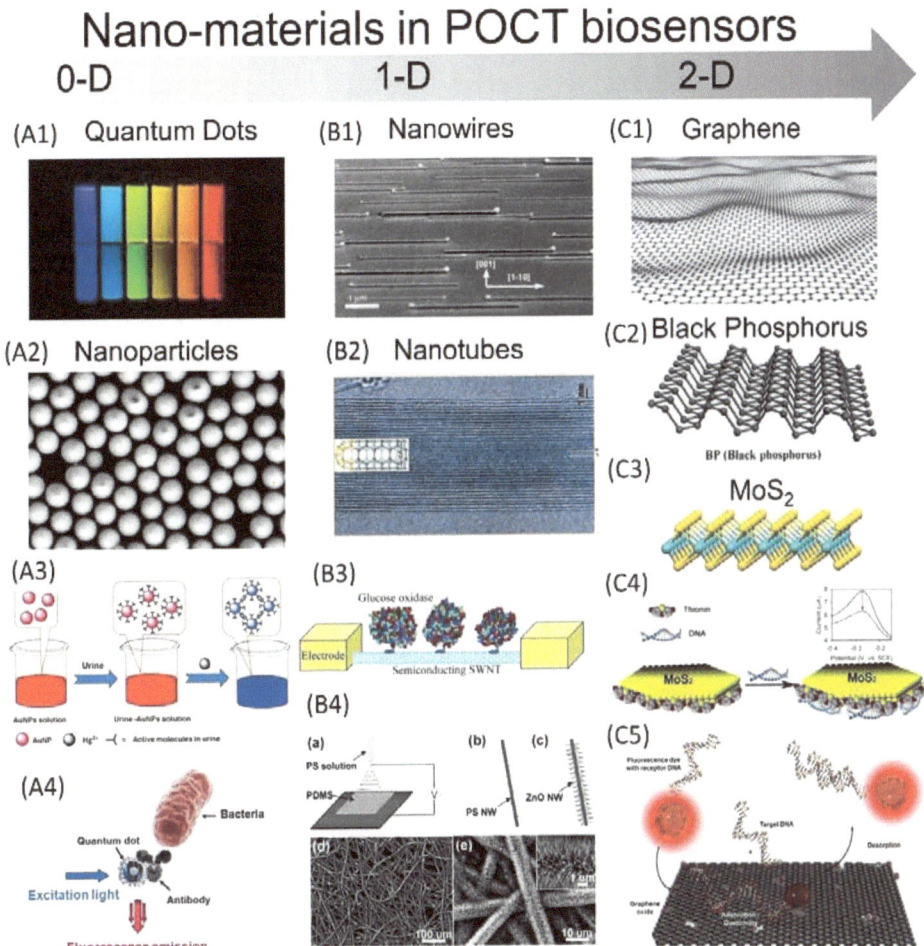

Fig. (19). Emerging nanomaterials for POCT biosensors: from 0D to 2D: (**A1**) QDs showing different colors; (b) SEM image of nanoparticles; (**A3**) Colorimetric sensing of Hg^+ ions in urine using AuNPs; (**A4**) Detection using the change in emission spectrum of QDs [99]; (**B1**) SEM image of horizontal GaAs nanowires grown *via* MOCVD; (**B2**) Transmission electron microscope image of carbon nanotubes; (**B3**) Single-walled semiconductor carbon nanotube used as a pH sensor once functionalized with redox enzyme glucose oxidase (GO_x) [100]; (B4) ZnO nanowires attached to the polystyrene nanowires to form a hierarchical structure for wearable sensors [97]; (**C1**) Illustration of monolayer graphene; (**C2**) Illustration of monolayer black phosphorus; (**C3**) Illustration of monolayer MoS_2; (**C4**). Direct DNA detection below the ppb level based on MoS_2 electrochemical sensors [98]; (**C5**) Highly efficient graphene-based FRET biosensors developed for DNA sensing. When the receptor DNA is absorbed on the surface of graphene oxide, the fluorescence is quenched. After hybridization with the analyte DNA, the dye is released and the fluorescence is re-established [80] (reprinted with permission from [77]; copyright 2014 National Biotechnology).

Detecting Smaller Biological Targets

With the advancement of micro/nanofabrication technologies, it is possible to manipulate smaller targets such as bacteria, exosomes, and proteins with unprecedented accuracy and achieve detection with a higher sensitivity, enabling POCT. Traditionally, without the use of microfluidics, sample treatment requires large amounts of samples and intense professional labor. However, with the use of microfluidics, liquid sample processing can be automated and simplified. Moreover, considerably fewer samples are required for analysis. For example, exosomes have considerable potential for early cancer diagnosis [101], as they are very stable and are abundant in blood, urine, saliva, breast milk, semen, ascites fluid, amniotic fluid, and cerebrospinal fluid. The concentration of exosomes in blood is approximately $10^5 \, \text{mL}^{-1}$ compared with the $10–100 \, \text{mL}^{-1}$ for circulating tumor cells (CTCs). Traditional methods of isolating exosomes include the steps of ultracentrifugation and density-gradient separation. However, ultracentrifugation is time-consuming (>4 h) and results in co-purification with nonexosomal or microvesicle debris. Density-gradient separation cannot separate exosomes from viruses or microvesicles, because they have similar buoyant densities. Both methods require expensive laboratory equipment and highly trained technicians.

Micro/nanofabrication techniques have considerable potential to improve the isolation of exosomes and microvesicles. New isolation technologies enabled by micro/nanofabrication are shown in Fig. (**20**). A microfluidic channel with ciliated micropillars has been fabricated with advanced micro/nanofabrication methods. When a liquid sample containing exosomes is injected, exosomes can fit into the small gaps between nanowires, thus enabling their isolation from cell debris and proteins, as shown in Fig. (**20a**) [102]. Fig. (**20b**) shows microdevices with acoustic generators to assist the separation of exosomes from larger extracellular vehicles (EVs). Fig. (**20c**) shows a nanoscale deterministic lateral displacement (DLD) array that combines microfabrication for producing microchannels and nanofabrication for producing nanopillar arrays, to separate exosomes [103]. Fig. (**20d**) shows acoustic devices that can separate exosomes [104]. An acoustic nanofilter is used to isolate nanoscale vesicles from cell culture media.

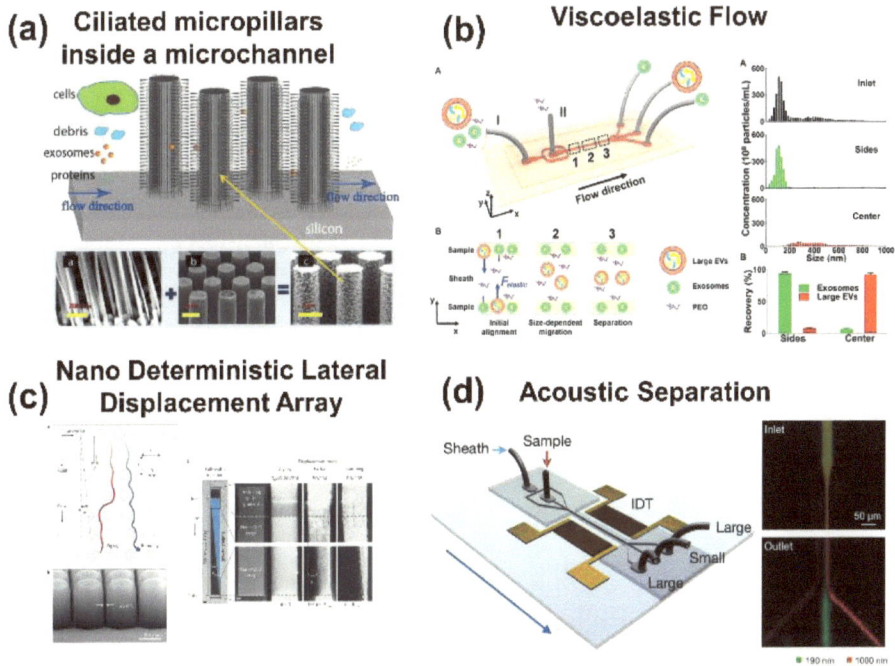

Fig. (20). Micro/nanofabrication for exosome isolation.

Evolution into Wearable POCT Sensors

Wearable sensing technologies are a future trend for POCT sensors because they provide easy access and constant physical and biochemical measurement, which are crucial for disease monitoring and therapy. Wearable sensors are not limited to be worn on wrists [105] similar to wearing a watch; they can be worn on various body locations such as teeth, eyes [106], chest [107], fingers [108], feet [109], ankles [110], ears [111], waist [112], and fingernails [113], as shown in Fig. (**21**).

Fig. (21). Wearable POCT sensors for various parts of a human body.

The motivation for developing sensors to be worn on different parts of the body is twofold. The first motivation is the demand for disease monitoring. For example, diabetes patients lose sense in their toes and cannot feel ulcers. Force sensing and temperature sensing are required on their shoes to compensate for their lost sense. Second, some sensors are to be worn without disturbing the daily activities of the wearer and some parts of the body are better for anchoring sensors with less movement and noise, such as ears [114].

System-level Integration of Sensors, Circuits, Cloud, and Artificial Intelligence

As shown in Fig. (**22**), micro/nanofabrication can revolutionize POCT technology. In the first stage, samples need to be acquired from a human body. Microneedles can assist in blood extraction [115, 116], and a recent reported paper has demonstrated that microscale hydrophobic/hydrophilic patterns could improve the efficiency of sweat collection from people, even during physical exercises [117]. In the second stage, the targets to be tested, such as CTCs, exosomes, and DNAs, are to be isolated. In the case of exosomes, a nano deterministic lateral displacement (nanoDLD) array can isolate exosomes, and micro/nano hierarchical structures can enable the capture of exosomes. In the third stage of detection, several technologies such as electrical, mechanical, and optical techniques utilize micro/nanofabrication. Even after diagnosis, therapy can be realized *via* drug delivery through the implanted devices [118]. In the future, systems integrating all these functions will be helpful to realize a fully functional POCT technology. Biochemical and physical sensors can be used in conjunction with big data, cloud computing, and artificial intelligence for better diagnosis and treatment at the point of care.

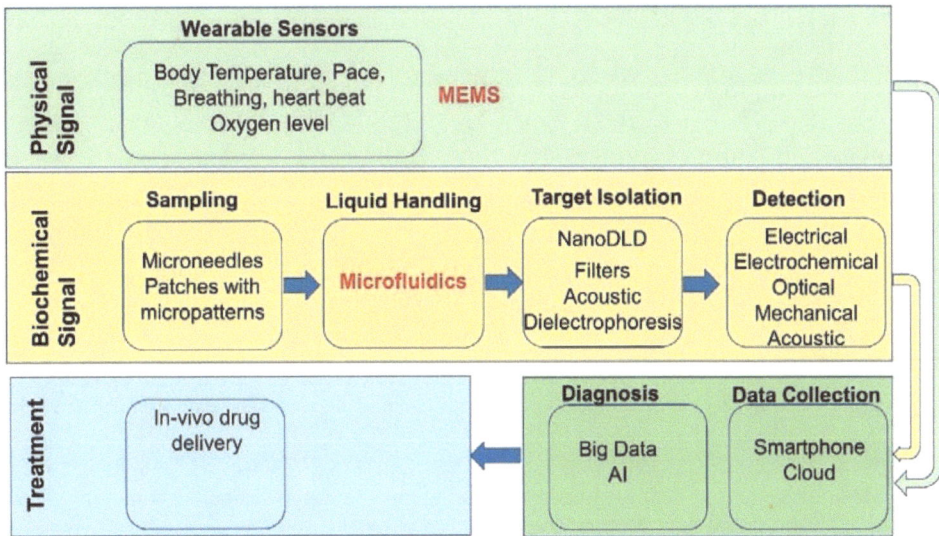

Fig. (22). System-level POCT.

CONCLUSION

In this book chapter, we first introduced the basics of micro/nanofabrication and listed the representative technologies widely used for POCT sensors. Then, we briefly introduced the common substrate materials used for constructing POCT sensors, considering quartz and paper as two representative materials. Finally, we discussed four development trends of POCT sensors from a micro/nanofabrication perspective. Micro/nanofabrication technologies are expected to revolutionize the IVD/POCT sensor industry because of their mass-production capability and cost benefits. Moreover, micro/nanofabricated sensors can be potentially integrated into a chip with a microelectronic circuit and communication module. Thus, future IVD/POCT biosensors can be readily configured to provide real-time patient monitoring and offer timelier and higher-quality diagnoses, which can significantly improve the efficiency of therapy.

CONSENT FOR PUBLICATION

Not applicable.

CONFLICT OF INTEREST

The authors confirm that this chapter contents have no conflict of interest.

ACKNOWLEDGMENTS

This work was supported by the National Natural Science Foundation of China (No. 61974128, No. 31770107, and No. 21874116), the Natural Science Foundation of Zhejiang Province (No. LY19F040007), Fundamental Research Funds for the Central Universities (No. 2-2050205-19-361), and Tang's Foundation. The work was also supported in part by the Zhejiang University/University of Illinois at Urbana-Champaign Institute and was led by Principal Supervisor Dr. Huan Hu.

REFERENCES

[1]   Hierlemann A, *et al*. Microfabrication techniques for chemical/biosensors. Proc IEEE 2003; 91: 839-63.
        [http://dx.doi.org/10.1109/JPROC.2003.813583]

[2]   Song CS, *et al*. Bottom-up copper electroplating using transfer wafers for fabrication of high aspect-ratio through-silicon-vias. Microelectron Eng 2010; 87: 510-3.
        [http://dx.doi.org/10.1016/j.mee.2009.06.029]

[3]   Li X, *et al*. Highly sensitive H2S sensor based on template-synthesized CuO nanowires. RSC Advances 2012; 2: 2302-7.
        [http://dx.doi.org/10.1039/c2ra00718e]

[4]   Li X, Bohn PW. Metal-assisted chemical etching in HF/H(2)O(2) produces porous silicon. Appl Phys Lett 2000; 77: 2572-4.

[http://dx.doi.org/10.1063/1.1319191]

[5]   Li XL. Metal assisted chemical etching for high aspect ratio nanostructures: A review of characteristics and applications in photovoltaics. Curr Opin Solid State Mater Sci 2012; 16: 71-81.
[http://dx.doi.org/10.1016/j.cossms.2011.11.002]

[6]   Park K, Millet LJ, Kim N, *et al.* Measurement of adherent cell mass and growth. Proc Natl Acad Sci USA 2010; 107(48): 20691-6.
[http://dx.doi.org/10.1073/pnas.1011365107] [PMID: 21068372]

[7]   Xie HK, Fedder GK. A CMOS-MEMS lateral-axis gyroscope 14th Ieee International Conference on Micro Electro Mechanical Systems, Technical Digest. 162-5.

[8]   Xia Y, Whitesides GM. Soft Lithography. Angew Chem Int Ed Engl 1998; 37(5): 550-75.
[http://dx.doi.org/10.1002/(SICI)1521-3773(19980316)37:5<550::AID-ANIE550>3.0.CO;2-G]
[PMID: 29711088]

[9]   James J, Goluch ED, Hu H, Liu C, Mrksich M. Subcellular curvature at the perimeter of micropatterned cells influences lamellipodial distribution and cell polarity. Cell Motil Cytoskeleton 2008; 65(11): 841-52.
[http://dx.doi.org/10.1002/cm.20305] [PMID: 18677773]

[10]   You JB, Kang K, Tran TT, *et al.* PDMS-based turbulent microfluidic mixer. Lab Chip 2015; 15(7): 1727-35.
[http://dx.doi.org/10.1039/C5LC00070J] [PMID: 25671438]

[11]   Joensson HN, Uhlén M, Svahn HA. Droplet size based separation by deterministic lateral displacement-separating droplets by cell--induced shrinking. Lab Chip 2011; 11(7): 1305-10.
[http://dx.doi.org/10.1039/c0lc00688b] [PMID: 21321749]

[12]   Holm SH, Beech JP, Barrett MP, Tegenfeldt JO. Separation of parasites from human blood using deterministic lateral displacement. Lab Chip 2011; 11(7): 1326-32.
[http://dx.doi.org/10.1039/c0lc00560f] [PMID: 21331436]

[13]   Yamaguchi Y, *et al.* Development of a poly-dimethylsiloxane microfluidic device for single cell isolation and incubation. Sens Actuators B Chem 2009; 136: 555-61.
[http://dx.doi.org/10.1016/j.snb.2008.11.052]

[14]   Cui S, Liu Y, Wang W, Sun Y, Fan Y. A microfluidic chip for highly efficient cell capturing and pairing. Biomicrofluidics 2011; 5(3): 32003-320038.
[http://dx.doi.org/10.1063/1.3623411] [PMID: 22662028]

[15]   Kang D-K, *et al.* Rapid detection of single bacteria in unprocessed blood using Integrated Comprehensive Droplet Digital Detection Proceedings of the National Academy of Sciences of the United States of America 2014; 106: 14195-200.
[http://dx.doi.org/10.1038/ncomms6427]

[16]   Brouzes E, Medkova M, Savenelli N, *et al.* Droplet microfluidic technology for single-cell high-throughput screening. Proc Natl Acad Sci USA 2009; 106(34): 14195-200.
[http://dx.doi.org/10.1073/pnas.0903542106] [PMID: 19617544]

[17]   Huebner A, Srisa-Art M, Holt D, *et al.* Quantitative detection of protein expression in single cells using droplet microfluidics. Chem Commun (Camb) 2007; (12): 1218-20.
[http://dx.doi.org/10.1039/b618570c] [PMID: 17356761]

[18]   Jang M, *et al.* Droplet-based Digital PCR System for Detection of Single-cell Level of Foodborne Pathogens. Biochip J 2017; 11: 329-37.
[http://dx.doi.org/10.1007/s13206-017-1410-x]

[19]   Delamarche E, Bernard A, Schmid H, Michel B, Biebuyck H. Patterned delivery of immunoglobulins to surfaces using microfluidic networks. Science 1997; 276(5313): 779-81.
[http://dx.doi.org/10.1126/science.276.5313.779] [PMID: 9115199]

[20] du Roure O, *et al.* Microfabricated arrays of elastomeric posts to study cellular mechanics. Microfluidics, Biomems, and Medical Microsystems Ii 2004; 5345: 26-34.
[http://dx.doi.org/10.1117/12.530688]

[21] Tan JL, Tien J, Pirone DM, Gray DS, Bhadriraju K, Chen CS. Cells lying on a bed of microneedles: an approach to isolate mechanical force. Proc Natl Acad Sci USA 2003; 100(4): 1484-9.
[http://dx.doi.org/10.1073/pnas.0235407100] [PMID: 12552122]

[22] James J, Goluch ED, Hu H, Liu C, Mrksich M. Subcellular curvature at the perimeter of micropatterned cells influences lamellipodial distribution and cell polarity. Cell Motil Cytoskeleton 2008; 65(11): 841-52.
[http://dx.doi.org/10.1002/cm.20305] [PMID: 18677773]

[23] Cerf A, Cau JC, Vieu C. Controlled assembly of bacteria on chemical patterns using soft lithography. Colloids Surf B Biointerfaces 2008; 65(2): 285-91.
[http://dx.doi.org/10.1016/j.colsurfb.2008.04.016] [PMID: 18556179]

[24] Picone R, Ren X, Ivanovitch KD, Clarke JD, McKendry RA, Baum B. A polarised population of dynamic microtubules mediates homeostatic length control in animal cells. PLoS Biol 2010; 8(11)e1000542
[http://dx.doi.org/10.1371/journal.pbio.1000542] [PMID: 21103410]

[25] Lin BJ. Deep uv lithography. J Vac Sci Technol 1975; 12: 1317-20.
[http://dx.doi.org/10.1116/1.568527]

[26] Wagner C, Harned N. EUV LITHOGRAPHY Lithography gets extreme. Nat Photonics 2010; 4: 24-6.
[http://dx.doi.org/10.1038/nphoton.2009.251]

[27] Chen YF. Nanofabrication by electron beam lithography and its applications: A review. Microelectron Eng 2015; 135: 57-72.
[http://dx.doi.org/10.1016/j.mee.2015.02.042]

[28] Craighead HG. Nanoelectromechanical systems. Science 2000; 290(5496): 1532-6.
[http://dx.doi.org/10.1126/science.290.5496.1532] [PMID: 11090343]

[29] Li WD, *et al.* Combined helium ion beam and nanoimprint lithography attains 4 nm half-pitch dense patterns. J Vac Sci Technol B 2012; 30.
[http://dx.doi.org/10.1116/1.4758768]

[30] Ward BW, *et al.* Helium ion microscope: A new tool for nanoscale microscopy and metrology. J Vac Sci Technol B 2006; 24: 2871-4.
[http://dx.doi.org/10.1116/1.2357967]

[31] Yanik AA, *et al.* Integrated nanoplasmonic-nanofluidic biosensors with targeted delivery of analytes. Appl Phys Lett 2010; 96.
[http://dx.doi.org/10.1063/1.3290633]

[32] Hu H, *et al.* Tip-Based Nanofabrication for Scalable Manufacturing. Micromachines (Basel) 2017; 8: 90.
[http://dx.doi.org/10.3390/mi8030090]

[33] Garcia R, Knoll AW, Riedo E. Advanced scanning probe lithography. Nat Nanotechnol 2014; 9(8): 577-87.
[http://dx.doi.org/10.1038/nnano.2014.157] [PMID: 25091447]

[34] Sheehan PE, *et al.* Nanoscale deposition of solid inks *via* thermal dip pen nanolithography. Appl Phys Lett 2004; 85: 1589-91.
[http://dx.doi.org/10.1063/1.1785860]

[35] Szoszkiewicz R, Okada T, Jones SC, *et al.* High-speed, sub-15 nm feature size thermochemical nanolithography. Nano Lett 2007; 7(4): 1064-9.
[http://dx.doi.org/10.1021/nl070300f] [PMID: 17385937]

[36]   Yan Y, Hu Z, Zhao X, Sun T, Dong S, Li X. Top-down nanomechanical machining of three-dimensional nanostructures by atomic force microscopy. Small 2010; 6(6): 724-8.
[http://dx.doi.org/10.1002/smll.200901947] [PMID: 20166110]

[37]   Song JQ, *et al.* Fabrication of gold nanostructures on graphite using atomic force microscope. Molecular Crystals and Liquid Crystals Science and Technology Section a-Molecular Crystals and Liquid Crystals 1997; Vol. 294: p. 51.

[38]   Garcia R, *et al.* Local oxidation of silicon surfaces by dynamic force microscopy: Nanofabrication and water bridge formation. Appl Phys Lett 1998; 72: 2295-7.
[http://dx.doi.org/10.1063/1.121340]

[39]   Piner RD, Zhu J, Xu F, Hong S, Mirkin CA. "Dip-Pen" nanolithography. Science 1999; 283(5402): 661-3.
[http://dx.doi.org/10.1126/science.283.5402.661] [PMID: 9924019]

[40]   Hu H, Cho H, Somnath S, Vakakis AF, King WP. Silicon nano-mechanical resonators fabricated by using tip-based nanofabrication. Nanotechnology 2014; 25(27)275301
[http://dx.doi.org/10.1088/0957-4484/25/27/275301] [PMID: 24960625]

[41]   Chou SY, *et al.* Nanoimprint lithography. J Vac Sci Technol B Microelectron Nanometer Struct Process Meas Phenom 1996; 14: 4129-33.
[http://dx.doi.org/10.1116/1.588605]

[42]   Guo LJ. Nanoimprint lithography: Methods and material requirements. Adv Mater 2007; 19: 495-513.
[http://dx.doi.org/10.1002/adma.200600882]

[43]   Zhuo Y, Hu H, Chen W, *et al.* Single nanoparticle detection using photonic crystal enhanced microscopy. Analyst (Lond) 2014; 139(5): 1007-15.
[http://dx.doi.org/10.1039/C3AN02295A] [PMID: 24432353]

[44]   Chen W, Long KD, Lu M, *et al.* Photonic crystal enhanced microscopy for imaging of live cell adhesion. Analyst (Lond) 2013; 138(20): 5886-94.
[http://dx.doi.org/10.1039/c3an01541f] [PMID: 23971078]

[45]   Gallegos D, Long KD, Yu H, *et al.* Label-free biodetection using a smartphone. Lab Chip 2013; 13(11): 2124-32.
[http://dx.doi.org/10.1039/c3lc40991k] [PMID: 23609514]

[46]   Liang C, Qu T, Cai J, Zhu Z, Li S, Li WD. Wafer-scale nanopatterning using fast-reconfigurable and actively-stabilized two-beam fiber-optic interference lithography. Opt Express 2018; 26(7): 8194-200.
[http://dx.doi.org/10.1364/OE.26.008194] [PMID: 29715788]

[47]   Bagheri S, *et al.* Large-Area Low-Cost Plasmonic Perfect Absorber Chemical Sensor Fabricated by Laser Interference Lithography. ACS Sens 2016; 1: 1148-54.
[http://dx.doi.org/10.1021/acssensors.6b00444]

[48]   Gisbert Quilis N, Lequeux M, Venugopalan P, *et al.* Tunable laser interference lithography preparation of plasmonic nanoparticle arrays tailored for SERS. Nanoscale 2018; 10(21): 10268-76.
[http://dx.doi.org/10.1039/C7NR08905H] [PMID: 29790495]

[49]   Campbell M, Sharp DN, Harrison MT, Denning RG, Turberfield AJ. Fabrication of photonic crystals for the visible spectrum by holographic lithography. Nature 2000; 404(6773): 53-6.
[http://dx.doi.org/10.1038/35003523] [PMID: 10716437]

[50]   Mohamed MS, *et al.* Analysis of Highly Sensitive Photonic Crystal Biosensor for Glucose Monitoring. Appl Comput Electromagn Soc J 2016; 31: 836-42.

[51]   Chang TY, Huang M, Yanik AA, *et al.* Large-scale plasmonic microarrays for label-free high-throughput screening. Lab Chip 2011; 11(21): 3596-602.
[http://dx.doi.org/10.1039/c1lc20475k] [PMID: 21901194]

[52]   Das A, Mao C, Cho S, Kim K, Park W. Over 1000-fold enhancement of upconversion luminescence

using water-dispersible metal-insulator-metal nanostructures. Nat Commun 2018; 9(1): 4828.
[http://dx.doi.org/10.1038/s41467-018-07284-w] [PMID: 30446644]

[53] Parisi A, Cino AC, Busacca AC, Cherchi M, Riva-Sanseverino S. Integrated Optic Surface Plasmon Resonance Measurements in a Borosilicate Glass Substrate. Sensors (Basel) 2008; 8(11): 7113-24.
[http://dx.doi.org/10.3390/s8117113] [PMID: 27873918]

[54] Vulto P, *et al.* A full-wafer fabrication process for glass microfluidic chips with integrated electroplated electrodes by direct bonding of dry film resist Journal of Micromechanics and Microengineering 2009; 19: 077001.
[http://dx.doi.org/10.1088/0960-1317/19/7/077001]

[55] Kinser ER, *et al.* Nanopatterned Bulk Metallic Glass Biosensors Acs Sensors. 2017; 2: pp. 1779-87.
[http://dx.doi.org/10.1021/acssensors.7b00455]

[56] Shekhawat G, Tark SH, Dravid VP. MOSFET-Embedded microcantilevers for measuring deflection in biomolecular sensors. Science 2006; 311(5767): 1592-5.
[http://dx.doi.org/10.1126/science.1122588] [PMID: 16456038]

[57] Bonanno LM, DeLouise LA. Whole blood optical biosensor. Biosens Bioelectron 2007; 23(3): 444-8.
[http://dx.doi.org/10.1016/j.bios.2007.05.008] [PMID: 17720473]

[58] Engel J, *et al.* Development of polyimide flexible tactile sensor skin. J Micromech Microeng 2003; 13: 359-66.
[http://dx.doi.org/10.1088/0960-1317/13/3/302]

[59] Cunningham BT, Li P, Schulz S, *et al.* Label-free assays on the BIND system. J Biomol Screen 2004; 9(6): 481-90.
[http://dx.doi.org/10.1177/1087057104267604] [PMID: 15452334]

[60] Hu H, *et al.* Super flexible sensor skin using liquid metal as interconnect 2007 Ieee Sensors. 2007; 1-3: pp. 815-7.
[http://dx.doi.org/10.1109/ICSENS.2007.4388525]

[61] Zhao Y, *et al.* Highly Stretchable and Strain-Insensitive Fiber-Based Wearable Electrochemical Biosensor to Monitor Glucose in the Sweat Analytical Chemistry. 2019; 91: pp. 6569-76.
[http://dx.doi.org/10.1021/acs.analchem.9b00152]

[62] Cho N-J, *et al.* Quartz crystal microbalance with dissipation monitoring of supported lipid bilayers on various substrates Nature Protocols. 2010; 5: pp. 1096-106.
[http://dx.doi.org/10.1038/nprot.2010.65]

[63] Cooper MA, *et al.* Direct and sensitive detection of a human virus by rupture event scanning Nature Biotechnology. 2001; 19: pp. 833-7.
[http://dx.doi.org/10.1038/nbt0901-833]

[64] Kleo K, *et al.* Detection of vaccinia virus DNA by quartz crystal microbalance Analytical Biochemistry. 2011; 418: pp. 260-6.
[http://dx.doi.org/10.1016/j.ab.2011.07.016]

[65] Martinez AW, Phillips ST, Butte MJ, Whitesides GM. Patterned paper as a platform for inexpensive, low-volume, portable bioassays. Angew Chem Int Ed Engl 2007; 46(8): 1318-20.
[http://dx.doi.org/10.1002/anie.200603817] [PMID: 17211899]

[66] Fenton EM, Mascarenas MR, López GP, Sibbett SS. Multiplex lateral-flow test strips fabricated by two-dimensional shaping. ACS Appl Mater Interfaces 2009; 1(1): 124-9.
[http://dx.doi.org/10.1021/am800043z] [PMID: 20355763]

[67] Nie J, Liang Y, Zhang Y, Le S, Li D, Zhang S. One-step patterning of hollow microstructures in paper by laser cutting to create microfluidic analytical devices. Analyst (Lond) 2013; 138(2): 671-6.
[http://dx.doi.org/10.1039/C2AN36219H] [PMID: 23183392]

[68] Bruzewicz DA, Reches M, Whitesides GM. Low-cost printing of poly(dimethylsiloxane) barriers to

define microchannels in paper. Anal Chem 2008; 80(9): 3387-92.
[http://dx.doi.org/10.1021/ac702605a] [PMID: 18333627]

[69] Carrilho E, Martinez AW, Whitesides GM. Understanding wax printing: a simple micropatterning process for paper-based microfluidics. Anal Chem 2009; 81(16): 7091-5.
[http://dx.doi.org/10.1021/ac901071p] [PMID: 20337388]

[70] Dungchai W, Chailapakul O, Henry CS. A low-cost, simple, and rapid fabrication method for paper-based microfluidics using wax screen-printing. Analyst (Lond) 2011; 136(1): 77-82.
[http://dx.doi.org/10.1039/C0AN00406E] [PMID: 20871884]

[71] Abe K, Suzuki K, Citterio D. Inkjet-printed microfluidic multianalyte chemical sensing paper. Anal Chem 2008; 80(18): 6928-34.
[http://dx.doi.org/10.1021/ac800604v] [PMID: 18698798]

[72] Yamada K, Henares TG, Suzuki K, Citterio D. Paper-based inkjet-printed microfluidic analytical devices. Angew Chem Int Ed Engl 2015; 54(18): 5294-310.
[http://dx.doi.org/10.1002/anie.201411508] [PMID: 25864471]

[73] Li X, Tian J, Nguyen T, Shen W. Paper-based microfluidic devices by plasma treatment. Anal Chem 2008; 80(23): 9131-4.
[http://dx.doi.org/10.1021/ac801729t] [PMID: 19551982]

[74] Olkkonen J, Lehtinen K, Erho T. Flexographically printed fluidic structures in paper. Anal Chem 2010; 82(24): 10246-50.
[http://dx.doi.org/10.1021/ac1027066] [PMID: 21090744]

[75] Chitnis G, Ding Z, Chang CL, Savran CA, Ziaie B. Laser-treated hydrophobic paper: an inexpensive microfluidic platform. Lab Chip 2011; 11(6): 1161-5.
[http://dx.doi.org/10.1039/c0lc00512f] [PMID: 21264372]

[76] Martinez AW, Phillips ST, Whitesides GM. Three-dimensional microfluidic devices fabricated in layered paper and tape. Proc Natl Acad Sci USA 2008; 105(50): 19606-11.
[http://dx.doi.org/10.1073/pnas.0810903105] [PMID: 19064929]

[77] Martinez AW, Phillips ST, Whitesides GM, Carrilho E. Diagnostics for the developing world: microfluidic paper-based analytical devices. Anal Chem 2010; 82(1): 3-10.
[http://dx.doi.org/10.1021/ac9013989] [PMID: 20000334]

[78] Park C, Han YD, Kim HV, Lee J, Yoon HC, Park S. Double-sided 3D printing on paper towards mass production of three-dimensional paper-based microfluidic analytical devices (3D-μPADs). Lab Chip 2018; 18(11): 1533-8.
[http://dx.doi.org/10.1039/C8LC00367J] [PMID: 29748672]

[79] He Y, Gao Q, Wu WB, Nie J, Fu JZ. 3D Printed Paper-Based Microfluidic Analytical Devices. Micromachines (Basel) 2016; 7: 7.
[http://dx.doi.org/10.3390/mi7070108] [PMID: 30404282]

[80] Holzinger M, *et al.* Nanomaterials for biosensing applications: a review Frontiers in Chemistry. 2014; 2. 2014-August-27 2014.

[81] Biju V. Chemical modifications and bioconjugate reactions of nanomaterials for sensing, imaging, drug delivery and therapy. Chem Soc Rev 2014; 43(3): 744-64.
[http://dx.doi.org/10.1039/C3CS60273G] [PMID: 24220322]

[82] Hao E, Schatz GC, Hupp JT. Synthesis and optical properties of anisotropic metal nanoparticles. J Fluoresc 2004; 14(4): 331-41.
[http://dx.doi.org/10.1023/B:JOFL.0000031815.71450.74] [PMID: 15617376]

[83] Aldewachi H, Chalati T, Woodroofe MN, Bricklebank N, Sharrack B, Gardiner P. Gold nanoparticle-based colorimetric biosensors. Nanoscale 2017; 10(1): 18-33.
[http://dx.doi.org/10.1039/C7NR06367A] [PMID: 29211091]

[84]   Du J, Zhu B, Chen X. Urine for plasmonic nanoparticle-based colorimetric detection of mercury ion. Small 2013; 9(24): 4104-11.
[http://dx.doi.org/10.1002/smll.201300593] [PMID: 23813852]

[85]   Resch-Genger U, Grabolle M, Cavaliere-Jaricot S, Nitschke R, Nann T. Quantum dots *versus* organic dyes as fluorescent labels. Nat Methods 2008; 5(9): 763-75.
[http://dx.doi.org/10.1038/nmeth.1248] [PMID: 18756197]

[86]   Zhu H, Sikora U, Ozcan A. Quantum dot enabled detection of Escherichia coli using a cell-phone. Analyst (Lond) 2012; 137(11): 2541-4.
[http://dx.doi.org/10.1039/c2an35071h] [PMID: 22396952]

[87]   Bruno JG, Phillips T, Carrillo MP, Crowell R. Plastic-adherent DNA aptamer-magnetic bead and quantum dot sandwich assay for Campylobacter detection. J Fluoresc 2009; 19(3): 427-35.
[http://dx.doi.org/10.1007/s10895-008-0429-8] [PMID: 19052851]

[88]   Kuang H, Cui G, Chen X, *et al.* A one-step homogeneous sandwich immunosensor for Salmonella detection based on magnetic nanoparticles (MNPs) and quantum Dots (QDs). Int J Mol Sci 2013; 14(4): 8603-10.
[http://dx.doi.org/10.3390/ijms14048603] [PMID: 23609493]

[89]   RAPID DETECTION OF LISTERIA MONOCYTOGENES USING QUANTUM DOTS AND NANOBEADS-BASED OPTICAL BIOSENSOR. Journal of Rapid Methods & Automation in Microbiology 2007; 15: 67-76.
[http://dx.doi.org/10.1111/j.1745-4581.2007.00075.x]

[90]   Murphy-Pérez E, Arya SK, Bhansali S. Vapor-liquid-solid grown silica nanowire based electrochemical glucose biosensor. Analyst (Lond) 2011; 136(8): 1686-9.
[http://dx.doi.org/10.1039/c0an00977f] [PMID: 21369619]

[91]   Zafar S, *et al.* Silicon Nanowire Field Effect Transistor Sensors with Minimal Sensor-to-Sensor Variations and Enhanced Sensing Characteristics Acs Nano. 2018; 12: pp. 6577-87.
[http://dx.doi.org/10.1021/acsnano.8b01339]

[92]   Barsan MM, Ghica ME, Brett CM. Electrochemical sensors and biosensors based on redox polymer/carbon nanotube modified electrodes: a review. Anal Chim Acta 2015; 881: 1-23.
[http://dx.doi.org/10.1016/j.aca.2015.02.059] [PMID: 26041516]

[93]   Lim ZH, *et al.* A facile approach towards ZnO nanorods conductive textile for room temperature multifunctional sensors. Sens Actuators B Chem 2010; 151: 121-6.
[http://dx.doi.org/10.1016/j.snb.2010.09.037]

[94]   Hu H, *et al.* Bio-inspired silicon nanospikes fabricated by metal-assisted chemical etching for antibacterial surfaces. Appl Phys Lett 2017; 111: •••.
[http://dx.doi.org/10.1063/1.5003817]

[95]   Sabri YM, Ippolito SJ, Tardio J, Bansal V, O'Mullane AP, Bhargava SK. Gold nanospikes based microsensor as a highly accurate mercury emission monitoring system. Sci Rep 2014; 4: 6741.
[http://dx.doi.org/10.1038/srep06741] [PMID: 25338965]

[96]   Dorvel BR, Reddy B Jr, Go J, *et al.* Silicon nanowires with high-k hafnium oxide dielectrics for sensitive detection of small nucleic acid oligomers. ACS Nano 2012; 6(7): 6150-64.
[http://dx.doi.org/10.1021/nn301495k] [PMID: 22695179]

[97]   Xiao X, *et al.* High-Strain Sensors Based on ZnO Nanowire/Polystyrene Hybridized Flexible Films Advanced Materials 2011; 23: 5440.
[http://dx.doi.org/10.1002/adma.201103406]

[98]   Wang T, Zhu R, Zhuo J, Zhu Z, Shao Y, Li M. Direct detection of DNA below ppb level based on thionin-functionalized layered MoS2 electrochemical sensors. Anal Chem 2014; 86(24): 12064-9.
[http://dx.doi.org/10.1021/ac5027786] [PMID: 25391335]

[99]   Yasmin J, *et al.* Biosensors and their applications in food safety: a review. J Biosyst Eng 2016; 41: 240-54.
[http://dx.doi.org/10.5307/JBE.2016.41.3.240]

[100] Besteman K, *et al.* Enzyme-coated carbon nanotubes as single-molecule biosensors. Nano Lett 2003; 3: 727-30.
[http://dx.doi.org/10.1021/nl034139u]

[101] Shao H, Chung J, Balaj L, *et al.* Protein typing of circulating microvesicles allows real-time monitoring of glioblastoma therapy. Nat Med 2012; 18(12): 1835-40.
[http://dx.doi.org/10.1038/nm.2994] [PMID: 23142818]

[102] Wang Z, Wu HJ, Fine D, *et al.* Ciliated micropillars for the microfluidic-based isolation of nanoscale lipid vesicles. Lab Chip 2013; 13(15): 2879-82.
[http://dx.doi.org/10.1039/c3lc41343h] [PMID: 23743667]

[103] Wunsch BH, Smith JT, Gifford SM, *et al.* Nanoscale lateral displacement arrays for the separation of exosomes and colloids down to 20 nm. Nat Nanotechnol 2016; 11(11): 936-40.
[http://dx.doi.org/10.1038/nnano.2016.134] [PMID: 27479757]

[104] Lee K, Shao H, Weissleder R, Lee H. Acoustic purification of extracellular microvesicles. ACS Nano 2015; 9(3): 2321-7.
[http://dx.doi.org/10.1021/nn506538f] [PMID: 25672598]

[105] Li N, Bedell S, Hu H, *et al.* Single Crystal Flexible Electronics Enabled by 3D Spalling. Adv Mater 2017; 29(18): •••.
[http://dx.doi.org/10.1002/adma.201606638] [PMID: 28230918]

[106] Rim YS, Bae SH, Chen H, *et al.* Printable Ultrathin Metal Oxide Semiconductor-Based Conformal Biosensors. ACS Nano 2015; 9(12): 12174-81.
[http://dx.doi.org/10.1021/acsnano.5b05325] [PMID: 26498319]

[107] Hwang S-W, *et al.* Biodegradable Elastomers and Silicon Nanomembranes/Nanoribbons for Stretchable, Transient Electronics, and Biosensors Nano Letters. 2015; 15: pp. 2801-8.
[http://dx.doi.org/10.1021/nl503997m]

[108] Sempionatto JR, Mishra RK, Martín A, *et al.* Wearable Ring-Based Sensing Platform for Detecting Chemical Threats. ACS Sens 2017; 2(10): 1531-8.
[http://dx.doi.org/10.1021/acssensors.7b00603] [PMID: 29019246]

[109] Seesaard T, *et al.* A Smart Sniffing Shoes Based on Embroidered Sensor Array 2013 10th International Conference on Electrical Engineering/Electronics, Computer, Telecommunications and Information Technology (Ecti-Con).
[http://dx.doi.org/10.1109/ECTICon.2013.6559483]

[110] Kim S, *et al.* SwellFit: Developing A Wearable Sensor for Monitoring Peripheral Edema Proceedings of the 52nd Hawaii International Conference on System Sciences.
[http://dx.doi.org/10.24251/HICSS.2019.468]

[111] Poh MZ, Swenson NC, Picard RW. Motion-tolerant magnetic earring sensor and wireless earpiece for wearable photoplethysmography. IEEE Trans Inf Technol Biomed 2010; 14(3): 786-94.
[http://dx.doi.org/10.1109/TITB.2010.2042607] [PMID: 20172836]

[112] Bourke AK, van de Ven P, Gamble M, *et al.* Evaluation of waist-mounted tri-axial accelerometer based fall-detection algorithms during scripted and continuous unscripted activities. J Biomech 2010; 43(15): 3051-7.
[http://dx.doi.org/10.1016/j.jbiomech.2010.07.005] [PMID: 20926081]

[113] Sakuma K, Abrami A, Blumrosen G, *et al.* Wearable Nail Deformation Sensing for Behavioral and Biomechanical Monitoring and Human-Computer Interaction. Sci Rep 2018; 8(1): 18031.
[http://dx.doi.org/10.1038/s41598-018-36834-x] [PMID: 30575796]

[114] He DD, Winokur ES, Sodini CG. An Ear-Worn Vital Signs Monitor. IEEE Trans Biomed Eng 2015; 62(11): 2547-52.
[http://dx.doi.org/10.1109/TBME.2015.2459061] [PMID: 26208264]

[115] Zhang P, *et al.* Design and fabrication of MEMS-based microneedle arrays for medical applications. Microsyst Technol 2009; 15: 1073-82.
[http://dx.doi.org/10.1007/s00542-009-0883-5]

[116] Lee K, *et al.* Drawing Lithography: Three-Dimensional Fabrication of an Ultrahigh-Aspect-Ratio Microneedle Advanced Materials 2010; 22: 483.
[http://dx.doi.org/10.1002/adma.200902418]

[117] Li G, Mo X, Law WC, Chan KC. Wearable Fluid Capture Devices for Electrochemical Sensing of Sweat. ACS Appl Mater Interfaces 2019; 11(1): 238-43.
[http://dx.doi.org/10.1021/acsami.8b17419] [PMID: 30516364]

[118] LaVan DA, *et al.* Small-scale systems for *in vivo* drug delivery Nature Biotechnology. 2003; 21: pp. 1184-91.
[http://dx.doi.org/10.1038/nbt876]

CHAPTER 3

Basic and Advanced Electrochemical Technology for Biosensing Applications

Tien-Chun Tsai, Neil Adrian P. Ondevilla and Hsien-Chang Chang[*]

Department of Biomedical Engineering, National Cheng Kung University, Tainan, 70101, Taiwan

Abstract: Electrochemical biosensors combine a molecular recognition concept involving the use of biosensors to sensitively detect target analytes with an attractive electrochemistry technique to analyze a biological sample due to the direct conversion of a biological event to an electronic signal. The strength of electrochemical biosensors allows sensitive, label-free biosensing with highly temporal resolution using a miniature instrument. This chapter commences with a fundamental introduction of the electrochemical principles, as well as providing a technological comparison between general voltammetric measurements, including cyclic voltammetry (CV), differential pulse voltammetry (DPV), and square wave voltammetry (SWV). It continues with a broad, detailed description of various electrochemical applications ranging over ion-selective electrodes, an enzyme-catalyzed / non-enzymatic glucose sensor, an aptamer-based biosensor (aptasensor), and a genosensor for nucleic acids. This chapter provides readers with a good insight into the usefulness, performance, and properties of electrochemical biosensors with many examples.

Keywords: Aptamer, Electrochemical sensors, Genosensor, Glucose sensor, Ion-selective electrodes.

INTRODUCTION

Numerous (micro)sensors based on electrochemical techniques have drawn a significant amount of attention to biomedical analysis applications, including non-invasive determinations of biomarkers in biological fluid [1], real-time monitoring of cellular exocytosis [2], and implantable recording in basic animal studies [3]. In contrast to various conventional techniques involving immunohistological staining, mass spectroscopy, and high-performance liquid chromatography (HPLC), electrochemical (micro)sensors provide some attractive advantages for biomedical diagnoses, such as label-free recording, great sensitivity, extremely high temporal resolution, and miniaturized device design.

[*] **Corresponding author Hsien-Chang Chang:** Department of Biomedical Engineering, National Cheng Kung University, Tainan 70101, Taiwan; E-mail: hcchang@mail.ncku.edu.tw

Han-Sheng Chuang & Yi-Ping Ho (Eds.)

Electrochemistry combines electrical effects with chemistry. The transducers used in this process consist of potentiometric, voltammetric, conductometric, and FET-based sensors [4]. With regards to the theory of electrochemical techniques, a three-electrode system is generally applied: The working electrode, where the redox reaction of the electroactive analytes is taking place at an adaptive potential, is measured relative to the reference electrode, through which no current flows, with the circuit being completed by the counter electrode (Fig. **1**). Two categories of procedures occur at the surface of the sensing electrodes: A given electrode-solution interface on the working electrode will show that capacitance always exists in the electrical double layer between the electrode and the bulk solution because such reactions are thermodynamically or kinetically unfavorable [5]. This procedure is called a non-faradaic process, which cannot be ignored in the electrochemical recording. In addition to the charging current brought about by the non-faradaic process, another reaction suggests that electrons are transferred across the electrode-solution interface to produce a current as the detectable signal at the adaptive potential. Electron transfer results from the redox reaction (*i.e.*, oxidation or reduction) of electroactive analytes. Since such a reaction is based on Faraday's law, which states that the amount of a chemical reaction (the mass of the substance deposited or liberated) is proportional to that of the electricity passed, which is called the faradaic process [5].

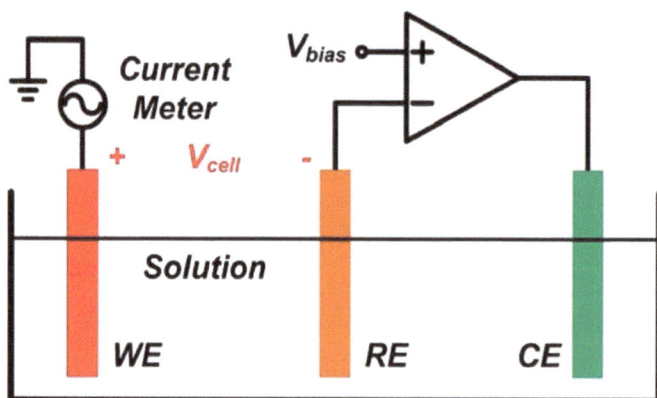

Fig. (1). Conceptual drawing of the electrochemical three-electrode system. Reprinted with permission from Ref [8].

Electrochemical biosensors have attracted increasing attention due to their notable advantages, such as being highly sensitive and accurate analytical tools able to achieve low detection limits, as well as the possibility of being used in real samples. They are also noticed for their robustness, cost-effectiveness, and ease of portability [6]. The disadvantages of electrochemical biosensors are related to the available choices for their bio-receptors and include the effects of pH, temperature, and ionic strength on the binding capacity of the bio-receptors, especially in the case of proteins and enzymes [7].

Electrochemical Techniques

Electrochemical biosensors combine a molecular recognition concept involving the use of biosensors to sensitively detect target analytes with an attractive electrochemistry technique to analyze a biological sample due to the direct conversion of a biological event to an electronic signal. These electrochemical methods that are commonly integrated with biosensors can be classified into voltammetry, potentiometry, and amperometry. The general feature of voltammetry is based on a varying potential, which is applied to the working electrode with respect to the reference electrode to find the potential ranges of an oxidizable or reducible species in the supporting electrolyte. The responsive current is contributed by the background current as well as the redox current resulting from the oxidative or reductive reaction in the electroactive molecules. Various electroactive analytes with different suitable potentials can be distinguished by their peak positions in the oxidation and the reduction reaction. Therefore, the resulting voltammogram is related to the chemical identity of various analytes and their concentrations and provides powerful qualitative and quantitative assessments for electroactive species [9].

Linear Sweep Voltammetry (LSV), Cyclic Voltammetry (CV) and Fast-Scan Cyclic Voltammetry (FSCV)

Voltammetry, applied with the potential scans used to record the resulting current, is the most important and widespread technique among various electrochemical methods now being used for biosensing applications. Specifically, the unstirred potential sweep methods, *i.e.* linear sweep voltammetry (LSV) and cyclic voltammetry (CV), represent the most widely used diagnostic tool for studying electrode processes. The difference between LSV and CV is that LSV is only a single sweep. However, the potential sweep in CV is inverted to form a single cycle or multiple cycles. The working principle of sweep voltammetry is the application of a continuous potential scan across the electrode–solution interface. The resulting current observed in the voltammogram depends on the mass transport (*i.e.* the diffusion of analytes from the bulk of the solution to the electrode) and charge transfer kinetics (*i.e.* the efficiency of electron transfer across the electrode–solution interface). Hence, current–potential curves are capable of giving detailed information regarding the kinetics of electron transfer associated with the electrochemical reaction taking place on the electrode surface.

CV has become a powerful technique for the evaluation of the initial electrochemical studies on developing systems. However, it is not applicable for carrying out a quantitative analysis because the resulting current involves not only the faradaic current from the redox reaction of the analytes but also the random capacitive (non-faradaic) current from the electrical double layer. Considering the reaction kinetics at the electrode surface, the existence of a charging current, which results from the double-layer capacitance in electrochemical measurements, cannot be ignored, where the charging current will be much larger than the faradaic current due to the redox of electroactive analytes at very low concentrations. The response of an ideal polarized electrode system is considered to be an *RC* circuit, which is represented by solution resistance (R_s) and double-layer capacitance (C_d) in series and charge transfer resistance (R_{ct}) in parallel. When applying a potential step of magnitude (E), the behavior of the charging current (i) with time (t) is given [5] by

$$i = \frac{E}{R_s} e^{\frac{-t}{R_s C_d}} \qquad (1)$$

Therefore, an exponentially decaying current has a time constant, $\tau = R_s C_d$, that corresponds to a potential step input. When a potential is applied to a working electrode for oxidation of target analytes, Cottrell's equation predicts that the electrochemical theory of the oxidative current will decay with time [5]:

$$i_{ox}(t) = n \cdot F \cdot A \cdot C_0 (D_0/\pi t)^{1/2} \qquad (2)$$

where i_{ox} is the oxidative current of the target analytes (*i.e.* Faradaic current); n is the number of electrons involved in the oxidation reaction; F is the Faraday constant; A is the area of the working electrode; C_0 is the analyte concentration in the bulk solution; D_0 is the diffusion coefficient, and t is the recording time. According to eqs. (1) and (2), the capacitive current decays with $e^{-t/RC}$ faster than the faradaic current during a period $t^{1/2}$ when applying a potential pulse.

In addition, another major shortcoming of CV measurement is the relatively poor temporal resolution because one scan often takes longer than several seconds. In contrast to the poor temporal resolution in CV scans, fast-scan cyclic voltammetry (FSCV), which is alternatively compatible with a kHz sampling rate, can record signals on a time scale of milliseconds and enables the real-time monitoring of neurotransmitters released from living cells [10]. The development of the FSCV technique has led to a much higher temporal resolution than CV scanning. During

FSCV operation, the applied potential is typically swept at scan rates faster than 100 V/s in the form of a triangular waveform, thus achieving temporal resolution on a millisecond scale [11]. In addition, FSCV is a potential-sweep technique; thus, target analytes and interfering agents with different redox potentials can be distinguished based on their peak current positions within the applied potential window. Nevertheless, a disadvantage of FSCV operating at high scan rates is that the background current greatly exceeds the redox current from the electrolyzed molecules. The background current, resulting primarily from the charging of the double layer around the electrode surface, has an amplitude that is directly proportional to the scan rate of the voltammetric detection. In contrast, the faradaic current produced from the redox reaction of electroactive species is proportional to merely the square root of the scan rate [5]. Therefore, Fig. (2) presents a recent study in which an analog background subtraction technique was proposed to minimize the impact of large background signals; consequently, signals of very small redox currents could be monitored [12].

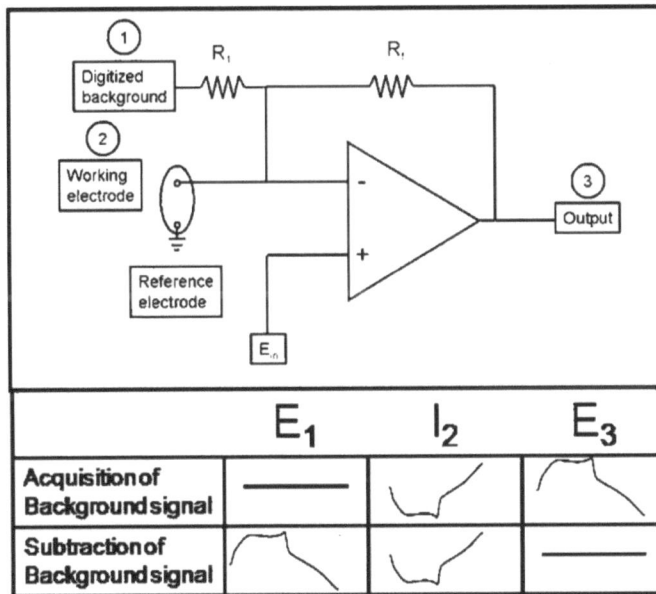

Fig. (2). Electronic setup for analog background subtraction. The background is subtracted as a two-step process, where the first step is the acquisition of the background signal. The waveform is applied to E_{in} while the other input (E_1) is disconnected, and the current at the working electrode (I_2) is transduced to a voltage (E_3). In the second step, the background signal is subtracted. The triangular waveform is applied to E_{in} while the background signal recorded during the first step (E_3) is applied to input (E_1). The current obtained at the working electrode (I_2) is canceled out at the summation point, resulting in a flat signal at the output (E_3). (Reprinted with permission from Ref [12]. Copyright 2008, American Chemical Society).

Differential Pulse Voltammetry (DPV) and Square Wave Voltammetry (SWV)

Based on the different decay rates for the charging current and the redox current, the differential pulse voltammetry (DPV) technique was initially developed to significantly eliminate the contribution of capacitive current by current sampling at the start and at the end of the applied pulse. As shown in Fig. (**3**), DPV mode provides a non-oxidative potential, V_A, (*i.e.* pre-pulse) to generate the charging current. The potential V_B (*i.e.* measuring pulse) that follows V_A can induce the oxidation of the target analytes to generate both the charging current and the oxidative current. Eventually, the measured current in DPV consists almost solely of the redox current of the target analytes by subtracting the capacitive current from that between the end of both the pre-pulse and measuring pulse. This makes it possible to substantially increase the signal–to–noise ratio (SNR), resulting in better sensitivity as well as a lower detection limit within the optimum parameters. However, the major drawback of the DPV technique is that it is limited by a poor temporal resolution, *i.e.* much longer analysis times of 2–4 min in each measurement, since the long pulse period for one full potential cycle is often required to be between 0.5 and 5 s under typical conditions.

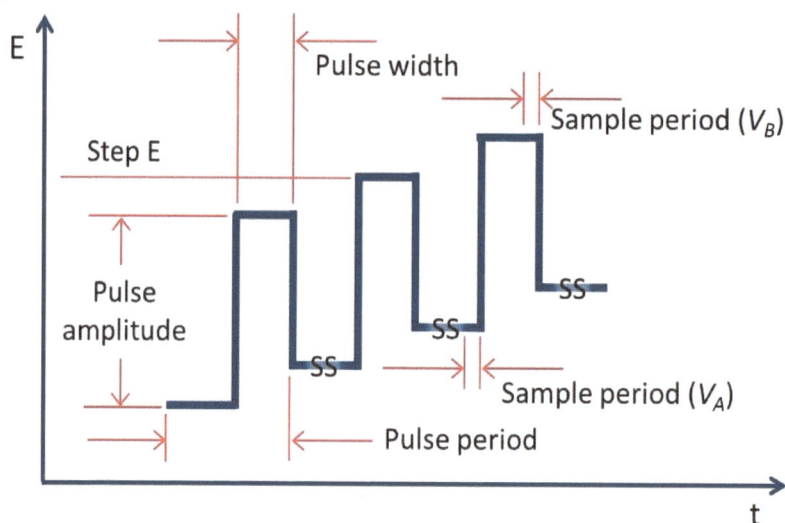

Fig. (3). The potential differential pulse voltammetry (DPV) waveform consists of small pulses superimposed upon a staircase waveform. The redox current of analytes could can be measured by subtracting the capacitive current from that between the end of both pre-pulse (V_A) and the measuring pulse (V_B). SS indicates a steady-state potential, where a negligible electrolysis occurs after the end of each pulse. This steady-state potential is changed steadily in small increments to compensate for the change in the bulk concentration of the sample, which results in a new initial concentration profile on the electrode surface, where it is reduced during the waiting period at some rate less than the maximum [5].

The application of square wave voltammetry (SWV) has become very popular in the last decade. It is much more sensitive than the other voltammetric techniques. As schematically illustrated in Fig. (**4A**), the potential SWV waveform, similar to that of DPV, applies a square wave that is superimposed on a staircase ramp. The total net current ($I_t = I_f\text{-}I_b$) is subtracted by sampling just before the end of each forward (I_f) and backward (I_b) pulse. Furthermore, the main strength of the SWV technique is that reduced scanning time can be found, with high effective scan rates of as high as 1 V/s, whereas DPV normally scans with kinetically slow processes, *i.e.* slow sweep rates between 1 and 10 mV/s. Fig. (**4B**) displays a reversible reaction. Owing to the fact that the I_t is much larger than either the forward or backward component, the sensitivity of SWV is usually higher than that of DPV. Thus, SWV is employed more often than DPV in pharmaceutical analyses because of its greater sensitivity and fast response [13].

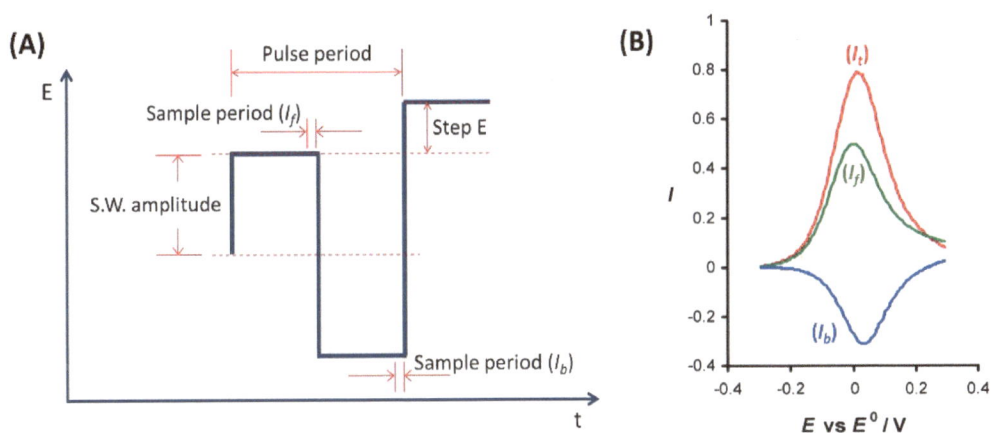

Fig. (4). (**A**) The potential square wave voltammetry (SWV) waveform is applied to measure the total net current ($I_t = I_f\text{-}I_b$) from the redox of analytes calculated between the end of both the forward (I_f) and backward pulse (I_b). (**B**) The total net current comprises the forward and backward currents. (Reprinted with permission from Ref [14]. Copyright 2013, American Chemical Society).

Ion-Selective Electrodes

Ion-selective electrodes (ISEs) are potentiometric sensors that have been conventionally defined as a zero-current technique that measures the potential across an interface. This technique is based on the principle of measuring the electromotive force (EMF) of a concentration cell [4]. The change in EMF measured by potentiometric devices is proportional to the logarithm of the ionic concentration. In practice, mixtures of several interfering ions coexist in a real sample. As regards sensing platforms ranging from the pharmaceutical chemistry to environmental pollutants, ISEs typically use an ionophore (*i.e.* an ion-selective membrane) to ensure selectivity toward a specific ion of interest. A large number of published studies have demonstrated the function of ion-selective membranes using carbon pastes and polyvinyl chloride (PVC) as well as unique ionophores specifically designed for the target ions. Carbon paste electrodes (CPEs) have attracted interest due to their stable response, renewability, and low Ohmic resistance [15, 16].

CPE-Based Potentiometric Sensors

CPE-based sensors are typically fabricated using graphite powder dispersed in a non-conductive mineral oil, causing an unpredictable influence from the contaminants in the mineral oil [17]. Carbon nanotubes (CNTs) incorporated with a selective agent are becoming increasingly useful in membrane composition to enhance the sensing capability of a targeted species. The unique physicochemical properties in CNTs, such as an ordered structure and high mechanical strength, high electrical and thermal conductivity, metallic or semi-metallic behavior, and large surface area, have already attracted interest. For example, a potentiometric sensor was made up of paraffin oil, graphite powder, multi-walled CNTs (MWCNTs), and *N*-(1-thia-2-ylmethylene)-1,3-benzothiazole-2-amine (TBA) as the ionophore for Ho^{3+} sensing [18]. TBA shows a special interaction toward Ho^{3+} among common alkali, alkali earth, and transition metal ions. The membrane in another novel Er^{3+}-selective sensor was fabricated with MWCNTs and *N'*-(--hydroxy-1,2-diphenylethylidene) benzohydrazide (HDEBH) [17]. This study demonstrated the incorporation of room temperature ionic liquids (RTIL), instead of the commonly used mineral oil, as well as the use of MWCNTs to enhance sensitivity.

PVC Membrane-Containing Sensors

PVC-based composite membranes have also been proven to be preferable materials for ISEs due to their simple construction, which suggests widespread applications ranging from both cations and anions. Exposure to high Al^{3+} ion levels can interfere with the metabolism of phosphorus, leading to a variety of bone lesions. Meanwhile, some recent evidence also suggests that Al^{3+} ions are related to the pathology of Parkinson's disease (PD), as well as Alzheimer's disease (AD) [19]. Hence, quantitative detection of Al^{3+} in the environment, medicine, and foodstuff has attracted great interest. A potentiometric electrode that consists of PVC and *N,N'*-propanediamide bis(2-salicylideneimine) (NPBS) matrix membrane allows for the selective sensing of Al^{3+} ions [20]. The excellent selectivity of the proposed sensor towards Al^{3+} ions in this study mainly resulted from the coordinate interaction between NPBS and Al^{3+} ions. The nitrogen (N) and oxygen (O) atoms in NPBS could be considered as electron donors, which coordinate metal ions as electron acceptors. This developed sensor afforded superior sensing performance compared with other sensing techniques, thus making it feasible for the potentiometric titration of Al^{3+} ions in real samples. In the case of anionic detection, a PVC-based sensor was incorporated with triazolophane as the ionophore for halide sensing [21]. The results indicated that cyclic compounds in triazolophane containing 1,2,3-triazole units can act as host molecules to interact strongly with halides, as shown in Fig. (5). The various compositions of the membranes were further evaluated to optimize the concentrations between the ionophore, plasticizer, and lipophilic additives in order to achieve the best selectivity toward Cl^- and Br^- ions. In summary, the lipophilicity of the plasticizer was found to have a great impact on the electrode response. On the other hand, the concentration of the lipophilic additives was recognized to be critical for optimal response. The utility of a triazolophane-incorporated with a PVC-based sensor was also proven by the quantification of Br^- ions in horse serum samples.

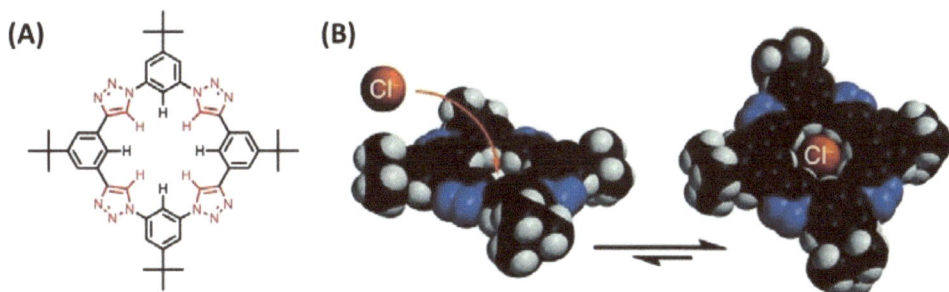

Fig. (5). (a) Triazolophane and (b) representative model of the interaction between triazolophane and Cl^- ions. (Reprinted with permission from Ref [21]. Copyright 2010, American Chemical Society).

Electrochemical Glucose Sensor

Quantitative monitoring of blood glucose has great clinical significance in the diagnosis and management of diabetes mellitus, which is one of the global health issues that result in risks of heart disease, kidney failure, and blindness. Hyperglycemia resulting from insulin deficiency is defined by blood glucose levels higher than the normal range of about 130 mg/dL in an empty stomach or above 180 mg/dL within 2 hours after the start of a meal [22]. Among various techniques, such as absorptiometry (and reflectometry), fluorescence, and surface plasmon resonance (SPR), electrochemical glucose sensors based on an enzyme-catalyzed reaction still dominate the glucose sensing industry, particularly with advanced developments in homecare, point-of-care tests (POCTs), and continuous glucose monitoring (CGM). The requirements for glucose meter systems is set by the International Organization for Standardization (ISO). The first ISO standard for the self-monitoring blood glucose (SMBG) systems was published in 2003 (*i.e.* ISO 15197: 2003). The latest standard set stringently in 2013 (*i.e.* ISO 15197:

2013) ensures higher accuracy and consistency of results for individual subjects with diabetes. Table **1** summarizes the minimum accuracy criteria in SMBG systems for the above-mentioned versions. The higher stringency for minimum accuracy criteria published in the ISO 15197: 2013 version is described as follows:

- Three different lots of testing strips must now be evaluated individually and combined;
- 99% of results must fall within zones A+B of a Consensus Error Grid (CEG) (Fig. **6**);
- 95% of results <100 mg/dL must fall within ±15% of the reference method;
- 95% of results <100 mg/dL must fall within ±15 mg/dL of the reference method;
- Scatter plots must be produced.

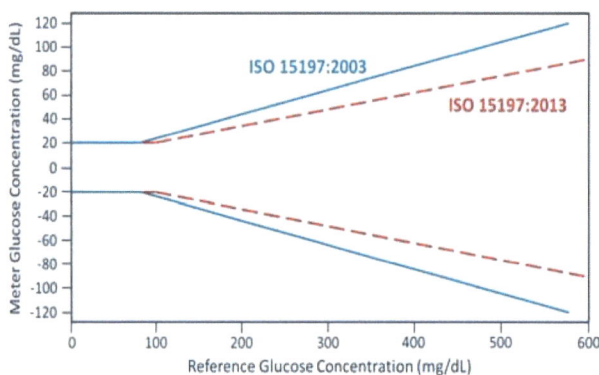

Fig. (6). Consensus Error Grid (CEG) for SMBG systems according to ISO 15197: 2003 (solid blue line) and ISO 15197: 2013 (broken red line) [23].

Table 1. Minimum accuracy criteria for SMBG systems according to ISO 15197: 2003 and ISO 15197: 2013 standards [23].

ISO 15197	Relative Number of Results	At Blood Glucose Concentrations	Within	CEG Zones
2003	95%	<75 mg/dL	±15 mg/dL	99% of results within CEG zones A + B
		<75 mg/dL	±20%	
2013	95%	<100 mg/dL	±15 mg/dL	
		<100 mg/dL	±15%	

Enzymatic Glucose Sensors

To date, the glucose meters based on the enzyme catalysis and amperometric methods are most commonly applied for SMBG and CGM systems. Glucose oxidase (GOx) is most widely utilized in commercialized glucose sensors in order to involve the electro-oxidation of glucose because of its low cost and high specificity. Since Clark and Lyons initially proposed the concept of enzymatic glucose electrodes in 1962 [24], an enormous amount of efforts has been focused on improvements in GOx-based amperometric biosensors for the purpose of achieving higher blood glucose determination accuracy, as shown in Fig. (**7**). Three generations of amperometric glucose biosensors involving GOx-based catalysis are described as follows:

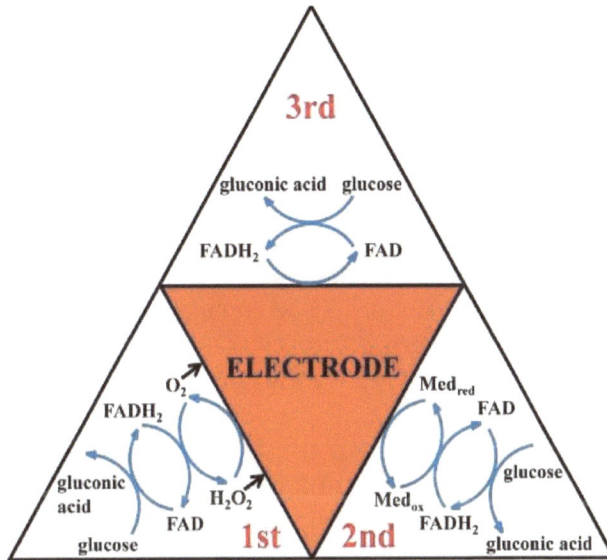

Fig. (7). Summary of enzymatic glucose oxidation mechanisms, presented as the first, second, and third generation sensors. (Reprinted with permission from Ref [22]. Copyright 2013, Royal Society of Chemistry).

First Generation

Clark and Lyons used a thin layer of GOx entrapped over an O_2-semipermeable dialysis membrane to enzymatically oxidize glucose in the presence of O_2, as shown in Eq. (3). According to Eq. (4), the consumption of O_2 was monitored using a platinum (Pt) cathode and used as the signal for indirect glucose quantification [2].

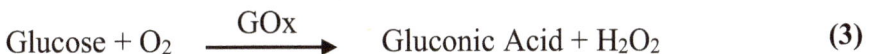

$$\text{Glucose} + O_2 \xrightarrow{\text{GOx}} \text{Gluconic Acid} + H_2O_2 \qquad (3)$$

$$O_2 + 4H^+ + 4e^- \xrightarrow{\quad E \quad} 2H_2O \qquad (4)$$

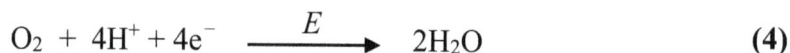

The current response of the first-generation glucose electrodes is directly proportional to the O_2 concentration in the samples; thus the amount of O_2 plays a critical role in the quantification of glucose levels. However, the fact that the normal O_2 level is about 1 order of magnitude lower than the physiological concentration of blood glucose should be considered. In the case of the first-generation amperometric glucose biosensors, the effect of an oxygen deficit greatly reduces the sensitivity to glucose at higher levels [25]. Previous studies have demonstrated poly(chlorotrifluorethylene) oil/GOx-coated CPEs [26] or an air diffusion biocathode (*i.e.* CueO from *Escherichia coli*) using O_2 directly from air [27] can be designed to increase the O_2 supply.

In addition, the accuracy and precision of a GOx-immobilized electrode based on O_2 consumption were significantly affected by the varying amounts of background O_2 in solution. A smart method was proposed to employ two working electrodes, where one of them was immobilized with GOx [28]. The accuracy of glucose determination was therefore improved by measuring the current differences for the electro-oxidation of O_2 in the solution. To conquer the limitation due to highly variable amounts of O_2 in background, the first amperometric glucose sensor based on the detection of H_2O_2 products under GOx catalysis (shown in eqs. (3) and (5)) was developed by Guilbault and Lubrano [29]. However, many coexisting electro-active species, such as ascorbic acid, uric acid, and dopamine, are present in biological fluids, which can be co-oxidized during electro-oxidation of produced H_2O_2 at a relatively high potential (*i.e.* +0.3~+0.8 V *vs.* SCE, commonly at about 0.6 V *vs.* SCE).

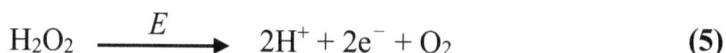

$$H_2O_2 \xrightarrow{\quad E \quad} 2H^+ + 2e^- + O_2 \qquad (5)$$

All of these contribute to the current responses simultaneously, resulting in insufficient selectivity and accuracy of the amperometric glucose determination. Considerable effort has been applied to improving the anti-interferent ability of first-generation glucose sensors. Two main strategies to minimize these interferences have been proposed: (1) decreasing the H_2O_2-oxidized potential by incorporating various catalysts co-immobilized around enzyme, such as Prussian blue (PB) [30 - 32], poly(toluidine blue O) (TBO) [33], and horseradish peroxidase (HRP) [34, 35] and (2) immobilizing GOx through a perm-selective membrane (*e.g.*, cellulose acetate, polyaniline, and polypyrrole) or a semipermeable film (*e.g.*, nafion, poly(vinylpyridine), and poly(ester-sulfonic acid)), which could inhibit the electroactive interfering species while retaining sufficient H_2O_2 or O_2 on the electrode surface [36, 37].

Second Generation

Two flavin adenine dinucleotide (FAD) cofactors that strongly bind to GOx act as the redox active centers within GOx and can be reduced to $FADH_2$ upon the enzymatic catalysis of glucose, as shown in Eq. (6). In fact, the $FADH_2$ is buried at a depth of about 13–15 Å below the electrode-contacting periphery of its glycoprotein, which implies that the rate of direct electron tunneling from the $FADH_2$ within GOx to the electrode surface is too slow to be measured in the absence of electron transfer mediators [38]. The second-generation glucose biosensors adopt artificial mediators, such as ferrocyanide/ferricyanide, hydroquinone, and ferrocene, to overcome the inherent limitations of oxygen deficits, especially in the detection of a high glucose level. These electron mediators may facilitate electron transfer efficiency by shuttling electrons from the active enzymatic center to the electrode surface [39]. The enzymatic catalysis in second-generation amperometric glucose sensors consists of the following three steps: (a) The electrons transfer from glucose to the two FAD reaction centers within GOx, which are reduced to $FADH_2$ (Eq. (6)); (b) the electrons transfer from the $FADH_2$ centers to the artificial mediators, and thus the oxidative state mediators (Med_{ox}) transform to reduced state mediators (Med_{red}) (Eq. (7)); (c) the electrons finally transfer through the artificial mediators to the electrode at an oxidized potential (Eq. (8)). In the second-generation biosensing mode, the current signals acquired by the oxidation of Med_{red} are proportionally related to the glucose concentration.

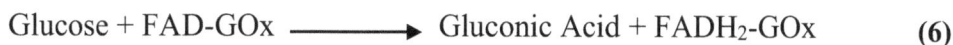

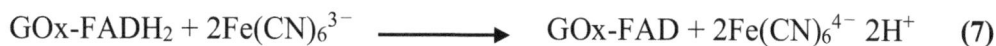

$$\text{Glucose} + \text{FAD-GOx} \longrightarrow \text{Gluconic Acid} + \text{FADH}_2\text{-GOx} \qquad (6)$$

$$\text{GOx-FADH}_2 + 2\text{Fe(CN)}_6^{3-} \longrightarrow \text{GOx-FAD} + 2\text{Fe(CN)}_6^{4-}\ 2\text{H}^+ \qquad (7)$$

$$2Fe(CN)_6{}^{4-} \xrightarrow{\quad E \quad} 2Fe(CN)_6{}^{3-} + 2e^- \qquad (8)$$

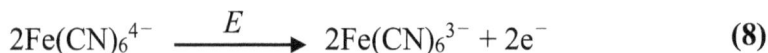

Considering the efficient interaction between electron mediators and FAD/FADH$_2$, GOx redox active centers are necessary to achieve an effective shuttle of electrons between GOx and the sensing electrode. The artificial mediator can either be dissolved in the liquid phase, which can diffuse toward the enzymatic active core [25], or it can be immobilized by being anchored directly to the GOx [40] or entrapped with GOx in a polymer film [41]. Unfortunately, soluble mediators cannot be applied in implantable sensors [42]. Although the solution-state mediators ideally react with the enzyme faster than with O$_2$ in solution, the effect of dissolved O$_2$ competing with the electron mediators is a possibility, thus reducing the efficiency of electron transfer between the redox active cores in GOx and the sensing electrode [43]. Various alternative attempts for tailoring the mediators in enzyme-containing films have been suggested. For example, the artificial mediators chemically bound to the polymer backbone have been widely employed to fabricate GOx-based glucose biosensors. In one case, the MWCNTs immobilized with GOx and a ferrocene derivatized poly(allylamine) (PAAm) redox polymer using electrostatic self-assembly were reported to form supra-molecular organized multilayers, leading to the development of a reagentless biosensor [44]. Another study also reported that the mediators were directly bound to polysiloxane to allow the close contact between the FAD/FADH$_2$ GOx centers and the immobilized mediators, which made it possible to overcome the issue of the soluble mediators diffusing between the bulk solution and the electrode surface [42]. In summary, achieving the direct electron transformation of enzymes depends closely on the distance between the redox-active mediators and the sensing electrode, and thus, the stable immobilization of the mediators with enzymes compared with the solution-state mediators, which indicates higher electron-exchange efficiency between co-immobilized mediators and enzymes.

Third Generation

Third-generation enzymatic glucose biosensors mainly comprise direct electron transfer between the GOx and the sensing electrode, instead of natural or artificial mediators. As mentioned previously, the inherent limitation in achieving the direct electron transfer between the sensing electrode and an enzyme can be attributed to the large protein in which the redox active center is entrapped. In recent years, remarkable advancements in the development of nano- and porous materials have greatly increased the electrode surface areas necessary to encompass the enzymes. This ideal biosensing model, based on the construction of various nano-materials (*e.g.,* metallic nanoparticles [45], graphene [46], CNT [47], and phosphorene [48]) onto the electrode surface, allows the direct electron transfer upon enzymatic oxidation without the complications of mediators. In addition, nano-materials (such as CNT-TiO$_2$ composite) rather than electron transfer mediators are promising to diminish the interferences from other electroactive species, owing to the determination of glucose at lower redox potentials of around -0.3 V and -0.5 V *vs.* Ag/AgCl, respectively [49].

Wang *et al.* constructed a unique hollow nanostructured Pt decorated multiwall carbon nanotube (HPt-CNT) composites over the glassy carbon electrode (GCE) by direct casting [50]. Based on the electrostatic adsorption and covalent modification, negatively-charged l-cysteine (l-cys) and positively-charged poly(diallydimethylammonium) chloride (PDDA)-covered gold nanoparticles (PDDA-Au) were attached on the electrode surface, allowing excellent covalent immobilization of GOx over the nanostructure layer resulting in the enhancement of the electrode response toward glucose. The results showed an apparent Michaelis–Menten constant (K_m^{app}) value of 4.14 mM using Lineweaver-Burk plots, indicating that the immobilized GOx on the electrode retained higher enzymatic activity. Qiu and co-workers also introduced a simple, sensitive strategy for detecting glucose by means of immobilizing GOx *via* physical adsorption onto a nanostructured Au thin film on GCE (GOx/Au/GCE) [51]. This as-prepared thin film was composed of a porous, biocompatible, and highly conductive platform, thus facilitating electron transfer between the redox active center of GOx and the sensing electrode, as determined through the use of CV scans. The enzymatic activity was estimated to determine the glucose concentration with a K_m^{app} value of 15.6 µM. Another interesting protocol suggested by Gao *et al.* is the fabrication of a nano-complex of GOx and hydroxyl fullerenes (HFs) by simple mixing, casting it onto a GCE followed by a chitosan membrane for protection [52]. The K_m^{app} value of the proposed glucose biosensor was calculated to be 694 µM.

Non-enzymatic Glucose Sensors

In spite of the fact that enzyme-based systems are dominating the glucose biosensor industry thus far, their applications remain commercially challenged. To overcome high O$_2$ dependency in the first generation, second-generation sensors have incorporated immobilized mediators to achieve O$_2$ independence and a lower amperometric potential in order to minimize interference from electroactive species. Nevertheless, these electrodes still suffer from lower reproducibility and higher cost due to the more complicated fabrication necessary for mass production. Also, third-generation glucose biosensors based on mesoporous nanomaterials are still in the development stage although numerous approaches suggest that these novel materials show potential.

In addition, another common problem is insufficient stability attributed to the nature of the enzymes involved in such systems, which seriously affects sensing performance. Even though GOx is quite stable compared to other enzymes, glucose sensors immobilized with GOx are always exposed to harsh conditions during fabrication, storage, and use. One published review suggested that possible thermal and chemical deformation of GOx will lead to a quick loss of its activity below pH=2 and above pH=8, as well as at temperatures over 40°C [53]. In addition to rigorous temperature and pH requirements necessary for sterilization during fabrication, the responses of glucose sensors are affected by environmental humidity as well [54]. Both high and low humidity are significantly harmful to immobilized enzymes and artificial mediators in use and can also affect their storage periods. This is why enzyme-free glucose biosensors always receive high interest.

Under Neutral Conditions

The use of non-enzymatic electrodes as glucose biosensors potentially moves the next generation forward in terms of the quantification of glucose levels. Instead of an enzymatic catalysis for glucose, continued efforts to realize the concept of non-enzymatic electrodes are mainly devoted to the efficient electro-oxidation of the glucose in the samples. According to some early studies on the electrochemical oxidation of glucose on a platinum surface in a neutral phosphate buffer (PB) solution, it was agreed that glucose was oxidized electrochemically *via* dehydrogenation at the C1 carbon [55, 56]. The β-form is the most reactive species among the different anomeric forms of glucose molecules due to the appropriate geometric orientation of the hydrogen atom bound to the anomeric carbon [57]. As shown in the cyclic voltammogram in Fig. (**8A**), a platinum-based working electrode was used as a reversible hydrogen electrode (RHE) to electrochemically detect glucose in the absence of an enzyme. The hydrogen region in which glucose produces the unique behavior of electrochemical oxidation could be observed between 0.15 V and 0.35 V *vs.* RHE [58]. In the presence of glucose, the relatively high current peaks that appeared below 0.35 V were associated with the adsorbed hydrogen atoms upon glucose electro-oxidation in the hydrogen region. The reaction was associated with the hemiacetal group in the adsorbed glucose, where either hydrogen adsorption or desorption took place, as illustrated in Fig. (**8B**). The cyclic voltammogram also exhibited a double layer region ranging from 0.4 V to 0.8 V *vs.* RHE [59]. The oxidation peak current within the double layer region decreased when anions or organic species, such as glucono-δ-lactone (*i.e.* the product of glucose oxidation), were adsorbed. In addition, the voltammetric behavior involving the reaction of glucose on the produced platinum oxide layer was found to be higher than the 1.1 V *vs.* RHE in the oxide region. The lactone-type product would thus be decomposed further due to oxidation [60].

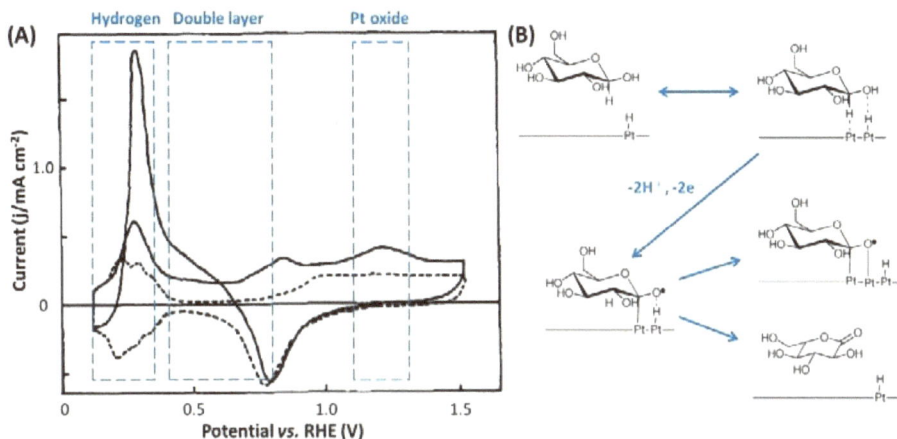

Fig. (8). (**A**) Cyclic voltammograms in the absence (dotted line) and presence (solid line) of 0.1 M glucose in PB solution at pH 7.5 showing three potential regions where glucose is electrochemically oxidized on a platinum electrode. (**B**) Elementary steps of the non-enzymatic glucose oxidation on a platinum surface in PB solution in the potential window of the hydrogen region, where hydrogen adsorption or desorption occurs (summarized and redrawn from figures in Ref [58].).

Under Basic Conditions

A previous study explored the electrochemical oxidation of glucose in a platinum working electrode line solution [61]. Different from the hydrogen adsorption that occurs in neutral solutions, the chemisorption of glucose on bare platinum initially yields adsorbed intermediates formed by dehydrogenation of the glucose anomeric carbon at low potentials. The adsorbed dehydrated intermediates are then further oxidized as weakly adsorbed gluconate, either linked by two oxygens in hydrogen regions below 0.3 V *vs.* RHE or by only one oxygen in the 0.3 V < *E* < 0.6 V double layer region. The adsorption strength of the intermediates tended to weaken when the applied potential was increased. At potentials higher than 0.6 V, the adsorbed dehydrogenated intermediates were oxidized to form glucono-δ-lactone without cleavage of the C-O-C bond. The glucono-δ-lactone slowly desorbed from the platinum surface and eventually became gluconate as a result of hydrolysis under basic conditions.

Under Acidic Conditions

In comparison with the electrochemical behavior in neutral or basic media, the small oxidative peaks in the cyclic voltammogram exhibited poor reactivity to glucose under acidic conditions [57]. A mechanistic study intended to explore glucose oxidation in 0.1 M $HClO_4$ confirmed that glucose oxidation is highly dependent on the surface planes of platinum. The isotope effect indicates that the rate-determining step involves the oxidation of the hydrogen atom bound to C1 carbon on two planes, *i.e.* Pt(111) and Pt(100), where the effect of one is different when the two are combined. According to the results of the linear sweep voltammogram, the amplitude of a single anodic peak in the Pt(111) plane was obviously larger compared with those of the double peaks for both Pt(111) and Pt(100). These findings indicated that the binding strength of the intermediates to the platinum surface are quite different. Glucono-δ-lactone was preferably adsorbed on Pt(111) whereas CO was bound to Pt(100). However, a clear mechanism has not been proposed yet according to related works on the electrochemical oxidation of glucose under acidic conditions [62].

Other Enzyme-Catalyzed Biosensor

Electrochemical methods based on horseradish peroxidase (HRP) have been extensively developed due to their fast response, high selectivity, and high sensitivity. 3,3'-5,5'-tetramethylbenzidine (TMB) is commonly used as a chromogenic substrate for HRP-based detection systems. It was first introduced by Bos, *et al.* in 1981 [63]. Fig. (**9**) shows that the oxidation of TMB by HRP/H_2O_2 is a well-known process, where a blue-colored complex product is first generated, which upon the addition of sulfuric acid, will turn yellow [64].

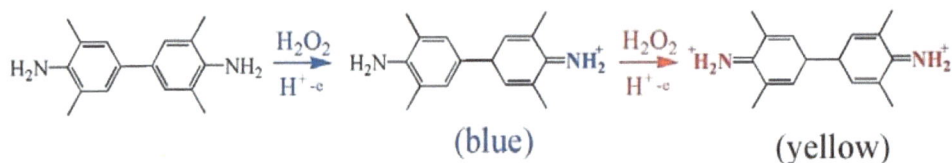

(blue)   (yellow)

Fig. (9). The TMB oxidation reaction. (Reprinted with permission from Ref [64]. Copyright 2014, PLOS).

There have been a number of works utilizing the electrochemical behavior mentioned above, one of which is the work of Mach, *et al.* for the detection of urogenital schistosomiasis in urine samples, as shown in Fig. (**10**) [65]. In this work, a capture probe was bound to the surface of the working electrode *via* gold-thiol linkage. The sample, assumed to contain the target analyte, was mixed with a detector probe and then added to the electrode surface. The detector probe had a fluorescein tag on its terminal end for further reaction. If the target was present in the sample, a complex containing the capture probe, target, and detector probe was formed. HRP-conjugated anti-fluorescein was then added into the complex followed by the addition of the TMB substrate. The electrochemical reaction mediated by the HRP was then measured amperometrically, where the acquired signal was proportional to the quantity of the target in the sample.

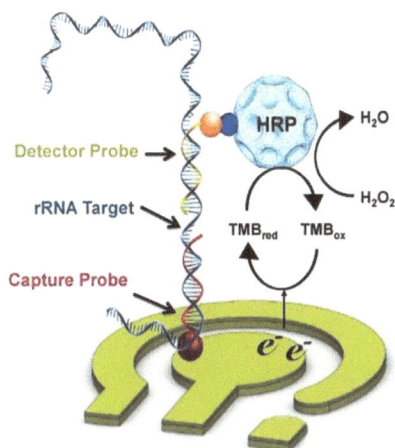

Fig. (10). Biosensor-based molecular detection of a urinary pathogen. (Reprinted with permission from Ref [65]. Copyright 2015, PLOS).

Nucleic Acid-Based Biosensors

Immunoassays are bioanalytical methods where a quantitative analysis depends on the reaction of the binding of the target (antigen) with an antibody. They have been widely used in many important areas of pharmaceutical analyses because of their inherent specificity, high-throughput, and high sensitivity in the analysis of wide range of analytes in biological samples [66]. However, the use of antibodies as bio-receptors leads to difficulties, especially during their development process. The process typically begins with the injection of the purified antigen. Small molecules will not provide an immune response, which prevents them from being viable targets for traditional antibody production. It is also difficult to generate antibodies to a highly toxic compound because they are initially produced in a living animal [67]. Because of these limitations, nucleic acid-based biosensors have attracted increasing attention since they provide many advantages over the use of antibodies, with the use of nucleic acid (DNA or RNA) as the bio-receptor. Nucleic acid-based biosensors can be classified into two types: aptasensors and genosensors.

Aptamer-Based Biosensors (Aptasensor)

Since their discovery in 1990, aptamers have attracted considerable attention in the areas of biosensor development [68]. Aptamers are oligonucleotides, either single-stranded DNA (ssDNA) or RNA, which can bind to a specific target molecule with high affinity and specificity [69]. They offer many advantages over antibodies, including relatively easy production, high affinity and specificity, easy chemical modification, and high stability. They also have high affinities for some ligands that are not recognized by antibodies, such as ions and small molecules. Thus, aptamers are regarded as promising alternatives to antibodies in bioanalytical fields.

Aptamers are selected *in vitro* through a typical method known as the Systematic Evolution of Ligands by EXponential enrichment (SELEX). Once selected, they can be synthesized with high reproducibility and purity from commercial sources. They have been recently considered as highly promising bio-recognition elements for biomarker detection. They undergo a conformational change when reacting with their targets where such a structural change makes it possible to omit additional labeling processes during target binding monitoring. Because of their given attributes, aptamers are expected to become an alternative to antibodies. In addition to the intrinsic advantages of biosensors, aptamer-based biosensors (aptasensor) offer the advantage of reusability over antibodies. In addition, their small size and flexibility allow efficient immobilization at high densities, which is of vital importance in multiplexing miniaturized systems.

Systematic Evolution of Ligands Through Exponential Enrichment (SELEX)

SELEX is a process in which aptamers with high affinity for a desired target are selected from a random oligonucleotide library, as illustrated in Fig. (**11**) [70]. Non-binding aptamers are discarded, and aptamers that bind to the proposed target are expanded through an iterative process. Positive and negative selection are done in order to improve the selectivity of the resulting aptamer candidates. Multiple rounds of SELEX are usually employed to increase the toughness of aptamer selection. This process usually yields around 10^6 aptamer sequences. Identifying the best candidates is a specialized process employing a variety of analytical techniques.

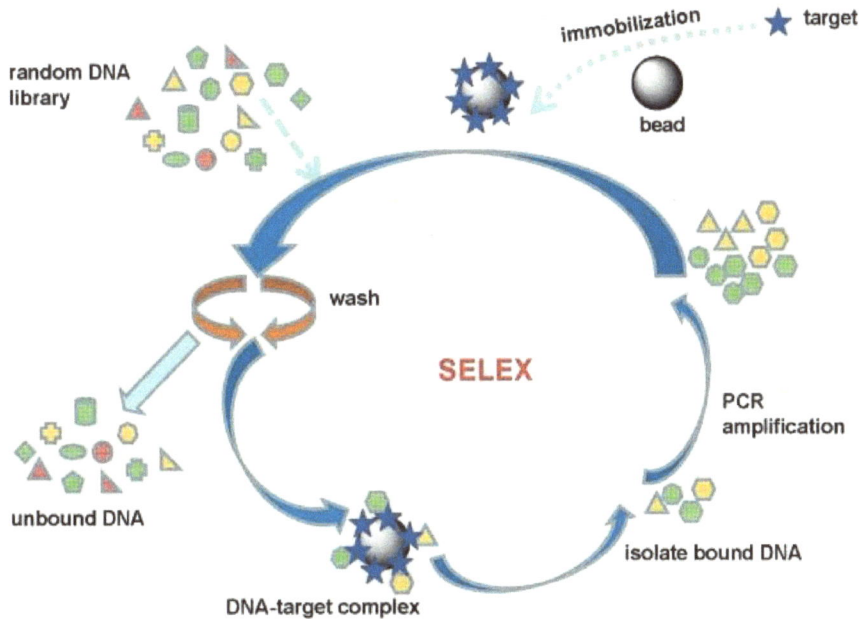

Fig. (11). Scheme for the systematic evolution of ligands using the exponential enrichment (SELEX) process. (Reprinted with permission from Ref [70]. Copyright 2014, Royal Society of Chemistry).

The SELEX process begins with the chemical synthesis of a single-stranded DNA library, which consists of random sequences at the center flanked by defined primer binding sites at each 5'- and 3'-terminus. Structurally constrained libraries contain oligonucleotides with stable regions, which help aptamers to fold according to a specific secondary structure. Libraries based on a known sequence are constructed by inserting known sequences in the central part of the oligonucleotide [71]. Once the library is generated, it is incubated with the target. Some oligonucleotides in the library will recognize the target. These oligonucleotides will then be the aptamers. The unbound sequences will be filtered out of the solution through elution. Due to the separation of aptamers from a specific nucleotide, they are amplified by either a polymerase chain reaction (PCR), in the case of single-stranded DNA (ssDNA) aptamers, or by its real-time counterpart, RT-PCR, in the case of RNA aptamers [72]. Consequently, the products of the amplification process are used as a new sub-library for the next selection round.

After SELEX, redundant and useless nucleotides can be deleted through a process called aptamer truncation. There are many strategies that involve aptamer truncation, which have been tested to minimize aptamer sequences without damaging their binding ability. Most of these strategies can be predicted based on computational biology. Some of the strategies to achieve efficient selection include the use of structure simulations and target docking algorithms, as well as partial fragmentation [73 - 75].

Sensing Mechanisms

Aptamers often undergo significantly conformational changes upon target binding, which causes them to have a very high affinity with their target molecules [76]. The ssDNA typically has a complex secondary structure due to many intra-molecular base pairing opportunities, which imparts increased stability to the folded complex. This conformational change is sensitive to a variety of environmental factors, including pH and temperature. As a result, aptamers can be selected to be responsive to any one or a combination of these factors. Some aptamers undergo conformational changes that can be converted into a current signal from the electroactive indicators anchored at the terminal [77]. Signal generation occurs upon a large binding-induced conformational change in an indicator-labeled aptamer upon target binding. Such aptamers offer great flexibility in the design of novel biosensors and lead to high detection sensitivity and selectivity.

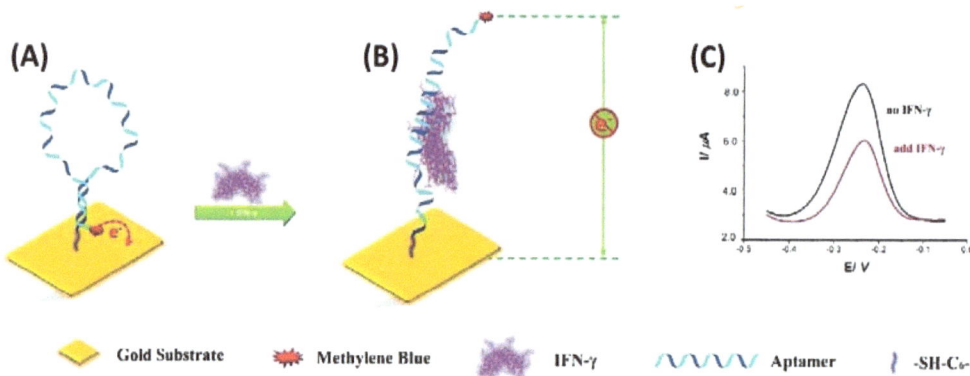

Fig. (12). (**A** and **B**) Schematic of electrochemical aptasensor for interferon (IFN)-γ based on target-induced aptamer unfolding. (**C**) The faradaic currents in the absence and presence of IFN-γ were measured using SWV. (Reprinted with permission from Ref [78]. Copyright 2010, American Chemical Society).

Liu *et. al* modified gold electrodes with methylene blue (MB) labeling aptamers and demonstrated electrochemical detection for interferon (IFN)-γ [78]. As schematically illustrated in Fig. (**12**), this study involved the self-assembly of a thiolated aptamer with a hairpin structure on a gold electrode. A thiolated hairpin structure of an aptamer at the 5'-end, which allowed self-assembly on gold electrodes, was anchored with the electroactive MB at its 3'-end, which was in close proximity to the electrode surface. Based on the target-induced unfolding sensing mechanism, the hairpin conformation was changed once the IFN-γ attached with the aptamers specifically. Then, MB moved away from the electrode surface, which lowered the electron-transfer efficiency.

Other studies based on the folding of target-induced aptamers have been conducted to investigate the selectivity and sensitivity of detection of the blood clotting enzyme, thrombin. In the absence of the target, the aptamer is thought to remain relatively unfolded, which allows the immobilized indicator at the end to collide with the electrode and transfer electrons. Upon thrombin binding, two events possibly take place: Either the electron transfer is inhibited, or its rate of reaction is increased. A previous study published by Xiao and co-workers indicated that electron transfer is inhibited upon the specific attachment of thrombin with an aptamer, which is presumably due to a binding-induced conformational change in the aptamer that significantly alters its electron tunneling distance and/or pathway [79]. It is assumed that the aptamer is in equilibrium with its unfolded state and its folded binding-competent G-quadruplex conformation and that this conformation is the only state in which the target can bind. Therefore, upon binding, the equilibrium is shifted to this state, which in turn produces the acquired signal. This electrochemical aptasensor has been described to be reagent-free, reusable, and selective for employing directly in blood. However, it suffers from limitations associated with having a "signal-off" architecture because it inhibits signal generation. Contaminants that degrade the aptamer or its redox label can give rise to "false positives" that are difficult to distinguish from signals arising from the binding of authentic analytes [80].

This concern is raised in another study, conducted by almost the same group, which focused on the increase in the electrochemical signal of the aptasensor upon target binding. This so called "signal-on" architecture can overcome the limitations in the previously described sensor. Fig. (**13**) illustrates an aptasensor based on the concept of the signal-on mechanism. The short MB-tagged oligonucleotides hybridize with both the thrombin-binding site of the original aptamer and the sequence that attaches the aptamer to the electrode surface. Thrombin binding stabilizes the secondary G-quadruplex structure of the aptamer, which in turn releases the tagged nucleotide, allowing it to collide with the electrode surface to produce a detectable current [80].

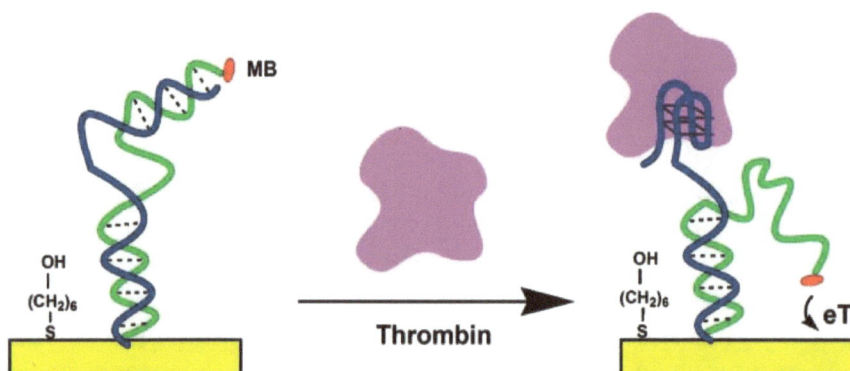

Fig. (13). Scheme for the alternative G-quadruplex conformation of an ssDNA aptamer stabilized by thrombin binding, allowing the MB tag at the end of the flexible aptamer to collide with the gold electrode surface. (Reprinted with permission from Ref [80]. Copyright 2005, American Chemical Society).

Electrochemical Genosensors

A genosensor is a type of biosensor that is specifically used to detect nucleic acids for which its recognition process is based on the complementary base pairing principle. Complementary sequences can be synthesized and immobilized on the sensor surface if the target nucleic acid sequence is known. This detection method is a suitable tool for the analysis of DNA in the determination of certain diseases [81]. Electrochemical genosensors can be either DNA-based or aptamer-based. DNA-based electrochemical genosensors utilize a small sequence of oligonucleotides, known as probes, as the bioreceptor immobilized on the transducer surface, while aptamer-based electrochemical genosensors use aptamers [82]. Due to their affinity, these oligonucleotide sequences recognize an analyte by complementarity-making duplexes. Electrochemical DNA-based genosensors can be coupled with nanoparticles or nanocomposites to improve both oligonucleotide sequence immobilization on the transducer surface and sensitivity to hybridization. The following discussion focuses on the development of DNA-based electrochemical genosensors.

microRNAs

microRNAs (miRNAs) are small non-coding RNAs that play an important role in the post-transcriptional regulation of gene expression in which they bind to complementary sequences on target messenger RNA transcripts, which often results in translational repression and gene silencing. It has been shown that *lin-4* RNA is the origin of miRNAs, the most abundant class of small regulatory RNAs [83]. This was first discovered through genetic screening of the nematode, *Caenorhabditis elegans*. A number of miRNAs are known for their functions in various processes, including cell proliferation, cell death, fat metabolism, neuronal patterning, hematopoietic differentiation, immunity, and control of leaf and flower development [84]. Most miRNA genes are found in the intergenic regions and contain their own miRNA gene promoters and regulatory units.

miRNAs have an effect on the development of cancer, in which they are either increased (upregulated) or decreased (downregulated) in cancer cells. They bind to mRNAs before translation to proteins that switch genes on and off [72]. miRNAs also have a role in heart diseases [85]. In diseased human hearts, expression levels of specific miRNAs change, which indicates their involvement in cardiomyopathies. miRNAs also regulate the nervous system, in which neural miRNAs are involved at various stages of synaptic development, including dendritogenesis, synapse formation, and synapse maturation [86].

Because of their short and highly homologous sequences, and also due to their low concentrations, wide dynamic range, large variations in base composition, and secondary structure, the detection of miRNAs is considered to be a great challenge. Currently, there are several analytical methods that have been developed for the detection of miRNAs. These methods include northern blot analyses, microarrays, RT-PCR, *in situ* hybridization, bioluminescence-based methods, fluorescence correlation spectroscopy, surface-enhanced Raman spectroscopy, surface Plasmon resonance spectroscopy, and high-throughput sequencing techniques [87]. Electrochemical approaches serve as suitable point-of-care diagnostics and multiplexed platform for fast, simple, and inexpensive nucleic acid analyses. Because of their high affinity for binding with their complementary sequence, they are the normal target in detection methods using electrochemical genosensors.

Capture Probe

DNA-based electrochemical genosensors utilize a small sequence of oligonucleotides, known as probes, as the bioreceptor immobilized on the electrode surface. These so-called capture probes can be classified into two categories: capture probes with signal probes and those without signal probes.

Capture Probe with a Signal Probe

As an oligonucleotide capture probe is immobilized on the surface of an electrode, the target analyte with complementary base pairs can be hybridized onto it. Signal probes can then be added to acquire a better electrochemical signal. A simple, sensitive, and label-free method using oligonucleotide encapsulated silver nanoclusters (Ag-NCs) as effective electrochemical probes has been described for miRNA biosensing [88]. Ag-NC anchored probes produce an electrochemical signal in response to a reduction in H_2O_2 (Fig. **14A**). Electrochemical detection using DPV has a limit of detection of 67 fM and a linear range of five orders of magnitude. The Ag-NC-based approach provides a novel avenue by which to detect miRNAs with high sensitivity and selectivity while avoiding laborious label and signal amplification. Another approach has been reported to immobilize enzymes at the terminal of signal probes for highly sensitive potentiometric detection of DNA hybridization [89]. As schematically illustrated in Fig. (**14B**), a low-volume solid-contact silver ISE was used to monitor the depletion of silver ions induced by the biocatalytic reaction of an alkaline-phosphatase enzyme probe. The resultant potential change given by the Ag^+-ISE indicated a limit of detection of 50 fM. This process holds great promise for monitoring various bio-affinity assays.

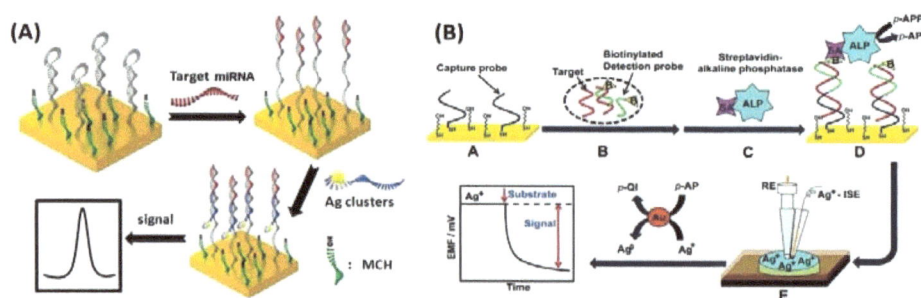

Fig. (14). (**A**) Illustration of electrochemical detection for miRNA using oligonucleotide encapsulated Ag-NCs and (**B**) representation of potentiometric detection for DNA hybridization. (Reprinted with permissions from [88, 89]. Copyrights 2012 and 2009, American Chemical Society).

Capture Probe without a Signal Probe

The other category of capture probe is the one without signal probes. However, the capture probe incorporates a redox label at the end, commonly methylene blue, to induce the electrochemical signal upon hybridization with the target nucleic acids. This indicator could also be nanoparticles. In this category, it is important to consider the conformations of the capture probe. Similar to the concept of folding and unfolding on the ssDNA aptamer, the capture probe exists in two conformations, the stem-loop and the linear conformation.

Incorporating an electroactive indicator at the end of capture probe forms the stem-loop conformation. The indicator is close to the electrode surface, resulting in a strong electrochemical signal before hybridization with the target analyte. Upon hybridization between the capture probe and the target nucleic acid, the conformation of the capture probe changes to a straight structure, which causes the indicator to be far from the electrode surface and in turn produces a lower signal. The linear conformation, on the other hand, already has the redox label far from the electrode, so the electrochemical signal will not depend on the distance of the label to the electrode surface. However, it will depend on the dynamics of the capture probe, which is dampened during the hybridization due to the limited flexibility of the probe-target complex, which in turn leads to a reduction in the electrochemical signal. A study using alternating current voltammetry, (ACV), CV, and DPV, was conducted to explore the sensor performance of electrochemical genosensors conjugated with either the stem-loop probe or linear probe [90]. The stem-loop probe exhibited good sensor performance compared with the linear probe when using ACV and CV. Using DPV, however, both sensors performed optimally under most pulse widths. In addition, when using longer pulse widths, both sensors behaved as "signal-on" sensors, which is generally more attractive for sensor applications.

Application of Solution-State Probe

A single nucleotide polymorphism (SNP) is a genetic change or variation that can occur in any individual's DNA sequence. These variations between individuals are thought to confer susceptibility to disease and determine responses to therapy. Therefore, SNPs have serious potential in diagnostic fields [91]. Electrochemical approaches are usually the preferred type of analysis used for the detection of microorganisms since they require minimal instrumentation and can be easily integrated with microelectronics into a chip-based format [92]. A label-based electrochemical analysis typically requires immobilization of a probe on the electrode sensing layer, like the one discussed in the previous section, but the reproducible modification of capture probes in the fabrication of electrochemical sensors is often a considerable challenge. An alternative strategy was proposed by Ahmed *et al.*, in which capture probe immobilization on the electrode surface could be avoided, as illustrated in Fig. (**15**). When the electroactive indicator (Hoechst 33258) intercalated into double-stranded DNA (dsDNA), *i.e.* the hybridization of the solution-state capture probe and target ssDNA, fewer free indicators on the electrode surface [93]. The resulting anodic peak current of the dsDNA-indicator complex decreased in proportion to the dsDNA titration. This decrease in the peak current can be regarded as the binding of the indicator with the dsDNA, which inhibits the electron transfer reaction. This shows that even without the immobilization of a capture probe, a signal can still be produced.

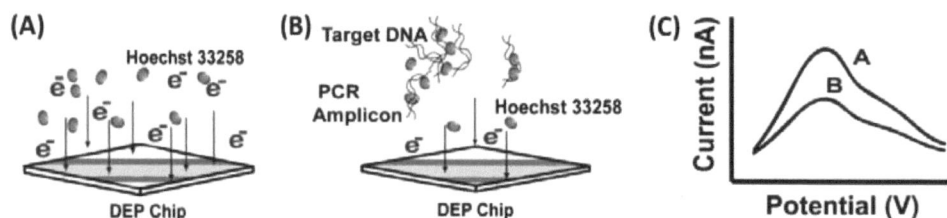

Fig. (15). Sensing mechanism for electrochemical DNA detection using a disposable electrochemical printed (DEP) chip without probe immobilization. (**A**) Higher electron-transfer efficiency from solution-state indicators (Hoechst 33258) to the sensor surface in the absence of dsDNA; (**B**) restrictions in Hoechst 33258 toward the electrode surface during the formation of the dsDNA-indicator complex, and (**C**) decrements in electrochemical responses after adding dsDNA. (Reprinted with permission from [93]. Copyright 2007, Royal Society of Chemistry).

CONCLUDING REMARKS

Electrochemical (micro)sensors, which are considered to be powerful tools, have been widely applied in various fields for fundamental cellular/animal studies and practical *in vitro* diagnoses, such as studies of protein-protein interactions, real-time cellular recording, neural signal transmission, diagnosis of viral infections, biomolecular detection, and nucleic acid screening. Electrochemical biosensors provide some attractive benefits in bio-sensing applications, involving label-free recording, great sensitivity, extremely high temporal resolution, and miniaturized device design. However, some challenges in terms of accuracy and reproducibility in mass production remain for future advancement of electrochemical biosensors. Notwithstanding these challenges, it is believed that innovative integration with actuator-based techniques and the continuous modeling of simple sensing mechanisms will continue to play a significant role in advancing electrochemical biosensors.

CONSENT FOR PUBLICATION

Not applicable.

CONFLICT OF INTEREST

The authors confirm that this chapter contents have no conflict of interest.

ACKNOWLEDGEMENTS

This work is partially funded by the Ministry of Science and Technology, Taiwan (MOST 108-2218-E-006-001 and MOST 108-2811-E-006-509).

REFERENCES

[1] Tsai TC, Huang FH, Chen JJJ. Selective detection of dopamine in urine with electrodes modified by gold nanodendrite and anionic self-assembled monolayer. Sens Actuators B Chem 2013; 181(0): 179-86.
[http://dx.doi.org/10.1016/j.snb.2013.01.081]

[2] Vickrey TL, Condron B, Venton BJ. Detection of endogenous dopamine changes in Drosophila melanogaster using fast-scan cyclic voltammetry. Anal Chem 2009; 81(22): 9306-13.
[http://dx.doi.org/10.1021/ac901638z] [PMID: 19842636]

[3] Tsai TC, Guo CX, Han HZ, *et al.* Microelectrodes with gold nanoparticles and self-assembled monolayers for *in vivo* recording of striatal dopamine. Analyst (Lond) 2012; 137(12): 2813-20.
[http://dx.doi.org/10.1039/c2an16306c] [PMID: 22577657]

[4] Eggins BR. Chemical sensors and biosensors, Ando DJ. England: John Wiley & Sons Ltd. 2002.

[5] Bard AJ, Faulkner LR. Electrochemical methods: Fundamentals and applications. 2nd ed., N.J.: John Wiley & Sons Ltd. 2001.

[6] El Harrad L, Bourais I, Mohammadi H, Amine A. Recent advances in electrochemical biosensors based on enzyme inhibition for clinical and pharmaceutical application. Sensors (Basel) 2018; 18(1): 164.
[http://dx.doi.org/10.3390/s18010164] [PMID: 29315246]

[7] Kumar H. Neelam. Enzyme-based electrochemical biosensors for food safety: a review. Nanobiosensors in Disease Diagnosis 2016; 5: 29-39.
[http://dx.doi.org/10.2147/NDD.S64847]

[8] Wang WS, Kuo WT, Huang HY, Luo CH. Wide dynamic range CMOS potentiostat for amperometric chemical sensor. Sensors (Basel) 2010; 10(3): 1782-97.
[http://dx.doi.org/10.3390/s100301782] [PMID: 22294899]

[9] Michael AC, Borland LM. Electrochemical methods for neuroscience. Boca Raton: Taylor & Francis Group 2007.

[10] Robinson DL, Hermans A, Seipel AT, Wightman RM. Monitoring rapid chemical communication in the brain. Chem Rev 2008; 108(7): 2554-84.
[http://dx.doi.org/10.1021/cr068081q] [PMID: 18576692]

[11] Phillips PEM, Wightman RM. Critical guidelines for validation of the selectivity of *in-vivo* chemical microsensors. Trends Analyt Chem 2003; 22(8): 509-14.
[http://dx.doi.org/10.1016/S0165-9936(03)00907-5]

[12] Hermans A, Keithley RB, Kita JM, Sombers LA, Wightman RM. Dopamine detection with fast-scan cyclic voltammetry used with analog background subtraction. Anal Chem 2008; 80(11): 4040-8.
[http://dx.doi.org/10.1021/ac800108j] [PMID: 18433146]

[13] Ozkan SA, Kauffmann JM, Zuman P. Electroanalysis in biomedical and pharmaceutical sciences. Springer-Verlag Berlin Heidelberg 2015.
[http://dx.doi.org/10.1007/978-3-662-47138-8]

[14] Mirceski V, Laborda E, Guziejewski D, Compton RG. New approach to electrode kinetic measurements in square-wave voltammetry: amplitude-based quasireversible maximum. Anal Chem 2013; 85(11): 5586-94.
[http://dx.doi.org/10.1021/ac4008573] [PMID: 23642036]

[15] Javanbakht M, Eynollahi Fard S, Abdouss M, *et al.* A biomimetic potentiometric sensor using molecularly imprinted polymer for the cetirizine assay in tablets and biological fluids. Electroanalysis 2008; 20(18): 2023-30.
[http://dx.doi.org/10.1002/elan.200804284]

[16] Goyal RN, Oyama M, Gupta VK, *et al.* Sensors for 5-hydroxytryptamine and 5-hydroxyindole acetic

acid based on nanomaterial modified electrodes. Sens Actuators B Chem 2008; 134(2): 816-21.
[http://dx.doi.org/10.1016/j.snb.2008.06.027]

[17]　Norouzi P, Sarmazdeh ZR, Faridbod F, *et al.* Er^{3+} carbon paste electrode based on new nano-composite. Int J Electrochem Sci 2010; 5: 367-76.

[18]　Faridbod F, Ganjali MR, Larijani B, *et al.* Ho^{3+} carbon paste sensor based on multi-walled carbon nanotubes: Applied for determination of holmium content in biological and environmental samples. Mater Sci Eng C 2010; 30(4): 555-60.
[http://dx.doi.org/10.1016/j.msec.2010.02.004]

[19]　Paik SR, Lee JH, Kim DH, Chang CS, Kim J. Aluminum-induced structural alterations of the precursor of the non-A β component of Alzheimer's disease amyloid. Arch Biochem Biophys 1997; 344(2): 325-34.
[http://dx.doi.org/10.1006/abbi.1997.0207] [PMID: 9264546]

[20]　Ma YH, Yuan R, Chai YQ, *et al.* A new aluminum(III)-selective potentiometric sensor based on *N,N'*-propanediamide bis(2-salicylideneimine) as a neutral carrier. Mater Sci Eng C 2010; 30(1): 209-13.
[http://dx.doi.org/10.1016/j.msec.2009.10.005]

[21]　Zahran EM, Hua Y, Li Y, Flood AH, Bachas LG. Triazolophanes: a new class of halide-selective ionophores for potentiometric sensors. Anal Chem 2010; 82(1): 368-75.
[http://dx.doi.org/10.1021/ac902132d] [PMID: 19994863]

[22]　Chen C, Xie Q, Yang D, *et al.* Recent advances in electrochemical glucose biosensors: A review. RSC Advances 2013; 3(14): 4473-91.
[http://dx.doi.org/10.1039/c2ra22351a]

[23]　Freckmann G, Schmid C, Baumstark A, Rutschmann M, Haug C, Heinemann L. Analytical performance requirements for systems for self-monitoring of blood glucose with focus on system accuracy: Relevant differences among ISO 15197:2003, ISO 15197:2013, and current FDA recommendations. J Diabetes Sci Technol 2015; 9(4): 885-94.
[http://dx.doi.org/10.1177/1932296815580160] [PMID: 25872965]

[24]　Clark LC Jr, Lyons C. Electrode systems for continuous monitoring in cardiovascular surgery. Ann N Y Acad Sci 1962; 102(1): 29-45.
[http://dx.doi.org/10.1111/j.1749-6632.1962.tb13623.x] [PMID: 14021529]

[25]　Sekretaryova AN, Vokhmyanina DV, Chulanova TO, Karyakina EE, Karyakin AA. Reagentless biosensor based on glucose oxidase wired by the mediator freely diffusing in enzyme containing membrane. Anal Chem 2012; 84(3): 1220-3.
[http://dx.doi.org/10.1021/ac203056m] [PMID: 22206508]

[26]　Wang J, Lu F. Oxygen-rich oxidase enzyme electrodes for operation in oxygen-free solutions. J Am Chem Soc 1998; 120(5): 1048-50.
[http://dx.doi.org/10.1021/ja972759p]

[27]　Kontani R, Tsujimura S, Kano K. Air diffusion biocathode with CueO as electrocatalyst adsorbed on carbon particle-modified electrodes. Bioelectrochemistry 2009; 76(1-2): 10-3.
[http://dx.doi.org/10.1016/j.bioelechem.2009.02.009] [PMID: 19345156]

[28]　Updike SJ, Hicks GP. The enzyme electrode. Nature 1967; 214(5092): 986-8.
[http://dx.doi.org/10.1038/214986a0] [PMID: 6055414]

[29]　Guilbault GG, Lubrano GJ. An enzyme electrode for the amperometric determination of glucose. Anal Chim Acta 1973; 64(3): 439-55.
[http://dx.doi.org/10.1016/S0003-2670(01)82476-4] [PMID: 4701057]

[30]　Ohnuki H, Saiki T, Kusakari A, Endo H, Ichihara M, Izumi M. Incorporation of glucose oxidase into Langmuir-Blodgett films based on Prussian blue applied to amperometric glucose biosensor. Langmuir 2007; 23(8): 4675-81.
[http://dx.doi.org/10.1021/la063175g] [PMID: 17367170]

[31] Chen C, Fu Y, Xiang C, *et al.* Electropolymerization of preoxidized catecholamines on Prussian blue matrix to immobilize glucose oxidase for sensitive amperometric biosensing. Biosens Bioelectron 2009; 24(8): 2726-9.
[http://dx.doi.org/10.1016/j.bios.2008.12.016] [PMID: 19167205]

[32] Zhao W, Xu JJ, Shi CG, Chen HY. Multilayer membranes via layer-by-layer deposition of organic polymer protected Prussian blue nanoparticles and glucose oxidase for glucose biosensing. Langmuir 2005; 21(21): 9630-4.
[http://dx.doi.org/10.1021/la051370+] [PMID: 16207046]

[33] Yao YL, Shiu KK. Low potential detection of glucose at carbon nanotube modified glassy carbon electrode with electropolymerized poly(toluidine blue O) film. Electrochim Acta 2007; 53(2): 278-84.
[http://dx.doi.org/10.1016/j.electacta.2007.04.007]

[34] Willner I, Katz E. Integration of layered redox proteins and conductive supports for bioelectronic applications. Angew Chem Int Ed Engl 2000; 39(7): 1180-218.
[http://dx.doi.org/10.1002/(SICI)1521-3773(20000403)39:7<1180::AID-ANIE1180>3.0.CO;2-E] [PMID: 10767010]

[35] Stein EW, Volodkin DV, McShane MJ, Sukhorukov GB. Real-time assessment of spatial and temporal coupled catalysis within polyelectrolyte microcapsules containing coimmobilized glucose oxidase and peroxidase. Biomacromolecules 2006; 7(3): 710-9.
[http://dx.doi.org/10.1021/bm050304j] [PMID: 16529405]

[36] Emr SA, Yacynych AM. Use of polymer films in amperometric biosensors. Electroanalysis 1995; 7(10): 913-23.
[http://dx.doi.org/10.1002/elan.1140071002]

[37] Moussy F, Jakeway S, Harrison DJ, Rajotte RV. *In vitro* and *in vivo* performance and lifetime of perfluorinated ionomer-coated glucose sensors after high-temperature curing. Anal Chem 1994; 66(22): 3882-8.
[http://dx.doi.org/10.1021/ac00094a007] [PMID: 7810896]

[38] Hecht HJ, Kalisz HM, Hendle J, Schmid RD, Schomburg D. Crystal structure of glucose oxidase from Aspergillus niger refined at 2.3 A resolution. J Mol Biol 1993; 229(1): 153-72.
[http://dx.doi.org/10.1006/jmbi.1993.1015] [PMID: 8421298]

[39] Rahman MM, Ahammad AJS, Jin JH, Ahn SJ, Lee JJ. A comprehensive review of glucose biosensors based on nanostructured metal-oxides. Sensors (Basel) 2010; 10(5): 4855-86.
[http://dx.doi.org/10.3390/s100504855] [PMID: 22399911]

[40] Schuhmann W, Ohara TJ, Schmidt HL, *et al.* Electron transfer between glucose oxidase and electrodes via redox mediators bound with flexible chains to the enzyme surface. J Am Chem Soc 1991; 113(4): 1394-7.
[http://dx.doi.org/10.1021/ja00004a048]

[41] Rajagopalan R, Aoki A, Heller A. Effect of quaternization of the glucose oxidase "wiring" redox polymer on the maximum current densities of glucose electrodes. J Phys Chem 1996; 100(9): 3719-27.
[http://dx.doi.org/10.1021/jp952160g]

[42] Hale PD, Inagaki T, Karan HI, *et al.* A new class of amperometric biosensor incorporating a polymeric electron-transfer mediator. J Am Chem Soc 1989; 111(9): 3482-4.
[http://dx.doi.org/10.1021/ja00191a084]

[43] Toghill KE, Compton RG. Electrochemical non-enzymatic glucose sensors: A perspective and an evaluation. Int J Electrochem Sci 2010; 5: 1246-301.

[44] Deng L, Liu Y, Yang G, *et al.* Molecular "wiring" glucose oxidase in supramolecular architecture. Biomacromolecules 2007; 8(7): 2063-71.
[http://dx.doi.org/10.1021/bm061049l] [PMID: 17563113]

[45] Holland JT, Lau C, Brozik S, Atanassov P, Banta S. Engineering of glucose oxidase for direct electron

transfer via site-specific gold nanoparticle conjugation. J Am Chem Soc 2011; 133(48): 19262-5.
[http://dx.doi.org/10.1021/ja2071237] [PMID: 22050076]

[46]   Kang X, Wang J, Wu H, Aksay IA, Liu J, Lin Y. Glucose oxidase-graphene-chitosan modified
       electrode for direct electrochemistry and glucose sensing. Biosens Bioelectron 2009; 25(4): 901-5.
       [http://dx.doi.org/10.1016/j.bios.2009.09.004] [PMID: 19800781]

[47]   Patolsky F, Weizmann Y, Willner I. Long-range electrical contacting of redox enzymes by SWCNT
       connectors. Angew Chem Int Ed Engl 2004; 43(16): 2113-7.
       [http://dx.doi.org/10.1002/anie.200353275] [PMID: 15083459]

[48]   Pumera M. Phosphorene and black phosphorus for sensing and biosensing. Trends Analyt Chem 2017;
       93: 1-6.
       [http://dx.doi.org/10.1016/j.trac.2017.05.002]

[49]   Si P, Ding S, Yuan J, Lou XW, Kim DH. Hierarchically structured one-dimensional TiO_2 for protein
       immobilization, direct electrochemistry, and mediator-free glucose sensing. ACS Nano 2011; 5(9):
       7617-26.
       [http://dx.doi.org/10.1021/nn202714c] [PMID: 21866956]

[50]   Wang Y, Yuan R, Chaia Y, *et al.* Direct electron transfer: Electrochemical glucose biosensor based on
       hollow Pt nanosphere functionalized multiwall carbon nanotubes. J Mol Catal, B Enzym 2011; 71(3):
       146-51.
       [http://dx.doi.org/10.1016/j.molcatb.2011.04.011]

[51]   Qiu C, Wang X, Liu X, *et al.* Direct electrochemistry of glucose oxidase immobilized on
       nanostructured gold thin films and its application to bioelectrochemical glucose sensor. Electrochim
       Acta 2012; 67: 140-6.
       [http://dx.doi.org/10.1016/j.electacta.2012.02.011]

[52]   Gao YF, Yang T, Yang XL, *et al.* Direct electrochemistry of glucose oxidase and glucose biosensing
       on a hydroxyl fullerenes modified glassy carbon electrode. Biosens Bioelectron 2014; 60: 30-4.
       [http://dx.doi.org/10.1016/j.bios.2014.04.005] [PMID: 24768859]

[53]   Wilson R, Turner APF. Glucose oxidase: An ideal enzyme. Biosens Bioelectron 1992; 7(3): 165-85.
       [http://dx.doi.org/10.1016/0956-5663(92)87013-F]

[54]   Park S, Boo H, Chung TD. Electrochemical non-enzymatic glucose sensors. Anal Chim Acta 2006;
       556(1): 46-57.
       [http://dx.doi.org/10.1016/j.aca.2005.05.080] [PMID: 17723330]

[55]   de Mele MFL, Videla HA, Arvía AJ. Comparative study of the electrochemical behaviour of glucose
       and other compounds of biological interest. Bioelectrochem Bioenerg 1982; 9(4): 469-87.
       [http://dx.doi.org/10.1016/0302-4598(82)85006-X]

[56]   de Mele MFL, Videla HA, Arvía AJ. Potentiodynamic study of glucose electro□oxidation at bright
       platinum electrodes. J Electrochem Soc 1982; 129(10): 2207-13.
       [http://dx.doi.org/10.1149/1.2123476]

[57]   Largeaud F, Kokoh KB, Beden B, *et al.* On the electrochemical reactivity of anomers: Electrocatalytic
       oxidation of α- and β-d-glucose on platinum electrodes in acid and basic media. J Electroanal Chem
       (Lausanne Switz) 1995; 397(1): 261-9.
       [http://dx.doi.org/10.1016/0022-0728(95)04139-8]

[58]   Ernst S, Heitbaum J, Hamann CH. The electrooxidation of glucose in phosphate buffer solutions: Part
       I. Reactivity and kinetics below 350 mV/RHE. J Electroanal Chem Interfacial Electrochem 1979;
       100(1): 173-83.
       [http://dx.doi.org/10.1016/S0022-0728(79)80159-X]

[59]   Ernst S, Heitbaum J, Hamann CH. The electrooxidation of glucose in phosphate buffer solutions:
       Kinetics and reaction mechanism. Phys Chem 1980; 84(1): 50-5.
       [http://dx.doi.org/10.1002/bbpc.19800840111]

[60]   Sakamoto M, Takamura K. Catalytic oxidation of biological components on platinum electrodes modified by adsorbed metals: Anodic oxidation of glucose. Bioelectrochem Bioenerg 1982; 9(5): 571-82.
[http://dx.doi.org/10.1016/0302-4598(82)80033-0]

[61]   Beden B, Largeaud F, Kokoh KB, *et al.* Fourier transform infrared reflectance spectroscopic investigation of the electrocatalytic oxidation of D-glucose: Identification of reactive intermediates and reaction products. Electrochim Acta 1996; 41(5): 701-9.
[http://dx.doi.org/10.1016/0013-4686(95)00359-2]

[62]   Popović KĐ, Tripković AV, Adžić RR. Oxidation of D-glucose on single-crystal platinum electrodes: A mechanistic study. J Electroanal Chem (Lausanne Switz) 1992; 339(1): 227-45.
[http://dx.doi.org/10.1016/0022-0728(92)80454-C]

[63]   Bos ES, van der Doelen AA, van Rooy N, Schuurs AHWN. 3,3'-5,5'-Tetramethylbenzidine as an Ames test negative chromogen for horse-radish peroxidase in enzyme-immunoassay. J Immunoassay 1981; 2: 187-204.
[http://dx.doi.org/10.1080/15321818108056977] [PMID: 7047570]

[64]   Liu Y, Zhu G, Yang J, Yuan A, Shen X. Peroxidase-like catalytic activity of Ag_3PO_4 nanocrystals prepared by a colloidal route. PLoS One 2014; 9(10)e109158
[http://dx.doi.org/10.1371/journal.pone.0109158] [PMID: 25271632]

[65]   Mach KE, Mohan R, Patel S, Wong PK, Hsieh M, Liao JC. Development of a Biosensor-Based Rapid Urine Test for Detection of Urogenital Schistosomiasis. PLoS Negl Trop Dis 2015; 9(7)e0003845
[http://dx.doi.org/10.1371/journal.pntd.0003845] [PMID: 26134995]

[66]   Darwish IA. Immunoassay Methods and their Applications in Pharmaceutical Analysis: Basic Methodology and Recent Advances. Int J Biomed Sci 2006; 2(3): 217-35.
[PMID: 23674985]

[67]   Ansar W, *et al.* Monoclonal antibodies: a tool in clinical research. Indian Journal of Clinical Medicine 2013; 4: 9-21.
[http://dx.doi.org/10.4137/IJCM.S11968]

[68]   Ellington AD, Szostak JW. *In vitro* selection of RNA molecules that bind specific ligands. Nature 1990; 346(6287): 818-22.
[http://dx.doi.org/10.1038/346818a0] [PMID: 1697402]

[69]   Chen Z, Chen L, Ma H, Zhou T, Li X. Aptamer biosensor for label-free impedance spectroscopy detection of potassium ion based on DNA G-quadruplex conformation. Biosens Bioelectron 2013; 48: 108-12.
[http://dx.doi.org/10.1016/j.bios.2013.04.007] [PMID: 23665159]

[70]   Zhou W, Huang PJ, Ding J, Liu J. Aptamer-based biosensors for biomedical diagnostics. Analyst (Lond) 2014; 139(11): 2627-40.
[http://dx.doi.org/10.1039/c4an00132j] [PMID: 24733714]

[71]   Ku TH, Zhang T, Luo H, *et al.* Nucleic acid aptamers: An emerging tool for biotechnology and biomedical sensing. Sensors (Basel) 2015; 15(7): 16281-313.
[http://dx.doi.org/10.3390/s150716281] [PMID: 26153774]

[72]   O'Donnell KA, Wentzel EA, Zeller KI, Dang CV, Mendell JT. c-Myc-regulated microRNAs modulate E2F1 expression. Nature 2005; 435(7043): 839-43.
[http://dx.doi.org/10.1038/nature03677] [PMID: 15944709]

[73]   Green LS, Jellinek D, Jenison R, Ostman A, Heldin CH, Janjic N. Inhibitory DNA ligands to platelet-derived growth factor B-chain. Biochemistry 1996; 35(45): 14413-24.
[http://dx.doi.org/10.1021/bi961544+] [PMID: 8916928]

[74]   Zhou J, Soontornworajit B, Snipes MP, Wang Y. Structural prediction and binding analysis of hybridized aptamers. J Mol Recognit 2011; 24(1): 119-26.

[http://dx.doi.org/10.1002/jmr.1034] [PMID: 21194122]

[75]   Shigdar S, Qiao L, Zhou SF, *et al*. RNA aptamers targeting cancer stem cell marker CD133. Cancer Lett 2013; 330(1): 84-95.
[http://dx.doi.org/10.1016/j.canlet.2012.11.032] [PMID: 23196060]

[76]   Song S, Wang L, Li J, *et al*. Aptamer-based biosensors. Trends Analyt Chem 2008; 27(2): 108-17.
[http://dx.doi.org/10.1016/j.trac.2007.12.004]

[77]   Ogasawara D, Hachiya NS, Kaneko K, Sode K, Ikebukuro K. Detection system based on the conformational change in an aptamer and its application to simple bound/free separation. Biosens Bioelectron 2009; 24(5): 1372-6.
[http://dx.doi.org/10.1016/j.bios.2008.07.082] [PMID: 18809306]

[78]   Liu Y, Tuleouva N, Ramanculov E, Revzin A. Aptamer-based electrochemical biosensor for interferon gamma detection. Anal Chem 2010; 82(19): 8131-6.
[http://dx.doi.org/10.1021/ac101409t] [PMID: 20815336]

[79]   Xiao Y, Lubin AA, Heeger AJ, Plaxco KW. Label-free electronic detection of thrombin in blood serum by using an aptamer-based sensor. Angew Chem Int Ed Engl 2005; 44(34): 5456-9.
[http://dx.doi.org/10.1002/anie.200500989] [PMID: 16044476]

[80]   Xiao Y, Piorek BD, Plaxco KW, Heeger AJ. A reagentless signal-on architecture for electronic, aptamer-based sensors via target-induced strand displacement. J Am Chem Soc 2005; 127(51): 17990-1.
[http://dx.doi.org/10.1021/ja056555h] [PMID: 16366535]

[81]   Uliana CV, Riccardi CS, Yamanaka H. Diagnostic tests for hepatitis C: recent trends in electrochemical immunosensor and genosensor analysis. World J Gastroenterol 2014; 20(42): 15476-91.
[http://dx.doi.org/10.3748/wjg.v20.i42.15476] [PMID: 25400433]

[82]   Goumi YE. Electrochemical genosensors: Definition and fields of application. Int J Biosens Bioelectron 2017; 3(5): 353-5.
[http://dx.doi.org/10.15406/ijbsbe.2017.03.00080]

[83]   Johnson BN, Mutharasan R. Biosensor-based microRNA detection: techniques, design, performance, and challenges. Analyst (Lond) 2014; 139(7): 1576-88.
[http://dx.doi.org/10.1039/c3an01677c] [PMID: 24501736]

[84]   Wahid F, Shehzad A, Khan T, Kim YY. MicroRNAs: synthesis, mechanism, function, and recent clinical trials. Biochim Biophys Acta 2010; 1803(11): 1231-43.
[http://dx.doi.org/10.1016/j.bbamcr.2010.06.013] [PMID: 20619301]

[85]   Zhao Y, Ransom JF, Li A, *et al*. Dysregulation of cardiogenesis, cardiac conduction, and cell cycle in mice lacking miRNA-1-2. Cell 2007; 129(2): 303-17.
[http://dx.doi.org/10.1016/j.cell.2007.03.030] [PMID: 17397913]

[86]   Beveridge NJ, Gardiner E, Carroll AP, Tooney PA, Cairns MJ. Schizophrenia is associated with an increase in cortical microRNA biogenesis. Mol Psychiatry 2010; 15(12): 1176-89.
[http://dx.doi.org/10.1038/mp.2009.84] [PMID: 19721432]

[87]   Labib M, Berezovski MV. Electrochemical sensing of microRNAs: avenues and paradigms. Biosens Bioelectron 2015; 68: 83-94.
[http://dx.doi.org/10.1016/j.bios.2014.12.026] [PMID: 25562735]

[88]   Dong H, Jin S, Ju H, *et al*. Trace and label-free microRNA detection using oligonucleotide encapsulated silver nanoclusters as probes. Anal Chem 2012; 84(20): 8670-4.
[http://dx.doi.org/10.1021/ac301860v] [PMID: 22985191]

[89]   Wu J, Chumbimuni-Torres KY, Galik M, Thammakhet C, Haake DA, Wang J. Potentiometric detection of DNA hybridization using enzyme-induced metallization and a silver ion selective electrode. Anal Chem 2009; 81(24): 10007-12.

[http://dx.doi.org/10.1021/ac9018507] [PMID: 19908886]

[90]   Lai RY, Walker B, Stormberg K, Zaitouna AJ, Yang W. Electrochemical techniques for characterization of stem-loop probe and linear probe-based DNA sensors. Methods 2013; 64(3): 267-75.
[http://dx.doi.org/10.1016/j.ymeth.2013.07.041] [PMID: 23933234]

[91]   Guttmacher AE, Collins FS. Genomic medicine--a primer. N Engl J Med 2002; 347(19): 1512-20.
[http://dx.doi.org/10.1056/NEJMra012240] [PMID: 12421895]

[92]   Pavlovic E, Lai RY, Wu TT, *et al.* Microfluidic device architecture for electrochemical patterning and detection of multiple DNA sequences. Langmuir 2008; 24(3): 1102-7.
[http://dx.doi.org/10.1021/la702681c] [PMID: 18181654]

[93]   Ahmed MU, Idegami K, Chikae M, *et al.* Electrochemical DNA biosensor using a disposable electrochemical printed (DEP) chip for the detection of SNPs from unpurified PCR amplicons. Analyst (Lond) 2007; 132(5): 431-8.
[http://dx.doi.org/10.1039/b615242b] [PMID: 17471389]

CHAPTER 4

Semiconductor Biosensors Based on Nanowire Field-Effect Transistors

Lester U. Vinzons[1] and Shu-Ping Lin[1,2,*]

[1] *Graduate Institute of Biomedical Engineering, National Chung Hsing University, Taichung, Taiwan*

[2] *Research Center for Sustainable Energy and Nanotechnology, National Chung Hsing University, Taichung, Taiwan*

Abstract: Semiconductor nanowire field-effect transistors (FETs) have attracted great interest as biosensors for point-of-care testing (POCT) because they allow label-free, real-time, ultrasensitive detection using devices that are compact, low power, and easily integrable with on-chip electronic systems. In the past twenty years, these devices have seen significant breakthroughs in various aspects of device development, such as design, fabrication, and surface functionalization, as well as in diagnostic applications, having demonstrated femtomolar detection of DNA, RNA, proteins, and small molecules. In this chapter, we highlight notable advancements in nanowire-based FET biosensors in the past decade, focusing, in particular, on biomarker detection using silicon, indium oxide and zinc oxide nanowire FET devices. Recent developments include new CMOS-compatible fabrication techniques, unconventional device configurations and detection schemes, coatings to enhance sensing stability, novel bioreceptor elements and surface modification schemes for sensitivity enhancement, as well as sample processing and portable readout systems. Furthermore, we also include studies that have used nanowire FETs in concert with pattern recognition methods for disease diagnosis using exhaled breath. The growing body of research indicates that practical solutions to long-standing issues are at hand, bringing nanowire-FET biosensors ever closer to adoption in real-world POCT applications.

Keywords: Biosensor, Biomarker, Diagnosis, Field effect, Indium oxide, Nanowire, Nanomaterial, Point of care, Sensor, Silicon, Semiconductor, Transistor, Zinc oxide.

INTRODUCTION

The past fifty years bore witness to paradigm shifts in healthcare as epitomized in the concepts of early disease detection [1], predictive, preventative, and person-

---

* **Corresponding author Shu-Ping Lin:** Graduate Institute of Biomedical Engineering, National Chung Hsing University, Taichung, Taiwan; Tel: +886-4-2284-0733 Ext: 652; Fax: +886-4-2285-2422; E-mail: splin@dragon.nchu.edu.tw

alized medicine [2], patient self-management [3], home telehealth [4], and global health [5]. Point-of-care testing (POCT) has played an integral role in the realization of these healthcare trends by providing quick, easy, and reliable disease diagnosis and prognosis [6 - 9]. POCT involves *in vitro* diagnostic tests conducted near the patient in a healthcare facility or at home for monitoring patient self-care [10]. It improves clinical decision making, increases patient adherence, and enhances patient satisfaction, leading to improved clinical outcomes and overall cost reduction [11]. An ideal POCT device should be **A**ffordable, **S**ensitive, **S**pecific, **U**ser-friendly, **R**apid and robust, **E**quipment-free and **D**eliverable to end-users ("ASSURED") [12, 13]. However, current conventional methods for biomarker detection such as enzyme-linked immunosorbent assay (ELISA), not only lack the sensitivity for early disease detection but also utilize labeling and fluorescent imaging, making them time-consuming and requiring bulky and expensive equipment [14, 15]. Due to these limitations, massive research efforts have been carried out in the past decades on electrical biosensors—devices that use biochemical reactions mediated by biological elements, such as enzymes and immunosystems, to detect chemicals using electrical signals [16]. These devices are highly attractive for POCT due to their high sensitivity, specificity, simplicity, and miniaturization [14]. Furthermore, they allow real-time analysis and are suitable to be combined with microarray, microfluidic, and telemetry technologies [15].

Among the different types of electrical biosensors, those that are based on the ion-sensitive field-effect transistor (ISFET) are one of the most popular devices [17]. Demonstrated by Bergveld in 1970 [18], the ISFET is basically a metal–oxide–semiconductor field-effect transistor (MOSFET) whose metal gate has been removed and with the distinguishing feature of having a threshold voltage that can be modified through the electrolyte/oxide interfacial potential [19]. Aside from fast responses and high sensitivities, ISFET-based biosensors, being a product of silicon microfabrication technologies, are also amenable to miniaturization, batch processing, and on-chip circuit integration, hence promising the realization of low-cost, portable bioanalytical systems [17, 20]. Furthermore, the exposed SiO_2 can be easily functionalized with biorecognition elements [20], while the sensitivity can be optimized by adjusting the gate voltage(s) [21]. These advantages have spurred the design of various types of ISFET-based biosensors in the past decades, such as enzyme-modified FETs, immunologically modified FETs, and DNA-modified FETs [17, 22].

Mirroring the trend in high-performance transistors and thin-film transistors [23], nanomaterials are increasingly being used as the channel of FET-based biosensors to surpass the sensitivity limits of the classical bulk-silicon-based ISFETs [24, 25]. Nanomaterials are suitable for the ultrasensitive detection of biomolecules due to their large surface-to-volume ratios and comparable dimensions with biological entities. A large surface-to-volume ratio means that a large proportion of the constituent atoms of material is located close to the material's surface, allowing the properties of the material to be strongly influenced by minor perturbations in the environment [26]. The dimensions of nanomaterials ($\approx$1–100 nm) are also comparable in size scale to most biological entities, such as nucleic acids, proteins, viruses, and cells [27]. This enables a few number of biological components to affect a large proportion of the nanomaterial, hence resulting in a large change in the material's characteristics. Since the first demonstration of nanomaterial-based sensing of biomolecules by Lieber's group [28] almost two decades ago, a plethora of studies have utilized semiconductor nanomaterials in FET detection platforms for biomarker detection [26, 29 - 33], exemplifying the promise of these devices for disease diagnosis. Nano-biosensors allow the direct, label-free, real-time, electronic detection of a wide range of biological and chemical species with high sensitivity and specificity [24]. Since these biosensors are configured as FETs and resistors, which are typical electronic components, they can be readily integrated with electronic signal processing systems [24] for the development of advanced but portable POCT devices.

In this chapter, we review the notable developments in the field of nanomaterial-based FET biosensing of disease biomarkers in the past decade (since 2009). We limit the included papers and discussions on nanowire biosensors since this device category has a longer history and has been thoroughly explored by many research groups, thereby including significant advancements that are applicable as well to FETs based on other semiconducting nanomaterials, such as carbon nanotubes, graphene, and MoS_2. The majority of the articles cited in the chapter involve silicon nanowire (SiNW) FETs, which reflects its share of publications in the literature on nanowire FET biosensors. This is to be expected because SiNW FETs are the natural progression of silicon-based ISFET technology, and hence share with traditional ISFETs their inherent advantage of benefitting from mature semiconductor processing technologies [26]. Aside from SiNWs, a number of developments based on the n-type semiconducting metal oxides indium oxide (In_2O_3) and zinc oxide (ZnO) are also included. These materials are next in popularity to SiNWs as inorganic nanowire channels in FET biosensors. The chapter is divided into two parts: in the first part, we discuss the most important concepts underlying the operation of nanowire FET biosensors and highlight major factors that must be considered in biosensing applications; in the second part, we describe recent developments in nanowire-FET-based biosensing which we deem relevant to biomarker detection and could pave the way towards practical, accurate, and reliable POCT devices in the future.

NANOWIRE FET BIOSENSORS: THE BASICS

Basic Design and Mechanism

The architecture of a typical nanowire FET is basically the same as that of an ISFET [17, 24, 26, 29] (Fig. **1a**): there are three terminals—drain, source, and gate, with the drain and source terminals flanking the nanowire channel and the gate immersed in an electrolyte surrounding the channel; the surface of the channel exposed to the solution is covered with a dielectric layer. Functionally, these parts serve the following purposes [24, 26, 27]: the channel acts as the path for the current (drain current), which is modulated by the electrolyte/dielectric interfacial potential (surface potential); the drain and source are the terminals where the electromotive force (drain–source voltage) for this current is applied; the liquid gate, which is ideally a reference electrode, is used to apply the potential (gate voltage) that determines the operating region of the transistor; and the dielectric serves as the substrate for the attachment of biorecognition molecules. In contrast with an ISFET, a nanowire FET has three important differences: first, there is a permanent structurally defined semiconducting channel in the nanowire FET—the nanowire—instead of an electrically induced thin channel; second, the bulk silicon (wafer) is not a necessary component of the device [34, 35]; and, the gate terminal can be applied *via* the back of the device channel, *e.g.*, using the silicon wafer, in which a dielectric layer isolates the bulk silicon from the source, drain, and nanowire [28].

Bound molecules on the surface of the nanowire modulate the surface potential of the channel through their polarity [36]. Changes in the surface potential alter the charge carrier density in the channel through electrostatic gating, resulting in changes in the measured conductance or drain current [26, 27, 29]. This electrostatic gating can be exerted by the analyte directly *via* the charges or dipole moments in the analyte [24, 34, 37], or indirectly *via* analyte-induced changes in charged surface states of a molecular monolayer or changes in the dielectric medium near the nanowire surface [38, 39]. The change in conductance ΔG of a nanowire due to a surface-charge density σ_S can be qualitatively described by $\Delta G = \mu \sigma_S P/L$, where μ is the carrier mobility, P is the perimeter of the nanowire supporting the surface charge, and L is the nanowire length [40]. Since the initial conductance is given by $G_0 = e\mu n_0 A/L$, where e is the elementary charge, n_0 is the carrier density, and A is the nanowire cross-sectional area, the nanowire response or sensitivity to the surface charge perturbation can be qualitatively described by the following expression [40]:

$$S = \frac{\Delta G}{G_0} = \frac{\sigma_S P}{e n_0 A} \tag{1}$$

For a cylindrical nanowire with radius r, the ratio P/A in eq. (1) can be replaced with $2/r$. Therefore, sensitivity expression becomes $S = (2\sigma_S)/(en_0 r)$. This clearly shows that the sensitivity of a nanowire biosensor increases as the radius is decreased, or equivalently, as the surface-to-volume ratio is increased [41]. Note that even though the carrier mobilities of nanowire semiconductors are lower than their bulk counterparts [42, 43], the mobility will ultimately only affect the signal change (*e.g.*, ΔG), but not the device sensitivity due to the absence of the mobility parameter in eq. (1) [44]. (Nevertheless, mobility fluctuations do affect the device performance due to the induced noise, as explained in the Noise section below.) How the current in the nanowire channel is affected by the surface potential depends on whether electrons or holes are the majority carriers in the channel [24, 26, 27] (Fig. **1b**): if the majority carriers are electrons (n-type channel), a positive surface potential leads to carrier accumulation and an increase in current, while a negative potential results in carrier depletion and a decrease in current; the reverse is true for a p-type channel.

Device Fabrication

Nanowire FET biosensors are fabricated using either bottom–up or top–down approach [26, 27]. In bottom–up fabrication (Fig. **1c**), nanowires are synthesized by chemical vapor deposition (CVD). For SiNWs, CVD is often performed *via* vapor–liquid–solid approach with gold nanoparticles (AuNPs) as catalysts and SiH_4 as the reactant [28, 45 - 49]. Doping with boron (p-type) or phosphorus (n-type) is carried out by mixing B_2H_6 or PH_3 in the reactant flow [46, 50]. A similar AuNP-catalyzed CVD method is commonly used for the growth of In_2O_3 nanowires, where the In vapor is generated by laser ablation of an InAs target [51 - 53]. For ZnO nanowires and nanorods, CVD with or without a catalyst can be used, with the zinc vapor generated by heating of Zn powder [54 - 56]. CVD of In_2O_3 and ZnO nanowires is performed under a constant flow of O_2 and an inert gas (Ar or N_2). After synthesis, the nanowires are then transferred to the device wafer by large-scale nanowire-positioning techniques, such as contact printing [49, 57], electric-field-directed assembly [58], and flow alignment [28, 59]. Source and drain contacts are typically patterned on the wafer after nanowire transfer. The nanowires are usually randomly aligned between the source and drain [60], although it is possible to exactly align the contacts to the nanowires by using electron-beam (e-beam) lithography [28, 61]. Bottom–up fabrication is theoretically simple and results in high-quality, monocrystalline nanowires. However, well-controlled transfer of aligned nanowires and reproducible formation of electrical contacts for mass fabrication remain challenging [62, 63].

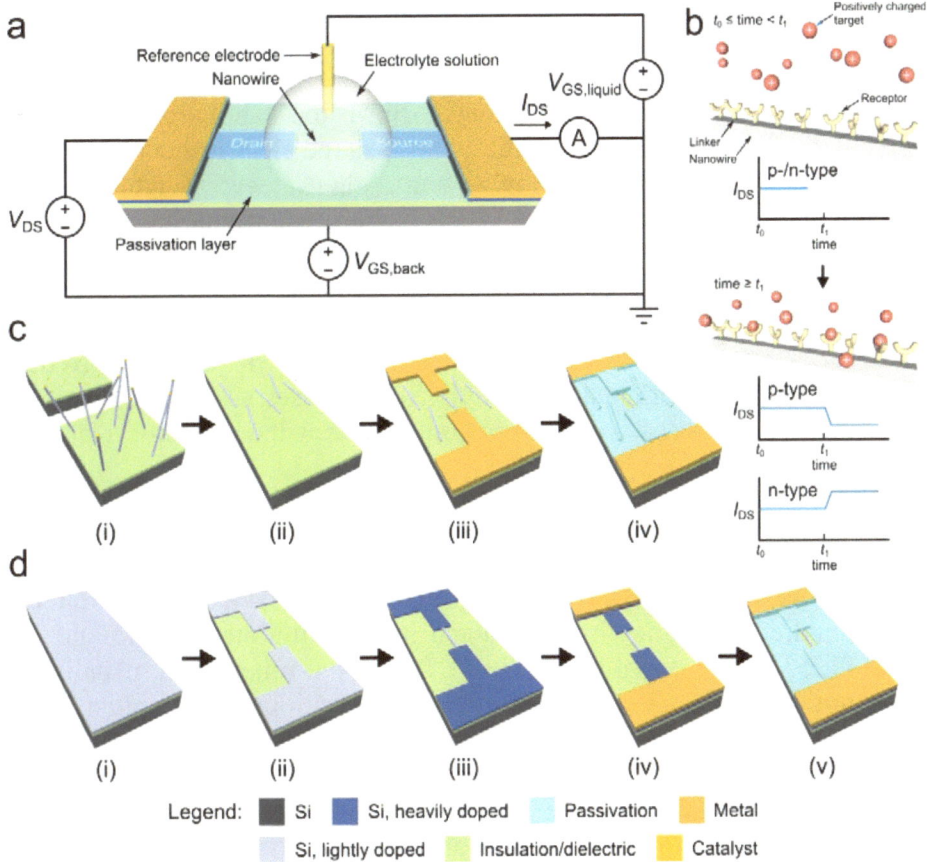

Fig. (1). Design, sensing response, and fabrication of nanowire FET biosensors. (a) Basic nanowire FET architecture and biosensing setup. (b) Current response of p-type and n-type nanowire FETs upon binding of a positively charged molecule to the immobilized receptor. (c) Typical fabrication process for a SiNW FET using the bottom–up approach: (i) nanowire synthesis using chemical vapor deposition catalyzed by metal nanoparticles (gold spheres); (ii) transfer and alignment of nanowires on the device substrate; (iii) patterning and deposition of metal source and drain contacts; and (iv) deposition of a passivation layer over the device, except on the nanowire channel and contact pads. (d) Typical fabrication process for a SiNW FET using the top–down approach: (i) formation of nanometer-thick Si device layer; (ii) patterning and etching of silicon to form the SiNW and source and drain contacts; (iii) doping of source and drain terminals; (iv) patterning and deposition of metal contact pads; and (v) deposition of a passivation layer over the device, except on the nanowire channel and contact pads. Symbols: V_{DS}, drain–source voltage; $V_{GS,liquid}$, liquid gate–source voltage; $V_{GS,back}$, back gate–source voltage; I_{DS}, drain–source current.

Top–down fabrication is used to fabricate SiNW FETs using standard semiconductor processing technologies (Fig. **1d**). Typically, SiNWs are defined on ultrathin silicon-on-insulator (SOI) wafers whose device layer is $\leq$ 100-nm thick. The nanowire etch mask may be patterned to sub-10 nm widths using serial techniques, such as e-beam lithography [64, 65], or to sub-50 nm widths using wafer-scale techniques, such as deep-UV (DUV) lithography [66 - 68], while the micrometer-scale mask for the electrical contacts may be patterned using conventional UV lithography [64, 69]. Then, dry etching (reactive-ion etching or RIE) of the SOI device layer is performed to form the nanowires [64, 67, 68]. Alternatively, the mask for the nanowires, as well as the electrical contacts, can be patterned using UV lithography, and then wet etching using tetramethylammonium hydroxide (TMAH) is performed on the SOI device layer with (100) orientation [70, 71]. Top–down-fabricated nanowire devices have the following advantages [66]: (1) high uniformity and reproducibility; (2) high yield; (3) excellent scalability and manufacturability; and (4) allows direct integration with other electrical circuits. However, the top–down approach requires specialized, expensive equipment and complex processes as well as costly SOI wafers [72, 73]. The use of wet etching, on the other hand, is not a preferred process in the semiconductor industry [73].

Bottom–up-fabricated nanowire FETs have cylindrical nanowire channels with typical diameters of ≈20–60 nm and lengths of ≈2–4 μm [28, 47 - 49]. They may be configured as either single- or multiple-nanowire devices, with the latter containing hundreds of nanowires contacted by interdigitated source and drain terminals [49, 53]. Top–down nanowire FETs, on the other hand, usually have nanowires with rectangular or trapezoidal cross-sections with dimensions of around 20–150 nm [64, 65, 67, 68, 70, 71]. The channel is typically tens of micrometers long and often consists of only a single nanowire. For SiNWs, the doping concentrations used in the literature vary greatly, with some of the nanowires being undoped [74, 75], while others having doping densities as high as 10^{15}–10^{19} atoms/cm^3 [64, 65]. Source and drain contacts to the nanowires are typically made of metal thin films (*e.g.*, Ti adhesive layer with Au contact) for bottom–up-fabricated devices and degenerately doped silicon (10^{19}–10^{20} atoms/cm^3) for top–down devices. Although most studies utilizing nanowires contacted by "source" and "drain" terminals refer to these devices as FETs, not all of them apply a gate voltage during detection experiments, resulting in a configuration that resembles a resistor more than a transistor device (Table **1**). Nevertheless, we include both types of configurations here as both utilize the field effect as the signal transduction mechanism.

Surface Functionalization

A bare inorganic nanowire surface is not that useful for biochemical detection, aside from pH sensing, because it does not have the capability to recognize the target molecule. This is why the nanowire must be "functionalized" by modifying its surface with the appropriate biorecognition element for the molecule of interest

[27, 29]. The biorecognition element for biomarker detection is usually either a single-stranded DNA for DNA/RNA detection or an antibody for protein biomarker detection. These biorecognition elements must be able to bind with their corresponding targets with high affinity and selectivity so that high sensitivity and specificity can be achieved by the biosensor. The functionalization of nanowires is typically done by covalent attachment of the biorecognition units onto the nanowire surface [26, 27, 29]. Such chemical grafting of DNA probes and antibodies, however, is not that straightforward because of the lack of appropriate functional groups on the nanowire surface that can react with existing end groups on the DNA and antibody molecules. Fortunately, semiconducting nanowires are usually covered by an oxide layer which can form hydroxyl groups in the air or after an activation treatment. These hydroxyl groups can react with various types of linker molecules, enabling the formation of a self-assembled monolayer (SAM) on the nanowire surface [76]. This SAM of linker molecules possesses functional groups which react with corresponding end groups on the biorecognition elements *via* well-known crosslinker chemistries.

Table 1. Notable NW FET-based biosensors of disease biomarkers reported in the past decade.

NW Synthesis/Fabrication	Material; NW#; $l \times w \times t$ or $l \times \varnothing$	Linker; Recognition Element	Detection Configura-tion; Signal	Target Analyte (Disease)	Detection Range; Limit of Detection	Detection medium	Ref
DNA and RNA							
E-beam lithography, dry etching of SOI wafer	Si; 1; 2 μm × 60 nm × 50 nm	APTES + GA; DNA	FET; gate voltage	BRAF^{V599E} gene (cancers)	10 fM – 10 nM; 0.88 fM	PBS, 0.01 M	[125]
DUV lithography, dry etching of poly-Si, dry oxidation	Si; 1; 200 μm × 20 nm × 40 nm	APTES + GA; PNA	Resistor; resistance	miRNA (cancer and other diseases)	1 fM – 1 nM; 1 fM	SSC, 0.01×	[67]
Poly-Si sidewall spacer technique	Si; 2; 2 μm × 80 nm × n.i.	APTES + GA; DNA	Resistor; current	Avian influenza virus H5 DNA	1 fM – 10 pM; n.i.	PBS, 0.01 M	[77]
DUV lithography with PR O$_2$ plasma ashing, dry etching of SOI wafer, oxidation and BOE	Si; 1; 500 nm × 50 nm × 50 nm	AuNPs; DNA	Resistor; current	Breast cancer DNA (breast cancer)	1 pM – 100 nM; 1 pM	n.i.	[126]
DUV lithography, dry etching of SOI wafer, oxidation	Si; 1; 90 μm × 50–60 nm × n.i.	APTES + GA; morpholino	Resistor; conductance	DNA (depends on the specific gene)	100 fM – 1 pM; 100 fM	SSC, 0.01×	[127]
UV lithography, anisotropic wet etching of SOI wafer	Si; 1; 6 μm × 20 nm × n.i.	APTES; DNA	FET; current	DNA (depends on the specific gene)	1 fM – 1 nM; 1 fM	PBS, 0.1×	[71]
					0.1 fM – 10 nM; 0.1 fM	PBS, 0.01×	[100]
E-beam lithography, anisotropic wet etching of SOI wafer	Si; 1; n.i. × 100 nm × 30 nm	Poly-L-lysine (on HfO$_2$); DNA	FET; threshold voltage	miR-10b DNA analog (breast cancer)	100 fM – 1 μM; 1 fM	SSC, 0.02×	[128]
Poly-Si sidewall spacer technique	Si; 2; 3 μm × 70 nm × n.i.	APTES + GA; DNA	FET; current	DNA (depends on the specific gene)	1 fM – 10 nM; 1 fM	n.i.	[75]
UV lithography, anisotropic wet etching of SOI wafer	Si; 1; 25 μm × 20 nm × n.i.	APTES; DNA (+ post-binding rolling circle amplification)	Resistor; current	Hepatitis B virus DNA	1 fM – 100 pM; 50 aM	Phi29 DNA polymerase reaction buffer, 0.1×	[129]

(Table 1) cont.....

UV lithography, anisotropic wet etching of SOI wafer	Si; 1; 16 μm × 80 nm × n.i.	APTES; DNA	FET; current	miR-21, miR-205 (cancers)	0.1 fM – 1 nM; 1 zeptomole	PBS, 0.01×	[130]
				miR-205 (cancers)	100 fM – 1 nM; 100 fM	Human serum, 100%	
E-beam lithography, dry etching of SOI wafer, oxidation	Si; 1; 400 μm × 20 nm × 30 nm	APTES + GA; DNA	Resistor; current, conductance	Dengue virus DNA	10 fM – 10 μM; 2 fM	n.i.	[131]
Proteins and Peptides							
Au-assisted CVD	Si; 1; 1.5 μm × Ø n.i.	APDES + SA; RNA aptamer	Resistor; current	VEGF (cancers)	104 pM – 52 nM; 104 pM	PBS	[132]
Au-assisted CVD	Si; 1; 2 μm × Ø n.i.	TMSPA; antibody	FET; conductance	PSA (prostate cancer)	1.5 fM – 15 pM; 1.5 fM	n.i.	[21]
Au-assisted CVD	Si; 1; n.i. × Ø30–60 nm	APTMS + MBS; GSH–GST–calmodulin	Resistor; conductance	cTnI (acute myocardial infarction)	10 nM – 1 μM; 7 nM	PS, 0.1×, with 100 μM Ca²⁺	[48]
DUV lithography, dry etching of SOI wafer, oxidation	Si; 1; 90 μm × 50–60 nm × n.i.	APTES + GA; antibody	Resistor; resistance	CK-MB, CK-MM, cTnT (acute myocardial infarction)	100 fg/mL – 1 ng/mL; 100 fg/mL	PBS, 0.01×	[68]
UV lithography, anisotropic wet etching of SOI wafer	Si; 1; 5 μm × 80 nm × 53 nm	APTES + GA; antibody	FET; current	cTnI (acute myocardial infarction)	0.092–46 ng/mL; 0.092 ng/mL	PBS, 0.1×	[133]
Au-assisted CVD	Si; 1; 2 μm × Ø n.i.	APTES + GA; F(ab')₂ antibody fragment	FET; conductance (calibrated)	cTnT (acute myocardial infarction)	20 pM – 4.7 nM; < 2 pM	Untreated serum	[104]
Poly-Si sidewall spacer technique with highly anisotropic dry etch	Si; n.i.; n.i. × 95 nm × 95 nm	APTES; antibody	FET; conductance	Interleukin-8, tumor necrosis factor alpha (inflammation)	10 fM – 10 nM; 10 fM	PS, 0.1 mM	[73]
E-beam lithography, dry etching of SOI wafer	Si; 25; 40 μm × 100 nm × 100 nm (square-wave pattern)	TESBA; DNA–AuNP–peptide complex	Resistor; conductance	Matrix metalloproteinase-2 (cancers)	100 fM – 10 nM; 100 fM	n.i.	[93]
UV lithography, anisotropic wet etching of SOI wafer	Si; 1; 10 μm × 60 nm × n.i.	APTES + GA; antibody	FET; current	hTSH (hyper/hypothyroidism)	0.02–30 mIU/L; 0.02 mIU/L	PBS, 0.01×	[134]
0.35-μm commercial CMOS process	Si; 1; n.i. × 625 nm × 167 nm	APTES + GA; antibody	Resistor; voltage in a Wheatstone bridge	cTnI (acute myocardial infarction)	320 fM – 320 pM (7.6 pg/mL – 7.6 ng/mL); 320 fM	PBS, 0.01×	[135]
PR ashing (lithography type n.i.), dry etching of bulk-Si wafer (anisotropic and isotropic)	Si; 1; 800 nm × 50 nm × 100 nm (underlap length = 200 nm)	Silica-binding protein; antigen	Underlap FET; current	Anti-avian influenza virus antibody	0.4–4 μg/mL; 144.7 ng/mL	n.i.	[136]
UV lithography, dry etching of PR, etching of poly-Si (dry or wet n.i.)	Si; 1; 2 μm × 150 nm × 50 nm	APTES + GA; antibody (on magnetic graphene sheets)	FET; current	Apolipoprotein A II (bladder cancer)	19.5 pg/mL – 1.95 μg/mL; 6.7 pg/mL	PBS, 0.5 mM	[137]
E-beam lithography, dry etching of SOI wafer	Si; n.a.; 10 μm × 50 nm × 100 nm (honeycomb pattern)	APTES + GA; antibody	FET; current	cTnI (acute myocardial infarction)	5–200 pg/mL; 5 pg/mL	PBS, 0.01×	[78]
Au-assisted CVD	Si; hundreds; 3 μm × Ø20 nm	APTMS + MBS; DNA aptamer	FET; gate voltage	Neuropeptide Y (cancer)	10 nM – 2.5 μM; n.i.	PBS, 0.1×	[138]

(Table 1) cont.....

E-beam lithography, wet etching of SOI wafer	Si; 8; 10 μm × 150 nm × 40 nm	APTES + GA; antibody	FET; conductance	Cytokeratin-19 (disseminated or circulating tumor cells)	25 fM – 25 nM; 80 fM (3.2 pg/mL) 0.1–1000 MCF-7 cells/mL; 0.01 cells/mL or 1 cell/10⁷ lymphoid cells	PBS, 0.01×	[65]
Au-assisted CVD	Si; 1; 2 μm × Ø20 nm	APDMES + GA; antibody	FET; current	Cancer antigen 15-3 (breast cancer)	0, 55, 135, 535 pM; n.i.	Sodium phosphate buffer, 155 μM	[139]
Lithography, dry etching of SOI wafer	Si; 20; 8 μm × 50 nm × 100 nm	APTES + GA; antibody	FET; current	PSA (prostate cancer)	1–100 ng/mL; 90 pg/mL	n.i.	[140]
E-beam lithography, dry etching of SOI wafer	Si; 1; 3 μm × 100 nm × 110 nm	GOPS-SH + AuNPs; antibody half-fragment	FET; current	PSA (prostate cancer)	23 fg/mL – 500 ng/mL; 23 fg/mL (0.7 fM)	PBS, 0.01×	[141]
E-beam lithography, wet etching of SOI wafer	Si; 1; 1 μm × 505 nm × n.i.	None; silane boronic acid ester	FET; current	FSH (menopause)	1 fM – 1 pM; 0.72 fM 1 fM – 1 pM; 1.1 fM	PBS, n.i. PBS with 20% serum	[142]
UV lithography, dry etching of poly-Si	Si; 1000; 30 μm × 120 nm × 50 nm	APTMS + GA; antibody	FET; current	CEACAM1 (cancers)	21.6 ng/mL (135 pM) – 50 μg/mL (250 nM)	n.i.	[143]
				CEACAM5 (cancers)	18 ng/mL (100 pM) – 50 μg/mL (220 nM)		
Au-assisted laser ablation CVD	In₂O₃; many (no. n.i.); 2.5 μm × Ø n.i.	6-phosphono-hexanoic acid + BMPH; antibody mimic protein	FET; current	Nucleocapsid (SARS)	0.6–10 nM; n.i.	PBS, 0.01×, with 44 μM BSA	[87]
Au-assisted laser ablation CVD	In₂O₃; many (no. n.i.); 2.5 μm × Ø n.i.	3-phosphono-proprionic acid; antibody	FET; current	CA-125 (ovarian cancer)	0.1–100 U/mL; 0.1 U/mL	Filtered blood, 0.01×	[53]
				IGF-II (ovarian cancer)	8–200 ng/mL; 8 ng/mL	Filtered blood, desalted	
Thermal evaporation	ZnO; 1; μm × Ø100 nm	Aminated polymer-like amorphous carbon; antibody	FET; current	Alpha-fetoprotein (liver cancer)	10–10,000 ng/mL; n.i.	PBS, 0.01 M	[144]
Solution-phase growth on seed layer	ZnO; many (no. n.i.); 1.54 μm × Ø228 nm (vertical array in vertical FET configuration)	MTS + GMBS; antibody	High-frequency heterodyne; mixing current at modulation frequency	Hepatitis B surface antigen	20 aM – 1 pM; 20 aM	PBS, 0.1 M	[85]
Small Molecules							
Au-assisted CVD	Si; 1; 4 μm × Ø n.i.	APTES + GA; antibody	Resistor; conductance	8-iso-prostaglandin F₂ₐ (lung oxidative stress)	10–80 pg/mL; n.i.	Exhaled breath condensate, 0.01×	[145]
Au-assisted CVD	Si; 1; 2 μm × Ø20–30 nm	APTMS; 4-carbox-phenylboronic acid	FET; gate voltage	Dopamine (PD, neuroblastoma, pheochromo-cytoma)	1 fM – 1 pM; 1 fM	PBS, 0.01×	[146]
Au-assisted CVD	Si; hundreds; 3 μm × Ø20–30 nm	APTMS + MBS; DNA aptamer	FET; gate voltage, conductance	Dopamine (PD, neuroblastoma, pheochromo-cytoma)	10 pM – 10 nM; n.i. 100 pM – 25 nM; n.i.	PBS, 0.1× PBS, 0.1×	[49] [138]

(Table 1) cont.....

Au-assisted CVD	Si; many (up to 10³); n.i. × Ø20 nm	APTES; glucose oxidase	FET; current	Glucose (diabetes)	0, 0.5, 0.75, 1 mM; n.i.	Phosphate citrate buffer, 0.05 M	[147]
Solution-phase growth on seed layer	ZnO; many (no. n.i.); n.i. (vertical array)	None; cholesterol oxidase	FET; current	Cholesterol (coronary heart disease, atherosclerosis)	1 µM – 45 mM; 50 nM	PBS, 0.1 M	[148]
Viruses							
Au-assisted CVD	Si; 1; 4 µm × Ø n.i.	APTES + GA; antibody	Resistor; conductance	Influenza A virus H3N2	$1.7 \times 10^2 – 1.7 \times 10^4$ viruses/µL; 1.7×10^2 viruses/µL	Exhaled breath condensate, 0.01×	[145]
Gases and Vapors							
Au-assisted CVD	Si; 1; 2 µm × Ø60 nm	None; hexyltrichloro-silane	Cross-reactive FET; current or conductivity	Hexane, octane, decane (cancers, neurodegenerative diseases)	19–250 ppm (hexane), 52–200 ppm (octane), 4–110 ppm (decane); n.i.	Air, 15% relative humidity	[149]
Au-assisted CVD	Si; multiple (no. n.i.); 2 µm × Ø40 nm	APTES; acyl chlorides (7 kinds)	Cross-reactive FET + ANN; V_{TH}, μ_h, SS + ANN output vector	Hexane, octane, decane, ethanol, cyclohexanone (cancers) + 6 other VOCs	VOC partial pressure/vapor pressure = 0.01, 0.02, 0.04, 0.08; n.i.	n.i.	[150]
E-beam lithography, dry etching of SOI wafer	Si; n.a.; n.i. × 30 nm × 100 nm (honeycomb pattern)	None; SnO₂ film	Resistor; resistance	NO (asthma)	100 ppm (others n.i.); 1 ppm	Dry air	[151]
Au-assisted CVD	Si; multiple (no. n.i.); 2 µm × Ø40 nm	None; TPS	Cross-reactive FET; area under the time curve of V_{TH}, μ_h, current at $V_{GS} = 0$	2-propenenitrile, 6-methyl-5-hepten-2-one, furfural (gastric cancer)	50–150 ppb, 5–150 ppb, 5–500 ppb, respectively; 50 or 5 ppb	Dry N₂	[152]
Au-assisted CVD	Si; multiple (no. n.i.); 2 µm × Ø40 nm	None, APTES + acyl chloride, or TTPS; TTPS, TPS, APTES, BPTS, heptanoyl chloride, anthracene	Cross-reactive FET; V_{TH}, μ_h, current at various V_{GS}	2-propenenitrile, 6-methyl-5-hepten-2-one, furfural (gastric cancer); Pentane (asthma and COPD); Heptane, decane, 2-methylpentane, 2-ethyl-1-hexanol, propanal, pentanal, acetone (lung cancer)	Varies per target (see ref)	n.i.	[153]

Symbols: *l*, length; *w*, width; *t*, thickness; Ø, diameter; V_{TH}, threshold voltage; μ_h, hole mobility; SS, subthreshold swing; V_{GS}, gate–source voltage. Abbreviations: NW, nanowire; e-beam, electron beam; SOI, silicon on insulator; DUV, deep ultraviolet; PR, photoresist; BOE, buffered oxide etch; UV, ultraviolet; CVD, chemical vapor deposition; CMOS, complementary metal–oxide–semiconductor; APTES, (3-aminopropyl)triethoxysilane; GA, glutaraldehyde; PNA, peptide nucleic acid; AuNP, Au nanoparticle; APDES, (3-aminopropyl)diethoxysilane; SA, succinic anhydride; APDMES, (3-aminopropyl)-dimeth-l-ethoxysilane; TMSPA, 3-(trimethoxysilyl)propyl aldehyde; MBS, 3-maleimidobenzoic acid *N*-hydroxysuccinimide ester; GSH, glutathione; GST, glutathione S-transferase; TESBA, 3-(triethoxysilyl)butylaldehyde; GOPS-SH, thiolated 3-glycidopropyltriethoxysilane; BMPH, *N*-(--maleimidopropionic acid) hydrazide; MTS, 3-mercaptopropyltrimethoxysilane; GMBS, *N*-γ-maleimidobutyryl-oxysuccinimide ester; APTMS, (3-aminopropyl)trimethoxysilane; ; TPS, trichloro(phenethyl)silane; TTPS, trichloro(3,3,3-trifluoropropyl)silane; BPTS, 3-bromopropyl trichlorosilane; FET, field-effect transistor; ANN, artificial neural network; miRNA, microRNA; VEGF, vascular endothelial growth factor; PSA, prostate-specific antigen; cTnI, cardiac troponin I; CK-MB, creatine kinase isoenzyme MB; CK-MM, creatine kinase isoenzyme MM; cTnT, cardiac troponin T; hTSH, human thyroid stimulating hormone; FSH, follicle-stimulating hormone; CEACAM, carcinoembryonic antigen-related cell adhesion molecule; SARS, severe acute respiratory syndrome; CA-125, cancer antigen 125; IGF-II, insulin growth factor II; PD, Parkinson's disease; VOC, volatile organic compound; COPD, chronic obstructive pulmonary disease; PBS, phosphate buffered saline; SSC, saline-sodium citrate; PS, phosphate solution; BSA, bovine serum albumin; n.i., not indicated; n.a., not applicable.

Among the most widely used linker molecules for the formation of SAMs on oxide surfaces of silicon-based FET biosensors are silanes [17, 27, 29]. The alkoxysilane agent (3-aminopropyl)triethoxysilane (APTES) is the most commonly used linker on SiNW-based biosensors [65, 67, 68, 71, 73, 75, 77, 78], followed by (3-aminopropyl)trimethoxysilane (APTMS) [48, 49]. The reaction of these aminosilanes with the surface hydroxyl groups occurs in four steps [79]: first, the alkoxy groups undergo hydrolysis; then, condensation occurs, forming silane oligomers; this is followed by hydrogen bonding of the surface hydroxyl groups with the remaining hydrolyzed alkoxy group of the silane; finally, a covalent bond forms upon drying or curing. This reaction is typically performed in the solution phase, where the silane is dissolved at ≈2% concentration in 95% ethanol, although vapor-phase modification is also performed. After modification with APTES or APTMS, the surface is coated with amine groups. At this point, biorecognition molecules containing carboxyl groups can be directly conjugated to the amine-modified surface *via* activation of the carboxyl groups by the zero-length crosslinker 1-ethyl-3-(3-dimethylaminopropyl)carbodiimide (EDC) assisted by *N*-hydroxysuccinimide (NHS) [71, 73], which results in the formation of an amide bond between the linker and the receptor molecule [80]. Despite the shorter linker length when using EDC–NHS conjugation, many groups still opt to use glutaraldehyde as a bridge between the aminosilanes and the biorecognition molecule [65, 67, 68, 75, 77, 78]. This may be due to the simpler procedure involved in glutaraldehyde crosslinking: simple immersion in an aqueous solution of around 2.5% glutaraldehyde followed by incubation with the receptor containing amine groups, *versus* two-step EDC–NHS conjugation in different buffers of the optimal pH. The formation of covalent bond between glutaraldehyde and amine groups is believed to be facilitated by the hemiacetal cyclic conformations of glutaraldehyde in both monomer and polymer form, wherein nucleophilic substitution of the amine group with the hydroxyl group of glutaraldehyde occurs [81]. In cases when a dense aminosilane/glutaraldehyde modification is formed, subsequent immobilization of receptor molecules may occur through hydrophobic, ionic exchange, and covalent interactions [81].

For ZnO nanowire biosensors, the starting linker molecules usually employed for functionalization are also alkoxysilanes [82 - 85]. For In_2O_3 nanowires, on the other hand, the most commonly used linkers are phosphonate derivatives [52, 53, 86 - 88], although silanes can be used as well [89 - 91]. The binding of phosphonic acids to metal oxides occurs through heterocondensation with surface hydroxyl groups, forming bidentate or tridentate binding modes [92]. Following the surface modification of ZnO and In$_2$O$_3$ nanowires with silanes or phosphonates, subsequent conjugation steps, as described above for SiNWs, can be performed to immobilize bioreceptors onto the sensor surface.

After conjugation of the biorecognition elements, the nanowire surface is typically blocked with bovine serum albumin (BSA) [65, 78, 87], polyethylene glycol (PEG) [68, 93], or Tween 20 [53, 65] to prevent nonspecific binding of untargeted proteins in complex fluids, which would cause false signals and/or loss of sensitivity in the FET device. In order to enable multiplexed detection of different biomarkers in a single chip, various bioreceptors are usually immobilized on different clusters of sensors in the nanowire FET chip using robotic spotting technology [47, 68, 94].

Factors Affecting Sensitivity

Nanowire Characteristics

The sensitivity of a nanowire biosensor is dependent on the nanowire diameter, number, length, and doping concentration [40, 62, 95]. Sensitivity increases as the width or diameter of nanowires decreases due to larger surface-to-volume ratios, resulting in a more significant effect of surface charges on the carrier density in the nanowire [62, 95]. For nanowires with widths larger than ~150 nm, changes in threshold voltage and conductance are almost negligible [62]. Device sensitivity is highest for single-nanowire devices and decreases as the number of nanowire increases because of competitive analyte binding in multi-nanowire devices, leading to analyte depletion in very dilute solutions [95]. Devices with shorter nanowires were predicted to have higher sensitivities [40]; however, experimental studies have shown that sensitivity, in fact, increases with channel length due to the diminished effect of contact resistance in longer nanowires [96, 97]. Finally, lower sensitivities and higher detection limits were observed for SiNWs with higher doping concentration (10^{19} *versus* 10^{17} atoms/cm^3) [95]. This is because of the stronger screening effect of charge carriers in highly doped nanowires [21], a phenomenon known as Thomas–Fermi screening.

The surface chemistry of nanowires has a significant effect on their performance as biosensors. The 1–2-nm-thick native oxide on a SiNW surface may degrade the sensor performance due to dielectric screening of the charged species or the presence of Si/SiO$_2$ interfacial densities of states [98, 99]. Removal of the native oxide from the SiNWs results in improved FET characteristics in solution and enhanced sensitivity to DNA detection, with an increase in the limit of detection by two orders of magnitude as well as an increase in the dynamic range [99]. The density of immobilized capture molecules may also affect the sensitivity of a FET biosensor in a non-monotonic manner as can be seen in the tradeoff between probe number and hybridization efficiency in DNA sensors [100]. Due to steric hindrance and electrostatic repulsion between DNA molecules, the extent of current change decreases when the probe density exceeds the optimal concentration [100].

The sensitivity of nanowire FET biosensors can also be enhanced by applying a liquid-gate bias such that the FET operates in the subthreshold (depletion) regime as opposed to the linear regime. This is because, in the subthreshold regime, there is low carrier concentration such that the carrier screening length (Thomas–Fermi screening length) is long relative to the nanowire radius; surface charges can thus affect the entire nanowire volume and cause large percentage changes in electrical parameters and improved detection limits [21]. Increased sensitivity of a nanowire FET device in the subthreshold regime is also observed when a back-gate voltage is applied [100].

Debye Screening

Aside from the intrinsic characteristics of the nanowire FET and its gate dielectric, extrinsic factors, such as the distance of the charged molecule from the nanowire surface and the ionic strength of the detection medium, also play a significant role in determining the effective sensitivity of the device. The nanowire–target separation is usually determined by the length of the functionalization molecule. This distance decreases the gating potential exerted by the charged molecule on the nanowire volume, resulting in an exponential decrease in device response [101]. However, in electrolytic media, this gating effect is also affected by the ionic strength of the solution due to the ionic screening of the biomolecular charges by counter ions in the solution [102 - 104]. The counter ions form an electrical double layer around the charged species, resulting in an exponentially decaying electrostatic potential with distance from the charge, a phenomenon referred to as Debye screening. The characteristic distance which defines the exponential decrease in potential is known as the Debye length, which is given by

$$\lambda_D = \sqrt{\frac{\varepsilon_0 \varepsilon_r k_B T}{2 N_A e^2 I}} \tag{2}$$

where ε_0 is the permittivity of free space, ε_r is the relative permittivity of the medium, k_B is the Boltzmann constant, T is the absolute temperature, N_A is Avogadro's number, and I is the ionic strength of the buffer solution. It can be seen from eq. (2) that a solution of higher ionic strength results in a smaller λ_D, which means a faster decrease of potential with distance. Common physiological samples, such as blood and urine, have ionic strengths greater than 100 mM ($\lambda_D \approx$ 0.7–2.2 nm), which severely impedes detection using large receptors such as antibodies [104]. This limitation imposed by Debye screening has impelled researchers to perform additional processes for sensing in biosamples, such as pre-capture sample desalting [47] or post-capture washing and subsequent detection in low-ionic-strength buffers [105].

Taking into consideration the effect of Thomas–Fermi screening and Debye screening, Sørensen *et al.* [41] analytically derived a more complete model to estimate the sensitivity of cylindrical nanowire biosensors. Their model adds the dimensionless functions Γ and Γ_l, with values between zero and unity, to the sensitivity equation in eq. (1), such that for a surface-charge density supported by a functionalization layer with molecules of length l, eq. (1) becomes $S = (\sigma_S P \Gamma \Gamma_l)/(e n_0 A)$. For the idealized case of an ultrathin oxide layer and a dilute carrier density, *i.e.*, Thomas–Fermi length $>> r$, $\Gamma \approx n_0^{1/3}$ [41]. Moreover, for a nanowire radius $r >> l$, $\Gamma_l \approx 2/(1 + \exp(l/\lambda_D))$ [106]. Therefore, the analytical model of Sørensen *et al.* becomes

$$S = \frac{\Delta G}{G_0} = \frac{2\sigma_S P}{e n_0^{2/3} A \left[1 + \exp\left(\frac{l}{\lambda_D} \right) \right]}$$ (3)

The expression in eq. (3) is consistent with experimental results showing that device sensitivity decreases with increasing doping concentration (carrier density) [95] and nanowire–target distance [101] and increases with longer Debye lengths [103].

The critical importance of Debye screening has been further highlighted in a study by Shoorideh and Chui [107]. Using both analytical methods and computer simulation, they concluded that, given negligible charge screening in the nanowire (*i.e.*, Thomas–Fermi length $>> r$ and subthreshold region of operation), it is not necessarily diameter reduction that leads to higher sensitivity but the overall concavity of the structure. They introduce the concept of surface-area-to-Deye-volume ratio, which must be increased in order to reduce screening by counter ions. This ratio increases with the cross-sectional area for concave structures but decreases with the cross-sectional area for convex structures. Thus, a convex structure such as a cylindrical nanowire will have diminished sensitivity when its diameter is decreased, contradicting the widely held belief that sensitivity increases with increasing surface-to-volume ratios. The reason why experimental studies observe an increase in sensitivity for reduced nanowire diameters, the authors argue, is that nanowires lying on an insulator with captured biomolecules on the nanowire surface as well as the immediate vicinity on the insulator form a concave structure at the nanowire–insulator junction whose effect dominates as the nanowire cross-sectional area is decreased.

Noise

Aside from the sensitivity of device, noise is an important parameter to be considered in biosensor design and evaluation since it is a major determining factor in the limit of detection of these devices. In particular, the limit of detection is defined as the minimum analyte concentration that yields a discriminable signal above the noise, typically, a signal-to-noise ratio (SNR) = 3. As MOSFETs approach the nanometer size range, however, low-frequency noise becomes more pronounced [108] due to two main phenomena, namely, random telegraph signal (RTS) noise and $1/f$ noise [109]. The former involves the capture and emission of electrons by carrier traps at the interface of the semiconductor and the oxide, resulting in a Coulomb potential and the consequent scattering of charge carriers in the channel [110, 111]. The latter, on the other hand, is caused by an inherent mobility fluctuation in the bulk of the semiconductor due to lattice scattering [112]. Due to their effect on the carriers, RTS noise is commonly referred to as carrier number fluctuation, while $1/f$ noise as carrier mobility fluctuation. The voltage noise power spectral density at the gate S_{VG} due to RTS noise can be expressed using the following model [113, 114]:

$$S_{V_G} = \frac{d_t k_B T e^2 N_{ot}}{fWLC_{ox}^2} \quad (4)$$

where d_t is the tunneling attenuation distance, N_{ot} the oxide trap density per unit area, W the channel width, and C_{ox} the gate oxide capacitance per unit area. On the other hand, the normalized drain current power spectral density $S_{I_{DS(1/f)}} / I^2_{DS}$ due to mobility fluctuation is given by Hooge's empirical equation [115]:

$$\frac{S_{I_{DS(1/f)}}}{I^2_{DS}} = \frac{\alpha_H}{Nf} \quad (5)$$

where α_H is Hooge's parameter and is a noise figure of merit of a given material and N is the total carrier number in the system. When $N < (4\alpha_H\pi)^{-1}$, RTS noise will dominate over $1/f$ noise in the device [109]. Aside from noise due to carrier trapping and lattice scattering, thermal noise due to random thermal motion of charge carriers also exists as a frequency-independent noise floor:

$$S_{I_{DS}(\text{thermal})} = \frac{4k_\text{B}T}{R} \tag{6}$$

where R is the resistance of the channel. However, thermal noise power is usually below that of RTS noise and $1/f$ noise in the low-frequency range [116, 117], where nanowire FET biosensors are operated.

Ghibaudo *et al.* [118] have derived the expression for the drain current power spectral density due to carrier number fluctuations and the correlated mobility fluctuations:

$$S_{I_{DS}(\text{total})} = \left(1 + \alpha\mu_0 C_{ox}\frac{I_{DS}}{g_m}\right)^2 g_m^2 S_{V_G} \tag{7}$$

where α is the Coulombic scattering coefficient, μ_0 is the low-field mobility, and g_m is the MOSFET transconductance. Since S_{V_G} is inversely related to the dimensions of the MOSFET channel area ($W{\times}L$) from eq. (4), it is expected that the overall noise will increase as the channel is scaled down to the nanometer regime, as in the case of nanowire FETs. However, the study by Lee *et al.* [119] showed the opposite trend, *i.e.*, the current noise power decreased as the nanowire diameter was reduced. The authors attributed this noise reduction to a volume inversion effect, wherein the drain current flows mostly in the middle portion of the nanowire, away from the semiconductor–oxide interface where carrier trap-induced noise occurs. A similar approach has been pursued by other researchers by employing both liquid and back-gate biasing [120] and using a depletion mode configuration [121]. Another strategy is to avoid or minimize the formation of carrier traps in the first place by using wet etching instead of plasma etching for the formation of the nanowire [122] or by utilizing a metal–silicon (Schottky junction) gate [123].

Despite efforts to minimize low-frequency noise, the sensing performance will still be dictated by the SNR, which, for a FET biosensor can be expressed as [124]

$$\text{SNR} = \frac{\Delta I}{\delta i} = \frac{g_m{\times}\Delta V}{\sqrt{\text{BW}}{\times}\sqrt{S_{I(f=1\,\text{Hz})}}} \tag{8}$$

where ΔI is the measured current response, δi the current noise, ΔV the change in surface potential due to analyte binding, BW a bandwidth-related quantity that depends on the largest and smallest sampled frequencies, and $S_{I(f=1\ Hz)}$ the power spectral density of the current noise at $f = 1$ Hz. Therefore, in order to decrease the detection limit, any measure to reduce the noise should not adversely affect the device transconductance [124].

Measurement Setup

Biomolecular detection using nanowire FETs typically requires an electronic detection instrumentation, a solution delivery or containment system, and the chip containing the nanowire FET devices. In proof-of-concept experiments, the chips are usually in the form of wafer dice (*i.e.*, not packaged) and electrical contacts are established using probe stations [67, 78] or wire bonding to printed circuit boards [71]. The detection system depends on the electrical parameters to be used for analytical measurements. For probing changes in the DC electrical properties of nanowire FETs, researchers usually employ source measure units or a semiconductor parameter analyzer, which can measure the drain current in response to sweeps of the gate voltage or drain voltage [53, 70, 71, 77, 78]. From the resulting $I–V$ plots, parameters such as drain current at a given voltage, threshold voltage, and resistance/conductance can be extracted and used for creating calibration curves for quantification of analytes. Other researchers use a resistor-like configuration of the nanowires for sensing experiments and measure changes in the AC conductance or resistance of the nanowire using a lock-in amplifier and a preamplifier [28, 47 - 49, 94].

Simple manual pipetting of analyte solutions onto nanowire FET biosensors can be performed [49], provided that solution evaporation is not a serious problem [29]. However, a majority of researchers opt to flow analyte solutions through a microfluidic channel (usually made of polydimethylsiloxane) [28, 47 - 49, 61, 94] to demonstrate the real-time detection capability of the biosensors. Some researchers prefer a macroscale sample holder over a microfluidic channel as a sample holder can serve as a mixing cell to facilitate faster responses by avoiding the restrictive laminar flow in microfluidic channels [53, 70]. Aside from demonstrating real-time detection, these flow systems allow the nanowire devices to overcome one important shortcoming inherent in nanoscale biosensors, which is the significantly smaller detection area available. By constraining the liquid in a microscale volume and/or facilitating mixing of solutions, the probability of the analyte molecules encountering the nanowire surface is significantly increased. Nevertheless, in situations where such flow systems are impractical, analyte preconcentration can be performed using integrated sample filtration and purification systems (as discussed below).

During the demonstration of the biosensing capability of prototypical nanowire devices, target biomolecules are usually dissolved in solutions of low ionic strength (*e.g.*, 0.01× PBS, $\lambda_D \approx 7.3$ nm; see Table **1**), unless special measures are taken to overcome Debye screening in high-ionic-strength solutions (also discussed in the following sections).

RECENT DEVELOPMENTS

In the pioneering work by Lieber's group in 2001 [28], the capability of nanowire devices to sense protein–protein interactions at low concentrations and in a label-free, real-time manner was demonstrated using CVD-synthesized SiNWs, showing the promise of these devices for rapid, highly sensitive disease diagnosis. Three years later, SiNW devices were applied to the ultrasensitive and selective sensing of DNA, achieving detections down to tens of femtomolar (by Lieber's group [61] and another group employing top–down-fabricated devices [64]). Moreover, Lieber's group reported the detection of single viruses and multiplexed detection of two different viruses on the same chip [94]. This idea of multiplexed detection was extended by Lieber's group in 2005 to the protein cancer biomarkers prostate-specific antigen (PSA), PSA-α1-antichymotrypsin, carcinoembryonic antigen (CEA), and mucin-1, achieving a detection limit of 50 fg/mL in 1 μM PBS and 0.9 pg/mL in desalted serum [47]. Likewise, Li *et al.* [52] showed the ability of In_2O_3 nanowire devices to detect PSA in concentrations as low as 5 ng/mL. Using TMAH wet etching instead of RIE, Stern *et al.* [70] obtained SiNW FETs with enhanced sensing performance, sensitive enough to detect antibodies down to 100 fM (in 1 mM buffer).

The brief account in the previous paragraph shows the significant developments in nanowire-FET-based biosensors applied to biomarker detection in the years 2001–2008. (For a more detailed discussion of the relevant studies in this period, please refer to the review article by Curreli *et al.* [27].) In this section, we present notable works done on nanowire FET devices from 2009 to date that have the potential to impact greatly future FET-based POCT devices. Table **1** shows a summary of selected nanowire FET devices reported in the past decade that were applied to the analytical detection of various biomolecules and chemicals for disease diagnosis. It can be seen that great improvements have been made in the detection limit of the devices, reaching sub-femtomolar levels for DNA and tens of fg/mL for PSA (0.01× PBS) using top–down-fabricated SiNW biosensors. Furthermore, SiNW FETs have also been applied to the sensing of volatile organic compounds (VOCs) for diagnosis *via* exhaled breath. In the subsections that follow, we delve into the different approaches proposed by various research groups that have allowed them to achieve such sensitivity enhancements as well as address other long-standing issues that hinder the widespread adoption of nanowire FET biosensors in POCT applications.

Low-Cost Top–Down Fabrication of SiNWs

UV and DUV Lithography

Instead of using serial patterning techniques, such as e-beam lithography, in top–down fabrication of SiNW FETs, the use of wafer-scale, parallel patterning processes, such as UV and DUV lithography is desirable for higher throughput and less expensive equipment. Ryu *et al.* [126] made use of DUV lithography and O_2 plasma ashing to pattern the photoresist mask for the dry etching of a SOI device layer. Afterwards, the dimensions of the formed SiNW were further reduced through repeated oxidation and wet etching using a buffered oxide etch, achieving a final width of 50 nm. The SiNW devices were successfully applied to the picomolar detection of breast cancer DNA. A similar fabrication process was utilized by Zhang *et al.* [127] to form 70-nm-wide SiNWs for the detection of DNA in the range of hundreds of femtomolar. Instead of using expensive SOI wafers, Agarwal *et al.* [154] performed DUV lithography and dry etching on poly-silicon deposited on a typical Si test wafer, followed by oxidation of the resulting Si "fins" to form SiNWs. The fabricated SiNWs, having typical width × height dimensions of 20 nm × 40 nm, were applied to microRNA (miRNA) detection using peptide nucleic acid hybridization, achieving a detection limit of 1 fM and single-nucleotide-polymorphism discrimination ability [67]. We have also used poly-silicon thin film to fabricate the SiNW FETs in our lab [155, 156]; however, instead of DUV lithography, we used conventional i-line photolithography, dry etching, and subsequent nanowire width reduction using dry oxidation of the poly-SiNW followed by hydrofluoric-acid wet etching. FET devices with 280- and 70-nm-wide SiNWs were successfully applied to the sensing of PSA [155] and monitoring of cells [156]. Chen *et al.* [137] also used i-line lithography coupled with dry etching to fabricate 150-nm-wide poly-SiNWs for sensing bladder cancer biomarker apolipoprotein A II from urine samples.

Sidewall Spacer Technique

A simple and low-cost fabrication process for poly-SiNW FET using neither e-beam nor DUV lithography was also proposed by Lin *et al.* [157]. This process, called the sidewall spacer technique, involves the following main steps (Fig. **2a**): first, an oxide dummy gate is formed, which serves as the template for nanowire formation; then, a poly-Si layer is conformally coated on the substrate by CVD and annealing; finally, a reactive plasma etch removes the poly-Si over the substrate except those at the dummy gate sidewalls (and masked source and drain areas), leading to the formation of a pair of self-aligned SiNW channels. Lin *et al.* [77] used this technique to fabricate SiNW FETs with 80-nm-wide nanowires and applied them as DNA biosensors for the sensitive and specific detection of the avian influenza (AI) virus H5 DNA. Wenga *et al.* [75] also used the sidewall spacer technique to fabricate 70-nm-wide SiNWs in a FET configuration where the dummy gate is utilized as a functional "step-gate". The resulting devices were used to detect DNA hybridization down to 1-fM concentration. Hakim *et al.* [73] utilized the same technique but with a highly anisotropic reactive-ion etch for fine control of the nanowire width. The resulting SiNWs had a cross-section with dimensions of 95 nm × 95 nm and with a shape of a rectangle, instead of a quarter circle (Figs. **2b** and **2c**). The fabricated poly-SiNW FETs were applied for the detection of inflammatory markers interleukin-8 and tumor necrosis factor-alpha with a detection limit of 10 fM for both.

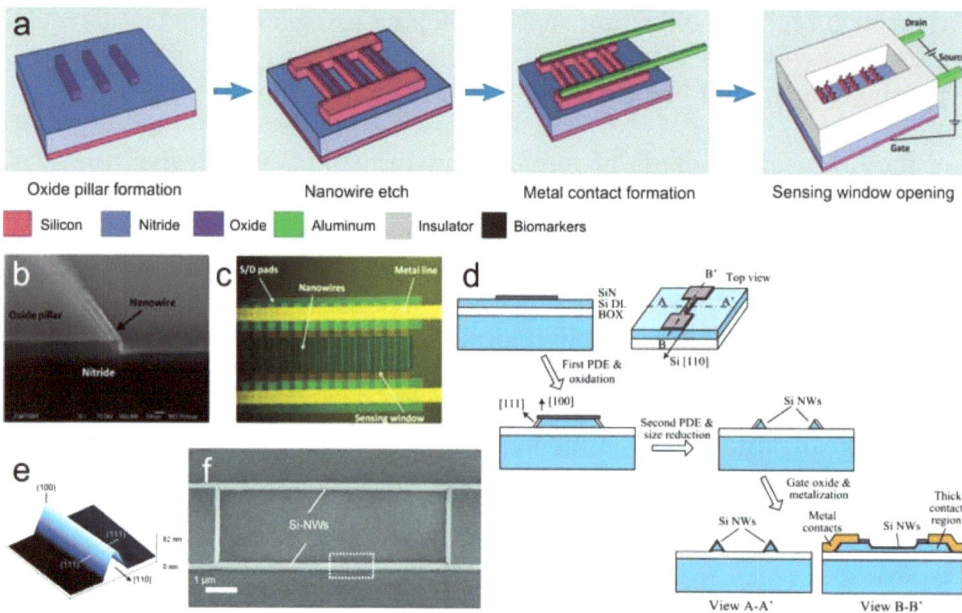

Fig. (2). Simple CMOS-compatible fabrication of SiNW devices. (a) Top–down fabrication of poly-SiNW biosensor using sidewall spacer technique, consisting of oxide pillar formation, etching to form SiNWs, metal contact formation, and insulation deposition and sensing window opening. (b, c) Scanning electron micrograph of a poly-SiNW and optical micrograph of a poly-SiNW device, respectively, formed by the sidewall spacer technique. (d) Top–down fabrication of SiNW devices using conventional lithography and anisotropic wet etching comprising four steps: lithographic patterning and etching of SiN mask; anisotropic wet etching of silicon followed by oxidation; another anisotropic wet etching of silicon; and SiNW oxidation and formation of metal contacts. (e, f) Atomic force micrograph and scanning electron micrograph of SiNWs formed by the anisotropic wet etching. Panels (a–c) adapted with permission from [73]; copyright 2012 American Chemical Society. Panels (d–f) reprinted with permission from [72]; copyright 2009 American Chemical Society. Abbreviations: DL, device layer; BOX, buried oxide; PDE, plane-dependent wet etching.

Anisotropic Wet Etching

The use of dry etching for top–down fabrication of SiNWs usually results in rough surfaces that lead to ion accumulation and reduction in device performance [70, 133]. Therefore, a number of research groups have proposed the use of anisotropic wet etching with TMAH on ultrathin (100) SOI wafers to form the nanoscale width of SiNWs. Since TMAH etches Si (111) planes more slowly than other planes, the wet etch smooths rough edges in non-(111) planes and leaves smooth sidewalls with (111) surfaces ideal for organic monolayer formation [70]. Kong *et al.* [133] utilized this wet etching technique with photolithography to fabricate 80-nm-wide SiNW devices for the sensitive detection of cardiac troponin I (cTnI) down to 0.092 ng/mL. Chen *et al.* [72] designed a fabrication process based on conventional lithography and TMAH wet etching of a (100) SOI device layer to obtain SiNW devices with sub-30-nm widths (Fig. **2d**). The process starts with a microlithography step to pattern a silicon nitride (SiN) mask, which defines the separation of the two SiNWs to be formed as well as the shape of the contacts. Then, anisotropic wet etching is performed using TMAH, forming slanted Si sidewalls at both sides of the SiN mask. A protective thermal oxide is then formed on the exposed sidewalls. A second microlithography step is performed to pattern another SiN mask over the contact areas. Then, a second anisotropic wet etch forms the two SiNWs with isosceles-triangle cross-sections. Finally, thermal oxidation is performed to passivate the freshly etched Si sidewalls. This fabrication process allows the independent control of the lateral dimensions of the SiNWs (10–200 nm) from the contacts and creates SiNWs with all-(111) surfaces (Figs. **2e** and **2f**). Using a similar technique, Gao *et al.* fabricated an analogous device albeit with only one SiNW ($\approx$ 20 nm in width) per FET and applied it to the femtomolar to sub-femtomolar detection of DNA [71, 100, 129] and multiplexed selective detection of AI virus DNA subtypes H1N1 and H5N1 [71]. This device has also been applied to the detection of the thyroid disease biomarker human thyroid stimulating hormone (hTSH) [134] and cancer-associated miRNAs miR-21 and miR-205 [130]. Sensing of hTSH in optimized buffer (0.01× phosphate buffered saline, PBS) showed a detection range from 0.02 to 30 mIU/L, while measurement of miR-21 and miR-205 in the same buffer exhibited detection from 0.1 fM to 1 nM with a calculated detection limit of 1 zeptomole (~600 copies of miRNA) and single-base-mismatch discrimination.

FET Design and Configuration

Dual Gating

A double-gate FET design was proposed to enhance the device sensitivity of top–down fabricated SiNW FET biosensors [158]. The two gates flank the nanowire along its axis and allow the application of symmetric/asymmetric biases (Fig. **3a**). Since the SiNW channel is p-type, while the source and drain terminals are n-type, application of more positive gate voltages results in the formation of an electron channel in the nanowire near the corresponding gate terminal which serves as the path for current flow. Using anti-AI virus antibody detection as a proof-of-concept, it was found that, when a bias greater than the threshold voltage for the double-gate mode (*i.e.*, same voltage is applied to the two gates) is applied to the second gate, the subthreshold slope, threshold voltage, and drain current changes dramatically upon capture of anti-AI based on the transfer curve where the first gate is swept. Such sensitivity is greater than that of the case where the second gate is floating, which is the configuration of the conventional single-gate SiNW FET (Figs. **3b** and **3c**). This increase in sensitivity was attributed to the diminished control of the swept gate (first gate) over the electron channel as the channel transfers to the second-gate side, thereby allowing the charged molecules to affect the current flow to a greater extent.

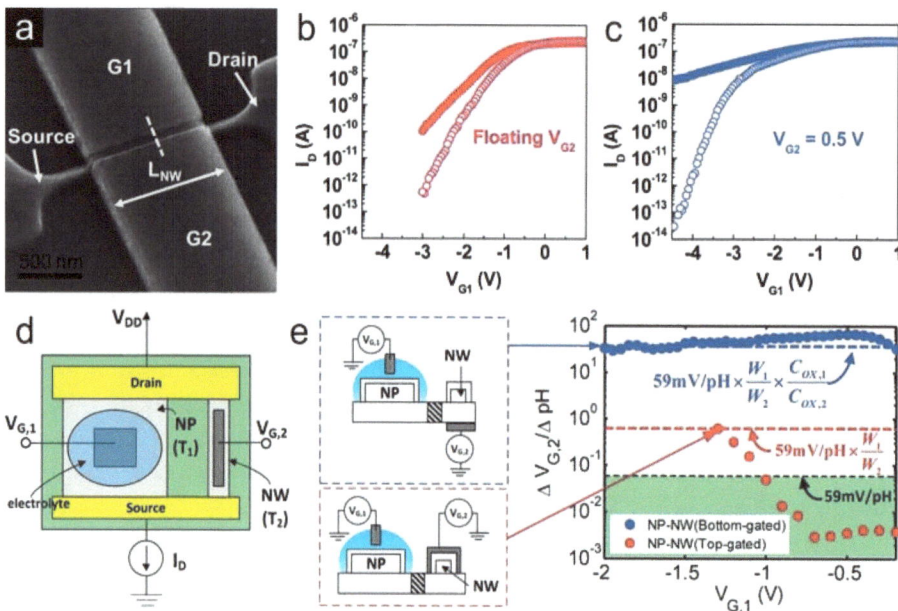

Fig. (3). FET designs for enhanced sensitivity. **(a)** Scanning electron micrograph of the double-gate SiNW FET showing gate 1 (G1) and gate 2 (G2). **(b, c)** I_D–V_{G1} graphs of the double-gate SiNW FET after immobilization of avian influenza (AI) antigen (filled circles) and capture of anti-AI antibody (hollow circles) for floating V_{G2} and $V_{G2} = 0.5$ V, respectively. Note that $V_{G2} = 0.5$ V is greater than the threshold voltage obtained when the same voltage is applied to G1 and G2. **(d)** Schematic diagram of the coupled nanoplate (NP)–nanowire (NW) FET sensor. (e) Measured pH sensitivity (circles) of the coupled NP–NW sensor for two different NW gate bias configurations: bottom gate (blue) and top gate (red). The dashed lines show the theoretical estimates, while the green region indicates the sensitivity regime below the classical Nernst limit. Panels (a–c) reprinted with permission from [158]; copyright 2010 American Chemical Society. Panels **(d)** and **(e)** reprinted with permission from [159]; copyright 2012 American Chemical Society. Symbols: G1, gate 1; G2, gate 2; L_{NW}, nanowire length; I_D, drain current; V_{G1}, voltage at G1; V_{G2}, voltage at G2; V_{DD}, drain voltage; T_1, sensor transistor; T_2, transducer transistor; $V_{G,1}$, gate voltage at T_1; $V_{G,2}$, gate voltage at T_2; NP, nanoplate; NW, nanowire; W_1, channel width of T_1; W_2, channel width of T_2; $C_{OX,1}$, gate oxide capacitance of T_1; $C_{OX,2}$, gate oxide capacitance of T_2.

A similar increase in sensitivity was demonstrated for pH sensing in a SiNW FET device with a top aluminum oxide (Al_2O_3) anti-leakage layer, except that here the dual gates were applied *via* the electrolyte (liquid gate) and the substrate (back gate) [160]. When pH sensing was performed at constant back-gate voltages while the liquid-gate potential was swept, the changes in threshold voltage were around 45–59 mV/pH. On the other hand, when the liquid-gate voltage was held constant and the back-gate potential was swept, the resulting sensitivities varied from a few mV/pH to 220 mV/pH, which greatly exceeds the Nernst limit of 59.5 mV/pH at room temperature. Using a simple capacitance model, the authors explained that this unexpected dramatic enhancement in pH sensitivity when the back-gate voltage was swept is due to the high nanowire oxide capacitance compared with the back-gate capacitance. The simultaneous use of a liquid gate and back gate can also be adopted to achieve the optimal SNR in different operation regimes [120]. In a p-type SiNW FET, applying a more negative back-gate potential (~ –10 V) at a liquid-gate voltage of around 0 V increases the transconductance of the device due to the movement of the conducting channel away from the gate oxide, where scattering is higher, towards the bulk volume of the SiNW. Analysis of the low-frequency flicker ($1/f$) noise in different operation regimes with the drain current held constant also shows lower spectral density when more negative back-gate voltages are applied. Further analysis of the SNR which takes into consideration both transconductance and low-frequency noise sources ($f = 1$ Hz – 10 kHz) reveals that the saturation mode of operation (high drain–source voltage) yields higher SNR values than the linear mode (low drain–source voltage) due to the saturation of the drain current (and flicker noise) while the transconductance still changes proportionally with the drain voltage. Note, however, that in both modes, the application of a negative back-gate voltage enhances the SNR due to the reduction of surface noise. This strategy of biasing a SiNW FET in the saturation regime and applying a back-gate potential has the potential to improve the detection limit in biosensing applications.

Nanoplate–Nanowire Transistor Pair

Instead of using a double-gate FET configuration, Go *et al.* [159] used an integrated silicon nanoplate–nanowire transistor pair to surpass the Nernst limit for pH sensors (Fig. **3d**). Amplification of the Nernst sensitivity by double-gated FETs is done *via* the measurement of the pH-dependent shift in gate voltage at a constant current as the back-gate voltage is swept. As was seen above [160], the lower capacitance of the back gate compared to that of the nanowire oxide allowed the large shifts in voltage. This is because such lowered capacitance reduces the capacity of the back-gate voltage to modulate the current; hence, larger voltage shifts are required to attain the same current levels. Go *et al.* hypothesized that a similar effect can be obtained by reducing the width:length ratio of the channel where the second gate voltage is applied. This scaling effectively reduces the extent of gate-modulated current change by increasing the channel resistance. Hence, the authors decoupled the sensor and transducer components of their FET device, where the nanoplate serves as the former and the nanowire—having drastically smaller width:length ratio—acts as the latter. They found that a back-gated SiNW transducer results in a sensitivity of ≈36 V/pH, while a top-metal-gated one has a sensitivity of ≈0.613 V/pH (Fig. **3e**). The authors suggest that further improvements can be achieved by employing a transducer channel material with a considerably lower mobility than the sensor channel. With due consideration to possible reductions in dynamic range [159], this unique hybrid architecture and detection scheme can be adopted for biosensors to achieve ultrasensitive biomarker detection.

Nanopore FET

With the goal of achieving direct, high-throughput, single-molecule DNA sequencing, Xie *et al.* [161] constructed a SiNW–nanopore FET sensor that consists of a silicon nitride membrane with *trans* and *cis* reservoirs above and below the membrane, respectively, and a 200-nm channel SiNW FET at the *trans* side. The nanopore, which was created using a focused e-beam, is located at the edge of the nanowire and extends through the membrane support. The hybrid FET sensor exhibits conductance pulses that correspond with ionic current pulses during DNA translocation but only when the *trans* chamber contains a solution of lower ionic strength than the *cis* chamber. Due to the inconsistent conductance change direction with the charge of the DNA, the observed conductance changes were attributed to a new detection mechanism, which involves detection of local potential changes around the nanopore, enabled by the increased solution resistance at the *trans* chamber comparable to that of the nanopore and the negligible solution resistance at the *cis* chamber. The authors proposed that, by utilizing techniques for base-resolved ionic current detection and engineered protein nanopores [162, 163], practical DNA sequencing with multiplexing capabilities can be achieved with the nanowire–nanopore FET.

Underlap FET

A modified FET structure similar to the MOSFET was previously proposed in order to create a FET-based biosensor that eliminates the need for a solution gate, thus making the device fully compatible with CMOS fabrication [164]. This device has been referred to as the underlap FET and has the typical structure of metal/oxide gate on silicon, except that the gate does not entirely overlap with the channel (hence the name "underlap" FET). The uncovered channel region serves as the sensing area, where binding of biomolecules greatly modulates the channel current. Compared to the nanogap FET [165], the underlap FET provides a more open sensing area for a higher probability of biomolecular binding. Moreover, since each device has its own dedicated gate, unlike in the case of back-gated FETs, individual device gate control can be achieved for sensor arrays.

As an improvement to the underlap FET, Kim *et al.* [136] developed a nano-FET version called an underlap-embedded SiNW FET, wherein the bulk-Si channel has been replaced with a SiNW. Aside from the unique structure, they also proposed a low-cost and self-aligned fabrication procedure, wherein a bulk-Si wafer was used instead of a SOI substrate, and the source and drain terminals were formed after the underlap region has been defined. Using RIE with combined anisotropic and isotropic etching, a suspended SiNW was formed on the bulk silicon. Device isolation was achieved by channel-stop implantation and oxide deposition under the suspended SiNW. After forming a thermal oxide around the SiNW, two poly-Si gates with a spacing in between were patterned in a single step, thus defining the underlap region. High-concentration doping *via* large-angle tilted ion implantation was then performed. In this step, the gates cover the underlap region *via* a shadow effect; thus, the source and drain areas are formed in a self-aligned manner. This technique prevents the underlap length from critically depending on error-prone alignment steps. After modification of the device with antigens attached to silica-binding protein, selective detection of anti-AI virus antibody was successfully performed down to around 1 nM.

Vertically Aligned Nanorods

FET biosensors with semiconducting channels modified with vertically aligned nanostructures have been realized using ZnO [85, 148] due to the ease by which such nanostructures can be formed *in situ via* a bottom–up approach. The fabrication of the devices entails patterning a ZnO thin film as the seed layer either by sputtering or by sol–gel technique followed by the growth of the vertical array of ZnO nanorods in a solution containing zinc nitrate and hexamine [166]. The source and drain terminals can be patterned before or after the ZnO nanorod growth. Ahmad *et al.* [148] made use of the ZnO nanorod array as both a sensing material and enzyme immobilization matrix for the detection of cholesterol. In physiological pH, ZnO is positively charged, thereby facilitating the adsorption of negatively charged proteins or enzymes without the use of linker molecules. Application of sufficiently high positive potentials at the liquid gate results in the generation of protons due to the oxidation of hydrogen peroxide, one of the products of the reaction between cholesterol and the enzyme cholesterol oxidase. The acidification of the medium, in turn, increases the conductance of the n-type ZnO channel. Using this detection scheme, a wide dynamic range (1 μM – 45 mM) was achieved with a limit of detection of around 50 nM. Furthermore, despite the relatively high liquid potentials applied, insensitivity towards other electroactive species was observed.

In contrast with the lateral drain-to-source configuration of the ZnO nanorod FETs in the above study, Chakraborty *et al.* [85] employed a vertical orientation so that the electrical characteristics of the entire length of the vertical nanorods can be probed. To construct these vertically contacted devices, an interdigitated source electrode was first formed on the substrate. Then, a ZnO seed layer was deposited, followed by the growth of vertical ZnO nanorods in the solution phase. Afterwards, the drain electrode with interdigitated pattern was formed on top of the nanorod array. In order to enable sensitive detection in high-ionic-strength solutions (0.1 M PBS and serum), the authors utilized sensing in high-frequency heterodyne mode [167], which disrupts the electric double layer near the FET channel and hence enables the electric potential of charged biomolecules to affect the channel conductance. This detection scheme was implemented by applying a high-frequency voltage signal and a modulating reference signal at the drain and source terminals, respectively, and then detecting the mixing current at the modulating frequency at the drain terminal. When applied to the detection of hepatitis B surface antigen in 0.1 M PBS, a detection limit of 20 aM was achieved for a 1-MHz signal, while only 1 fM was obtained for the lateral FET configuration. This drastic improvement in the detection limit for the vertical configuration was attributed to the measurement of conductivity changes in both the nanorods and the seed layer—as compared to just the seed layer in the lateral configuration—which enables the detection of the gating effect by captured analytes in the entire nanorod array.

Reducing Device-to-Device Variations

Calibration by Transconductance

Device-to-device variation in biosensor performance is almost an unavoidable problem especially with bottom–up-fabricated FETs [168]. These inconsistencies make reliable, quantitative measurements difficult to achieve in practice and are one of the major roadblocks towards the commercialization of nanowire-based biosensors. Using liquid-gated FETs with CVD-synthesized In_2O_3 nanowire channels and the biotin–streptavidin system as a model, Ishikawa *et al.* [169] found that the transconductance and absolute response (*i.e.*, current change from baseline) of each device are linearly proportional. They then derived the "calibrated response" by dividing the absolute responses by the transconductance value at a given drain and gate voltage. Using the ratio of standard deviation to the mean as a measure of device-to-device variation, they found that the variation was 59% when using the absolute response and 16% for the calibrated response.

The proposed calibration method was also found to be superior to the oft-used normalization method, wherein the measured parameter is divided by the initial value, which gave a variation of 25%. Using a conventional transistor model, the authors showed that, for a biosensor with electrostatic gating as the dominant sensing mechanism, the calibrated response is effectively the equivalent potential change induced by the captured biomolecules at the gate. This potential is independent of intrinsic device characteristics and hence unaffected by device-to-device variations caused by inconsistencies in device fabrication.

Optical Self-Calibration

In order to avoid the cumbersome process of calibrating each device prior to biosensing application, Peretz-Soroka *et al.* [170] proposed an approach towards self-calibrating devices, which entails the use of photoactive switchable molecular recognition layers and ratiometric measurement of the electrical signals arising from the ground and excited states of these molecules. In their initial study, the authors demonstrated this concept with pH sensing through the use of the fluorescent pH indicator 8-hydroxypyrene-1,3,6-trisulfonyl chloride (HPTS) (Fig. **4a**). HPTS has a pK_a of ~7.3 in the ground state and thus becomes protonated and unprotonated below and above this pH value, respectively. When illuminated at 405 nm, the pK_a of HPTS becomes ~0.4; hence, HPTS molecules become highly acidic and expel their protons above this pH value. The varied extent of HPTS protonation in different pH environments and illumination conditions allows the differential modulation of the SiNW current. By calculating the ratio of the current response of the HPTS-modified SiNW FETs in the illuminated and dark conditions at a fixed pH value in different pH environments, precise pH responses were obtained among different devices (Figs. **4b** and **4c**), with device-to-device variations drastically smaller than transconductance-calibrated SiNW FETs. This optical self-calibration of SiNW devices can also be applied to other target biomolecules through the use of receptor photoacids or photobases responsive to other analytes.

Improved Fabrication Process

With the objective of addressing the root cause of variability among nanowire sensors, Zafar *et al.* [69] identified key issues in the top–down processing of SiNW FETs from SOI wafers in order to devise an improved, more rationalized fabrication procedure. From device simulations, the authors identified gate dielectric thickness variation over the nanowire and nanowire width as significant factors affecting the device parameters. In addition, through preliminary experiments, they found that the thickness of the materials in a SiO_2/HfO_2 gate dielectric stack also critically impacts device characteristics due to charge trapping. The final design specifications were a SiNW with a width of 30 nm and a length of 5 μm and a dual-layer gate dielectric consisting of 2 nm/3 nm-thick SiO_2/HfO_2. In terms of the fabrication process, the authors identified five objectives that must be met: (1) uniform SOI device layer thickness throughout the wafer; (2) minimal nanowire sidewall roughness for a Si/SiO_2 interface with low defect density; (3) optimal gate dielectric stack thickness with good uniformity over the nanowire; (4) well-aligned HfO_2 and nitride mask with the SiNW width; and (5) complete removal of the nitride mask. Particular attention was given to the optimization of e-beam lithography in order to obtain smooth nanowire sidewalls and minimize alignment errors between the HfO_2/SiN stack and the nanowire. The e-beam resist thickness (20 nm) was chosen such that it is sufficiently thin to reduce roughness, while the e-beam dose was optimized such that it is high enough to decrease sidewall roughness but low enough to achieve the small nanowire width. Moreover, e-beam exposure was divided into two parts: a sparse level for the nanowires and a dense level for the contact lines and probe pads. This is to minimize thermal drift effects that lead to misalignment between the HfO_2/SiN stack and the nanowire width (Figs. **4d** and **4e**). These design specifications and process improvements led to SiNW FETs with significantly less device-to-device variations (Fig. **4f**): 1.7% and 10% standard deviation in subthreshold swing and threshold voltage values as compared to 7% and 22.3%, respectively, before process enhancements. Calibration curves for pH sensing show exponential fits with 8.7% and 0.9% variability among devices before and after process optimization, respectively (Fig. **4g**). Furthermore, the mean peak sensitivity was calculated to be 2.21, which is near the theoretical limit of 2.303, with only 3% variability.

Surface Coating and Functionalization

Selective Surface Functionalization

Selective functionalization of the SiNW surface, as opposed to functionalization of the entire SiO_2-covered substrate, is important in order to ensure that low-concentration analytes will not be depleted by the substrate and thus reach the sensor surface. To achieve this for a bottom–up-processed SiNW FET device, Li *et al.* [49, 146] performed APTMS modification of SiNWs before the photolithographic patterning of source and drain contacts. SiNWs synthesized by Au-catalyzed CVD were exposed to thermally vaporized APTMS to avoid aggregation resulting from solution-phase process. Surface chemical analysis of APTMS-modified SiNWs shows that the APTMS layer survives the device fabrication, which includes harsh processing steps, such as photoresist coating, organic solvent immersion, and annealing at 380 °C in forming gas [146]. Compared with a device wherein the surrounding oxide substrate was also modified, the selectively modified SiNW FETs exhibit faster response times and lower detection limits [146]. When applied to the detection of dopamine released from high-K$^+$-stimulated PC12 cells, only selectively modified devices show distinctive responses [146].

Selective functionalization for top–down-fabricated SiNW devices was previously achieved by localized Joule heating to selectively ablate an inert polymer passivation layer (polytetrafluoroethylene) on the nanowires [171]. Utilizing a fabrication- and linker-chemistry-based approach, Masood *et al.* [172] fabricated an all-(111) SiNW biosensor [72] and exploited the preferential alkyl and alkenyl monolayer formation on Si (111) surfaces to selectively functionalize the nanowires. First, an H-terminated silicon surface was formed by removal of the native oxide with 1% hydrofluoric acid and surface preparation with 40% ammonium fluoride. UV-initiated hydrosilylation was then performed with n-(--hexynyl)phthalimide precursor to form an alkenyl monolayer with pthalimide end groups. Using methylamine, the pthalimide groups were replaced with amine functional groups, which can then be used to attach biomolecules on the SiNW using various conjugation techniques. Oxide-passivated SiNW devices have been shown to have poorer FET characteristics and lower sensitivities than SiNWs with the oxide removed [99]. The study of Masood *et al.* also shows that SiNWs passivated with aminoalkenyl monolayers have higher sensitivities than those passivated with a 10-nm oxide layer. Therefore, methods to selectively functionalize oxide-free SiNWs will greatly help in further improving the performance of SiNW-based biosensors.

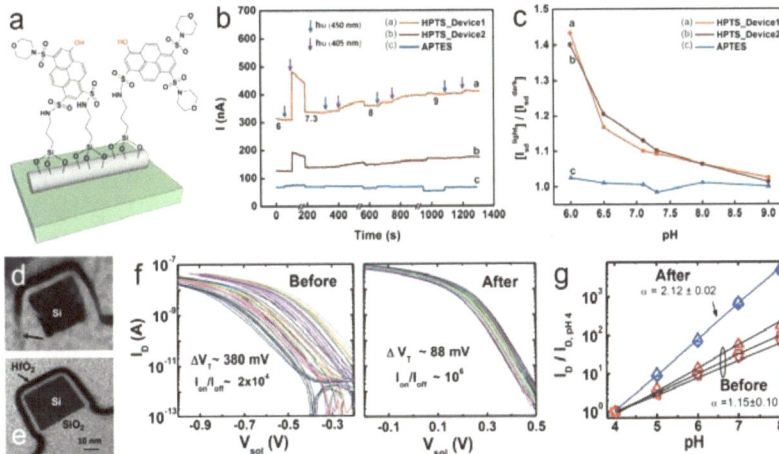

Fig. (4). Minimizing response variations among devices. (a) Schematic diagram of a SiNW modified with (3-aminopropyl)triethoxysilane (APTES) and an activated derivative of the photoactive molecule 1-hydroxypyrene-1,3,6-trisulfonate (HPTS) with exposed phenol functional groups. (b) Real-time pH monitoring using HPTS-modified (traces a and b) and APTES-modified SiNW FETs (trace c) with light irradiation at 405 nm (purple arrows) and 450 nm (blue arrows). (c) Calculated ratio of drain current at illuminated (405 nm) and dark conditions for different pH values measured from HPTS-modified and APTES-modified devices. (d, e) Transmission electron micrograph of SiNW cross-section before and after fabrication improvements, respectively. Part of the HfO_2 gate dielectric is removed in the former (shown by arrow). (f) Measured transfer curves from two device sets (70 FETs per set) corresponding to the before and after fabrication improvements conditions. (g) Measured pH calibration curves for devices fabricated before and after process enhancements. Solid lines indicate exponential curve fit to the data with the exponent represented by α. Panels (a–c) reprinted with permission from [170]; copyright 2013 American Chemical Society. Panels (d–g) reprinted with permission from [69]; copyright 2018 American Chemical Society. Symbols: $h\nu$, photon energy; I, current; I_{sd}, source–drain current; I_D, drain current; V_{sol}, solution-gate voltage; ΔV_T, threshold voltage range; I_{on}/I_{off}, on-current to off-current ratio; α, exponent of the exponential fit.

An electrochemical method was utilized by Mohd Azmi *et al.* [173] using an aryl diazonium linker molecule to selectively functionalize SiNW devices fabricated from SOI wafers by a top–down process. To prepare the SiNWs for chemical grafting, their surfaces were H-terminated *via* RIE in a CHF_3/Ar environment. Cyclic voltammetry was then performed to reduce 4-nitrobenzene diazonium molecules into nitrophenyl radicals, which, in turn, react with the H-terminated silicon atoms, resulting in the covalent attachment of nitrophenyls onto the SiNWs. Another reduction reaction was performed *via* constant-potential amperometry to convert the nitrophenyls into anilines, thereby changing the nitro groups into amine groups. Antibodies against 8-hydroxyguanosine, a biomarker for prostate cancer risk, were then attached to the SiNW surface by reacting their carboxyl groups with the amine groups of the aniline molecules, hence forming an amide bond. Using this functionalization scheme, silicon microwires with 3-µm diameter were used for the detection of 8-hydroxyguanosine in the concentration range of 1 ng/mL to 40 ng/mL. A similar electrochemical method has been employed for the selective functionalization of In_2O_3 nanowires using 4-(2,--dimethoxyphenyl)butyl-phosphonic acid [88]. Upon application of an oxidizing potential, the *p*-dimethoxyphenyl groups are converted to *p*-benzoquinone, which can readily react with thiol and amine groups of biomolecules.

A facile method for selective surface functionalization of SiNWs with the silane linker APTES was introduced recently by Mirsian *et al.* [140]. The procedure involves a combination of oxygen plasma treatment followed by silanization reaction in anhydrous toluene solvent instead of the typical 96% ethanol. With this process, the authors showed that it is possible to selectively functionalize top–down-fabricated SiNW arrays with APTES molecules without modifying the surrounding silicon oxide insulation layer, even without the use of any special chemicals or equipment. They explained that two key mechanisms are responsible for such selective functionalization: First, the oxygen plasma treatment eliminated most of the thin SiO_2 on the SiNWs while retaining the thicker SiO_2 on the substrate. Since silicon is activated by oxygen plasma better than SiO_2 [174], the oxide-free SiNWs are more reactive towards APTES than the surrounding substrate. Second, anhydrous organic solvents result in a preferential APTES growth orthogonal to the surface rather than parallel to it as in the case of APTES monolayer formation due to hydrolysis of ethoxy groups [175]. The selectively modified SiNW devices had a detection limit of 90 pg/mL, compared with 700 pg/mL for the non-selectively modified devices.

Optimization of Antibody Orientation

Aside from limiting the immobilization of receptors on nanowires, sensitivity improvement has been achieved by optimizing the orientation of antibodies immobilized on the nanowires through the use of an external electric field during the immobilization process [143]. This strategy is based on the fact that well-oriented antibodies have high binding affinities with their respective antigens [176]. It was hypothesized that the charge polarity of antibodies in aqueous solutions can be exploited to control their orientation during immobilization through the use of the externally applied electric field. Using CEA-related cell adhesion molecules 1 and 5 (CEACAM1 and CEACAM5) antibodies and atomic force microscopy force–volume mapping, stronger antigen–antibody binding forces were achieved at specific angles of the applied electric field: 135°/180° for CEACAM1 and 225°/270° for CEACAM5. When the same angles of electric field were applied during antibody immobilization on SiNW FETs, larger current changes (more than three-fold) and SNRs (more than two-fold) were obtained for both target antigens, resulting in a limit of detection of 135 pM (21.6 ng/mL) and 100 pM (18 ng/mL) for CEACAM1 and CEACAM5, respectively.

Stability in Aqueous Solutions

Silicon dioxide has been the preferred insulator in silicon-based chips over the years due to its facile controlled growth and stability (at least in air). However, in biosensing applications where it has to be immersed in aqueous solutions, the use of SiO_2 leads to hysteresis and decreased sensitivity due to water absorption that results in the formation of buried sites [177]. In order to mitigate stability issues of SiNW biosensors in fluid environments, Dorvel *et al.* [128] proposed the use of the high-k dielectric hafnium oxide (HfO_2) instead of silicon oxide as a passivation layer for the SiNW. High-*k* dielectrics allow thicker layers to be used while maintaining high capacitance, thereby reducing gate leakage without compromising device sensitivity. Using an optimized atomic layer deposition (ALD) process, HfO_2 was coated on e-beam and wet-etch-defined SiNWs. The resulting devices exhibit stable threshold voltage after the first 10 min, low device intrinsic noise, and low (800-pA), stable leakage current. DNA detection was carried out using HfO_2-coated SiNWs modified with poly-L-lysine and probe DNAs by electrostatic attraction. This non-covalent-bond functionalization results in horizontally lying DNA molecules, which brings the charges closer to the nanowire. Devices modified with lower-molecular-weight poly-L-lysine were able to detect DNA analogs of miR-10b down to 100 fM, with a theoretical detection limit of 1 fM.

SiNW sensors with stacked high-k dielectrics were developed in order to achieve better sensitivity and stability [178]. The 30-nm stack was composed of 5 nm/10 nm/15 nm SiO_2/HfO_2/Al_2O_3 (OHA) layers, where SiO_2 was grown by thermal oxidation and HfO_2 and Al_2O_3 were deposited by ALD. The metal oxides were expected to provide protection against hydration for the SiO_2 layer, with Al_2O_3 placed on top of HfO_2 due to its lower drift and hysteresis. Comparison of the pH sensing performance of the SiNW sensor with OHA thin film and a SiNW sensor with a single 30-nm SiO_2 layer shows higher output currents, higher pH sensitivity, smaller hysteresis, and lower drift for the OHA thin film sensor (Figs. **5a** and **5b**), showing its strong potential for ultrasensitive and stable biosensing.

pH- and Ion-Concentration-Independent Sensing

Despite allowing devices to achieve better sensitivity and stability, high-k dielectrics, such as HfO_2 and Al_2O_3, just as SiO_2, possess hydroxyl groups which make them sensitive to variations in pH and Cl^- ion concentration in the solution [179]. This makes sensing of a particular analyte difficult in a background of changing pH and Cl^- ion concentration. In order to address this issue, Wipf *et al.* [180] proposed the use of a thin gold coating over Al_2O_3-insulated SiNWs configured as liquid-gated FETs. Using the well-known thiol–gold conjugation chemistry, the gold surface was modified with SAMs of Na^+-selective 15-crown-5 ether with a dithiolane moiety (Fig. **5c**). Sensing with functionalized SiNWs and bare-gold SiNWs in solutions of varied pH and different NaCl and KCl concentrations shows that functionalized and bare-gold devices exhibit similar threshold voltage changes in response to pH and [KCl] but different changes in response to [NaCl]. Calculating the differential signal between the functionalized and bare-gold SiNWs results in a response to NaCl of –44 mV/dec and a response to KCl and pH of 0 mV/dec (Fig. **5d**). The unexpected responses of bare-gold SiNWs towards pH, NaCl, and KCl were attributed to the existence of a small number hydroxyl groups on the gold surface. However, these undesirable responses were retained by the functionalized gold-coated SiNWs, unlike functionalized oxide-coated SiNWs [181], thereby allowing its elimination by differential measurement and revealing the desired response towards the target analyte Na^+. The authors propose that this retention of responses towards pH and Cl^- is due to the thiol binding only at non-oxidized gold atoms, which left the hydroxyl groups unmodified (Fig. **5c**).

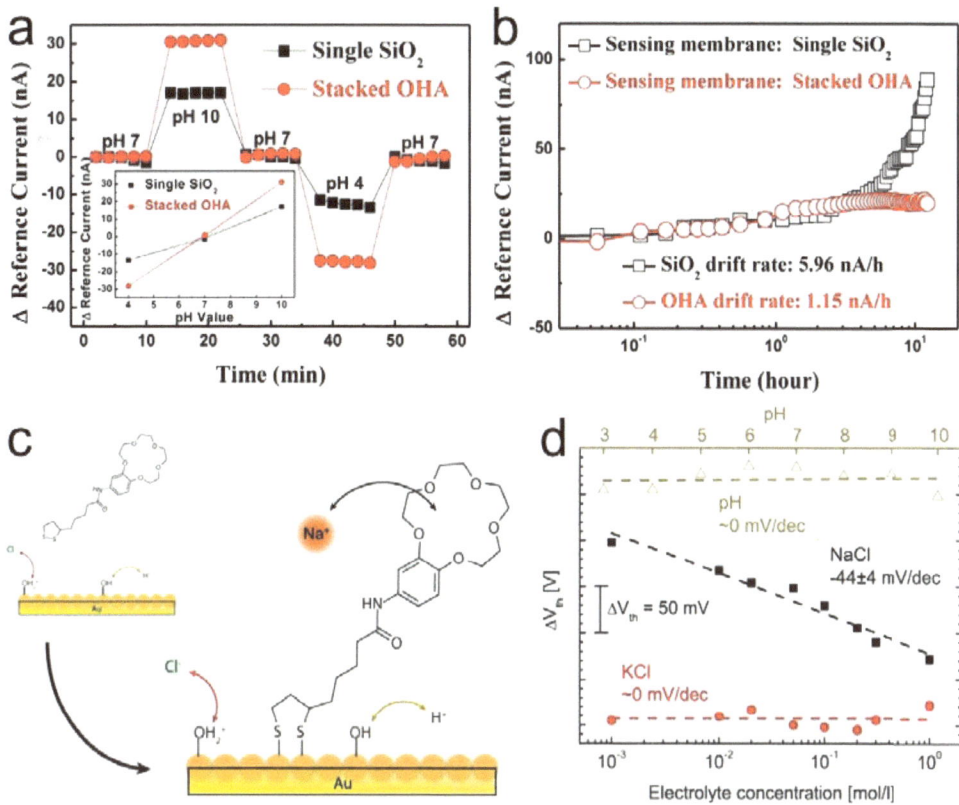

Fig. (5). Coatings for stable sensing in aqueous solutions. (a) Hysteresis of SiNW sensors with SiO_2 and $SiO_2/HfO_2/Al_2O_3$ (OHA) stacked dielectric in the pH cycle of 7-10-7-4-7. The inset shows the width of the hysteresis for the pH cycle. (b) Current drift with time for SiNW sensors with SiO_2 and OHA dielectric layers, measured for 12 h. (c) Proposed immobilization reaction of the sodium-selective crown ether on the SiNW gold coating: the thiol is believed to react only with gold atoms, hence the amount of hydroxyl groups is unchanged. (d) Differential threshold voltage (ΔV_{th}), obtained by subtracting the bare gold V_{th} value from the active 15-crown-5-modified gold V_{th} value, *versus* electrolyte concentration and pH. Panels (a) and (b) reprinted with permission from [178]; copyright 2013 American Chemical Society. Panels (c) and (d) reprinted with permission from [180]; copyright 2013 American Chemical Society.

Reusability

The development of a reusable nanowire biosensor will result not only in cost savings but also in less time and effort expended for surface functionalization and sensor calibration. Although it has been shown in flow measurement systems that antigen–antibody binding is reversible due to its noncovalent nature [28, 94], some target–probe systems are more difficult to reverse due to the relatively stronger bonds involved. DNA and RNA sensors, for instance, require denaturation of the hybridized target–probe strands in order to reuse the device. But such denaturation step usually has some limitations, such as failure to return the signal to the baseline [130] or decreasing sensor responses in subsequent hybridizations [182]. Furthermore, protein dissociation from an antibody by means of chaotic flow and control of ionic strength and pH [183] may be impractical for portable devices and may lead to antibody denaturation.

In order to achieve a reusable SiNW-FET biosensor for protein detection, Lin *et al.* [184] proposed the use of the reversible association–dissociation between glutathione (GSH) and glutathione S-transferase (GST) to reliably regenerate the nanowire surface. For the immobilization of GSH on the SiNW FET, an APTMS SAM was first grafted onto the nanowire, and then a second linker, 3-maleimidobenzoic acid *N*-hydroxysuccinimide ester (MBS), was used to bond GSH to APTMS. They demonstrated that a GSH-modified SiNW device, subsequently modified with GST and a biotin-tagged antibody against GST, shows distinct conductance changes upon exposure to streptavidin. After elution with 10 mM GSH, the SiNW conductance was restored to the pre-GST level, indicating successful detachment of the GST–aGST-biotin–streptavidin complex. Note that, despite the relatively long molecular chain starting from APTMS to the biotin–streptavidin complex (~15 nm), the SiNW could still detect streptavidin in the concentration range of 10–200 nM in $0.1\times$ phosphate solution. In a later study by the same group [48], GST-tagged calmodulin (CaM-GST) was bound to a GSH-modified SiNW FET to obtain a reusable CaM-modified SiNW biosensor capable of detecting cTnI in the range of 10 nM to 1 µM in the presence of Ca^{2+}.

Channel Gating within the Debye Length

As mentioned above, the sensitivity of nanowire biosensors can be enhanced by bringing the charged analyte closer to the nanowire surface. Aside from increasing the electric-field effect from the analyte, shorter distances may also bring the nanowire channel within the Debye length of the target molecule and hence reduce ion screening. The use of aptamers as the biorecognition element is one of the most viable strategies in positioning target biomolecules closer to the sensing surface. Aptamers are single-stranded oligonucleotides (DNA or RNA) or peptides that can bind to different molecules with high affinity and specificity. They are typically 1–2 nm in size, almost ten times smaller than antibodies; hence, they allow binding events to occur much closer to the FET channel [185]. The linker chemistry for binding aptamer probes on the FET surface depends on the available functional groups on the aptamers. In the case of thiolated DNA aptamers [49, 91, 138], a two-molecule linker is usually used (Fig. **6a**): first, an amine-terminated silane monolayer (*e.g.*, APTMS) is formed on the gate oxide; then, MBS is reacted with the amine group to impart maleimide groups to the sensor surface. These maleimide groups, in turn, crosslink with the thiol group of the aptamers, thereby immobilizing the aptamers to the sensor surface. Lee *et al.*

[132] demonstrated the first use of aptamers in SiNW-based sensors, enabling the detection of vascular endothelial growth factor down to 100 pM concentration. Using a DNA aptamer, Li *et al.* [49] was able to detect the small, weakly charged molecule dopamine down to 10 pM level (Fig. **6b**) with excellent selectivity against non-catecholamines and at least 10-fold better binding affinity over catecholamines epinephrine and norepinephrine. The same group [138] also demonstrated the detection of nanomolar levels of the cancer biomarker neuropeptide Y. In a recent study by Nakatsuka *et al.* [91], nanometer-thin In_2O_3 FETs modified with different kinds of DNA aptamers successfully detected small molecules having weak charges (dopamine and serotonin), neutral charge (glucose), or zero net charge (sphingosine-1-phosphate) in full-ionic-strength physiological solutions (*e.g.*, 1× PBS). This significant advancement in FET-based biosensing was enabled by the unique conformational changes of the aptameric stem loop induced by target binding that bring the negative charges of the aptamers closer to or farther from the FET channel, resulting in the modulation of the drain current.

Instead of using aptamers, Ishikawa *et al.* [87] utilized antibody mimic proteins (AMPs) on In_2O_3 NW FETs to detect nucleocapsid protein, a biomarker linked to severe acute respiratory syndrome (SARS). Just like aptamers, AMPs are also relatively small (2–5 nm) and can be engineered/evolved to have high binding affinity and selectivity. In the study, fibronectin-based AMP molecules with peptide sequences specific to nucleocapsid were immobilized on the In_2O_3 NW surface using two linker molecules: first, 6-phosphonohexanoic acid was deposited on the nanowire surface resulting in exposed carboxyl groups; these carboxyl groups were then activated with EDC and reacted with *N*-(--maleimidopropionic acid) hydrazide, resulting in maleimido groups that can then react with the thiol groups of the AMP. The functionalized devices were able to detect nucleocapsid in the concentration range of 0.6 to 10 nM in 0.01× PBS containing 44 μM BSA. Although sensing in high-ionic-strength solutions was not demonstrated, the authors were able to show a detection range comparable with ELISA but with a considerably reduced detection period (≈10 min).

In order to enable the detection of biomolecules in untreated biosamples, Elnathan *et al.* [104] used size-reduced antibody fragments as biorecognition elements in a SiNW FET for the capture proteins closer to the nanowire surface. F(ab')$_2$ and Fab antibody fragments against human cardiac troponin T (cTnT) and cTnI were bound onto the SiNWs *via* their free amine groups (lysine residues) through glutaraldehyde crosslinking with amine-modified nanowire surfaces. Sensing experiments show that F(ab')$_2$- and Fab-modified SiNW FETs show responses to 40 nM cTnT even in 1× PBS (Fig. **6c**). Furthermore, F(ab')$_2$-modified devices are capable of detecting < 0.1 pM of cTnT in undiluted, desalted human serum and >

0.2 nM in untreated, undesalted serum. In order to improve the detection limit in untreated samples, the SiNWs were modified with a lower surface density of F(ab')$_2$ fragments by decreasing the surface coverage of the glutaraldehyde crosslinker. The hypothesis was that well-separated crosslinker and Fab units can bend closer to the nanowire surface under flow conditions. It was found that a moderate surface density of F(ab')$_2$ fragments is able to push the detection limit down to < 2 pM. All experiments were also performed for cTnI, and similar results were obtained.

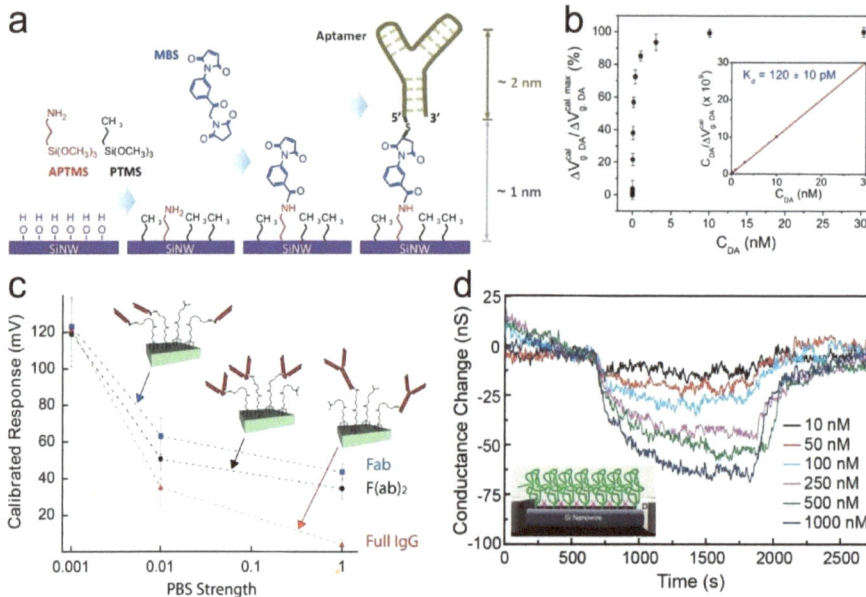

Fig. (6). Overcoming the Debye screening limitation. (a) Scheme for immobilization of aptamer on SiNWs: modification of the hydroxyl-terminated Si surface with (3-aminopropyl)trimethoxysilane (APTMS) (with propyltrimethoxysilane, PTMS, to modulate APTMS density), followed by the second linker molecule 3-maleimidobenzoic acid *N*-hydroxysuccinimide ester (MBS), and then attachment of the thiolated aptamer. (b) Calibration curve for dopamine detection using the calibrated shift in gate voltage ($\Delta V_{g,DA}^{cal}$) normalized to the saturated $\Delta V_{g,DA}^{cal}$ ($\Delta V_{g,DA}^{cal,max}$) as the sensing signal. The inset shows the fitted curve to the Langmuir adsorption isotherm model, giving a dissociation constant $K_d = 120 \pm 10$ pM for the aptamer–dopamine complex. (c) Calibrated response of SiNW-FET devices functionalized with full immunoglobulin G (IgG) antibody or antibody fragments F(ab)$_2$ or Fab against human cardiac troponin T (cTnT) for different ionic strengths of phosphate buffered saline (PBS). Responses were measured for 40 nM cTnT. (d) Real-time signal responses of a SiNW FET modified with (3-aminopropyl)triethoxysilane (APTES) and polyethylene glycol (PEG) to different concentrations of prostate-specific antigen in 100 mM phosphate buffer. The inset shows a schematic diagram for the APTES/PEG-modified SiNW FET with the magenta and green features representing the APTES and the PEG molecules, respectively. Panel (a) adapted with permission from [49]; copyright 2013 American Chemical Society. Panel (b) reprinted with permission from [49]; copyright 2013 American Chemical Society. Panel (c) adapted with permission from [104]; copyright 2012 American Chemical Society. Panel (d) adapted with permission from [186]; copyright 2015 American Chemical Society.

PEGylation to Suppress Debye Screening

The direct detection of biomolecules in physiological samples of high ionic strength is a great challenge for FET-based biosensors due to Debye screening. Although practical workarounds, such as desalting [47] and post-binding washing [105], have been devised to address this issue, these solutions require additional processing steps and preclude real-time detection. A promising approach has been proposed by Gao *et al.* [186] that does not entail complicated sample processing and additional device components. Their solution involves modifying the surface of a SiNW with long-chain silane-PEG (10 kDa) to alter the ionic environment near the SiNW surface and minimize Debye screening. The PEG was mixed in a solution with APTES in a 4:1 APTES/PEG ratio. APTES/PEG-modified SiNW FETs exhibited clear responses to PSA flow for phosphate buffer (PB) solutions with ionic strengths of 10, 50, 100, and 150 mM, whereas APTES-modified devices showed no response to PSA for solutions >10 mM PB. The responses of APTES/PEG-modified SiNW FETs to 100 nM PSA were 44 mV, 40 mV, and 28 mV in PB solutions with ionic strengths of 10 mM (Debye length 2.2 nm), 100 mM (0.67 nm), and 150 mM (0.54 nm), respectively. In 100 mM PB, well-defined responses were demonstrated by the APTES/PEG-modified device for PSA concentrations in the range of 10–1000 nM (Fig. **6d**). Since the physiological ionic strength is 100–200 mM, PEG-modification of nanowire FET biosensors represents a promising approach towards direct biomolecular detection in biological samples. The authors suggested that the increase in effective Debye length is due to the PEG-induced decrease in the dielectric constant near the nanowire surface [187, 188]; however, this is unlikely because the Debye length is directly related to the dielectric constant. Further studies need to be done to fully understand the signal enhancement caused by PEG [189].

Detection Methods

Frequency-Domain Detection

Frequency-domain electrical measurement was proposed as a complement to time-domain measurements using SiNW FETs based on the assumption that biomolecule binding affects the noise frequency spectra more significantly than other noise sources [190]. If this premise holds true, then the biomolecule-binding-associated Lorentzian function should manifest as a graph superimposed to the noise-related $1/f$ curve in the frequency spectrum. Measurements of the voltage noise spectra of anti-PSA-modified SiNWs during PSA flow in equilibrium conditions reveal curves with a distinct Lorentzian shape (*versus* the $1/f$ curve shape for blank solutions) up to 0.15 pM PSA (Figs. **7a** and **7b**), which is lower than the 5-pM detection limit in the time-domain measurement using the same device. Control experiments using the same anti-PSA-modified SiNWs with solutions containing cholera toxin subunit B show similar $1/f$ curves as the blank solutions, indicating that the noise spectra only show Lorentzian-shaped graphs when targeted binding occurs on the devices. Nevertheless, it should be noted that the features of the Lorentzian curves (*e.g.*, characteristic frequency) did not show any correlation with the PSA concentration; hence, the proposed frequency-domain detection only gives qualitative information about the target analyte.

Random Telegraph Signals

Highly miniaturized electronic devices such as those consisting of nanowires exhibit RTS noise, which is caused by the discrete switching of the device current due to random trapping and de-trapping of charge carriers in defect sites of the oxide near the nanowire channel [191, 192] (see Noise section above). The switching of the current between two levels is characterized by two time constants: the capture time constant τ_c, which is the average time a carrier spends in the free state before being captured in a trap, and the emission time constant τ_e, which is the average time a carrier spends in the captured state before being released from the trap. Due to the strong dependence of the capture time on the drain current [111], Li *et al.* [193] conjectured that the RTSs—usually deemed undesirable in electronic applications—can be exploited as a source of information in SiNW-FET-based biosensing. Using pH sensing as a test, they obtained the current spectral density (Fig. **7c**) and the time trace of the current switching (Fig. **7d**) at different pH values. From the spectra, the characteristic frequency f_0 of the Lorentzian curve can be obtained. From the time trace, a histogram of the current change was constructed from which two peaks can be seen, one for the free state count c_f and another for the captured state count c_c. Since $c_f/c_c = \tau_c/\tau_e$ for a given time trace, and since $f_0 = (2\pi\tau)^{-1}$, the values of τ_c and τ_e can be calculated from the relation $\tau = \tau_c\tau_e/(\tau_c + \tau_e)$. It was observed that τ_c is very sensitive to pH, while τ_e is only weakly dependent on it. In the pH range of 5.5 to 8.5, τ_c shows a 7.4-factor change, while the drain current only shows a 1.96-factor change (Fig. **7e**), demonstrating that detecting surface potential changes using RTSs results in higher sensitivity. The observation that $\tau_c \propto$ (drain current)$^{-3}$ was attributed to the Coulomb blockade effect [111, 192].

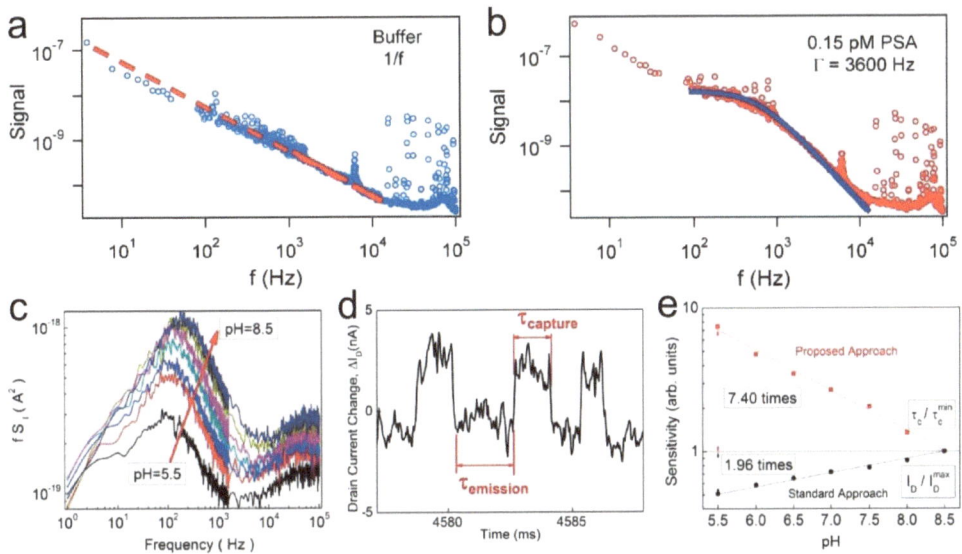

Fig. (7). Signal fluctuations as information source. (a) Power spectral density of voltage (blue circles) of a SiNW FET sensor modified with antibodies against prostate-specific antigen (PSA) in buffer solution showing a $1/f$ frequency dependence (red dashed line). (b) Power spectrum (red circles) of the same SiNW FET in a solution with 0.15 pM PSA showing a Lorentzian-shaped curve (blue line) with a characteristic frequency (Γ) of 3600 Hz. The unit for the y-axis in (a) and (b) is V^2/Hz. (c) Power spectral density of drain current of a SiNW FET multiplied by frequency at different pH values. (d) Random telegraph signals in a SiNW FET at pH 7.5 showing signal levels corresponding to the time spent by a carrier in the free state before capture by a trap in the gate dielectric, $\tau_{capture}$ or τ_c, and the time spent by a carrier in the captured state, $\tau_{emission}$ or τ_e. (e) Sensitivities towards pH calculated from the normalized τ_c and drain current I_D. Panels (a) and (b) reprinted with permission from [190]; copyright 2010 American Chemical Society. Panels (c–e) reprinted with permission from [193]; copyright 2014 American Chemical Society.

Antigen–Antibody Dissociation

A unique but simple detection method was proposed by Krivitsky *et al.* [139] to enable the real-time detection of antigens from complex, untreated samples in microfluidic systems. The analytical detection is carried out during the antigen–antibody dissociation temporal regime, after the target protein has bound to a high-affinity antibody immobilized on a SiNW FET and interfering chemical species have been flushed out from the sensing area using a low-ionic-strength "sensing" buffer. Due to the differing dissociation rates of the target antigen and the nonspecific species, the dissociation time window can be split into a transient fast-dissociation subregime due to the nonspecific species and a plateau-like slow-dissociation subregime attributed to the target biomolecules. For this method to be applicable in quantitative analyte measurements, however, three conditions must be met: (1) the dissociation kinetics of the antigen and the interfering entities must be sufficiently different; (2) ample time must be given for the antigen to bind to the antibody during the association regime; and (3) the fast and slow dissociation subregimes must be accurately delineated. The first requirement of a high-affinity antibody can be eased by using faster flow rates or fluid velocities, such that the nonspecific dissociation rate is effectively increased. The second condition can be satisfied by waiting for the device response to plateau in time before starting the flushing process. Nevertheless, the third condition is relatively difficult and impractical due to the requirement of an antigen-free reference sample. As a workaround, the authors included reference SiNW FETs modified with nonspecific proteins on the same microfluidic chip as the antibody-modified SiNW FETs to allow the simple delineation of the two dissociation subregimes during a single flow of the untreated, antigen-containing biosample. Using this proposed detection method, Krivitsky *et al.* were able to detect cancer antigen 15-3 in unprocessed serum samples in physiologically relevant concentrations. It is worth noting that the proposed method is quite different from the post-capture washing earlier proposed [105] in that the capture and washing steps are all integrated into a single microfluidic platform and that the detection window is optimally determined from the association and dissociation kinetics of the chemical species involved. This allows real-time detection without *ex situ* sample manipulation and with greatly shortened detection times (few minutes *versus* 45 min [105]).

Signal Amplification

Choi *et al.* [93] proposed a cleavage-based mechanism for the SiNW-FET biosensing of matrix-metalloproteinase-2 (MMP-2), a biomarker for different types of cancer, using negatively charged DNA–AuNP complexes coupled with a MMP-2-cleavable peptide sequence. When MMP-2 interacts with the peptide, the DNA–AuNP detaches from the SiNW, resulting in a large conductance change, which is at least 10-fold greater compared with the use of only the peptide sequence. Such large signal change was possible because the amount of negative charges contained in the DNA–AuNP complexes is considerably higher than that of the peptide sequence. Using this approach, the authors were able to achieve a detection sensitivity of 100 fM and a response time of 13 s. Aside from signal amplification, this cleavage-based detection scheme is advantageous because it eliminates the need for antibodies, which are costly and easily denatured; however, it only applies to analytes with the capability of inducing a detachment event upon reaction with the biorecognition molecule.

Gao *et al.* [129] approached the challenge of improving the detection limit in DNA sensing by drastically increasing the measured signal and thus the SNR of SiNW devices. To achieve this, they used the rolling circle amplification (RCA) technique, performed in two steps (Fig. **8a**): first, in a single step, target DNA is hybridized with the capture probe and the RCA primer, and then the primer is hybridized with the RCA template; second, the amplification reaction is carried out at room temperature by addition of Phi29 DNA polymerase and deoxynucleotides. The result of the RCA reaction is a long single-stranded DNA (ssDNA) attached to the target DNA molecules. This ssDNA contains a negatively charged phosphate backbone, thereby increasing the gating effect of the negative charges already present in the target DNA. RCA reaction after the capture of different concentrations of hepatitis B virus DNA resulted in nearly 100% increase in signal (Fig. **8b**) with a calculated SNR > 20 for 1-fM DNA after 700 s reaction time. The theoretical detection floor is thus 50 aM. Non-complementary and one-base-mismatched DNA resulted in considerably smaller signal change compared with the fully complementary target DNA.

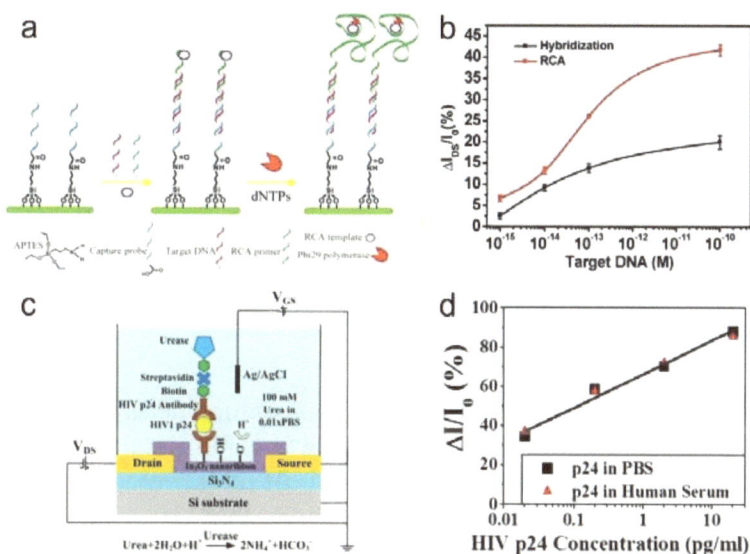

Fig. (8). Signal amplification to improve detection limits. (a) SiNW-based DNA detection with rolling circle amplification (RCA): The target DNA is captured by a DNA probe, which is immobilized on the SiNW by (3-aminopropyl)triethoxysilane (APTES). At the same time, hybridization of the RCA primer is carried out, followed by hybridization of the RCA template. Finally, addition of Phi29 polymerase with the deoxynucleotides attaches a long single-stranded DNA. (b) Change in drain–source current (I_{DS}) normalized to the initial current (I_0) corresponding to the hepatitis B virus DNA concentration for non-amplified detection and the RCA-amplified detection process shown in (a). (c) Schematic diagram of electronic enzyme-linked immunosorbent assay (ELISA) for the detection of human immunodeficiency virus type 1 (HIV1) p24 antigen using a top–down-fabricated In_2O_3 nanoribbon FET. The urea–urease enzyme reaction consumes hydrogen ions in the solution, causing a change in the pH, which can be detected by the FET. (d) Normalized current responses to different p24 concentrations in phosphate buffered saline (PBS) and in human serum facilitated by the electronic ELISA scheme shown in (c). Panels (a) and (b) adapted with permission from [129]; copyright 2013 American Chemical Society. Panels (c) and (d) reprinted with permission from [194]; copyright 2015 American Chemical Society.

Similar to the RCA technique for DNA detection, the method proposed by Aroonyadet *et al.* [194] aims to amplify the sensing signal during protein detection to enhance the effective sensitivity of the device. The idea is to use electronic ELISA based on urease enzyme activity to induce large pH changes in the solution that can be detected by pH-sensitive nano-FETs. The authors employed 20-nm-thick, amorphous In_2O_3 nanoribbon FETs fabricated using a CMOS-compatible top–down approach. The ELISA-based sensing was demonstrated on the detection of the p24 protein, a biomarker for human immunodeficiency virus type 1 infection. After the capture of the p24 antigen on antibody-functionalized devices, biotinylated secondary antibodies were bound to the p24 antigen followed by the attachment of streptavidin. Then, biotinylated urease enzyme was attached to the complex. Upon introduction of urea, urease catalyzes its hydrolysis, consuming hydrogen ions and decreasing the solution pH in the process (Fig. **8c**). Using this detection scheme, p24 was detected in the concentration range of 20 fg/mL (~250 viruses/mL) to 20 pg/mL in a starting solution of 1× PBS or human serum (Fig. **8d**), with a projected detection limit of 200 ag/mL. However, it must be noted that such sensitivity was attained with intermediate washing steps and final detection in urea solution (probably in a buffer of low ionic strength).

Towards Real-World POCT Applications

Sample Filtration and Purification

The complex composition of biosamples, such as blood serum, cell extracts, and urine, poses a great challenge in direct sensing with biological solutions. Blood, for example, can contain around 60–85 mg/mL of total protein with over 10,000 protein species in concentrations spanning more than 10 orders of magnitude [104]. With the target protein present in concentrations 10–11 orders of magnitude lower than other charged proteins in the blood, there is a great deal of background noise present, masking the signal from the low-concentration protein of interest [104]. Furthermore, biofouling due to non-specific binding of proteins on the active surface will severely degrade the selectivity and sensitivity of biosensors. Consequently, biomolecular separation and purification techniques are almost always required with any bioanalytical technique employing biosamples.

To address the complexity of detecting biomarkers in whole blood, Chang *et al.* [53] proposed a system with a simple custom-made microfilter that can be used with finger-prick blood (Fig. **9a**). The microfilter is coupled to an In_2O_3 nanowire biosensor which performs biomarker detection. The microfilter has a polycarbonate membrane with 400-nm pores, which filters out blood cells from 500 μL of clotted blood. In order to prevent signal loss due to nonspecific binding in diluted serum, antibody-functionalized nanowires were passivated with Tween 20. The feasibility of the biosensing system was demonstrated by detecting cancer antigen 125 (CA-125) and insulin growth factor II (IGF-II), which are biomarkers for epithelial ovarian cancer. In order to avoid Debye screening, the quasi-serum filtrate was diluted 100× (final ionic strength of 1.5 mM) before spiking it with CA-125. On the other hand, the quasi-serum filtrate was passed through a portable gravity desalting column before spiking it with IGF-II. The detection limit achieved with these methods were 0.1 U/mL for CA-125 (10 U/mL before dilution) (Fig. **9b**) and 8 ng/mL for IGF-II.

Stern *et al.* [195] proposed a two-stage device where the sensor, a Si nanoribbon FET, is separate from an upstream microfluidic purification chip (MPC), which in turn extracts and pre-concentrates target biomarkers from the blood. This compartmental design enhances the performance of the FET sensor by preventing biofouling and non-specific adsorption on the sensor surface, decreasing the required detection limit due to pre-concentration of the analyte, and obviating the Debye length screening issue by using a low-salt buffer (1 mM bicarbonate buffer) for detection. The main component of the MPC are the photocleavable crosslinkers which can be conjugated to primary antibodies *via* their amino group and bound to an avidin-functionalized MPC *via* their biotin group. After capturing biomarkers from the blood, the MPC is perfused with wash and sensing buffers. UV light irradiation releases the biomarker–antibody complex into the sensing buffer for subsequent binding with the secondary antibodies on the FET sensors downstream. Using the Si nanoribbon FETs, cancer antigens PSA and carbohydrate antigen 15.3 (CA15.3) were detected from 10 μL MPC-purified, spiked blood samples at concentrations as low as 2.0 ng/mL for PSA and 15 U/mL for CA15.3. The entire process takes less than 20 min.

A similar concept was proposed by Krivitsky *et al.* [183], except that the purification compartment is composed of vertically aligned SiNW arrays modified with the required antibody receptors. The SiNW arrays were fabricated using silver-assisted chemical etching with nanosphere lithography, resulting in highly porous nanowires for greatly increased effective surface area for the capture of biomolecules (Fig. **9c**). As with the device of Stern *et al.* [195], the SiNW-array purification unit also performs the functions of filtering (*i.e.*, removal of cellular components), protein separation and preconcentration, and desalting. However, it is simpler because photocleavable crosslinkers are not used and the same type of antibodies can be used in both purification and sensing compartments. Proteins captured by antibodies are released simply by making use of chaotic elution and by choosing the right antibody and solution ionic strength and pH. The preconcentrated proteins are released in a low-ionic-strength buffer and detected at a downstream SiNW sensor integrated in the same platform (Fig. **9d**).

Measurements using blood samples spiked with cTnT show successful detection below picomolar levels (Fig. **9e**) with a total assay time not exceeding 10 min.

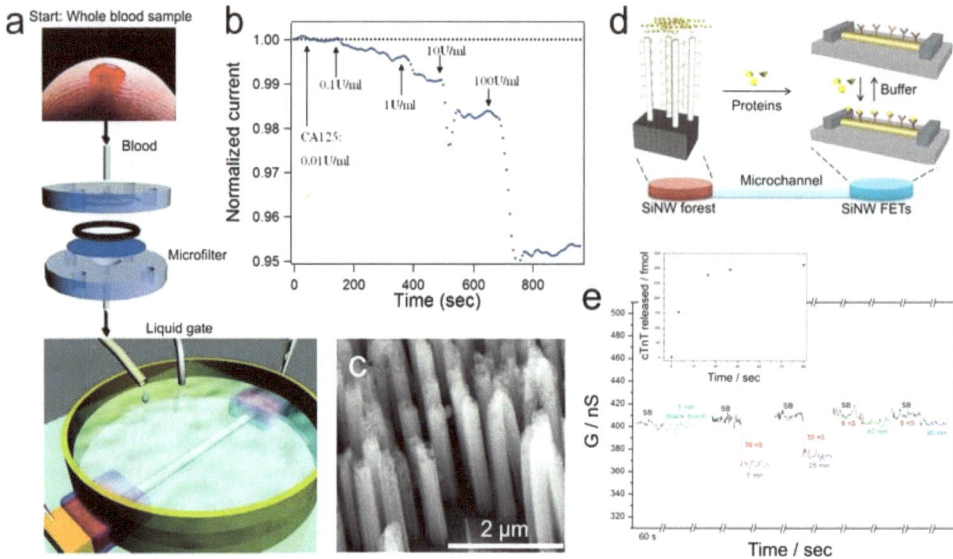

Fig. (9). Purification of blood samples for biosensing. (a) Schematic diagram of a system for whole-blood biomarker detection consisting of a microfilter for sample processing, a mixing cell for sample delivery, and an In_2O_3 nanowire device for biosensing. (b) Real-time sensing of cancer antigen 125 (CA125) in filtered, 100× diluted whole blood using the detection system in (a). (c) Scanning electron micrograph of vertically aligned porous SiNW arrays ("SiNW forest") for separation of biomarkers from whole blood. (d) Schematic diagram of a single-chip platform for whole-blood biomarker detection based on a SiNW-forest sample processing compartment and a SiNW-FET biosensing chamber. (e) Real-time detection of cardiac troponin T (cTnT) in spiked blood samples using the operation scheme shown in (d). Solutions alternated between blank sensing buffer (SB, 150 µM phosphate buffer) and cTnT-loaded SB from the elution. The inset shows the amount of cTnT released from the SiNW forest compartment as a function of elution time, which was subsequently detected by the SiNW FETs. Panels (a) and (b) reprinted with permission from [53]; copyright 2011 American Chemical Society. Panel (c) adapted with permission from [183]; copyright 2012 American Chemical Society. Panels (d) and (e) reprinted with permission from [183]; copyright 2012 American Chemical Society.

Zhang *et al.* [105] proposed a blood filtration chip and SiNW sensor chip that are integrated back-to-back in a single chip without any connecting tubes. The filter chip is designed to accept finger-prick blood and contains a pillar gap microstructure (< 0.8 µm), which removes the cell components from the blood *via* cross-flow filtration. As a proof-of-concept, a solution consisting of 2 µL of blood mixed and 198 µL of 1× PBS and spiked with either the cardiac biomarker cTnT, creatine kinase MM (CK-MM), or creatine kinase MB (CK-MB) was flowed through the filtration chip and onto the sensor chip surface. Sensing carried out in pure PBS buffer by differently modified SiNW devices allowed the specific detection of the biomarkers down to 1 pg/mL. The whole process took 45 min to complete.

Droplet Microfluidics

As pointed out in the previous section, microscale fluidic systems are important for handling and processing small volumes of biological samples so that analyte detection can be performed accurately by nanoscale biosensors. A notable advancement in microfluidic systems is the development of droplet-based or digital microfluidics, which allows liquid samples to be handled in isolated nano- to femtoliter droplets for parallel, precise, and automated operations [196]. Schütt et al. [147] demonstrated the integration of SiNW FET sensors in a microfluidic platform with water-in-oil emulsion droplets. Using droplet volumes of 1–10 nL, the authors found that droplet plugs with lengths slightly larger than the NW sensor are necessary to minimize the influence of oil–water interfaces in the sensor responses and to effectively probe the inner droplet environment. Droplets with pH values from 4 to 8 and different ionic concentrations resulted in sensor responses with good SNR, albeit with lower-than-expected sensitivity due to the formation of an oil film on the nanowire surface, which results in a weaker gate coupling. In order to test the system's feasibility for real-world biosensing applications, glucose detection was performed in droplets containing the enzyme glucose oxidase, which catalyzes the oxidation of glucose and results in a concomitant increase in pH. Obvious signal responses were observed in the glucose concentrations of 0, 0.5, 0.75, and 1 mM, demonstrating the promise of the nanowire sensor/droplet microfluidics platform for high-throughput bioassays.

Readout Systems

To achieve simple, fast, and simultaneous detection of multiple biomarkers in a portable format, Zhang et al. [68] designed an application-specific integrated circuit (ASIC)-based readout system for use with SiNW biosensors. The readout circuit makes use of a conventional resistance-to-frequency converter composed of a SiNW switch array, a current integrator, a comparator, and a ring voltage-controlled oscillator. The SiNW chip is placed on a "test jig," which is separate from the readout board and is connected to the latter *via* ribbon cables. This setup enables the realization of a more cost-effective design as the SiNW chip can be disposed of independent of the readout module. Detection of cardiac biomarkers in serum is performed as follows: first, the resistance of the antibody-modified SiNW is measured in 0.01× PBS; then, the SiNW devices are incubated with the serum sample; the devices are washed with 1× PBS to remove unbound proteins; finally, resistance measurements are performed in 0.01× PBS. Using this protocol with the readout ASIC, the biomarkers cTnT, CK-MB, and CK-MM were detected in the concentration range of 100 fg/mL to 1 ng/mL.

Yen *et al.* [135] presented a biosensor chip wherein the SiNW devices are fully integrated with other electronic modules, which include a microcontroller, a low-noise analog front-end circuit, a 10-bit analog-to-digital converter (ADC), a temperature sensor, and an on-off-key wireless transceiver. Although the system on chip does not feature multiplexed detection capabilities and the sensor cannot be independently disposed of, the chip's fully integrated design makes it more suitable in applications where portability is important. Each chip contains four SiNW devices, which are connected as resistors in a full Wheatstone bridge configuration to minimize the effects of external noise and fabrication process variations. Only two devices, which are located in one branch each and diagonally across each other, have their nanowires exposed to the sensing environment, while the other two function as reference resistors. The SiNW biosensors employ a unique bottom-gate-induced enhancement of target analyte binding. Unlike typical back-gated SiNW-FET configurations, where the back-gate potential is applied at the back of the Si wafer, the proposed design consists of a degenerately doped poly-Si as the bottom-gate under a lightly doped poly-SiNW, with an intervening 120-nm-thick oxide layer in between. The sensing protocol consists of first measuring the baseline signal in 0.01× PBS without a bottom-gate potential, and then binding of the target protein in serum with an applied bottom-gate potential, followed by washing and measuring the response signal in 0.01× PBS without a bottom-gate potential. This sensing scheme enabled the detection of cTnI biomarker in the range of 320 fM to 320 pM (or 7.6 pg/ml to 7.6 ng/ml).

A portable, battery-powered, handheld device capable of reading signals from a disposable SiNW-based biosensor card was developed by Mohd Azmi *et al.* [173]. The handheld device contains an electronic readout system consisting of a data acquisition circuit, a microcontroller with an internal 10-bit ADC, and a liquid-crystal display screen. The PIC-based microcontroller measures the resistance of the SiNWs *via* a voltage divider circuit and creates the display graphics. The device is also equipped with a battery-check mechanism to ensure that there is ample power for accurate biosensor characterization. The biosensor card comprises a copper board on which the SiNW chip is wire-bonded and connects to the handheld device *via* pressure contacts. The authors reported that qualitative detection of a biomarker can be performed by the readout system by comparing the SiNW resistance before and after analyte binding, although actual, validated readings from the handheld device were not shown.

Preliminary Clinical Validation

Testing nanowire biosensors on biological samples from actual patients is an important validation process towards the commercialization of the technology and its application in real-life medical diagnosis. Using poly-SiNW FETs modified with magnetic graphene loaded with antibody capture elements, Chen *et al.* [137] differentiated patients with bladder cancer from age-matched patients with hernia by detecting the protein biomarker apolipoprotein A II from urine samples. The urine samples were first cleared of cells and debris by centrifugation before introducing them to the sensing devices. In order to avoid the Debye screening problem and eliminate interfering species, the urine sample was removed from the device after target binding, and then thorough washing was performed. Measurement was performed in 0.5 mM PBS. It was found that the concentration of apolipoprotein A II in bladder cancer patients (late and advanced stage) is 29–344 ng/mL, which is significantly higher than the concentration of 0.425–9.47 ng/mL measured from hernia patients. The measured protein levels were also consistent with the results from a commercial human apolipoprotein immunoassay based on fluorescence detection.

Tran *et al.* [65] applied their SiNW FETs in the detection of circulating tumor cells (CTCs) in a stage IIIB colorectal cancer patient *via* the sensing of cytokeratin-19 from lysed blood mononuclear cells. Peripheral blood mononuclear cells were first isolated from the blood sample obtained from the patient and a healthy subject. Using imaging flow cytometry, the presence and absence of CTCs in patient blood and healthy blood, respectively, were confirmed. A total of 16 CTCs were detected in 4 mL of patient blood. The purified lysate used in the FET detection was obtained using a two-step lysing/extraction protocol: isolated mononuclear cells were ultrasonicated in a lysing buffer and centrifuged to precipitate the keratin proteins; the precipitates were then dissolved in a keratin solubilizing buffer containing urea and briefly ultrasonicated. The prepared samples were incubated with the antibody-functionalized SiNW devices. Then, as with the above study, the devices were thoroughly washed with PBS. Measurements were then performed in 0.01× PBS. The modified devices showed an average conductance increase of 8.9% for the patient blood sample, which is significantly different to the mean conductance increase of 2.9% for the healthy blood sample. Meanwhile, unmodified devices showed less than 2% conductance change in response to both samples.

A simple demonstration of real-time detection of the liver cancer biomarker alpha-fetoprotein in the serum of a liver carcinoma patient was performed by Ra *et al.* [144]. They used ZnO nanowire FETs, wherein the nanowire was coated with a polymer-like amorphous carbon for stability of the ZnO nanowire in aqueous solutions. By performing an NH_3 plasma treatment step, the polymer sheath was modified with amine groups for conjugation with the antibody. Serum samples were first diluted ten times with 10 mM PBS to increase the Debye length. Reproducible signal changes were exhibited by antibody-functionalized devices when serum and PBS were alternately flowed through the nanowire biosensor. On the other hand, no significant signal changes were seen from the bare devices for alternate flows of PBS and dilute patient serum.

Aside from the three studies above which used blood and urine as samples, a number of research groups working on diagnosis *via* exhaled breath have also utilized samples from human subjects to validate the diagnostic performance of their devices. The studies of some of these groups are discussed in the next section.

Breath Condensate and Gas-Phase Detection

Virus Detection from Breath Condensate

Disease diagnosis using exhaled breath condensate (EBC) is very attractive because it is fully noninvasive and the samples are easy to collect. Using EBC samples with SiNW biosensors, Shen *et al.* [145] demonstrated sensitive and selective detection of influenza A virus H3N2 within a few minutes. EBC collection was performed using a custom-made device with an ultralow-temperature-treated hydrophobic film. The collected EBC samples were diluted 100-fold in order to prevent signals due to impurities, such as chemicals and other microorganisms. Sensing with virus-spiked EBC shows that virus-antibody-modified SiNW devices exhibit conductance changes directly related to the viral load, with a lower limit of 170 viruses/μL. Tests with human subjects showing onset flu symptoms reveal that, in 90% of the cases, the positive/negative results of SiNW devices were consistent with the positive/negative results of quantitative reverse transcription polymerase chain reaction (RT-qPCR). With the total time from EBC collection to test results taking only 2 min, the SiNW-based sensor is shown to be ideal for rapid diagnosis of respiratory viral infections.

Gas Sensor with Decoupled Gas-Sensitive Medium

SiNW-based sensors have been applied to the detection of various gaseous molecules, including nitrogen oxide (NO) and ammonia (NH_3) [197], which can serve as biomarkers of asthma and liver dysfunction, respectively. In these sensors, the detection mechanism is based on a doping/de-doping effect caused by the donation or extraction of electrons to/from the channel by the reducing or oxidizing target gases. Many of the SiNW-based sensors configured as FETs were used bare [34, 198, 199]. This means that the SiNW serves as both the chemically reactive material and transducing component, which could lead to electrical stress and changes in electrical properties with time, as observed in one study [199]. The same can be said of metal-oxide chemiresistors for gas sensing [151]. In order to avoid electrical-stress-related baseline drift in gas sensors, Han *et al.* [151] proposed a FET-based gas sensor with a gas-sensitive region decoupled from the transistor channel. The chemically reactive material consists of a tin oxide (SnO_2) thin film, while the channel is made of silicon with a nanowire-honeycomb structure. Here, changes in the carrier concentration of the SnO_2 due to oxidation/reduction by gas molecules alter the film's extent of polarization with respect to the SiNW channel, hence modulating its electric-field gating effect. Since the bias (drain–source) voltage is only applied to the SiNW channel, the SnO_2 sensing film is not subjected to electrical stress. On the other hand, since the SiNW does not participate in charge-transfer reactions, a smaller bias voltage can be used, which means lower electrical stress, as well. The sensitivity of the SnO_2/SiNW FET towards NO was found to be two orders of magnitude greater than that of a SnO_2 chemiresistor because the FET was operated in the subthreshold region. Due to the lower electrical stress, no current drift was observed from the FET over a period of $\approx$30 hours. Another advantage of the proposed device is its normally-off operation due to the complementary doping of the SiNW and the source/drain terminals. This has two consequences: first, considerable current only flows in the presence of a reactive gas, resulting in very low total power consumption; second, the device only responds to either oxidizing gases or reducing gases, providing a level of selectivity even without any pattern recognition schemes.

Sensing Volatile Organic Compounds

Nonpolar breath VOCs, such as hexane, decane, and octane, can serve as useful biomarkers of various diseases, including cancer and neurodegenerative diseases [200]. However, SiNW FET sensors suffer low sensitivity towards nonpolar VOCs due mainly to poor functionalization coverage of the SiO_2 surface and lack of suitable surface-modification molecules [149]. Haick's group [149] approached this problem by modifying the SiNW surface with dense, hydrophobic, organic hexyltrichlorosilane (HTS) for passivation of the surface trap states at the air/SiO_2 interface. Nonpolar VOCs (hexane, octane, decane), polar VOCs (ethanol, butanol, hexanol), and water caused distinct changes in the conductivity of the HTS-modified SiNWs: nonpolar VOCs decreased the SiNW conductivity at high positive gate voltages; polar VOCs increased the conductivity of the SiNW at high negative voltages; and, water decreased the SiNW conductivity at high negative voltages. Using quartz crystal microbalance and spectroscopic ellipsometry, the authors concluded that the modulation of SiNW conductivity by the nonpolar VOCs is due to two indirect molecular gating effects [38]: (1) changes in the charged surface states at the SiO_2/monolayer interface owing to changes in the conformation of the HTS monolayer; and (2) changes in the dielectric near the SiNW surface due to condensation of the VOCs.

In two related studies from the same group [39, 201], the effects of the functional group and chain length of the organic monolayer surface modification on the sensing performance of SiNW FETs were investigated. It was found that larger changes in threshold voltage could be achieved for longer chain lengths of the molecular monolayer due to the greater number of adsorbed VOC molecules on the SiNW surface [201]. On the other hand, the functional group of the monolayer has a more significant effect on the shift direction of the threshold voltage compared with the chain length [39, 201]. In both studies, SiNW FETs modified with polar molecular layers exhibit responses toward both polar and nonpolar VOCs in a concentration-dependent manner [39, 201]. To be of any practical use, however, the SiNW devices should be able to discriminate among the different VOCs. Hence, Haick's group [202] applied discriminant function analysis (DFA) with leave-one-out cross-validation to determine the discriminative ability of differently modified SiNW FETs towards polar and nonpolar VOCs with a background of realistic humidity. They used nine different molecules to functionalize the SiNWs separately (resulting in nine unique sensors) and analyzed the signals using changes in three FET parameters, namely, threshold voltage, carrier mobility, and on current. While individual sensors were not sufficiently selective, combinations of the sensors were able to demonstrate accurate discrimination among the VOCs: all ten sensors (including the unmodified sensor) can differentiate between polar and nonpolar VOCs with 94% accuracy; specific subsets of sensors (*e.g.*, having different end groups or having different chain lengths) can discriminate among alcohols and among nonpolar VOCs with 100% and 83% accuracy, respectively; and all ten sensors can identify each VOC correctly from the pool of 12 VOCs with at least 83% accuracy. These results point to the possibility of using these sensors in concert for a VOC olfactory sensing system.

Artificial Intelligence

In order to demonstrate the feasibility of using SiNW FETs for real-world sensing of VOCs, Haick's group [150] utilized machine learning, specifically artificial neural network (ANN) models, with seven SiNW FET devices having different SAM modifications (Fig. **10a**) to try to identify and quantify eleven selected VOCs, five of which (hexane, octane, decane, ethanol, cyclohexanone) are known cancer biomarkers in the breath volatilome. The ANN models used were feed-forward multilayer perceptrons with input, hidden, and output layers [203] (Fig. **10b**). Four independent sensing parameters of the SiNW-FET devices—threshold voltage, hole mobility, on current, and subthreshold swing—were used as the input nodes, while the eleven VOCs were assigned at the output layer as dependent vectors in a ten-dimensional space. The goal was to use the unique combinations of parameter values as a fingerprint to discriminate among the various VOCs. The sigmoid function and the trainBR function were used as the ANN transfer function and training function, respectively. Using a learning data set obtained from sensing experiments, the model for each SiNW FET was trained and optimized. Based on the results obtained from the verification data set, four of the seven SiNW FETs are able to identify all the VOCs, with the device having a COOH functional group being the most accurate (Fig. **10c**). Moreover, the latter device was also shown to be able to differentiate among two- and three-component VOC mixtures. For the quantification of the VOCs, the same ANN models were used, except that the output layer represents the various VOC concentrations (VOC partial pressure/total pressure = 0.01, 0.02, 0.04, and 0.08). Optimization of the models was carried out using an experimental design based on the Box–Wilson central composite design (2^4 + star points) and a parameter selection based on the least mean prediction error. Optimization results show that each VOC has at least one SiNW FET with a mean prediction error < 10%; thus, it is possible to estimate the VOC concentration using a single molecularly modified SiNW FET device in conjunction with an ANN model.

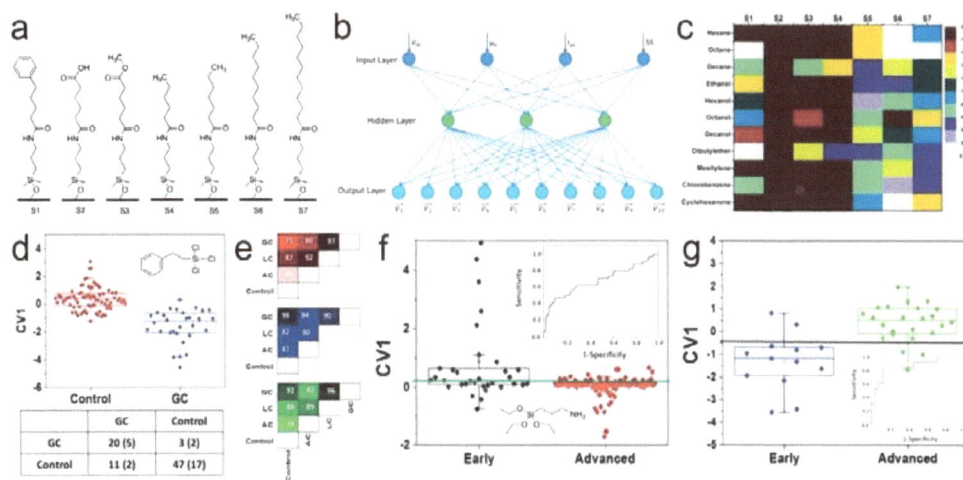

Fig. (10). Towards disease diagnosis *via* exhaled breath. (a) Examples of molecular layers for SiNW FET modification to obtain seven different sensors (S1–S7) for the detection of volatile organic compounds (VOCs): S1, 5-phenylvaleric chloride ($C_{11}H_{13}ClO$); S2, 1,4-butanedicarbonyl chloride ($C_6H_8Cl_2O_2$; acyl chloride group hydrolyzed during preparation); S3, methyl adipoyl chloride ($C_7H_{11}ClO_3$); S4, hexanoyl chloride ($C_6H_{11}ClO$); S5, heptanoyl chloride ($C_7H_{13}ClO$); S6, decanoyl chloride ($C_{10}H_{19}ClO$); and S7, dodecanoyl chloride ($C_{12}H_{23}ClO$). (b) Schematic diagram of an artificial neural network (ANN) model with three layers (input, hidden, and output) for identification of VOCs. (c) Heat map of the logarithm Euclidean distance at a VOC concentration of 0.08 (VOC partial pressure/total pressure). This Euclidean distance is the distance between the target vector and prediction vector and describes the recognition power of the sensors. (d) First canonical variable 1 (CV1) values from discriminant function analysis (DFA) of sensor data and classification confusion matrix from leave-one-out cross-validation for the control group *versus* gastric cancer (GC) group. Pattern recognition was carried out using breath analysis data from trichloro(phenethyl)silane (TPS)-modified SiNW FET devices. Values in brackets were obtained using blind analysis (test data set). (e)

Calculated sensitivity (red), specificity (blue), and accuracy (green) using leave-one-out cross-validation for binary comparisons between GC, lung cancer (LC), asthma and chronic obstructive pulmonary disease (AC), and control groups, classified using an ANN model. Breath analysis data were obtained using TPS-modified SiNW FETs. (f, g) CV1 values from DFA for stage classification of LC and GC, respectively. Data were obtained using (3-aminopropyl)triethoxysilane-modified SiNW FETs. The insets show receiver operating characteristic curves. Panels (a–c) reprinted with permission from [150]; copyright 2014 American Chemical Society. Panel (d) adapted with permission from [152]; copyright 2015 American Chemical Society. Panels (e–g) adapted with permission from [153]; copyright 2016 American Chemical Society. Symbols: V_{th}, threshold voltage; μ_h, hole mobility; I_{on}, on current; SS, subthreshold swing; v_1–v_{10}, VOC-encoding output vectors.

Diagnosis via Exhaled Breath

Using one of the molecular modifications in their previous study [202], Haick's group found in another study [152] that, with the aid of DFA, a single molecularly modified SiNW-FET biosensor can be used to identify patients with gastric cancer with high accuracy. The use of a simple pattern recognition method instead of ANN, which gives more accurate results but is also a lot more demanding computationally [204], was made possible by the judicious choice of the functionalization molecule. This molecule was trichloro(phenethyl)silane (TPS), a phenethyl-ended silane that is cross-reactive with different VOCs but shows stronger responses to gastric-cancer-related VOCs (2-propenenitrile, 6-methyl-5-hepten-2-one, and furfural) than confounding VOCs (2-ethyl-1-hexanol and nonanal) as compared to other molecular layers used in the study. The quantities used for VOC sensing were the area under the time curve of three FET electrical parameters, namely, threshold voltage, hole mobility, and current at zero gate voltage (subthreshold). Using parameter values obtained with breath samples from gastric cancer patients and healthy individuals, canonical variables were obtained from the DFA method for use in a patient-classification model. Using leave-one-out cross-validation with blind samples, the DFA model with inputs from TPS-modified sensors was able to discriminate gastric cancer patients from the control individuals with 71% sensitivity [= true positive/(true positive + false negative)], 89% specificity [= true negative/(true negative + false positive)], and 85% accuracy [= (true positive + true negative)/total] (Fig. **10d**). Discrimination between patients with early and advanced stages of gastric cancer was also attempted using the same methods; however, low specificity (67%) was obtained due to the small sample number for early-stage gastric cancer. It should also be noted that the devices were found to be relatively insensitive to confounding factors such as gender, tobacco consumption, and *H. pylori* infection, making them suitable for practical applications.

Taking their study a step further, Haick's group [153] combined molecularly modified SiNW FETs with ANN to discriminate between patients with gastric cancer (GC), lung cancer (LC), and non-cancerous lung disease (asthma and chronic obstructive pulmonary disease, AC), as well as healthy individuals (control). Six different molecular modifications with either polar or nonpolar functional groups were employed in the study, namely, TPS, trichloro(3,3,3-trifluoropropyl)silane, heptanoyl chloride, APTES, anthracene, and 3-bromopropyl trichlorosilane (for sensors 1–6 or S1–S6, respectively). The FET parameters utilized were threshold voltage, hole mobility, and drain current at different gate voltages. Binary classification was used to distinguish among the patient groups and healthy individuals, resulting in six classifiers (GC–LC, GC–AC, LC–AC, GC–control, LC–control, and AC–control). As there were six differently functionalized sensors, a total of 36 ANN models were created. In order to decrease the computational load of ANN modeling, a preliminary screening for FET parameters that would yield the best discrimination was first performed using Relief-F feature selection [205]. Then, ANN models consisting of multilayer perceptrons with input, hidden, and output layers were trained using breath samples from actual patients and healthy subjects to optimize the weights and network parameters of the model. The sigmoid function and the trainLM (Levenberg–Marquardt) function were used as the ANN transfer function and training function, respectively. Classification success was evaluated using leave-one-out cross-validation. Based on the results of the ANN-analyzed binary comparisons, S1, S3, and S5 have the highest overall classification scores. For example, S1 can correctly distinguish LC patients from healthy individuals with a sensitivity of 87%, specificity of 82%, and accuracy of 84% (Fig. **10e**). In separating LC from AC (cancer *versus* non-cancer) patients, S1 achieved a sensitivity of 92%, specificity of 80%, and accuracy of 89% (Fig. **10e**). When the binary classifications were made using DFA, the best results were obtained with S1, S3, and S4. Aside from patient classification, the authors also applied DFA to discriminate between early (stages 1 and 2) and advanced (stages 3 and 4) stages of LC and GC. (DFA was used instead of ANN because of the small sample size.) The best results were obtained using S4 (Figs. **10f** and **10g**), with an accuracy of 81% and 87% for LC and GC, respectively. The area under the receiver operating characteristic curves were calculated to be 0.68 for LC and 0.87 for GC (Figs. **10f** and **10g**). These results show that breath sensing with molecularly modified SiNW FETs and ANN or DFA models is a promising technique for noninvasive disease diagnosis.

SUMMARY AND OUTLOOK

Developments in various facets of nanowire-FET biosensing platforms in the past decade have brought this biosensor technology closer to real-world POCT applications. Top–down, wafer-scale patterning techniques such as DUV and UV lithography coupled with dry and wet etching of a SOI device layer, respectively, have been successfully employed to fabricate SiNW FETs that are capable of detecting femtomolar concentrations of DNA [71, 100, 127], RNA [130], and cardiac biomarkers [68]. Moreover, SiNW FETs fabricated using conventional UV lithography and dry etching of poly-Si thin films (*e.g.*, sidewall spacer technique [73, 157]) also showed femtomolar sensitivities in DNA and RNA detection [67, 75, 77]. With greatly improved fabrication processes aided by device simulations [69], sensitivities can be pushed to the theoretical limits and device-to-device sensing variations can be greatly minimized. These advancements make it possible to achieve highly sensitive devices with reproducible and scalable fabrication for low-cost, disposable biosensor chips.

Enhancement of device sensitivity and detection limit in nanowire FET biosensors has been pursued using various approaches: changes in device configuration [158 - 160], new detection modalities [85, 190, 193], selective surface functionalization [49, 88, 146, 171 - 173], shorter capture probes [49, 87, 104, 138], PEGylation [186], and signal amplification [93, 129, 194]. The use of dual gating with galvanostatic detection [158 - 160], frequency-domain detection [190, 193], and heterodyne detection [85] may be promising techniques for enhancing device sensitivity and overcoming the Debye screening limitation; however, they require complicated electronics, which may hinder the development of cheap, portable devices. Signal amplification using RCA for DNA/RNA detection [129] and electronic ELISA for protein detection [194] offer promising approaches to overcome low SNR and Debye screening; nevertheless, multiple reaction steps and reagent handling diminish the advantage of simple operation of FET-based biosensors. On the other hand, rational choice of surface modification procedures and bioreceptor units is, more often than not, sufficient in attaining the sensitivities needed for early disease detection. For top–down fabricated FET devices, electrochemical immobilization [173] or activation [88] of linker molecules is a versatile method for achieving selective surface modification of nanowires. Meanwhile, the use of novel bioreceptors such as antibody fragments [104] and aptamers [91] enable field-effect sensing in high ionic strength solutions. Aptamers are especially promising as they allow the detection of neutral or weakly charged molecules due to their ability to change conformation upon binding of the target analyte [91]. The challenge with these latter approaches is that the methods and materials for device preparation are more complex, which might increase costs. However, once the bioreceptor selection/synthesis and surface functionalization have been optimized and scaled up, the increases in per-device cost can be negligible. Co-modification with long-chain PEG [186] offers a facile way to suppress Debye screening and enhance device responses in high-ionic-strength solutions, as already demonstrated in a variety of FET devices, including dual-gate Si nanoribbon FET [206], extended-gate FET [207], carbon nanotube FET [189], and graphene FET [188, 208].

The introduction of miniature complementary modules for sample processing [53,

105, 183, 195] and electrical detection [68, 135, 173] are important developments towards portable nanowire biosensors with real biosamples, such as whole blood and urine. Micro-/nano-fabricated modules [105, 183, 195] for the filtration and purification of microliter volumes of sample liquids greatly simplify the sensitivity requirements of nanowire FET devices. However, the need for fluid actuation, sample dilution, and elution may result in relatively bulky devices with complex operation. These sample processing steps need to be completely automated if the diagnostic tests are to be self-administered by patients. Portable readout systems where SiNW devices are connected as disposable chips [68, 173] are highly desirable to avoid instability and biofouling issues arising from the repeated use of a single nanowire biosensor. Multiplexed detection among an array of SiNW devices has also been achieved for simultaneous detection of multiple biomarkers [68]. Nevertheless, these embodiments make use of the SiNW devices as resistor elements, *i.e.*, no gate voltage was applied, which prevents more precise control of the device sensitivity.

Despite the challenges mentioned above, the prospects of nanowire-FET biosensors in POCT applications look promising. Compared with other competitive techniques, such as PCR and surface plasmon resonance, nanowire-FET platforms are generally small-sized, easily calibrated, and compatible with microfluidics and handheld form factors [65]. Furthermore, they typically consume little power and occupy small footprints, allowing the creation of dense sensor arrays for multiplexed detection in small-volume samples [69, 168]. With the goal of meeting the ASSURED criteria for POCT devices, future nanowire-FET biosensors should focus on achieving low-cost, ultrasensitive devices with simple operation and capable of direct detection from biosamples (untreated blood, saliva, urine, sweat, *etc.*). From the developments made in the past decade, this means moving towards single-use devices fabricated with CMOS-compatible fabrication procedures and modified with short-length bioreceptor molecules. Future research should also capitalize on nanowire-FET-based biosensing *via* exhaled breath wherein samples can be obtained with ease and continuously for real-time monitoring [152, 153]. With more studies that involve clinical validation of the devices among actual patients, it is possible that these goals will be fulfilled within the next decade, if not sooner, and it is only a matter of time before the translation of nanowire-FET technology from bench to bedside (as well as to homes and communities) finally becomes reality.

CONSENT FOR PUBLICATION

Not applicable.

CONFLICT OF INTEREST

The authors confirm that this chapter contents have no conflict of interest.

ACKNOWLEDGEMENT

The authors would like to thank the Ministry of Science and Technology of Taiwan for the financial support under Contract Nos. MOST 107-2221-E-005-055- and MOST 108-2221-E-005-023-.

REFERENCES

[1]   Etzioni R, Urban N, Ramsey S, *et al.* The case for early detection. Nat Rev Cancer 2003; 3(4): 243-52.
        [http://dx.doi.org/10.1038/nrc1041] [PMID: 12671663]

[2]   Weston AD, Hood L. Systems biology, proteomics, and the future of health care: toward predictive, preventative, and personalized medicine. J Proteome Res 2004; 3(2): 179-96.
        [http://dx.doi.org/10.1021/pr0499693] [PMID: 15113093]

[3]   Holman H, Lorig K. Patient self-management: a key to effectiveness and efficiency in care of chronic disease. Public Health Rep 2004; 119(3): 239-43.
        [http://dx.doi.org/10.1016/j.phr.2004.04.002] [PMID: 15158102]

[4]   Koch S. Home telehealth--current state and future trends. Int J Med Inform 2006; 75(8): 565-76.
        [http://dx.doi.org/10.1016/j.ijmedinf.2005.09.002] [PMID: 16298545]

[5]   Koplan JP, Bond TC, Merson MH, *et al.* Towards a common definition of global health. Lancet 2009; 373(9679): 1993-5.
        [http://dx.doi.org/10.1016/S0140-6736(09)60332-9] [PMID: 19493564]

[6]   Lehmann CA. The future of home testing--implications for traditional laboratories. Clin Chim Acta 2002; 323(1-2): 31-6.
        [http://dx.doi.org/10.1016/S0009-8981(02)00181-X] [PMID: 12135805]

[7]   Yager P, Domingo GJ, Gerdes J. Point-of-care diagnostics for global health. Annu Rev Biomed Eng 2008; 10: 107-44.
        [http://dx.doi.org/10.1146/annurev.bioeng.10.061807.160524] [PMID: 18358075]

[8]   Rusling JF, Kumar CV, Gutkind JS, Patel V. Measurement of biomarker proteins for point-of-care early detection and monitoring of cancer. Analyst (Lond) 2010; 135(10): 2496-511.
        [http://dx.doi.org/10.1039/c0an00204f] [PMID: 20614087]

[9]   Akhmetov I, Bubnov RV. Assessing value of innovative molecular diagnostic tests in the concept of predictive, preventive, and personalized medicine. EPMA J 2015; 6: 19.
        [http://dx.doi.org/10.1186/s13167-015-0041-3] [PMID: 26425215]

[10]   Gubala V, Harris LF, Ricco AJ, Tan MX, Williams DE. Point of care diagnostics: status and future. Anal Chem 2012; 84(2): 487-515.
        [http://dx.doi.org/10.1021/ac2030199] [PMID: 22221172]

[11]   Price CP. Point of care testing. BMJ 2001; 322(7297): 1285-8.
        [http://dx.doi.org/10.1136/bmj.322.7297.1285] [PMID: 11375233]

[12]   Peeling RW, Holmes KK, Mabey D, Ronald A. Rapid tests for sexually transmitted infections (STIs): the way forward. Sex Transm Infect 2006; 82 (Suppl. 5): v1-6.
        [http://dx.doi.org/10.1136/sti.2006.024265] [PMID: 17151023]

[13]   St John A, Price CP. Existing and Emerging Technologies for Point-of-Care Testing. The Clinical biochemist Reviews 2014; 35(3): 155-67.

[14]   Wang J. Electrochemical biosensors: towards point-of-care cancer diagnostics. Biosens Bioelectron 2006; 21(10): 1887-92.
[http://dx.doi.org/10.1016/j.bios.2005.10.027] [PMID: 16330202]

[15]   Arruda DL, Wilson WC, Nguyen C, *et al.* Microelectrical sensors as emerging platforms for protein biomarker detection in point-of-care diagnostics. Expert Rev Mol Diagn 2009; 9(7): 749-55.
[http://dx.doi.org/10.1586/erm.09.47] [PMID: 19817557]

[16]   2014.https://goldbook.iupac.org/

[17]   Schöning MJ, Poghossian A. Recent advances in biologically sensitive field-effect transistors (BioFETs). Analyst (Lond) 2002; 127(9): 1137-51.
[http://dx.doi.org/10.1039/B204444G] [PMID: 12375833]

[18]   Bergveld P. Development of an ion-sensitive solid-state device for neurophysiological measurements. IEEE Trans Biomed Eng 1970; 17(1): 70-1.
[http://dx.doi.org/10.1109/TBME.1970.4502688] [PMID: 5441220]

[19]   Bergveld P. Thirty years of ISFETOLOGY: What happened in the past 30 years and what may happen in the next 30 years. Sens Actuators B Chem 2003; 88(1): 1-20.
[http://dx.doi.org/10.1016/S0925-4005(02)00301-5]

[20]   Yuqing M, Jianguo G, Jianrong C. Ion sensitive field effect transducer-based biosensors. Biotechnol Adv 2003; 21(6): 527-34.
[http://dx.doi.org/10.1016/S0734-9750(03)00103-4] [PMID: 14499153]

[21]   Gao XP, Zheng G, Lieber CM. Subthreshold regime has the optimal sensitivity for nanowire FET biosensors. Nano Lett 2010; 10(2): 547-52.
[http://dx.doi.org/10.1021/nl9034219] [PMID: 19908823]

[22]   Lee CS, Kim SK, Kim M. Ion-sensitive field-effect transistor for biological sensing. Sensors (Basel) 2009; 9(9): 7111-31.
[http://dx.doi.org/10.3390/s90907111] [PMID: 22423205]

[23]   Franklin AD. DEVICE TECHNOLOGY. Nanomaterials in transistors: From high-performance to thin-film applications. Science 2015; 349(6249): aab2750.
[http://dx.doi.org/10.1126/science.aab2750] [PMID: 26273059]

[24]   Patolsky F, Lieber CM. Nanowire nanosensors. Mater Today 2005; 8(4): 20-8.
[http://dx.doi.org/10.1016/S1369-7021(05)00791-1]

[25]   Nair PR, Alam MA. Performance limits of nanobiosensors. Appl Phys Lett 2006; 88(23): 233120.
[http://dx.doi.org/10.1063/1.2211310]

[26]   Chen K-I, Li B-R, Chen Y-T. Silicon nanowire field-effect transistor-based biosensors for biomedical diagnosis and cellular recording investigation. Nano Today 2011; 6(2): 131-54.
[http://dx.doi.org/10.1016/j.nantod.2011.02.001]

[27]   Curreli M, Rui Z, Ishikawa FN, *et al.* Real-Time, Label-Free Detection of Biological Entities Using Nanowire-Based FETs. IEEE Trans NanoTechnol 2008; 7(6): 651-67.
[http://dx.doi.org/10.1109/TNANO.2008.2006165]

[28]   Cui Y, Wei Q, Park H, Lieber CM. Nanowire nanosensors for highly sensitive and selective detection of biological and chemical species. Science 2001; 293(5533): 1289-92.
[http://dx.doi.org/10.1126/science.1062711] [PMID: 11509722]

[29]   Mu L, Chang Y, Sawtelle SD, Wipf M, Duan X, Reed MA. Silicon Nanowire Field-Effect Transistors—A Versatile Class of Potentiometric Nanobiosensors. IEEE Access 2015; 3: 287-302.
[http://dx.doi.org/10.1109/ACCESS.2015.2422842]

[30]   Nehra A, Pal Singh K. Current trends in nanomaterial embedded field effect transistor-based biosensor. Biosens Bioelectron 2015; 74: 731-43.
[http://dx.doi.org/10.1016/j.bios.2015.07.030] [PMID: 26210471]

[31]   Tran T-T, Mulchandani A. Carbon nanotubes and graphene nano field-effect transistor-based biosensors. Trends Analyt Chem 2016; 79: 222-32.
[http://dx.doi.org/10.1016/j.trac.2015.12.002]

[32]   Gan X, Zhao H, Quan X. Two-dimensional MoS_2: A promising building block for biosensors. Biosens Bioelectron 2017; 89(Pt 1): 56-71.
[http://dx.doi.org/10.1016/j.bios.2016.03.042] [PMID: 27037158]

[33]   Mao S, Chen J. Graphene-based electronic biosensors. J Mater Res 2017; 32(15): 2954-65.
[http://dx.doi.org/10.1557/jmr.2017.129]

[34]   McAlpine MC, Ahmad H, Wang D, Heath JR. Highly ordered nanowire arrays on plastic substrates for ultrasensitive flexible chemical sensors. Nat Mater 2007; 6(5): 379-84.
[http://dx.doi.org/10.1038/nmat1891] [PMID: 17450146]

[35]   Timko BP, Cohen-Karni T, Yu G, Qing Q, Tian B, Lieber CM. Electrical recording from hearts with flexible nanowire device arrays. Nano Lett 2009; 9(2): 914-8.
[http://dx.doi.org/10.1021/nl900096z] [PMID: 19170614]

[36]   Tisch U, Haick H. Nanomaterials for cross-reactive sensor arrays. MRS Bull 2011; 35(10): 797-803.
[http://dx.doi.org/10.1557/mrs2010.509]

[37]   Bashouti MY, Tung RT, Haick H. Tuning the electrical properties of Si nanowire field-effect transistors by molecular engineering. Small 2009; 5(23): 2761-9.
[http://dx.doi.org/10.1002/smll.200901402] [PMID: 19771570]

[38]   Paska Y, Stelzner T, Assad O, Tisch U, Christiansen S, Haick H. Molecular gating of silicon nanowire field-effect transistors with nonpolar analytes. ACS Nano 2012; 6(1): 335-45.
[http://dx.doi.org/10.1021/nn203653h] [PMID: 22176137]

[39]   Wang B, Haick H. Effect of functional groups on the sensing properties of silicon nanowires toward volatile compounds. ACS Appl Mater Interfaces 2013; 5(6): 2289-99.
[http://dx.doi.org/10.1021/am4004649] [PMID: 23452335]

[40]   Nair PR, Alam MA. Design Considerations of Silicon Nanowire Biosensors. IEEE Trans Electron Dev 2007; 54(12): 3400-8.
[http://dx.doi.org/10.1109/TED.2007.909059]

[41]   Sørensen MH, Mortensen NA, Brandbyge M. Screening model for nanowire surface-charge sensors in liquid. Appl Phys Lett 2007; 91(10): 102105.
[http://dx.doi.org/10.1063/1.2779930]

[42]   Gunawan O, Sekaric L, Majumdar A, *et al.* Measurement of carrier mobility in silicon nanowires. Nano Lett 2008; 8(6): 1566-71.
[http://dx.doi.org/10.1021/nl072646w] [PMID: 18444687]

[43]   Ford AC, Ho JC, Chueh Y-L, *et al.* Diameter-dependent electron mobility of InAs nanowires. Nano Lett 2009; 9(1): 360-5.
[http://dx.doi.org/10.1021/nl803154m] [PMID: 19143505]

[44]   De Vico L, Sørensen MH, Iversen L, *et al.* Quantifying signal changes in nano-wire based biosensors. Nanoscale 2011; 3(2): 706-17.
[http://dx.doi.org/10.1039/C0NR00442A] [PMID: 21173975]

[45]   Morales AM, Lieber CM. A laser ablation method for the synthesis of crystalline semiconductor nanowires. Science 1998; 279(5348): 208-11.
[http://dx.doi.org/10.1126/science.279.5348.208] [PMID: 9422689]

[46]   Cui Y, Duan X, Hu J, Lieber CM. Doping and Electrical Transport in Silicon Nanowires. J Phys Chem B 2000; 104(22): 5213-6.
[http://dx.doi.org/10.1021/jp0009305]

[47]   Zheng G, Patolsky F, Cui Y, Wang WU, Lieber CM. Multiplexed electrical detection of cancer

markers with nanowire sensor arrays. Nat Biotechnol 2005; 23(10): 1294-301.
[http://dx.doi.org/10.1038/nbt1138] [PMID: 16170313]

[48]   Lin TW, Hsieh PJ, Lin CL, *et al.* Label-free detection of protein-protein interactions using a calmodulin-modified nanowire transistor. Proc Natl Acad Sci USA 2010; 107(3): 1047-52.
[http://dx.doi.org/10.1073/pnas.0910243107] [PMID: 20080536]

[49]   Li BR, Hsieh YJ, Chen YX, Chung YT, Pan CY, Chen YT. An ultrasensitive nanowire-transistor biosensor for detecting dopamine release from living PC12 cells under hypoxic stimulation. J Am Chem Soc 2013; 135(43): 16034-7.
[http://dx.doi.org/10.1021/ja408485m] [PMID: 24125072]

[50]   Zheng G, Lu W, Jin S, Lieber CM. Synthesis and Fabrication of High-Performance n-Type Silicon Nanowire Transistors. Adv Mater 2004; 16(21): 1890-3.
[http://dx.doi.org/10.1002/adma.200400472]

[51]   Li C, Zhang D, Han S, Liu X, Tang T, Zhou C. Diameter-Controlled Growth of Single-Crystalline In2O3 Nanowires and Their Electronic Properties. Adv Mater 2003; 15(2): 143-6.
[http://dx.doi.org/10.1002/adma.200390029]

[52]   Li C, Curreli M, Lin H, *et al.* Complementary detection of prostate-specific antigen using In2O3 nanowires and carbon nanotubes. J Am Chem Soc 2005; 127(36): 12484-5.
[http://dx.doi.org/10.1021/ja053761g] [PMID: 16144384]

[53]   Chang H-K, Ishikawa FN, Zhang R, *et al.* Rapid, label-free, electrical whole blood bioassay based on nanobiosensor systems. ACS Nano 2011; 5(12): 9883-91.
[http://dx.doi.org/10.1021/nn2035796] [PMID: 22066492]

[54]   Chang P-C, Fan Z, Wang D, *et al.* ZnO Nanowires Synthesized by Vapor Trapping CVD Method. Chem Mater 2004; 16(24): 5133-7.
[http://dx.doi.org/10.1021/cm049182c]

[55]   Huang YH, Zhang Y, Liu L, Fan SS, Wei Y, He J. Controlled synthesis and field emission properties of ZnO nanostructures with different morphologies. J Nanosci Nanotechnol 2006; 6(3): 787-90.
[http://dx.doi.org/10.1166/jnn.2006.086] [PMID: 16573138]

[56]   Ra H-W, Choi DH, Kim SH, Im Y-H. Formation and Characterization of ZnO/a-C Core−Shell Nanowires. J Phys Chem C 2009; 113(9): 3512-6.
[http://dx.doi.org/10.1021/jp8085304]

[57]   Fan Z, Ho JC, Jacobson ZA, *et al.* Wafer-scale assembly of highly ordered semiconductor nanowire arrays by contact printing. Nano Lett 2008; 8(1): 20-5.
[http://dx.doi.org/10.1021/nl071626r] [PMID: 17696563]

[58]   Duan X, Huang Y, Cui Y, Wang J, Lieber CM. Indium phosphide nanowires as building blocks for nanoscale electronic and optoelectronic devices. Nature 2001; 409(6816): 66-9.
[http://dx.doi.org/10.1038/35051047] [PMID: 11343112]

[59]   Huang Y, Duan X, Wei Q, Lieber CM. Directed assembly of one-dimensional nanostructures into functional networks. Science 2001; 291(5504): 630-3.
[http://dx.doi.org/10.1126/science.291.5504.630] [PMID: 11158671]

[60]   Patolsky F, Zheng G, Lieber CM. Fabrication of silicon nanowire devices for ultrasensitive, label-free, real-time detection of biological and chemical species. Nat Protoc 2006; 1(4): 1711-24.
[http://dx.doi.org/10.1038/nprot.2006.227] [PMID: 17487154]

[61]   Hahm J-i, Lieber CM. Direct Ultrasensitive Electrical Detection of DNA and DNA Sequence Variations Using Nanowire Nanosensors. Nano Lett 2004; 4(1): 51-4.
[http://dx.doi.org/10.1021/nl034853b]

[62]   Elfström N, Juhasz R, Sychugov I, Engfeldt T, Karlström AE, Linnros J. Surface charge sensitivity of silicon nanowires: size dependence. Nano Lett 2007; 7(9): 2608-12.
[http://dx.doi.org/10.1021/nl0709017] [PMID: 17691849]

[63]   Tong HD, Chen S, van der Wiel WG, Carlen ET, van den Berg A. Novel top-down wafer-scale fabrication of single crystal silicon nanowires. Nano Lett 2009; 9(3): 1015-22.
[http://dx.doi.org/10.1021/nl803181x] [PMID: 19199755]

[64]   Li Z, Chen Y, Li X, Kamins TI, Nauka K, Williams RS. Sequence-Specific Label-Free DNA Sensors Based on Silicon Nanowires. Nano Lett 2004; 4(2): 245-7.
[http://dx.doi.org/10.1021/nl034958e]

[65]   Tran DP, Winter MA, Wolfrum B, *et al.* Toward Intraoperative Detection of Disseminated Tumor Cells in Lymph Nodes with Silicon Nanowire Field Effect Transistors. ACS Nano 2016; 10(2): 2357-64.
[http://dx.doi.org/10.1021/acsnano.5b07136] [PMID: 26859618]

[66]   Gao Z, Agarwal A, Trigg AD, *et al.* Silicon nanowire arrays for label-free detection of DNA. Anal Chem 2007; 79(9): 3291-7.
[http://dx.doi.org/10.1021/ac061808q] [PMID: 17407259]

[67]   Zhang GJ, Chua JH, Chee RE, Agarwal A, Wong SM. Label-free direct detection of MiRNAs with silicon nanowire biosensors. Biosens Bioelectron 2009; 24(8): 2504-8.
[http://dx.doi.org/10.1016/j.bios.2008.12.035] [PMID: 19188058]

[68]   Zhang GJ, Chai KTC, Luo HZH, *et al.* Multiplexed detection of cardiac biomarkers in serum with nanowire arrays using readout ASIC. Biosens Bioelectron 2012; 35(1): 218-23.
[http://dx.doi.org/10.1016/j.bios.2012.02.052] [PMID: 22459581]

[69]   Zafar S, D'Emic C, Jagtiani A, *et al.* Silicon Nanowire Field Effect Transistor Sensors with Minimal Sensor-to-Sensor Variations and Enhanced Sensing Characteristics. ACS Nano 2018; 12(7): 6577-87.
[http://dx.doi.org/10.1021/acsnano.8b01339] [PMID: 29932634]

[70]   Stern E, Klemic JF, Routenberg DA, *et al.* Label-free immunodetection with CMOS-compatible semiconducting nanowires. Nature 2007; 445(7127): 519-22.
[http://dx.doi.org/10.1038/nature05498] [PMID: 17268465]

[71]   Gao A, Lu N, Dai P, *et al.* Silicon-nanowire-based CMOS-compatible field-effect transistor nanosensors for ultrasensitive electrical detection of nucleic acids. Nano Lett 2011; 11(9): 3974-8.
[http://dx.doi.org/10.1021/nl202303y] [PMID: 21848308]

[72]   Chen S, Bomer JG, van der Wiel WG, Carlen ET, van den Berg A. Top-down fabrication of sub-30 nm monocrystalline silicon nanowires using conventional microfabrication. ACS Nano 2009; 3(11): 3485-92.
[http://dx.doi.org/10.1021/nn901220g] [PMID: 19856905]

[73]   Hakim MM, Lombardini M, Sun K, *et al.* Thin film polycrystalline silicon nanowire biosensors. Nano Lett 2012; 12(4): 1868-72.
[http://dx.doi.org/10.1021/nl2042276] [PMID: 22432636]

[74]   Hsiao CY, Lin CH, Hung CH, *et al.* Novel poly-silicon nanowire field effect transistor for biosensing application. Biosens Bioelectron 2009; 24(5): 1223-9.
[http://dx.doi.org/10.1016/j.bios.2008.07.032] [PMID: 18760914]

[75]   Wenga G, Jacques E, Salaün AC, Rogel R, Pichon L, Geneste F. Step-gate polysilicon nanowires field effect transistor compatible with CMOS technology for label-free DNA biosensor. Biosens Bioelectron 2013; 40(1): 141-6.
[http://dx.doi.org/10.1016/j.bios.2012.07.001] [PMID: 22841443]

[76]   Pujari SP, Scheres L, Marcelis ATM, Zuilhof H. Covalent surface modification of oxide surfaces. Angew Chem Int Ed Engl 2014; 53(25): 6322-56.
[http://dx.doi.org/10.1002/anie.201306709] [PMID: 24849332]

[77]   Lin CH, Hung CH, Hsiao CY, Lin HC, Ko FH, Yang YS. Poly-silicon nanowire field-effect transistor for ultrasensitive and label-free detection of pathogenic avian influenza DNA. Biosens Bioelectron 2009; 24(10): 3019-24.

[http://dx.doi.org/10.1016/j.bios.2009.03.014] [PMID: 19362813]

[78]   Kim K, Park C, Kwon D, *et al.* Silicon nanowire biosensors for detection of cardiac troponin I (cTnI) with high sensitivity. Biosens Bioelectron 2016; 77: 695-701.
[http://dx.doi.org/10.1016/j.bios.2015.10.008] [PMID: 26496224]

[79]   Witucki GL. A Silane Primer: Chemistry and Applications of Alkoxy Silanes. J Coatings Technology 1993; 65(822): 57-60.

[80]   Sehgal D, Vijay IK. A method for the high efficiency of water-soluble carbodiimide-mediated amidation. Anal Biochem 1994; 218(1): 87-91.
[http://dx.doi.org/10.1006/abio.1994.1144] [PMID: 8053572]

[81]   Barbosa O, Ortiz C, Berenguer-Murcia Á, Torres R, Rodrigues RC, Fernandez-Lafuente R. Glutaraldehyde in bio-catalysts design: a useful crosslinker and a versatile tool in enzyme immobilization. RSC Advances 2014; 4(4): 1583-600.
[http://dx.doi.org/10.1039/C3RA45991H]

[82]   Choi A, Kim K, Jung H-I, Lee SY. ZnO nanowire biosensors for detection of biomolecular interactions in enhancement mode. Sens Actuators B Chem 2010; 148(2): 577-82.
[http://dx.doi.org/10.1016/j.snb.2010.04.049]

[83]   Liu X, Lin P, Yan X, *et al.* Enzyme-coated single ZnO nanowire FET biosensor for detection of uric acid. Sens Actuators B Chem 2013; 176: 22-7.
[http://dx.doi.org/10.1016/j.snb.2012.08.043]

[84]   Fathil MFM, Md Arshad MK, Ruslinda AR, *et al.* Substrate-gate coupling in ZnO-FET biosensor for cardiac troponin I detection. Sens Actuators B Chem 2017; 242: 1142-54.
[http://dx.doi.org/10.1016/j.snb.2016.09.131]

[85]   Chakraborty B, Ghosh S, Das N, RoyChaudhuri C. Liquid gated ZnO nanorod FET sensor for ultrasensitive detection of Hepatitis B surface antigen with vertical electrode configuration. Biosens Bioelectron 2018; 122: 58-67.
[http://dx.doi.org/10.1016/j.bios.2018.09.019] [PMID: 30240967]

[86]   Curreli M, Li C, Sun Y, *et al.* Selective functionalization of In2O3 nanowire mat devices for biosensing applications. J Am Chem Soc 2005; 127(19): 6922-3.
[http://dx.doi.org/10.1021/ja0503478] [PMID: 15884914]

[87]   Ishikawa FN, Chang H-K, Curreli M, *et al.* Label-free, electrical detection of the SARS virus N-protein with nanowire biosensors utilizing antibody mimics as capture probes. ACS Nano 2009; 3(5): 1219-24.
[http://dx.doi.org/10.1021/nn900086c] [PMID: 19422193]

[88]   Zhang R, Curreli M, Thompson ME. Selective, electrochemically activated biofunctionalization of In2O3 nanowires using an air-stable surface modifier. ACS Appl Mater Interfaces 2011; 3(12): 4765-9.
[http://dx.doi.org/10.1021/am2012454] [PMID: 22039782]

[89]   Kim J, Rim YS, Chen H, *et al.* Fabrication of High-Performance Ultrathin In2O3 Film Field-Effect Transistors and Biosensors Using Chemical Lift-Off Lithography. ACS Nano 2015; 9(4): 4572-82.
[http://dx.doi.org/10.1021/acsnano.5b01211] [PMID: 25798751]

[90]   Rim YS, Bae S-H, Chen H, *et al.* Printable Ultrathin Metal Oxide Semiconductor-Based Conformal Biosensors. ACS Nano 2015; 9(12): 12174-81.
[http://dx.doi.org/10.1021/acsnano.5b05325] [PMID: 26498319]

[91]   Nakatsuka N, Yang K-A, Abendroth JM, *et al.* Aptamer-field-effect transistors overcome Debye length limitations for small-molecule sensing. Science 2018; 362(6412): 319-24.
[http://dx.doi.org/10.1126/science.aao6750] [PMID: 30190311]

[92]   Hotchkiss PJ, Jones SC, Paniagua SA, *et al.* The modification of indium tin oxide with phosphonic acids: mechanism of binding, tuning of surface properties, and potential for use in organic electronic

applications. Acc Chem Res 2012; 45(3): 337-46.
[http://dx.doi.org/10.1021/ar200119g] [PMID: 22011002]

[93]   Choi JH, Kim H, Choi JH, Choi JW, Oh BK. Signal enhancement of silicon nanowire-based biosensor for detection of matrix metalloproteinase-2 using DNA-Au nanoparticle complexes. ACS Appl Mater Interfaces 2013; 5(22): 12023-8.
[http://dx.doi.org/10.1021/am403816x] [PMID: 24164583]

[94]   Patolsky F, Zheng G, Hayden O, Lakadamyali M, Zhuang X, Lieber CM. Electrical detection of single viruses. Proc Natl Acad Sci USA 2004; 101(39): 14017-22.
[http://dx.doi.org/10.1073/pnas.0406159101] [PMID: 15365183]

[95]   Li J, Zhang Y, To S, You L, Sun Y. Effect of nanowire number, diameter, and doping density on nano-FET biosensor sensitivity. ACS Nano 2011; 5(8): 6661-8.
[http://dx.doi.org/10.1021/nn202182p] [PMID: 21815637]

[96]   Shin K-S, Pan A, On Chui C. Channel length dependent sensitivity of Schottky contacted silicon nanowire field-effect transistor sensors. Appl Phys Lett 2012; 100(12): 123504.
[http://dx.doi.org/10.1063/1.3696035]

[97]   Lee R, Kwon DW, Kim S, *et al.* Nanowire size dependence on sensitivity of silicon nanowire field-effect transistor-based pH sensor. Jpn J Appl Phys 2017; 56(12): 124001.
[http://dx.doi.org/10.7567/JJAP.56.124001]

[98]   Sham TK, Naftel SJ, Kim PSG, *et al.* Electronic structure and optical properties of silicon nanowires: A study using x-ray excited optical luminescence and x-ray emission spectroscopy. Phys Rev B 2004; 70(4): 045313.
[http://dx.doi.org/10.1103/PhysRevB.70.045313]

[99]   Bunimovich YL, Shin YS, Yeo W-S, Amori M, Kwong G, Heath JR. Quantitative real-time measurements of DNA hybridization with alkylated nonoxidized silicon nanowires in electrolyte solution. J Am Chem Soc 2006; 128(50): 16323-31.
[http://dx.doi.org/10.1021/ja065923u] [PMID: 17165787]

[100]   Gao A, Lu N, Wang Y, *et al.* Enhanced sensing of nucleic acids with silicon nanowire field effect transistor biosensors. Nano Lett 2012; 12(10): 5262-8.
[http://dx.doi.org/10.1021/nl302476h] [PMID: 22985088]

[101]   Zhang G-J, Zhang G, Chua JH, *et al.* DNA sensing by silicon nanowire: charge layer distance dependence. Nano Lett 2008; 8(4): 1066-70.
[http://dx.doi.org/10.1021/nl072991l] [PMID: 18311939]

[102]   Bergveld P. The future of biosensors. Sens Actuators A Phys 1996; 56(1): 65-73.
[http://dx.doi.org/10.1016/0924-4247(96)01275-7]

[103]   Stern E, Wagner R, Sigworth FJ, Breaker R, Fahmy TM, Reed MA. Importance of the Debye screening length on nanowire field effect transistor sensors. Nano Lett 2007; 7(11): 3405-9.
[http://dx.doi.org/10.1021/nl071792z] [PMID: 17914853]

[104]   Elnathan R, Kwiat M, Pevzner A, *et al.* Biorecognition layer engineering: overcoming screening limitations of nanowire-based FET devices. Nano Lett 2012; 12(10): 5245-54.
[http://dx.doi.org/10.1021/nl302434w] [PMID: 22963381]

[105]   Zhang GJ, Luo ZH, Huang MJ, Ang JJ, Kang TG, Ji H. An integrated chip for rapid, sensitive, and multiplexed detection of cardiac biomarkers from fingerprick blood. Biosens Bioelectron 2011; 28(1): 459-63.
[http://dx.doi.org/10.1016/j.bios.2011.07.007] [PMID: 21807497]

[106]   Vacic A, Criscione JM, Rajan NK, Stern E, Fahmy TM, Reed MA. Determination of molecular configuration by debye length modulation. J Am Chem Soc 2011; 133(35): 13886-9.
[http://dx.doi.org/10.1021/ja205684a] [PMID: 21815673]

[107]   Shoorideh K, Chui CO. On the origin of enhanced sensitivity in nanoscale FET-based biosensors. Proc

Natl Acad Sci USA 2014; 111(14): 5111-6.
[http://dx.doi.org/10.1073/pnas.1315485111] [PMID: 24706861]

[108] Valenza M, Hoffmann A, Sodini D, Laigle A, Martinez F, Rigaud D. Overview of the impact of downscaling technology on 1/f noise in p-MOSFETs to 90 nm. IEE Proc, Circ Devices Syst 2004; 151(2): 102-10.
[http://dx.doi.org/10.1049/ip-cds:20040459]

[109] Toita M, Vandamme LKJ, Sugawa S, Teramoto A, Ohmi T. Geometry and Bias Dependence of Low-Frequency Random Telegraph Signal and 1/f Noise Levels in MOSFETs. Fluct Noise Lett 2005; 05(04): L539-48.
[http://dx.doi.org/10.1142/S0219477505002999]

[110] Ralls KS, Skocpol WJ, Jackel LD, *et al.* Discrete Resistance Switching in Submicrometer Silicon Inversion Layers: Individual Interface Traps and Low-Frequency (1/f?) Noise. Phys Rev Lett 1984; 52(3): 228-31.
[http://dx.doi.org/10.1103/PhysRevLett.52.228]

[111] Lukyanchikova NB, Petrichuk MV, Garbar NP, Simoen E, Claeys C. RTS capture kinetics and Coulomb blockade energy in submicron nMOSFETs under surface quantization conditions. Microelectron Eng 1999; 48(1): 185-8.
[http://dx.doi.org/10.1016/S0167-9317(99)00367-6]

[112] Hooge FN, Kleinpenning TGM, Vandamme LKJ. Experimental studies on 1/f noise. Rep Prog Phys 1981; 44(5): 479-532.
[http://dx.doi.org/10.1088/0034-4885/44/5/001]

[113] Jayaraman R, Sodini CGA. 1/f noise technique to extract the oxide trap density near the conduction band edge of silicon. IEEE Trans Electron Dev 1989; 36(9): 1773-82.
[http://dx.doi.org/10.1109/16.34242]

[114] Rajan NK, Routenberg DA, Chen J, Reed MA. Temperature dependence of 1/f noise mechanisms in silicon nanowire biochemical field effect transistors. Appl Phys Lett 2010; 97(24): 243501.
[http://dx.doi.org/10.1063/1.3526382] [PMID: 21221250]

[115] Hooge FN. $1/f$ noise is no surface effect. Phys Lett A 1969; 29(3): 139-40.
[http://dx.doi.org/10.1016/0375-9601(69)90076-0]

[116] Reza S, Bosman G, Islam MS, Kamins TI, Sharma S, Williams RS. Noise in Silicon Nanowires. IEEE Trans NanoTechnol 2006; 5(5): 523-9.
[http://dx.doi.org/10.1109/TNANO.2006.880908]

[117] Bedner K, Guzenko VA, Tarasov A, *et al.* Investigation of the dominant 1/f noise source in silicon nanowire sensors. Sens Actuators B Chem 2014; 191: 270-5.
[http://dx.doi.org/10.1016/j.snb.2013.09.112]

[118] Ghibaudo G, Roux O, Nguyen-Duc C, Balestra F, Brini J. Improved Analysis of Low Frequency Noise in Field-Effect MOS Transistors. physica status solidi (a) 1991; 124(2): 571-81.

[119] Lee S, Baek C, Park S, *et al.* Characterization of Channel-Diameter- Dependent Low-Frequency Noise in Silicon Nanowire Field-Effect Transistors. IEEE Electron Device Lett 2012; 33(10): 1348-50.
[http://dx.doi.org/10.1109/LED.2012.2209625]

[120] Pud S, Li J, Sibiliev V, *et al.* Liquid and back gate coupling effect: toward biosensing with lowest detection limit. Nano Lett 2014; 14(2): 578-84.
[http://dx.doi.org/10.1021/nl403748x] [PMID: 24392670]

[121] Cho H, Kim K, Yoon J, Rim T, Meyyappan M, Baek C. Optimization of Signal to Noise Ratio in Silicon Nanowire ISFET Sensors. IEEE Sens J 2017; 17(9): 2792-6.
[http://dx.doi.org/10.1109/JSEN.2017.2674672]

[122] Rajan NK, Routenberg DA, Chen J, Reed MA. 1/f Noise of Silicon Nanowire BioFETs. IEEE Electron Device Lett 2010; 31(6): 615-7.

[http://dx.doi.org/10.1109/LED.2010.2047000]

[123] Chen X, Chen S, Hu Q, Zhang S-L, Solomon P, Zhang Z. Device Noise Reduction for Silicon Nanowire Field-Effect-Transistor Based Sensors by Using a Schottky Junction Gate. ACS Sens 2019; 4(2): 427-33.
[http://dx.doi.org/10.1021/acssensors.8b01394] [PMID: 30632733]

[124] Rajan NK, Duan X, Reed MA. Performance limitations for nanowire/nanoribbon biosensors. Wiley Interdiscip Rev Nanomed Nanobiotechnol 2013; 5(6): 629-45.
[http://dx.doi.org/10.1002/wnan.1235] [PMID: 23897672]

[125] Wu CC, Ko FH, Yang YS, Hsia DL, Lee BS, Su TS. Label-free biosensing of a gene mutation using a silicon nanowire field-effect transistor. Biosens Bioelectron 2009; 25(4): 820-5.
[http://dx.doi.org/10.1016/j.bios.2009.08.031] [PMID: 19765969]

[126] Ryu SW, Kim CH, Han JW, *et al.* Gold nanoparticle embedded silicon nanowire biosensor for applications of label-free DNA detection. Biosens Bioelectron 2010; 25(9): 2182-5.
[http://dx.doi.org/10.1016/j.bios.2010.02.010] [PMID: 20227871]

[127] Zhang GJ, Luo ZH, Huang MJ, Tay GK, Lim EJ. Morpholino-functionalized silicon nanowire biosensor for sequence-specific label-free detection of DNA. Biosens Bioelectron 2010; 25(11): 2447-53.
[http://dx.doi.org/10.1016/j.bios.2010.04.001] [PMID: 20435462]

[128] Dorvel BR, Reddy B Jr, Go J, *et al.* Silicon nanowires with high-k hafnium oxide dielectrics for sensitive detection of small nucleic acid oligomers. ACS Nano 2012; 6(7): 6150-64.
[http://dx.doi.org/10.1021/nn301495k] [PMID: 22695179]

[129] Gao A, Zou N, Dai P, *et al.* Signal-to-noise ratio enhancement of silicon nanowires biosensor with rolling circle amplification. Nano Lett 2013; 13(9): 4123-30.
[http://dx.doi.org/10.1021/nl401628y] [PMID: 23937430]

[130] Lu N, Gao A, Dai P, *et al.* CMOS-compatible silicon nanowire field-effect transistors for ultrasensitive and label-free microRNAs sensing. Small 2014; 10(10): 2022-8.
[http://dx.doi.org/10.1002/smll.201302990] [PMID: 24574202]

[131] Nuzaihan M N M, Hashim U, Md Arshad MK, *et al.* Electrical detection of dengue virus (DENV) DNA oligomer using silicon nanowire biosensor with novel molecular gate control. Biosens Bioelectron 2016; 83: 106-14.
[http://dx.doi.org/10.1016/j.bios.2016.04.033] [PMID: 27107147]

[132] Lee HS, Kim KS, Kim CJ, Hahn SK, Jo MH. Electrical detection of VEGFs for cancer diagnoses using anti-vascular endotherial growth factor aptamer-modified Si nanowire FETs. Biosens Bioelectron 2009; 24(6): 1801-5.
[http://dx.doi.org/10.1016/j.bios.2008.08.036] [PMID: 18835770]

[133] Kong T, Su R, Zhang B, Zhang Q, Cheng G. CMOS-compatible, label-free silicon-nanowire biosensors to detect cardiac troponin I for acute myocardial infarction diagnosis. Biosens Bioelectron 2012; 34(1): 267-72.
[http://dx.doi.org/10.1016/j.bios.2012.02.019] [PMID: 22386490]

[134] Lu N, Dai P, Gao A, *et al.* Label-free and rapid electrical detection of hTSH with CMOS-compatible silicon nanowire transistor arrays. ACS Appl Mater Interfaces 2014; 6(22): 20378-84.
[http://dx.doi.org/10.1021/am505915y] [PMID: 25338002]

[135] Pei-Wen Y, Che-Wei H, Yu-Jie H, *et al.* A device design of an integrated CMOS poly-silicon biosensor-on-chip to enhance performance of biomolecular analytes in serum samples. Biosens Bioelectron 2014; 61: 112-8.
[http://dx.doi.org/10.1016/j.bios.2014.05.010] [PMID: 24861571]

[136] Kim JY, Ahn JH, Moon DI, Park TJ, Lee SY, Choi YK. Multiplex electrical detection of avian influenza and human immunodeficiency virus with an underlap-embedded silicon nanowire field-

effect transistor. Biosens Bioelectron 2014; 55: 162-7.
[http://dx.doi.org/10.1016/j.bios.2013.12.014] [PMID: 24374298]

[137]   Chen HC, Chen YT, Tsai RY, *et al.* A sensitive and selective magnetic graphene composite-modified polycrystalline-silicon nanowire field-effect transistor for bladder cancer diagnosis. Biosens Bioelectron 2015; 66: 198-207.
[http://dx.doi.org/10.1016/j.bios.2014.11.019] [PMID: 25460902]

[138]   Banerjee S, Hsieh YJ, Liu CR, *et al.* Differential Releases of Dopamine and Neuropeptide Y from Histamine-Stimulated PC12 Cells Detected by an Aptamer-Modified Nanowire Transistor. Small 2016; 12(40): 5524-9.
[http://dx.doi.org/10.1002/smll.201601370] [PMID: 27551968]

[139]   Krivitsky V, Zverzhinetsky M, Patolsky F. Antigen-Dissociation from Antibody-Modified Nanotransistor Sensor Arrays as a Direct Biomarker Detection Method in Unprocessed Biosamples. Nano Lett 2016; 16(10): 6272-81.
[http://dx.doi.org/10.1021/acs.nanolett.6b02584] [PMID: 27579528]

[140]   Mirsian S, Khodadadian A, Hedayati M, Manzour-Ol-Ajdad A, Kalantarinejad R, Heitzinger C. A new method for selective functionalization of silicon nanowire sensors and Bayesian inversion for its parameters. Biosens Bioelectron 2019; 142: 111527.
[http://dx.doi.org/10.1016/j.bios.2019.111527] [PMID: 31344601]

[141]   Presnova G, Presnov D, Krupenin V, *et al.* Biosensor based on a silicon nanowire field-effect transistor functionalized by gold nanoparticles for the highly sensitive determination of prostate specific antigen. Biosens Bioelectron 2017; 88: 283-9.
[http://dx.doi.org/10.1016/j.bios.2016.08.054] [PMID: 27567265]

[142]   Lee M, Palanisamy S, Zhou BH, *et al.* Ultrasensitive Electrical Detection of Follicle-Stimulating Hormone Using a Functionalized Silicon Nanowire Transistor Chemosensor. ACS Appl Mater Interfaces 2018; 10(42): 36120-7.
[http://dx.doi.org/10.1021/acsami.8b11882] [PMID: 30256613]

[143]   Su D-S, Chen P-Y, Chiu H-C, Han C-C, Yen T-J, Chen H-M. Disease antigens detection by silicon nanowires with the efficiency optimization of their antibodies on a chip. Biosens Bioelectron 2019; 141: 111209.
[http://dx.doi.org/10.1016/j.bios.2019.03.042] [PMID: 31357174]

[144]   Ra HW, Kim JT, Khan R, *et al.* Robust and multifunctional nanosheath for chemical and biological nanodevices. Nano Lett 2012; 12(4): 1891-7.
[http://dx.doi.org/10.1021/nl204280d] [PMID: 22432910]

[145]   Shen F, Wang J, Xu Z, *et al.* Rapid flu diagnosis using silicon nanowire sensor. Nano Lett 2012; 12(7): 3722-30.
[http://dx.doi.org/10.1021/nl301516z] [PMID: 22731392]

[146]   Li BR, Chen CW, Yang WL, Lin TY, Pan CY, Chen YT. Biomolecular recognition with a sensitivity-enhanced nanowire transistor biosensor. Biosens Bioelectron 2013; 45: 252-9.
[http://dx.doi.org/10.1016/j.bios.2013.02.009] [PMID: 23500372]

[147]   Schütt J, Ibarlucea B, Illing R, *et al.* Compact Nanowire Sensors Probe Microdroplets. Nano Lett 2016; 16(8): 4991-5000.
[http://dx.doi.org/10.1021/acs.nanolett.6b01707] [PMID: 27417510]

[148]   Ahmad R, Tripathy N, Hahn YB. High-performance cholesterol sensor based on the solution-gated field effect transistor fabricated with ZnO nanorods. Biosens Bioelectron 2013; 45: 281-6.
[http://dx.doi.org/10.1016/j.bios.2013.01.021] [PMID: 23500376]

[149]   Paska Y, Stelzner T, Christiansen S, Haick H. Enhanced sensing of nonpolar volatile organic compounds by silicon nanowire field effect transistors. ACS Nano 2011; 5(7): 5620-6.
[http://dx.doi.org/10.1021/nn201184c] [PMID: 21648442]

[150] Wang B, Cancilla JC, Torrecilla JS, Haick H. Artificial sensing intelligence with silicon nanowires for ultraselective detection in the gas phase. Nano Lett 2014; 14(2): 933-8.
[http://dx.doi.org/10.1021/nl404335p] [PMID: 24437965]

[151] Han JW, Rim T, Baek CK, Meyyappan M. Chemical Gated Field Effect Transistor by Hybrid Integration of One-Dimensional Silicon Nanowire and Two-Dimensional Tin Oxide Thin Film for Low Power Gas Sensor. ACS Appl Mater Interfaces 2015; 7(38): 21263-9.
[http://dx.doi.org/10.1021/acsami.5b05479] [PMID: 26381613]

[152] Shehada N, Brönstrup G, Funka K, Christiansen S, Leja M, Haick H. Ultrasensitive silicon nanowire for real-world gas sensing: noninvasive diagnosis of cancer from breath volatolome. Nano Lett 2015; 15(2): 1288-95.
[http://dx.doi.org/10.1021/nl504482t] [PMID: 25494909]

[153] Shehada N, Cancilla JC, Torrecilla JS, *et al.* Silicon Nanowire Sensors Enable Diagnosis of Patients via Exhaled Breath. ACS Nano 2016; 10(7): 7047-57.
[http://dx.doi.org/10.1021/acsnano.6b03127] [PMID: 27383408]

[154] Agarwal A, Buddharaju K, Lao IK, Singh N, Balasubramanian N, Kwong DL. Silicon nanowire sensor array using top–down CMOS technology. Sens Actuators A Phys 2008; 145-146: 207-13.
[http://dx.doi.org/10.1016/j.sna.2007.12.019]

[155] Lin SP, Chi TY, Lai TY, Liu MC. Investigation into the effect of varied functional biointerfaces on silicon nanowire MOSFETs. Sensors (Basel) 2012; 12(12): 16867-78.
[http://dx.doi.org/10.3390/s121216867] [PMID: 23223082]

[156] Lin SP, Vinzons LU, Kang YS, Lai TY. Non-Faradaic electrical impedimetric investigation of the interfacial effects of neuronal cell growth and differentiation on silicon nanowire transistors. ACS Appl Mater Interfaces 2015; 7(18): 9866-78.
[http://dx.doi.org/10.1021/acsami.5b01878] [PMID: 25899873]

[157] Lin HC, Lee MH, Su CJ, Huang TY, Lee CC, Yang YS. A simple and low-cost method to fabricate TFTs with poly-Si nanowire channel. IEEE Electron Device Lett 2005; 26(9): 643-5.
[http://dx.doi.org/10.1109/LED.2005.853669]

[158] Ahn J-H, Choi S-J, Han J-W, Park TJ, Lee SY, Choi Y-K. Double-gate nanowire field effect transistor for a biosensor. Nano Lett 2010; 10(8): 2934-8.
[http://dx.doi.org/10.1021/nl1010965] [PMID: 20698606]

[159] Go J, Nair PR, Reddy B Jr, Dorvel B, Bashir R, Alam MA. Coupled heterogeneous nanowire-nanoplate planar transistor sensors for giant (>10 V/pH) Nernst response. ACS Nano 2012; 6(7): 5972-9.
[http://dx.doi.org/10.1021/nn300874w] [PMID: 22695084]

[160] Knopfmacher O, Tarasov A, Fu W, *et al.* Nernst limit in dual-gated Si-nanowire FET sensors. Nano Lett 2010; 10(6): 2268-74.
[http://dx.doi.org/10.1021/nl100892y] [PMID: 20499926]

[161] Xie P, Xiong Q, Fang Y, Qing Q, Lieber CM. Local electrical potential detection of DNA by nanowire-nanopore sensors. Nat Nanotechnol 2011; 7(2): 119-25.
[http://dx.doi.org/10.1038/nnano.2011.217] [PMID: 22157724]

[162] Clarke J, Wu H-C, Jayasinghe L, Patel A, Reid S, Bayley H. Continuous base identification for single-molecule nanopore DNA sequencing. Nat Nanotechnol 2009; 4(4): 265-70.
[http://dx.doi.org/10.1038/nnano.2009.12] [PMID: 19350039]

[163] Derrington IM, Butler TZ, Collins MD, *et al.* Nanopore DNA sequencing with MspA. Proc Natl Acad Sci USA 2010; 107(37): 16060-5.
[http://dx.doi.org/10.1073/pnas.1001831107] [PMID: 20798343]

[164] Lee K-W, Choi S-J, Ahn J-H, *et al.* An underlap field-effect transistor for electrical detection of influenza. Appl Phys Lett 2010; 96(3): 033703.

[http://dx.doi.org/10.1063/1.3291617]

[165] Im H, Huang X-J, Gu B, Choi Y-K. A dielectric-modulated field-effect transistor for biosensing. Nat Nanotechnol 2007; 2(7): 430-4.
[http://dx.doi.org/10.1038/nnano.2007.180] [PMID: 18654328]

[166] Vayssieres L. Growth of Arrayed Nanorods and Nanowires of ZnO from Aqueous Solutions. Adv Mater 2003; 15(5): 464-6.
[http://dx.doi.org/10.1002/adma.200390108]

[167] Kulkarni GS, Zhong Z. Detection beyond the Debye screening length in a high-frequency nanoelectronic biosensor. Nano Lett 2012; 12(2): 719-23.
[http://dx.doi.org/10.1021/nl203666a] [PMID: 22214376]

[168] Vacic A, Criscione JM, Stern E, Rajan NK, Fahmy T, Reed MA. Multiplexed SOI BioFETs. Biosens Bioelectron 2011; 28(1): 239-42.
[http://dx.doi.org/10.1016/j.bios.2011.07.025] [PMID: 21820303]

[169] Ishikawa FN, Curreli M, Chang H-K, *et al.* A calibration method for nanowire biosensors to suppress device-to-device variation. ACS Nano 2009; 3(12): 3969-76.
[http://dx.doi.org/10.1021/nn9011384] [PMID: 19921812]

[170] Peretz-Soroka H, Pevzner A, Davidi G, *et al.* Optically-gated self-calibrating nanosensors: monitoring pH and metabolic activity of living cells. Nano Lett 2013; 13(7): 3157-68.
[http://dx.doi.org/10.1021/nl401169k] [PMID: 23772673]

[171] Park I, Li Z, Pisano AP, Williams RS. Selective surface functionalization of silicon nanowires via nanoscale joule heating. Nano Lett 2007; 7(10): 3106-11.
[http://dx.doi.org/10.1021/nl071637k] [PMID: 17894518]

[172] Masood MN, Chen S, Carlen ET, van den Berg A. All-(111) surface silicon nanowires: selective functionalization for biosensing applications. ACS Appl Mater Interfaces 2010; 2(12): 3422-8.
[http://dx.doi.org/10.1021/am100922e] [PMID: 21090766]

[173] Mohd Azmi MA, Tehrani Z, Lewis RP, *et al.* Highly sensitive covalently functionalised integrated silicon nanowire biosensor devices for detection of cancer risk biomarker. Biosens Bioelectron 2014; 52: 216-24.
[http://dx.doi.org/10.1016/j.bios.2013.08.030] [PMID: 24060972]

[174] Alam AU, Howlader MMR, Deen MJ. The effects of oxygen plasma and humidity on surface roughness, water contact angle and hardness of silicon, silicon dioxide and glass. J Micromech Microeng 2014; 24(3): 035010.
[http://dx.doi.org/10.1088/0960-1317/24/3/035010]

[175] Ghorbanpour M, Falamaki C. A novel method for the fabrication of ATPES silanized SPR sensor chips: Exclusion of Cr or Ti intermediate layers and optimization of optical/adherence properties. Appl Surf Sci 2014; 301: 544-50.
[http://dx.doi.org/10.1016/j.apsusc.2014.02.121]

[176] Tajima N, Takai M, Ishihara K. Significance of antibody orientation unraveled: well-oriented antibodies recorded high binding affinity. Anal Chem 2011; 83(6): 1969-76.
[http://dx.doi.org/10.1021/ac1026786] [PMID: 21338074]

[177] Bousse L, Bergveld P. The role of buried OH sites in the response mechanism of inorganic-gate pH-sensitive ISFETs. Sens Actuators 1984; 6(1): 65-78.
[http://dx.doi.org/10.1016/0250-6874(84)80028-1]

[178] Bae TE, Jang HJ, Yang JH, Cho WJ. High performance of silicon nanowire-based biosensors using a high-k stacked sensing thin film. ACS Appl Mater Interfaces 2013; 5(11): 5214-8.
[http://dx.doi.org/10.1021/am401026z] [PMID: 23651227]

[179] Tarasov A, Wipf M, Stoop RL, *et al.* Understanding the electrolyte background for biochemical sensing with ion-sensitive field-effect transistors. ACS Nano 2012; 6(10): 9291-8.

[http://dx.doi.org/10.1021/nn303795r] [PMID: 23016890]

[180] Wipf M, Stoop RL, Tarasov A, *et al.* Selective sodium sensing with gold-coated silicon nanowire field-effect transistors in a differential setup. ACS Nano 2013; 7(7): 5978-83.
[http://dx.doi.org/10.1021/nn401678u] [PMID: 23768238]

[181] Tarasov A, Wipf M, Bedner K, *et al.* True reference nanosensor realized with silicon nanowires. Langmuir 2012; 28(25): 9899-905.
[http://dx.doi.org/10.1021/la301555r] [PMID: 22631046]

[182] Zheng C, Huang L, Zhang H, Sun Z, Zhang Z, Zhang G-J. Fabrication of Ultrasensitive Field-Effect Transistor DNA Biosensors by a Directional Transfer Technique Based on CVD-Grown Graphene. ACS Appl Mater Interfaces 2015; 7(31): 16953-9.
[http://dx.doi.org/10.1021/acsami.5b03941] [PMID: 26203889]

[183] Krivitsky V, Hsiung LC, Lichtenstein A, *et al.* Si nanowires forest-based on-chip biomolecular filtering, separation and preconcentration devices: nanowires do it all. Nano Lett 2012; 12(9): 4748-56.
[http://dx.doi.org/10.1021/nl3021889] [PMID: 22852557]

[184] Lin S-P, Pan C-Y, Tseng K-C, *et al.* A reversible surface functionalized nanowire transistor to study protein–protein interactions. Nano Today 2009; 4(3): 235-43.
[http://dx.doi.org/10.1016/j.nantod.2009.04.005]

[185] Song S, Wang L, Li J, Fan C, Zhao J. Aptamer-based biosensors. Trends Analyt Chem 2008; 27(2): 108-17.
[http://dx.doi.org/10.1016/j.trac.2007.12.004]

[186] Gao N, Zhou W, Jiang X, Hong G, Fu TM, Lieber CM. General strategy for biodetection in high ionic strength solutions using transistor-based nanoelectronic sensors. Nano Lett 2015; 15(3): 2143-8.
[http://dx.doi.org/10.1021/acs.nanolett.5b00133] [PMID: 25664395]

[187] Arnold K, Herrmann A, Pratsch L, Gawrisch K. The dielectric properties of aqueous solutions of poly(ethylene glycol) and their influence on membrane structure. Biochim Biophys Acta 1985; 815(3): 515-8.
[http://dx.doi.org/10.1016/0005-2736(85)90381-5] [PMID: 3995041]

[188] Gao N, Gao T, Yang X, *et al.* Specific detection of biomolecules in physiological solutions using graphene transistor biosensors. Proc Natl Acad Sci USA 2016; 113(51): 14633-8.
[http://dx.doi.org/10.1073/pnas.1625010114] [PMID: 27930344]

[189] Filipiak MS, Rother M, Andoy NM, *et al.* Highly sensitive, selective and label-free protein detection in physiological solutions using carbon nanotube transistors with nanobody receptors. Sens Actuators B Chem 2018; 255: 1507-16.
[http://dx.doi.org/10.1016/j.snb.2017.08.164]

[190] Zheng G, Gao XP, Lieber CM. Frequency domain detection of biomolecules using silicon nanowire biosensors. Nano Lett 2010; 10(8): 3179-83.
[http://dx.doi.org/10.1021/nl1020975] [PMID: 20698634]

[191] Kirton MJ, Uren MJ. Noise in solid-state microstructures: A new perspective on individual defects, interface states and low-frequency $(1/f)$ noise. Adv Phys 1989; 38(4): 367-468.
[http://dx.doi.org/10.1080/00018738900101122]

[192] Clément N, Nishiguchi K, Fujiwara A, Vuillaume D. One-by-one trap activation in silicon nanowire transistors. Nat Commun 2010; 1: 92.
[http://dx.doi.org/10.1038/ncomms1092] [PMID: 20981020]

[193] Li J, Pud S, Petrychuk M, Offenhäusser A, Vitusevich S. Sensitivity enhancement of Si nanowire field effect transistor biosensors using single trap phenomena. Nano Lett 2014; 14(6): 3504-9.
[http://dx.doi.org/10.1021/nl5010724] [PMID: 24813644]

[194] Aroonyadet N, Wang X, Song Y, *et al.* Highly scalable, uniform, and sensitive biosensors based on top-down indium oxide nanoribbons and electronic enzyme-linked immunosorbent assay. Nano Lett

2015; 15(3): 1943-51.
[http://dx.doi.org/10.1021/nl5047889] [PMID: 25636984]

[195] Stern E, Vacic A, Rajan NK, *et al.* Label-free biomarker detection from whole blood. Nat Nanotechnol 2010; 5(2): 138-42.
[http://dx.doi.org/10.1038/nnano.2009.353] [PMID: 20010825]

[196] Teh S-Y, Lin R, Hung L-H, Lee AP. Droplet microfluidics. Lab Chip 2008; 8(2): 198-220.
[http://dx.doi.org/10.1039/b715524g] [PMID: 18231657]

[197] Cao A, Sudhölter EJ, de Smet LC. Silicon nanowire-based devices for gas-phase sensing. Sensors (Basel) 2013; 14(1): 245-71.
[http://dx.doi.org/10.3390/s140100245] [PMID: 24368699]

[198] Talin AA, Hunter LL, Léonard F, Rokad B. Large area, dense silicon nanowire array chemical sensors. Appl Phys Lett 2006; 89(15): 153102.
[http://dx.doi.org/10.1063/1.2358214]

[199] Skucha K, Fan Z, Jeon K, Javey A, Boser B. Palladium/silicon nanowire Schottky barrier-based hydrogen sensors. Sens Actuators B Chem 2010; 145(1): 232-8.
[http://dx.doi.org/10.1016/j.snb.2009.11.067]

[200] Tisch U, Haick H. Arrays of Nanomaterial-Based Sensors for Breath Testing.Volatile Biomarkers. Boston: Elsevier 2013; pp. 301-23.
[http://dx.doi.org/10.1016/B978-0-44-462613-4.00016-7]

[201] Wang B, Haick H. Effect of chain length on the sensing of volatile organic compounds by means of silicon nanowires. ACS Appl Mater Interfaces 2013; 5(12): 5748-56.
[http://dx.doi.org/10.1021/am401265z] [PMID: 23725353]

[202] Ermanok R, Assad O, Zigelboim K, Wang B, Haick H. Discriminative power of chemically sensitive silicon nanowire field effect transistors to volatile organic compounds. ACS Appl Mater Interfaces 2013; 5(21): 11172-83.
[http://dx.doi.org/10.1021/am403421g] [PMID: 24144671]

[203] Basheer IA, Hajmeer M. Artificial neural networks: fundamentals, computing, design, and application. J Microbiol Methods 2000; 43(1): 3-31.
[http://dx.doi.org/10.1016/S0167-7012(00)00201-3] [PMID: 11084225]

[204] Blackard JA, Dean DJ. Comparative accuracies of artificial neural networks and discriminant analysis in predicting forest cover types from cartographic variables. Comput Electron Agric 1999; 24(3): 131-51.
[http://dx.doi.org/10.1016/S0168-1699(99)00046-0]

[205] Robnik-Šikonja M, Kononenko I. Theoretical and Empirical Analysis of ReliefF and RReliefF. Mach Learn 2003; 53(1): 23-69.
[http://dx.doi.org/10.1023/A:1025667309714]

[206] Ma S, Li X, Lee YK, Zhang A. Direct label-free protein detection in high ionic strength solution and human plasma using dual-gate nanoribbon-based ion-sensitive field-effect transistor biosensor. Biosens Bioelectron 2018; 117: 276-82.
[http://dx.doi.org/10.1016/j.bios.2018.05.061] [PMID: 29909199]

[207] Gutiérrez-Sanz Ó, Andoy NM, Filipiak MS, Haustein N, Tarasov A. Direct, Label-Free, and Rapid Transistor-Based Immunodetection in Whole Serum. ACS Sens 2017; 2(9): 1278-86.
[http://dx.doi.org/10.1021/acssensors.7b00187] [PMID: 28853283]

[208] Andoy NM, Filipiak MS, Vetter D, Gutiérrez-Sanz Ó, Tarasov A. Graphene-Based Electronic Immunosensor with Femtomolar Detection Limit in Whole Serum. Advanced Materials Technologies 2018; 3(12): 1800186.
[http://dx.doi.org/10.1002/admt.201800186]

CHAPTER 5

Fluorescence Biosensors

Huong T. Vu[1], Soonwoo Hong[1] and Hsin-Chih Yeh[1,2,*]

[1] *Department of Biomedical Engineering, The University of Texas at Austin, USA*

[2] *Department of Biomedical Engineering and Texas Materials Institutes, The University of Texas at Austin, USA*

Abstract: This chapter provides an overview of state of the art in fluorescence detection using molecular-sized biosensors. In the past three decades, a number of activatable or tunable fluorescence biosensors have been developed, including FRET sensors, intercalating dyes, electron transfer-based sensors, fluorescein-based sensors, split GFP, biarsenical-tetracysteine sensors, aptamer sensors, H-dimer sensors, lanthanide-based sensors, carbon nanotube sensors, quencher transfer/detachment, FRET binary probes and chameleon NanoCluster Beacons. Researchers have proposed various methods to increase the dynamic range, the specificity, and the sensitivity of the aforementioned sensors. The requirements for using fluorescence sensors in biomedical imaging are reviewed, which provide general guidance for readers to conduct medical diagnosis with these newly-developed biosensing technologies. The chapter concludes with a brief perspective into the future of fluorescence-based biosensing systems.

Keywords: Activatable sensors, Fluorescence techniques, Nanomaterials sensors, Turn-on sensors, Tunable sensors.

INTRODUCTION

Fluorescence technologies have revolutionized the way that complex biological and chemical systems are studied. They allow simple, real-time, highly sensitive, and environment-friendly imaging or detection of specific biomolecules or compounds, facilitating basic research in quantitative biology, analytical chemistry, and clinical medicine [1]. In the past 30 years, a remarkable advance in the instrumentation has enabled the direct observation of even a single fluorescent molecule at room temperature in aqueous solution [2]. At the same time, the development of new fluorescent probes, such as genetically encoded green fluorescence proteins, intercalating dyes, and cell-permeable fluorophores, have offered researchers unprecedented visual access to the inner workings of cells [3]

** **Corresponding author Hsin-Chih Yeh:** Department of Biomedical Engineering and Texas Materials Institutes, the University of Texas at Austin, USA; E-mail: tim.yeh@austin.utexas.edu*

Han-Sheng Chuang & Yi-Ping Ho (Eds.)

and even live animals [4]. Whereas a wide variety of organic dyes, fluorescent proteins, and semiconductor nanocrystals have been successfully commercialized and routinely used in the laboratory and clinical settings today, researchers are still on a quest to develop the next-generation fluorescent probes that are smaller, brighter, cheaper, and more photostable than the current fluorophores, while being genetically encodable, emission spectrum tunable, and nontoxic. To bypass the need for the tedious and labor-intensive "immobilization and wash" steps in many *in-vitro* bioassays, such as enzyme-linked immunosorbent assay (ELISA), a number of fluorescent probes have been turned into "fluorescence biosensors" that significantly light up or change color upon binding with their specific targets (Fig. **1**). Intercalating dyes, molecular beacons, binary probes and aptamer-based sensors are successful examples that have made a major impact on the biomedical research.

In this chapter, an overview of important fluorescence molecular biosensors developed in the past three decades is provided and their principles, functions, and the current use in biomedical diagnostics are discussed. It is emphasized that the focus of this chapter is on those chemical constructs whose fluorescence emissions can be tuned by fluorescence resonance energy transfer, electron transfer, constraint of the molecular movement, assembly of a fluorescent entity, and ligand effect "upon target recognition". Throughout the years various names have been given to these fluorescence biosensors by different researchers, including separation-free probes, turn-on probes, activatable probes, tunable probes, and multicolor probes. As long as the molecular construct has a "target recognition portion" and a "fluorescence signal transduction portion", and one of the fluorescence signatures (intensity, intermittency, spectrum, anisotropy, lifetime and duration) changes upon target binding, this molecular construct is called a fluorescence biosensor. While fiber optics-based sensors combined with fluorescence readouts are considered as fluorescence biosensors by some researchers [5], here only the molecular-sized biosensors are reviewed.

After a brief introduction of the basic concepts in fluorescence biosensors, this book chapter classifies fluorescence biosensors based on their signal-transduction mechanisms, readout formats, reporter types, and other features. Other than design principles and functions, major impacts made by individual biosensors in quantitative biology, analytical chemistry, and clinical medicine are also presented here. Emerging sensor materials, signal-amplification strategies, and the requirements for using fluorescence sensors in biomedical imaging are also discussed. The concluding remarks provide a perspective on past developments and future directions.

Basics of Molecular Biosensors and General Applications

Molecular sensors are molecular-level devices that can indicate the existence of their target molecules or the extent of target activities. Here targets can be biological entities, such as DNA, RNA, proteins, enzymes, small metabolites, cell membrane, organelles, and cancer cells; or chemical compounds, such as ions, heavy metals, gas molecules, and drug molecules. Target activities can be enzyme activities, molecular association or dissociation. The term "analyte" is used to collectively represent targets and target activities. A typical molecular sensor can be broken down into two portions: (i) the target capture and molecular recognition portion and (ii) the signal transduction portion (Fig. **1B**).

The target capture and recognition portion serves as a "receptor" which recognizes and binds to the analytes of interest. Common recognition portions for molecular biosensors include antibodies, membrane receptors, nucleic acids, aptamers, polymers, and small molecules. Mechanisms for capture and recognition include antigen-antibody binding, adsorption, nucleic acid hybridization, covalent and non-covalent attachments, and crosslinking. Analyte binding can alter physical properties of the recognition portion, such as conformational changes and electron redistributions, or trigger chemical reactions, such as reduction-oxidation (redox) reactions.

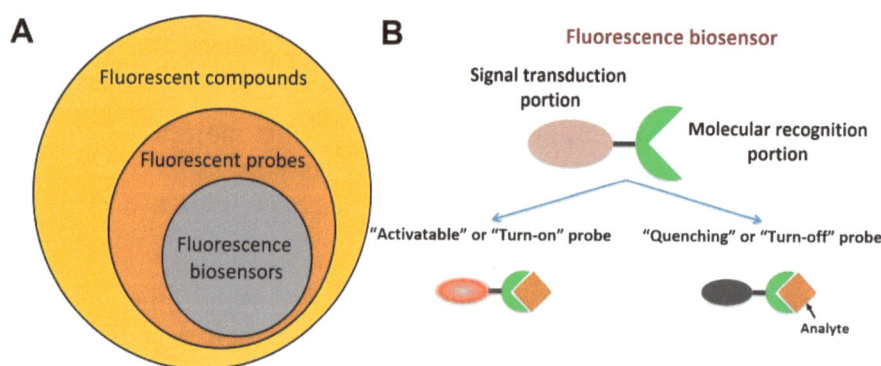

Fig. (1). (A) Among all the fluorescent compounds available today, only a portion of them are bright and stable enough to be used as fluorescent probes. Among all the fluorescent probes available, only a portion of them have interesting photophysical properties that can be employed as the basis for fluorescence biosensor development. **(B)** The essential components of a molecular-scale fluorescence biosensor (molecular recognition portion vs. signal transduction portion) and the two different sensing actions (turn-on vs. turn-off).

The effect of analyte binding is then transduced into readout signals by the signal transduction portion. In a typical fluorescence biosensor, the transduction portion is a fluorophore (or fluorophores) that converts analyte binding events into fluorescence emission. Table **1** provides the working principles and examples of five signal transduction mechanisms commonly used in today's fluorescence biosensors.

Table 1. Five different signal-transduction mechanisms and their corresponding biosensor examples.

Transduction Methods	Description of Actions	Biosensor Examples and References
Fluorescence resonance energy transfer (FRET)	Analyte binding changes the distance between donor and acceptor, generating "FRET signals". Here FRET signals can be acceptor emission or change in donor's lifetime.	Molecular beacons (MB) [6, 7] TaqMan probes [8-10] Cameleon sensors [11] Quantum dot-based sensors [12, 13] Hetero-FRET sensors [14, 15] Homo-FRET sensors [4]
Formation of fluorescent constructs	Analyte binding induces assembly of a fully functional fluorophore	Split GFP [16-18] Genetically encoded fluorescent protein sensors [19-22] H-dimer [23-27]
Photoinduced electron transfer (PET)	Analyte binding prevents electron transfer from an electron donor to a fluorophore, thus restoring fluorophore's emission.	Smart probes [28] Fluorescein-based probes [29-31]
Suppression of non-radiative pathways	Analyte binding restricts fluorophore's motion or increases viscosity in fluorophore's vicinity, suppressing non-radiative pathways of the fluorophore.	Intercalating dyes [32-40] FlAsH and ReAsH [41, 42] Aptamer-based sensors [43-49]
Ligand effects	Analyte binding changes the electronic structures of the fluorophore.	NanoCluster Beacons (NCB) [50-58] Carbon nanotube-based sensors [59]

Classification of Fluorescence Biosensors

Since all fluorescence properties, such as quantum yield, extinction coefficient, emission intermittency, anisotropy, lifetime, emission spectra, and emission duration, can be used as a basis for sensing, here fluorescence biosensors are classified by their readout formats (Table **2**). As the brightness of fluorophore can be easily read by a low-cost camera, many fluorescence sensors are based on the intensity reading, which is the product of fluorophore's quantum yield and extinction coefficient. However, many factors can bias fluorophore's intensity reading in a detector, including self-quenching of the fluorophore, electronic quantum yield of the detector, excitation intensity fluctuation, inner filter effect, solvent effect, photobleaching, and so on [1]. Consequently, intensity-based biosensors may have poor performance and give an ambiguous sensing result.

Table 2. Fluorescence biosensor classification based on their readout formats.

Readout Format	Biosensor Examples	References
Intensity	NanoCluster Beacons (NCB) Molecular beacons (MB) GCaMP	[50 - 58] [6, 7] [19]
Lifetime	Protein induced fluorescence enhancement (PIFE) sensors	[60]
Blinking	Cy5 blinking sensors	[61]
Emission spectra	Wavelength-shifting molecular beacons Cameleon Chameleon NanoCluster Beacons	[62] [11] [52]
Anisotropy	Aptamer-based biosensors	[63, 64]
Duration	Protein-DNA dissociation sensors, DNA sensors	[65, 66]

In contrast, the color-change or wavelength-shifting sensors can be less ambiguous in molecular sensing [11, 52, 62]. However, spectrum-change signals often have to be read by sophisticated tools, such as a fluorescence spectrometer or a microscope equipped with multiple excitation/detection channels. Similarly, fluorescence blinking (intermittency) is often on the microsecond time scale that requires sophisticated electronics for data acquisition and real-time interpretation [61]. As fluorescence lifetime is even on the nanosecond timescale [60], high-temporal resolution, single-photon-counting devices, such as an avalanche photodiode (APD) or a photomultiplier tube (PMT), combined with time-correlated single-photon counting (TCSPC) electronics, are often needed to detect time-resolved fluorescence [1]. Although the hardware requirements to read lifetime- or blinking-based sensing signals add cost to the detection, these sensors are less prone to the environmental factors, thus providing more robust sensing results. Please note that here we exclude the sensors whose readout format is "absorption spectrum change", as these sensors are often based on gold nanoparticles that are non-fluorescent [67]. They should be reviewed elsewhere [68]. Sensors that bind to target biomolecules can exhibit reduced rotational diffusion or translational diffusion, leading to a change in fluorescence anisotropy [63, 64] or fluorescence duration [65, 66]. Fluorescence duration change is often probed by a fluctuation analysis technique, such as fluorescence correlation spectroscopy (FCS) [69], which is well-reviewed in Rigler and Elson's book [70].

Commonly used fluorescent reports or fluorophores can be classified into 4 major groups – organic dyes, green fluorescent proteins (GFP), semiconductor quantum dots (QD) [71, 72], and fluorescent nanomaterials (such as noble metal nanoclusters [73, 74] or carbon nanotubes [59]) (Table **3**). Organic dyes, such as Alexa, Atto, Bodipy, and Cyanine dyes, are widely used today in fluorescence imaging due to their excellent brightness and photostability, but they remain non-specific unless conjugated to an antibody or other targeted ligand. While GFP represents a considerable step forward from organic dyes as they can be genetically encoded (fused to a protein of interest) and used to probe the inner workings of live cells [3], GFP are generally dim, environment-sensitive, and lack photostability. In addition, the size of GFP (27 kDa, 2.4×4.2 nm [75]) is much larger than that of organic dyes (typically < 1 kDa, smaller than 1 nm), which may alter the function of the fused target protein. Semiconductor QD are by far the most photostable fluorophores in the toolbox ($100\times$ more stable than organic dyes [71]) and are very bright (extinction coefficient $\sim 5 \times 10^5$ cm^{-1}M^{-1} [76]), but the commercially available QD often have a toxic core (cadmium) with an overall size of 15-20 nm, making them unsuitable for many cellular and tissue sensing applications. While emerging fluorescent nanomaterials, such as noble metal nanoclusters [73, 74] and carbon nanotubes [59], possess unique photophysical properties and have been made into fluorescence biosensors for special applications [50, 59], their cytotoxicity and non-specific interactions with cellular structures are largely unknown. Like QD, the sensors based on emerging nanomaterials are currently designed for *in-vitro* applications.

Table 3. Fluorescence biosensor classification based on their fluorescent reporters.

Types of Reporters	Description	References
Fluorescent proteins	Cameleon GCaMP Split GFP	[11] [19] [16 - 18]
Organic dyes	TG-βGal H-dimer sensors Aptamer sensors Intercalators	[14, 31] [23 - 27] [46, 47] [34]
Semiconductor quantum dots	Maltose sensors DNA sensors Protein beacons	[12] [13] [77]
Emerging fluorescent nanomaterials	NanoCluster Beacons DNA-SWNT divalent metal ion sensors	[50] [59]

Many other ways can be used to classify fluorescence biosensors; for instance, turn-on vs. turn-off, reversible vs. irreversible, genetically encodable vs. exogenous sensors (Table **4**). To use exogenous sensors inside live cells, a cell delivery method, such as electroporation, lipofection, microinjection, reversible permeabilization [78], and cell-penetrating peptides [79, 80], is often required. In this book chapter, the focus is on the fluorescence activation mechanisms. Understanding the detailed activation principles is important in both choosing the appropriate biosensors for specific applications and designing new sensors for future applications.

Table 4. Fluorescence biosensor classification based on three sensor features

Types	Description	References
Turn-on sensors	Split GFP Aptamer sensors	[16 - 18] [46, 47]
Turn-off sensors	Cl⁻ sensors	[81, 82]
Reversible sensors	Molecular beacons NanoCluster Beacons	[6, 7] [50]
Irreversible sensors	TaqMan	[8 - 10]
Genetically encodable sensors	Cameleons FlAsH	[11] [41]
Exogenous sensors	Dual molecular beacons	[78]

Advantages of the Activatability of Fluorescence Biosensors

Activatable fluorescence biosensors are unique in the field of *in-vitro* and *in-vivo* biosensing as they can be turned on upon target binding, but otherwise, remain undetectable. This activatability greatly improves the signal-to-background signals in target detection, making the removal of unbound sensors unnecessary. Activatable fluorescence biosensors are particularly important for live cell or tissue studies where removal of unbound sensors is difficult. One example is the Ca^{2+} sensor Cameleon that enables real-time observation of Ca^{2+} concentration dynamics in HeLa cells [11]. Activatable probes are also useful in the development of super-resolution microscopy techniques where the ability to turn on and off specific dyes at specific locations and times allows images to be taken with a greater resolution than the one imposed by the diffraction limit [83].

DESIGN PRINCIPLES OF ACTIVATABLE OR TUNABLE FLUORESCENCE BIOSENSORS

Until now, a number of activatable fluorescence biosensors have been developed, including FRET sensors [6, 11], intercalating dyes [34], electron transfer-based sensors [28], environment-sensitive Aequorea fluorescent proteins [84], split GFP [16, 18], biarsenical-tetracysteine sensors [41, 42], aptamer sensors [43 - 49], H-dimer sensors [23 - 27], and lanthanide-based sensors [85, 86]. Similarly, a number of tunable (*e.g.* color-switching) sensors have also been demonstrated, such as carbon nanotube sensors [59], quencher transfer/detachment [87, 88], FRET binary probes [89, 90], and chameleon NanoCluster Beacons [52]. Readers are also recommended to refer to review articles in fluorescence sensor development by Yeh [53], Kobayashi [4], Kolpashchikov [91], Vendrell [92], Kool [93], Li [94], Ranasinghe and Brown [95], and Ihara [96]. As shown in Table **1**, activation mechanisms can be categorized as follows: (1) FRET, (2) formation of fluorescent constructs, (3) photoinduced electron transfer, (4) suppression of non-radiative pathways, (5) and ligand effect. Here the most important fluorescence biosensors developed, based on each of these activation schemes, are discussed.

Fluorescence Resonance Energy Transfer (FRET)

Most fluorescence sensors employ FRET as their signal transduction mechanism (Fig. **2**). In FRET, the energy transfer efficiency from the donor to the acceptor is highly sensitive to the separation distance between them, following an inverse sixth power law due to the dipole-dipole interactions [1]. In a simple intramolecular FRET sensor design, a donor and an acceptor fluorophore can be labeled at the two ends of the target-binding domain on a sensor. When binding to the target, the target-binding domain undergoes a conformational change, bringing the two fluorophores in close proximity (typically < 10 nm, twice as the Förster distance), thus enabling FRET [11]. A similar strategy (target binding inducing donor-acceptor distance change) is also applied to the intermolecular FRET sensor design [97]. Upon donor excitation, the non-radiative resonance energy transfer can be detected as follows: (1) a decrease in the donor emission, (2) an increase in the acceptor emission, and (3) a decrease in donor lifetime. FRET signals can be used to precisely quantify target molecules, even down to the single-molecule level [98].

The FRET efficiency analysis comes with a number of benefits, such as being highly quantitatively reliable and correcting for many optical artifacts and differences in expression level of the FRET sensors. However, FRET sensors require a large conformational change upon target binding for sensing; therefore, they often suffer from either slow response or low FRET signals. Another limitation is the requirement of using FRET sensors at a low concentration. This is to avoid quenching the sensor donor by another sensor nearby (*i.e.* homoFRET or self-quenching). Some of the most famous and widely used FRET-based biosensors, starting with the important sensors for PCR amplicon detection, are discussed below.

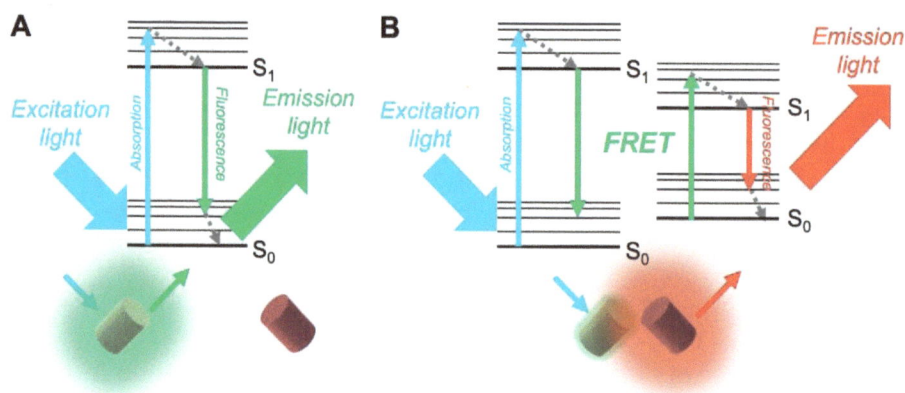

Fig. (2). Jablonski diagram of fluorescence resonance energy transfer (FRET). (**A**) When a donor fluorophore is far from an acceptor fluorophore, the energy transfer is prohibited and only the donor emits a fluorescence. (**B**) When the donor-acceptor distance is within twice the Förster radius (typically ~10 nm), non-radiative resonance energy transfer takes place and the acceptor emission is observed.

Intramolecular FRET-based Sensors

TaqMan

One major breakthrough in polymerase chain reaction (PCR) techniques is the replacement of *E. Coli* DNA polymerase with Thermus aquaticus (Taq) DNA polymerase that is thermostable over a wide range of temperatures during the PCR cycles, eliminating the need to add fresh enzyme every cycle [101]. Other than the superior thermostability, Taq polymerase has 5'-3' exonuclease activity that cleaves 5' terminal nucleotides of dsDNA into small mono- and oligonucleotides (Fig. **3**). Taking advantage of this exonuclease activity, Gelfand's group designed a FRET-based probe called TaqMan for closed-tube PCR product detection [8]. TaqMan is a DNA probe labeled with a fluorescent reporter and a quencher at its 3' and 5' ends (Fig. **3**). Due to the energy transfer process between the reporter and the quencher, this probe is initially dark. As Taq polymerase cleaves the TaqMan probe during the elongation step, reporters are separated from the quenchers and become highly emissive. By detecting the reporter signal, PCR products can be continuously monitored in a homogeneous assay. The probe design and the PCR setup were further improved by Lee [9], Williams [10], and Whitcombe [102], making TaqMan one of the gold-standard assays in pathogen identification. Readers are also recommended to refer to review articles in reporter-quencher pair selection by Johansson [103] or Lakowicz [1].

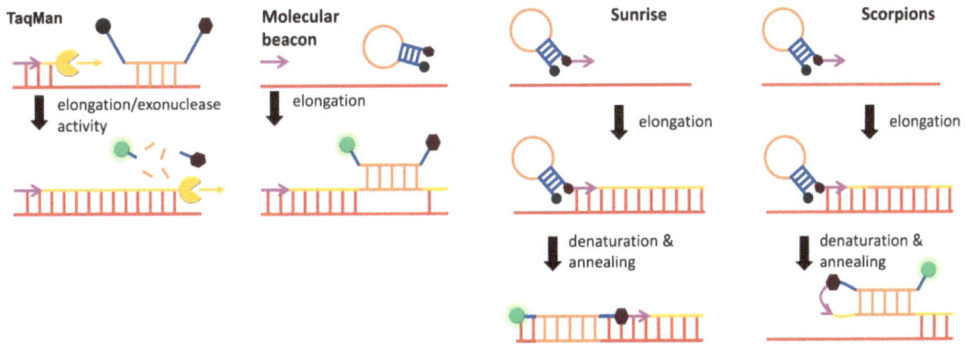

Fig. (3). Different PCR amplicon detection assays: TaqMan [8], molecular beacons [6], Sunrise [99], and Scorpions [100]. In PCR, the *Thermus aquaticus* (*Taq*) DNA polymerase cleaves the TaqMan probe during the elongation cycle, restoring the originally quenched fluorescence of the reporters. Molecular beacon is a stem-loop probe that fluoresces upon hybridization with the target DNA. Sunrise and Scorpions are two distinct tailed primer designs, in which the stem-loop structures open up upon primer-target hybridization (Sunrise) or primer's self-probing after elongation (Scorpions).

Molecular Beacons

Although TaqMan is a highly specific FRET probe for PCR amplicon detection, it requires enzymatic cleavage to unleash the fluorescence signal. A well-known non-enzymatic FRET sensor that fluoresces upon sensor-target hybridization is the molecular beacon (MB) developed by Tyagi and Kramer [6, 7] (Fig. **4**). In the unbound state (Fig. **4A**), MB has a stem-loop structure with a reporter and a quencher attached to its 5' and 3' ends, respectively. As the complementary target sequence lies in the loop segment, in the bound state (Fig. **4A**), the hairpin structure opens up, separating the reporter from the quencher and restoring its fluorescence. The sensor-target hybrid in the bound state is designed to be more thermostable than the hairpin structure in the unbound state. Hence, molecular beacons can detect specific nucleic acids in a homogenous solution without using any enzymes. Other than FRET, Tyagi also pointed out that the tendency of the reporter to bind to the quencher also has a strong influence on quenching efficiency (termed "contact quenching") [104].

Over the years, efforts have been made to enhance the activation ratios of MB and diversify their applications [105]. One improvement is the creation of a wavelength-shifting MB that has two dyes (a harvester and an emitter) conjugated to the 5' end of an MB [62]. This design allows the MB to strongly absorb the light in the wavelength range of the monochromatic light source by the harvester while emitting in the desired emission range of the emitter (Fig. **4B**).

Molecular beacons have been used in real-time PCR assays [106], DNA microarrays [107], and live-cell mRNA quantification assays [78]. The hairpin structure was also incorporated in the tailed primer designs, so-called Sunrise primer [99] and Scorpions primer [100], for PCR product detection (Fig. **3**). In the Sunrise primer design, the detection signal originates from the hybridization of the primer-extended product with its complementary strand. In contrast, the Scorpions primer is designed to target the extension product of the primer, the so-called self-probing amplicons. These tailed primer designs can more specifically distinguish true amplicons from any undesired amplification products, such as primer dimers, eliminating any false positives in a closed-tube reaction.

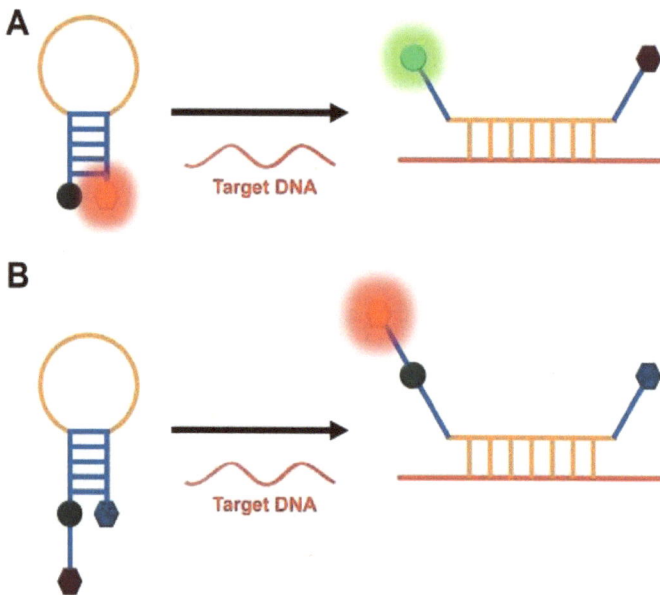

Fig. (4). (**A**) Schematic diagram of molecular beacon: (left) unbound-state and (right) bound-state of a molecular beacon. In the first MB design, the reporter (green circle) was fluorescein and the quencher (red hexagon) was DABCYL(4-[4'-dimethylaminophenylazo]benzoic acid [7]. (**B**) Schematic diagram of wavelength-shifting molecular beacon: (left) unbound state and (right) bound state. Using another FRET process between the harvester (green circle) and the emitter (red hexagon), this MB design allows fluorescein (the harvest) excitation at 488 nm and Texas Red (the emitter) emission at 615 nm [62].

Cameleon

Cameleon was the first genetically encoded calcium ion sensor (GECI) pioneered by Tsien [11], which consists of two variants of GFP (*e.g.* CFP and YFP) fused at the two termini of a Ca^{2+} binding domain (calmodulin, CaM, and M13, Fig. **5**). Cameleon sensor undergoes a conformational change upon Ca^{2+} binding to the calmodulin (CaM) element, bringing the two flanking FPs into close proximity and increasing the resonance energy transfer between them, thus alternating the wavelength of the emission signal. Hence, Cameleon's color corresponds to Ca^{2+} concentration, similar to a chameleon that alters its skin color in response to the environment.

With two decades of improvement [108], many Cameleon-like sensors are available today, enabling visualization and monitoring of Ca^{2+} levels in mitochondria [109] and in neurons and muscle cells of a transgenic animal [110 - 112]. Compared with other Ca^{2+} sensors that are not cell permeable and require microinjection for live-cell studies (*e.g.* fura-2 and indo-1 [113]), Cameleon and its derivatives are all genetically encodable and can be steadily generated in a specific compartment within live cells without the need of a delivery system. Unlike the single-emission sensors, such as GCaMP (see discussion below) [19], Cameleon sensor has the advantages of ratiometric sensing, which is particularly important in live-cell or tissue imaging as ratiometric imaging is less sensitive to the variations in optical path length, excitation intensity, and sensor concentration *in vivo*. However, like many other GFP-based sensors, Cameleon sensor has a long maturation time and a slow response to Ca^{2+} due to its large size. Thus, real-time monitoring of fast neural circuit dynamics inside neural cells still requires small-molecule Ca^{2+} sensors [114].

Following the design principle of Cameleon, many other genetically encoded sensors have been developed for detection of other target molecules in live cells, including Clomeleon (for Cl$^-$ sensing) [115], pHlameleon (for pH sensing) [116], and CUTie (for cAMP sensing) [117]. A similar design strategy has also been adopted to design fluorescence sensors to indicate programmed cell death via protease activity [118], image protein activity in live embryos [119], visualize small GTPases activity [120, 121], and reveal other activities inside cells [122 - 129].

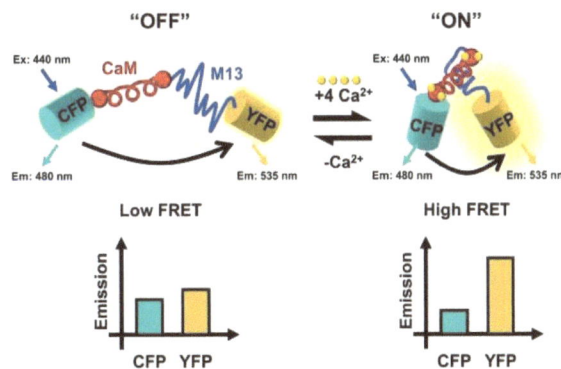

Fig. (5). Schematic diagram of the Cameleon sensor. Cameleon consists of two variants of GFP (*e.g.* CFP and YFP) fused at two termini of a Ca^{2+} binding domain (CaM and M13). When 4 Ca^{2+} ions bind to the CaM and M13 domain, Cameleon undergoes a conformational change, which brings the donor (CFP) closer to the acceptor (YFP) and enables FRET [138].

Intermolecular FRET-based Sensors

QD-based FRET Nanosensors

Semiconductor quantum dots (QD) have a number of advantages that make them superior contrast agents in fluorescence imaging, including size-tunable fluorescence emission due to quantum confinement effect, strong absorption in the UV range, narrow emission linewidth (1/3 of that of organic dyes), and great photostability (100-fold more stable than organic dyes). Soon after the first demonstration of QDs in biosensing and imaging [71, 72], QDs have been combined with various functional groups and organic dyes to make activatable biosensors [12, 77]. One example is the single-QD-based DNA sensor developed by Wang's group [13], which comprises of two target-specific DNA probes that are linked to Cy5 and biotin, respectively (Fig. **6**). When a target DNA strand is present, it is sandwiched by the two DNA probes and the resulting hybrid is captured by a streptavidin-coated QD. As multiple target-probe hybrids are captured by one QD, a strong FRET signal is seen. QD-based biosensors are often intermolecular FRET-based sensors (also called binary sensors [91]), where donor and acceptor are not on the same molecular construct. When properly designed, quantum dots offer the benefits of eliminating direct acceptor excitation, decreasing spectral overlap between donor and acceptor emission to reduce cross talk, maximizing donor emission and acceptor absorbance overlap, and allowing detection at a wavelength far away from the excitation wavelength to reduce background scattering and autofluorescence. Similar QD-FRET-based biosensors are developed for detection of proteins [77] and carbohydrates [12].

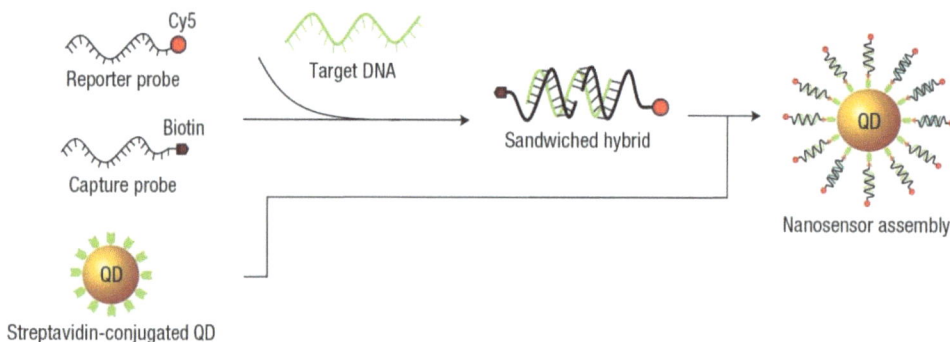

Fig. (6). Schematic diagram of QD-based FRET biosensors. In the presence of target DNAs, a nanosensor assembly can be formed. Reprinted from [13] with permission from Springer Nature.

Homo-FRET Sensors

Homo-FRET refers to resonance energy transfer between multiple identical fluorophores that are labeled on a single macromolecular construct [4], a phenomenon known as self-quenching (Fig. 7). Upon macromolecule digestion (*e.g.* in the lysosome), organic dyes are separated from each other and dequenched. Tumor-targeting proteins, such as avidin [130] and GSA [131], are the molecular construct examples that utilize multiple labeling, self-quenching, and lysosomal digestion as strategies for cancer cell imaging. Unlike hetero-FRET, homo-FRET uses only a single fluorescent probe, and therefore, the fluorophore should have sufficient spectral overlap between the emission and the absorption.

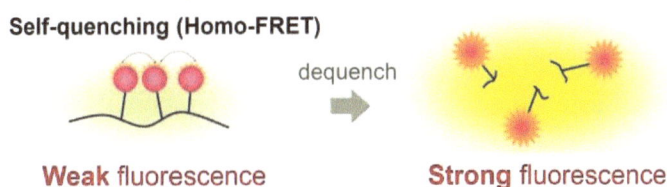

Fig. (7). Scheme for homo-FRET. When dequenched by certain macromolecule digestion processes in the lysosomes of the target cells, homo-FRET sensors can emit strong fluorescence. Reprinted from [4] with permission from the American Chemical Society.

Photoinduced Electron Transfer (PET)

Other than FRET, a number of electronic interactions also provide fluorescence quenching, including intersystem crossing, Dexter interactions, and photoinduced electron transfer [1]. As all these three quenching mechanisms have the same short-range distance dependence (most effective interaction distance between reporter and quencher to be within 0.2 nm), it is often difficult to know the true quenching mechanism behind a quenching experiment. Many reports even indicated that quenching could occur by a combination of these mechanisms. Here the focus is on photoinduced electron transfer (PET) as it has been used as the activation principle in designing many fluorescence sensors, such as smart probes [28] and fluorescein-based sensors [29, 30]. There are two key differences between FRET and PET. First, FRET is due to long-range dipolar interactions between excited donor and acceptor, while PET is due to short-range interactions between reporter and quencher (where either one of them can be the excited molecule and electron donor). Second, FRET can generate a strong acceptor emission (if the acceptor is not a quencher), while PET is usually associated with reporter quenching.

Smart Probes

In a PET example, an electron donor (D_p) can be excited and form an "electron-transfer complex" ($[D_p^+A_p^-]^*$) with an electron acceptor (A_p^-) that is in contact with the donor (Fig. **8A**). The electron-transfer complex has lower energy because the ability to donate and accept electrons alters when the donor is in the excited state and excitation provides the energy to drive charge separation. In PET, the terms donor and acceptor do not identify which species is reporter or quencher or which species is initially in the excited state. Sauer's group reported "smart probes" that use an oxazine dye JA242 as the reporter and intrinsic guanine bases as the quenchers in a molecular beacon configuration, where guanine bases serve as the electron donors and JA242 serves as the electron acceptor (Fig. **8B**) [28]. In the unbound state, the oxazine dye is quenched by the proximal guanine bases through PET. In the bound state, the formation of electron-transfer complex is prohibited, thus restoring the fluorescence. Using canonical nucleobases as the quenchers, smart probes have an advantage in the manufacturing cost.

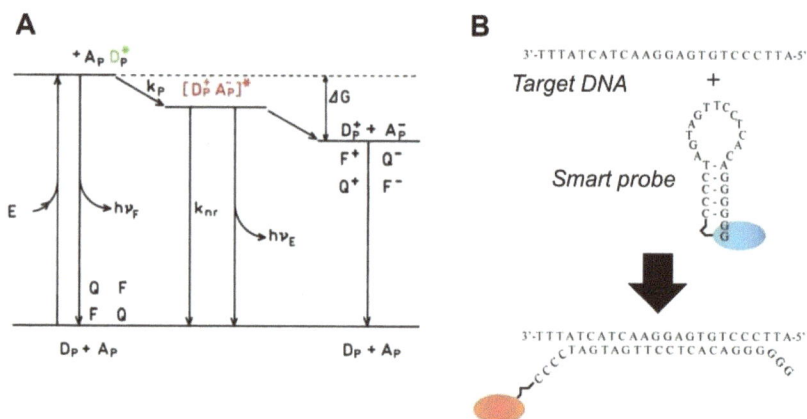

Fig. (8). (**A**) Energy diagram for photoinduced electron transfer (PET). Here both fluorophore (F) and quencher (Q) can be the electron donor. Reprinted from [1] with permission from Springer Nature. (**B**) Schematic diagram of the smart probe. Here the fluorescent reporter is the oxazine dye JA242, which can be quenched by proximal guanine bases due to PET—reprinted from [28] with permission from the American Chemical Society.

Fluorescein-based Sensors

As the fluorescence of fluorescein derivatives can be quenched by PET from a benzene moiety (electron donor) to the xanthene moiety (electron acceptor) [29, 30], Nagano and coworkers developed a cell-permeable β-galactosidase sensor, termed TG-βGal [31] (Fig. **9**). TG-βGal consists of a fluorescein derivative (TokyoGreen) and a mono-β-D-galactopyranoside. Hydrolysis of the β---galactopyranoside by β-galactosidase changes the HOMO energy level of the benzene moiety (electron donor) to be lower than that of the excited xanthene moiety (the fluorophore), thus inhibiting PET and restoring the sensor fluorescence. PET-based sensors have been adopted to facilitate tumor imaging in mice [4].

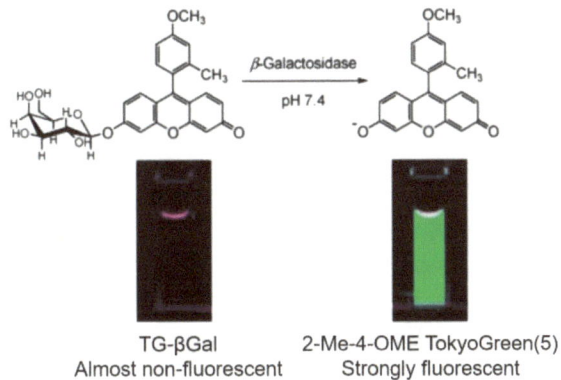

Fig. (9). Reaction scheme for TG-βGal sensor. Upon hydrolysis of the β-D-galactopyranoside on the TG-βGal sensor, the sensor is turned on and becomes highly fluorescent. Reprinted from [31] with permission from the American Chemical Society.

Formation of Fluorescent Constructs

Another design principle for activatable fluorescence sensors is the target-binding-induced formation of fluorescent constructs or destruction of non-fluorescent constructs. The formation of a fluorescent construct can take place both *in vitro* and *in vivo,* by simply combining two non-fluorescent fragments into a functional fluorescent entity, such as split GFP [16 - 18], or by changing the conformation of a misfolded version of fluorescent proteins into a well-folded version, such as GCaMP [19]. The destruction of a non-fluorescent construct can be the target-binding-induced dissociation of an H-dimer [23 - 27].

Split GFP

Split GFP shares the same operation concept as enzyme complementation sensors that were designed to probe protein-protein interactions [133 - 136]. An enzyme protein is dissected into two nonfunctional components, which can then reconstitute to form a functional structure. The two components are fused to two different proteins of interest, respectively, and are genetically encoded to be produced inside cells where the protein-protein interactions normally occur. Association between the investigated proteins brings the two nonfunctional components together, which then self-assemble to form a functional enzyme. Hence, interactions between proteins can be discerned based on the enzymatic activities. While these enzyme complementation sensors can provide significantly amplified target-specific signals, they require an additional step to read the enzymatic activities, for instance, by a biochemical, histochemical, colorimetric, chemiluminescent, or fluorescent means. Attempts were then made to apply the same complementary strategy to the fragments of fluorescent proteins, creating sensors which allow us to directly observe fluorescence signals upon protein association [137]. Waldo's group engineered to split GFP into two fragments of unequal sizes – a 15-amino-acid and a 214-amino-acid fragments [16], where the small fragment can serve as a small protein tag. Upon correct folding of the target protein, the tag is accessible for the complementary fragment to bind and form a functional GFP. For any reasons, such as misfolding or aggregation, the small GFP tag is inaccessible and complementation is prohibited. Hence, the split GFP sensor can be used as a protein solubility detector inside live cells [17]. Split GFP has been employed to tag RNA for RNA imaging (Fig. **10**) [132] and to study cell contacts and synapses in live neural cells [18].

GCaMP

GCaMP is a type of genetically encoded fluorescent protein sensor that is designed to visualize and monitor Ca^{2+} levels in live neuron and muscle cells [19]. Both Cameleon and GCaMP are normally referred to as GECI – genetically encoded calcium indicators [139]. In the GCaMP sensor, a GFP is engineered so that its N- and C-termini are fused to a Ca^{2+} binding unit composed of calmodulin (CaM) and CaM-binding region of chicken myosin light chain kinase (M13) (Fig. **11**). In the absence of Ca^{2+}, CaM and M13 are relatively disordered, keeping the circularly permuted fluorescent protein (cpEGFP) in a non-fluorescent state due to the solvent exposure of the chromophore. Upon Ca^{2+} binding, the CaM domain wraps around the M13 peptide, creating a new interface between the Ca^{2+} binding unit and the cpEGFP. This new interface alters the solvent environment around the chromophore, turning cpEGFP into a highly fluorescent protein [20]. GCaMP has been used to measure neural circuits in *C elegans* [21] and image neural activity in transgenic mice [22]. Whereas GECI, such as Cameleon and GCaMP, have been used for biological applications, they have shown limited utility in complex animals or mammals [139]. Due to this limitation, Fluo-8 AM, a cell-permeable Ca^{2+} indicator, has been used in cells from mammals and other species [140, 141].

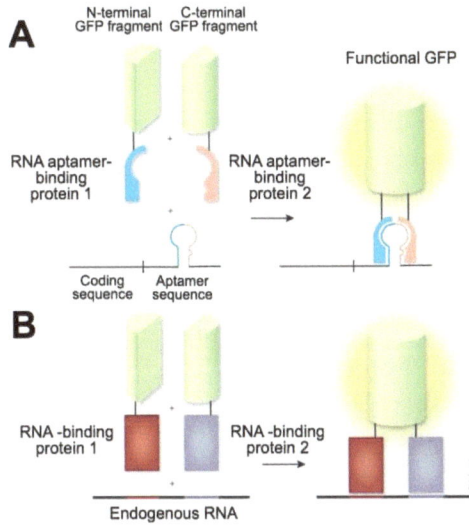

Fig. (10). (**A**) Each GFP fragment is fused to a split RNA aptamer-binding protein. When these fusion proteins bind together to the aptamer sequence, the GFP fragments self-assemble into a functional GFP. (**B**) Two RNA-binding proteins are engineered to bind to an endogenous RNA at the juxtaposition, reconstituting a functional GFP. Reprinted from [132] withpermission from Springer Nature.

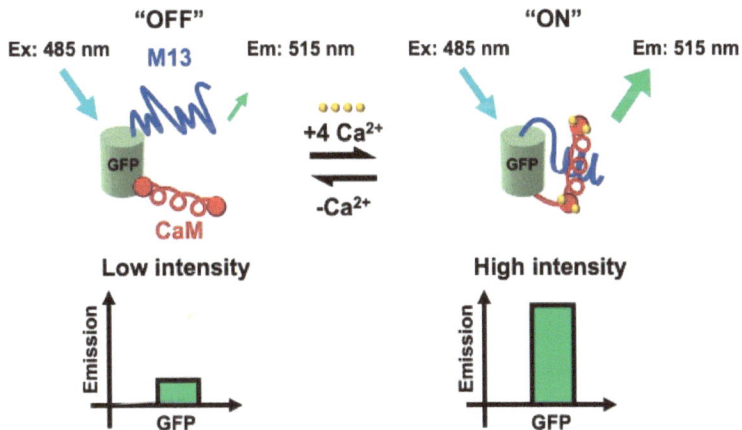

Fig. (11). Schematic diagram of GCaMP. GFP is fused to the calmodulin (CaM) and CaM-binding region of chicken myosin light chain kinase (M13). Upon Ca^{2+} binding, the CaM domain wraps around the M13, leading M13 to be ordered and resulting in the recovery of GFP fluorescence. Adapted from [138].

H-dimer

Fluorophores, such as cyanine dyes, rhodamine, and Bodipy derivatives, can form homodimers and homo-aggregates at relatively high concentrations (Fig. **12**). Due to the strong coupling of the transition dipoles of tightly packed dye molecules, these aggregates exhibit blue-shifted (H-aggregate) or red-shifted (J-aggregate) absorption spectra, which, in other words, quench monomer's original fluorescence [26, 27]. This self-quenching property of H-type or J-type aggregation is extremely useful in designing fluorescence sensors, including protein [24] and DNA sensors [23, 25] (Fig. **13**). In Fig. (**13B**), a closed conformation of the biotin(B)-NeutrAvidin(A) surface-immobilized two-piece MB(4a+4b) opens up with target 3a DNA, allowing single molecule fluorescence imaging because of a stronger fluorescence signal. Compared to the traditional FRET-based sensors, such as molecular beacons, H-dimer sensors allow for two fluorophores, instead of one, to be simultaneously turned on, providing a stronger fluorescence signal upon target binding.

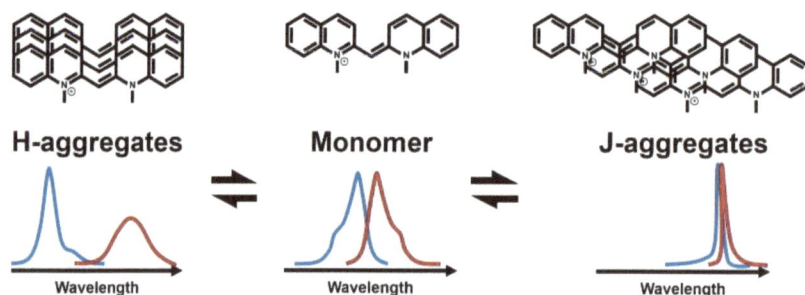

Fig. (12). H-aggregate and J-aggregate of fluorophores (cyanine dye). At relatively high molecular concentrations, fluorophores can form homo-aggregates, such as H-aggregates and J-aggregates. This formation change also causes the shift of absorbance spectra (bottom).

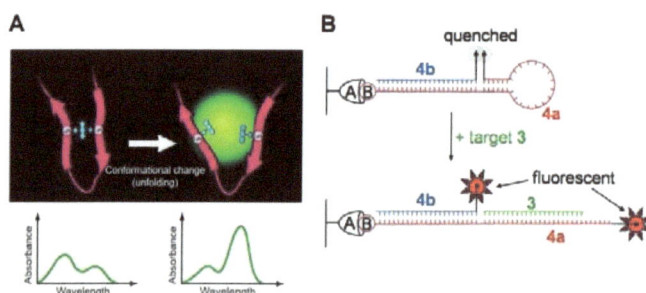

Fig. (13). H-dimer sensors. (**A**) Rhodamine 6G (R6G) or TAMRA form H-dimers with quenched monomer fluorescence. Target protein binding alters sensor's conformation, resulting in H-dimer dissociation and monomer fluorescence activation. (**B**) An H-dimer sensor designed for DNA sensing. Reprinted from [24] (**A**) and [23] (**B**) with permission from the American Chemical Society.

Suppression of Non-radiative Decay Pathways

Intercalating Dyes

The term "intercalation" was first introduced by Lerman, in 1961, while he examined the interactions between acridine derivatives and DNA [32]. Lerman found that the flat polycyclic compounds intercalate, or insert and stack, between basepairs by extension and unwinding of the deoxyribose-phosphate backbone. Although the use of mono intercalators in hybridization detection was demonstrated in 1980s [90], intercalating dyes did not make an impact in biological research until the invention of bis-intercalators. Compared to mono intercalators, bis-intercalators have a greater binding affinity with dsDNA and exhibit higher fluorescence enhancement after intercalation (more than 1000-fold enhancement for the TOTO dyes, Fig. 14) [33 - 35]. Fig. (**14D**) shows a peptide nucleic acid (PNA)-based light-up sensor. The excellent hybridization properties of PNA leads to the large fluorescence enhancement upon binding to target DNA. PNAs can also combine with forced intercalation probes, in which thiazole orange (TO) in FIT-PNA is coupled as base surrogate and high fluorescence is obtained only with matched DNA (Fig. **14E**) [143]. If TO dye and thiazole red (TR) dye are incorporated into two DNA/RNAs, they can serve as an interstrand energy transfer pair in DNA/RNA. (Fig. **14F**). Intercalation between base pairs effectively increases the local viscosity of the dye, which suppresses its non-radiative decay pathways by dampening its rapid intramolecular motion, leading to significantly enhanced dye fluorescence. Cyanine dyes as TOTO, TOPRO, and YOYO are common DNA dyes for fixed cells as they are not cell permeable. Efforts have been made to design new cyanine dyes with improved permeability for live cell imaging [145 - 147]. Instead of intercalating between base pairs, an asymmetrical cyanine dye, such as SYBR Green I and PicoGreen, binds to the minor groove of DNA, similar to Hoechst or DAPI dyes [37, 40], which also dampens dye's intramolecular motions and suppresses the non-radiative pathways [40].

FlAsH and ReAsH

Tsien's group introduced the biarsenical sensors and tetracysteine motifs for site-specific fluorescent labeling of recombinant proteins in live cells [41, 42]. The tetracysteine motif Cys-Cys-Xaa-Xaa-Cys-Cys (where Xaa is a non-cysteine amino acid) can be genetically fused within a target protein and be specifically recognized by a cell-permeable fluorescein derivative with two As(III) substituents, FlAsH, which fluoresces only after the arsenic binds to the cysteine thiols. The small size of EDT permits rotation of the aryl-arsenic bond and excited state quenching by vibrational deactivation, making FlAsH-EDT$_2$ complex non-fluorescent (Fig. **15**). In contrast, the FlAsH-peptide complex (which is much smaller than a GFP) evades such quenching because its more rigid conformation should hinder conjugation of the arsenic lone pair electrons with the fluorescein orbitals [41], leading to a 50,000-fold increase in fluorescence. Many analogues of FlAsH have been synthesized, such as ReAsH, showing applications in affinity chromatography, fluorescence anisotropy measurements, and electron-microscopic localization of tetracysteine-tagged proteins [42].

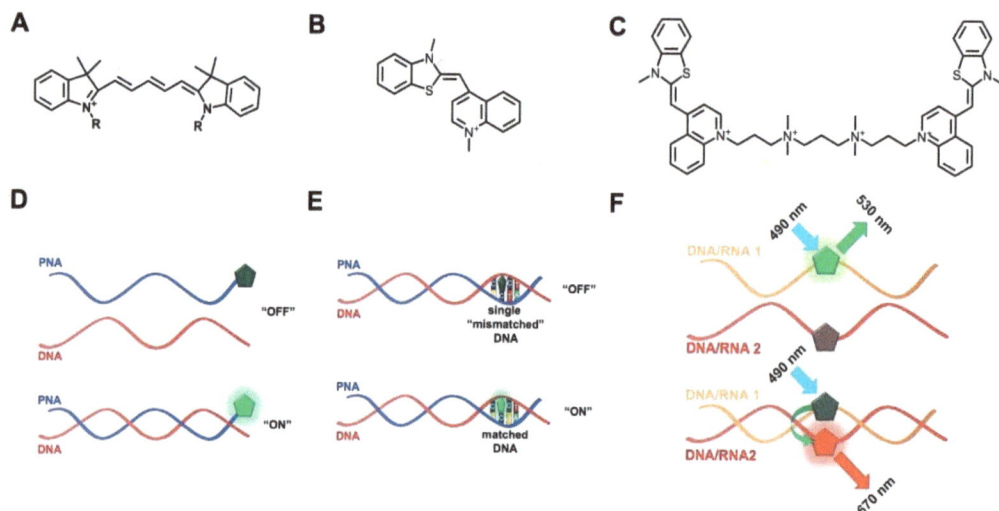

Fig. (14). Structures of symmetric and asymmetric cyanine dyes: (**A**) Cy5, (**B**) Thiazole Orange (TO), and (**C**) Thiazole Orange homodimer (TOTO). Schematic diagram of intercalating probes: (**D**) Light-up probes adapted from [142], (**E**) Forced intercalation (FIT) probes adapted [143], and (**F**) DNA/RNA traffic light probes adapted from [144].

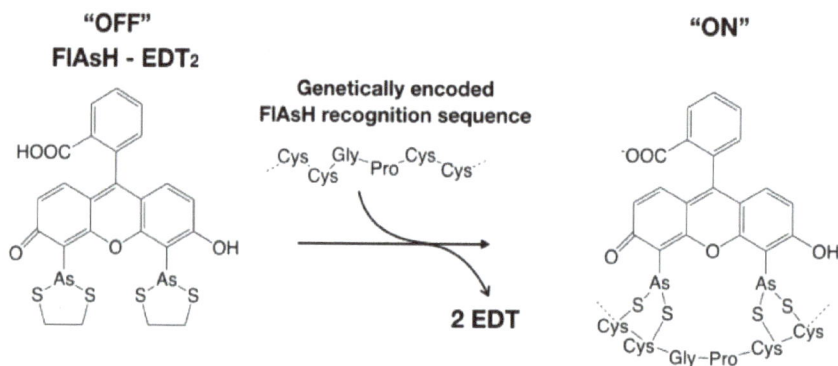

Fig. (15). Schematic of FlAsH. FlAsH-EDT$_2$ is non-fluorescent. Upon binding with the tetracystein tag, FlAsH-peptide complex recovers in fluorescence adapted from [41, 42].

Malachite Green and Spinach

Aptamers are a versatile platform for fluorescence sensor designs. Fluorophores, such as malachite green, when binding with their specific aptamers, exhibit a strong fluorescence enhancement (more than 2,000-fold) due to the suppression of fluorophore's vibration [45]. High viscosity and cold environment can also restrict fluorophore's vibration and enhance its fluorescence. Rather than using the GFP tagged MS2-coat protein binding system for mRNA imaging [148 - 150], Tsien proposed a more compact strategy to genetically tag RNA in live cells – fusing RNA to the shortest possible nucleotide sequences (*i.e.* aptamers) that can bind specific membrane-permeable dyes and strongly enhance their fluorescence [45]. Following the same concept, Jaffrey's group has created an aptamer-fluorophore complex, termed Spinach, for ribosomal RNA imaging in live cells [46]. In particular, in Jaffrey's system, the RNA aptamers switch on the fluorescence of GFP-like fluorophores, such as DMHBI. With directed evolution and high throughput fluorescence screening, increased fluorescence and rapid aptamer folding have been achieved [47]. Not limited to RNA sensing, more Spinach-based sensors have been created to detect the small-molecule metabolites, such as adenosine, ADP, S-adenosylmethionine, guanine, and GTP (Fig. **16**) [151], and the proteins such as streptavidin, thrombin, and MS2 coat protein (MCP) [152].

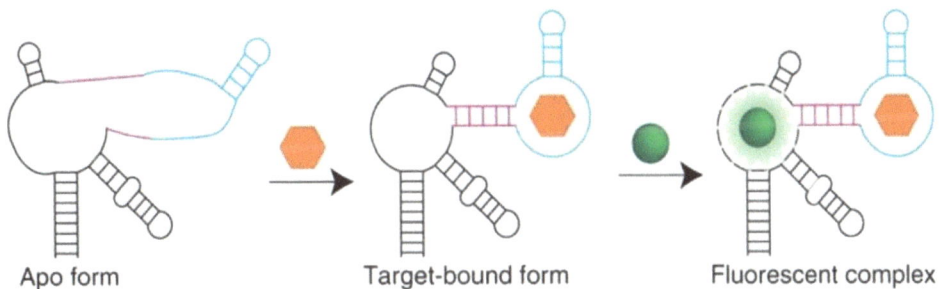

| Apo form | Target-bound form | Fluorescent complex |

Fig. (16). Spinach-based sensors. The sensor comprises Spinach (black), a transducer (pink), and target-binding aptamer (blue). Target (orange hexagon) binding to the aptamer promotes the stabilization of the transducer stem, enabling Spinach to fold and activate DFHBI (green ball) fluorescence. Reprinted from [152] with permission from Springer Nature.

Ligand Effects

NanoCluster Beacons

Although few-atom noble metal nanoclusters (a collection of 2-30 gold or silver atoms) were first prepared and studied in rare gas matrices, more than 5 decades ago [53], it was not until early 2000s when Dickson, Petty, and others started to use ligands, such as dendrimers [154] and DNA [73], as templates to synthesize fluorescent gold and silver nanoclusters in aqueous solution, opening the door to the use of noble metal nanoclusters as contrast agents in fluorescence imaging. Providing the missing link between atomic and nanoparticle behaviors in noble metals, few-atom gold or silver clusters possess many intriguing photophysical properties not before seen in organic dyes or semiconductor quantum dots [53, 155]. One unique property is the guanine-proximity-induced fluorescence activation phenomenon, discovered by Yeh and his coworkers on dark silver nanoclusters templated in DNA [50]. As the ensemble fluorescence enhancement by guanine proximity can be more than 1,500-fold [51], Yeh has turned this new fluorescence activation method into a variety of binary sensor designs, collectively termed NanoCluster Beacons (NCB, Fig. **17A**), for pathogenic DNA [50], SNP [52], enzymatic activity [57], and DNA methylation [56] detection. Whereas guanines often quench organic dyes, such as fluorescein due to photoinduced charge transfer [156], in NCB, a guanine-rich tail is used to enhance the silver cluster's fluorescence. The activation color of NCB highly depends on the template sequence and the activator sequence [51]. A palette of NCB (from green to deep red) has been created (Fig. **17B**) [55].

The atomic structures of silver nanoclusters in DNA are still under investigation. Gwinn's group proposed a rod shape for all fluorescent silver nanoclusters templated in DNA based on their mass spectrum data, in which a neutral silver core (gray balls) is surrounded by silver ions (blue balls) that bind with nucleobases (Fig. **17C**) [153]. Petty's group recently reported the first crystal structure of an emissive multinuclear silver cluster (Ag_8) bound to DNA to 0.93 Å resolution [157]. These first atomic details of a DNA-templated silver cluster fluorophore have enlightened many aspects of biological assembly, nanoscience, and metal cluster photophysics. Mechanisms for their interesting fluorescence activatability and tunability properties will soon be elucidated, opening new avenues for sensor development.

Carbon Nanotube-based Sensors

Strano's group demonstrated that single-walled carbon nanotubes (SWNT), wrapped with DNA (Fig. **18A**), could be placed inside whole blood, tissue, and live cells to detect harmful contaminants (such as Hg^{2+} ions) using a near-infrared light (785 nm) [59]. Double-stranded DNA can have conformation transition from the native, right-handed B form to the left-handed Z form upon interactions with certain cations (*e.g.* Hg^{2+}, Co^{2+}, Ca^{2+} and Mg^{2+}). Such a B-to-Z transition modulates the dielectric environment of SWNT (around which DNA is adsorbed) and decreases SWNT's near-IR emission (a ligand effect). As a result, this red-shifted fluorescence signal can be employed to detect divalent metal cations that bind to DNA and stabilize the Z form (Fig. **18B**). Whereas in whole blood and tissue, the presence of interfering absorbers of Hg^{2+} (free DNA, proteins, *etc.*) shifts the observed sensitivity to larger values (~3.5 mM in blood and ~8 mM in tissue), the DNA-SWNT sensors provide a unique way to detect the residual ions that are locally bound to the sensors in these heterogeneous media.

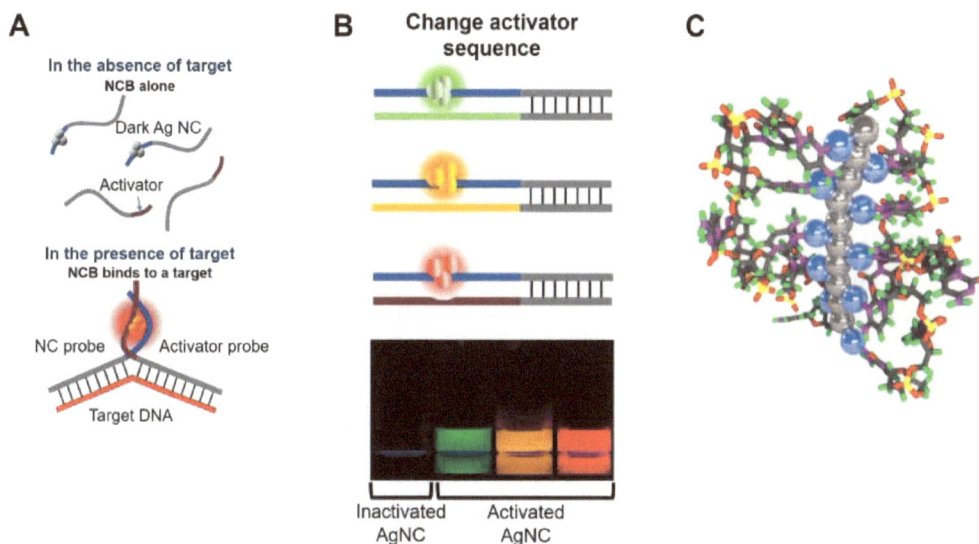

Fig. (17). (**A**) Schematic diagram of NanoCluster Beacons (NCB). In the absence of a target sequence, an NCB consists of an NC strand (with non-emissive Ag clusters) and an activator strand. NCB lights up tremendously in the presence of a target DNA. Reprinted from [50] with permission from the American Chemical Society. (**B**) The different activation colors can be produced by changing activator sequences (bottom strands). Reprinted from [53] with permission from The Royal Society of Chemistry. (**C**) Rod shape hypothesis. Neutral silver core (gray) is wrapped by base-bound Ag^+ ions (blue). Reprinted from [153] with permission from the Multidisciplinary Digital Publishing Institute.

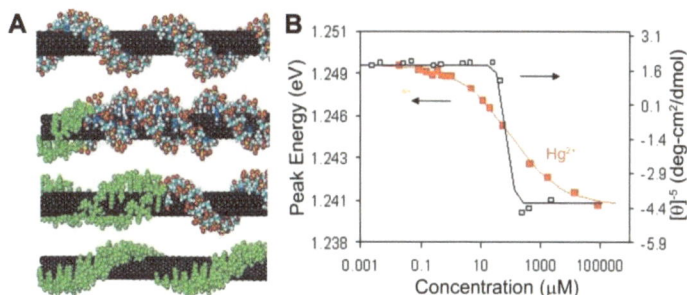

Fig. (18). (**A**) The transition of DNA secondary structure from the B form to the Z form on a single-called carbon nanotube. (**B**) A red curve and black curve show the emission energy and the ellipticity of the 285-nm versus Hg^{2+} concentrations, respectively. Reprinted from [59] with permission by The American Association for the Advancement of Science.

STRATEGIES TO ENHANCE FLUORESCENCE SIGNALS AND SPECIFICITY

While targeting binding triggers fluorescence property changes in the above biosensors, such changes are often insignificant. To increase the dynamic range and the sensitivity of fluorescence biosensors, a number of signal enhancement methods have been proposed.

Metastable Hairpin Sensors and Hybridization Chain Reaction

Nucleic acid circuits have emerged as a promising field with increasing importance for analytical applications [158]. One example is the hybridization chain reaction (HCR), which leads to strong signal amplification [159]. In one case of HCR, two DNA sensors initially form two metastable hairpins in solution (H1 and H2 in Fig. **19A**) [160]. Upon adding a target DNA to the system, H1 first binds with the target (Initiator I in Fig. **19A**) through toehold displacement and opens the hairpin to expose its H1 output domain. Hybridization of this H1 output domain to the input domain of H2 opens the hairpin to expose an H2 output domain identical in sequence to the target. Regeneration of the target sequence provides the basis for a chain reaction of alternating H1 and H2 polymerization steps, leading to the formation of a nicked double-stranded 'polymer' [160]. Not just for DNA detection, a similar concept can be used to detect small molecules, such as ATP through an aptamer-metastable hairpin sensor design [159]. Metastable sensors have been employed to simultaneously monitor the expression and localization of five different mRNAs in fixed zebrafish embryos [160].

By introducing a split DNAzyme to the metastable sensor design (that cleaves fluorescently quenched substrate after assembly), HCR can push the detection's sensitivity down to 10 fM (Fig. **19B**) [161]. However, similar to PCR, non-specific hybridization among the numerous metastable sensors can lead to the accumulation of background in HCR (or called circuit leakage) [158]. While systematically analyzing the origins of chain reaction leakage and designing cascaded HCA have yielded a nearly 600,000-fold signal amplification [162] with low leakage, the overall four-layer cascaded reactions required 12 hours to execute, making the cascaded HCR less useful for many diagnostic applications.

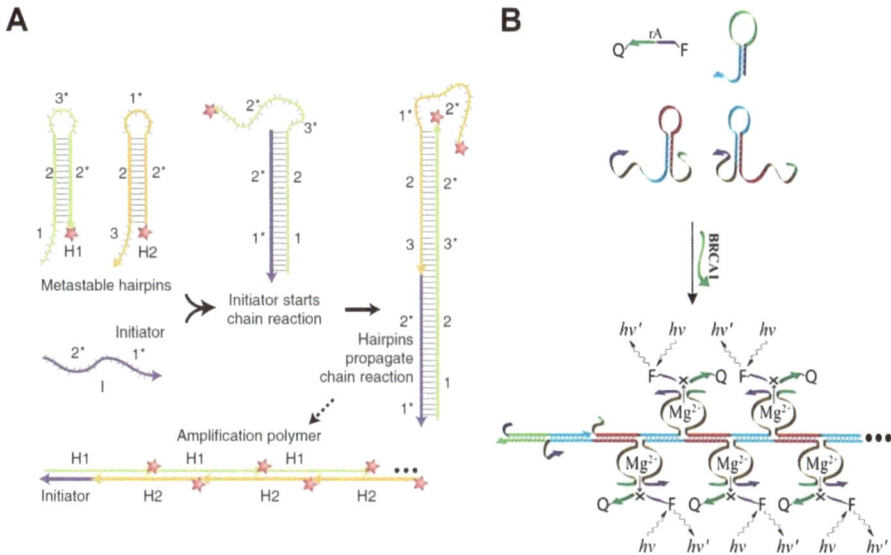

Fig. (19). (A) Schematic diagram of hybridization chain reaction (HCR). Initiator (I) is hybridized with a hairpin (H1) through toehold displacement, which leads H1 to open its '3* - 2*' segment. This I-H1 complex nucleates with another hairpin H2, opening '1* - 2*' segment, which can play a role as an initiator. This is the basis of a chain reaction amplification. Reprinted from [160] with the permission with Springer Nature. (B) Analysis of BRAC1 oncogene using probe hairpin and two functional hairpins. In the presence of BRCA1 oncogene and Mg^{2+}, the DNAzyme causes the cleavage of the substrate and leads to fluorescence emission. Q, F, and rA represent a quencher, fluorophore and ribonucleobase, respectively. Reprinted from [161] with permission by the American Chemical Society.

Multiple Labels and Fluorogenic Arrays

A straightforward way for signal amplification is through the binding of multiple fluorescence sensors (*e.g.* molecular beacons) to a target molecule that is sufficiently large, such as mRNA [163]. Natural genes can be engineered to have multiple molecular beacon binding sites for studying the mechanism of mRNA transport in different cell types. It was later found that the activatable sensor (molecular beacon) in this multiple-labeling strategy can be simply replaced by a cheaper linear DNA probe that always fluoresces (Fig. **20A**) [164], leading to a target signal way above the background signal given by the unbound, free-diffusing linear probes. However, using molecular beacons or linear probes in live cells requires a live-cell delivery method, such as the reversible permeabilization method with streptolysin O [78]. Without using any exogenous fluorescence sensors, intracellular mRNA imaging today is mostly done through the insertion of 24 copies of MS2-binding RNA hairpin into the untranslated region of target mRNA. Twenty-four MS2 coat proteins (fused with GFP) then bind with these hairpin motifs, giving the target mRNA a strong fluorescence signal that enables many mRNA studies in live cells [148 - 150]. mRNA can also be engineered to have multiple binding sites for activatable biosensors, such as split GFP and aptamer tags, to suppress the background noise [165]. Based on the same multiple-labeling amplification strategy, Vale's group developed a protein-scaffold system, termed SunTag, for imaging of single protein molecules in live cells [166] (Fig. **20B**). In particular, the dCas9-SunTag allows for imaging specific loci in genomic DNA in live cells [166].

Although multiple-labeling provides significant signal amplification, photobleaching of the labels still prevents long-term observation of target molecules in live cells. Liphardt's group recently created a fluorogenic array system whose 24 fluorescence sensors (GFP) not only fluoresce 26-fold stronger upon binding with the nanobodies but also can be replenished (bleached sensors replaced by functional sensors by tuning dissociation kinetics, Fig. **20C**) [167]. Combining activatability, signal amplification and fluorescence replenishment, fluorogenic array systems have extended the average tracking duration of single histone H2B to ~13 minutes in live U2OS cells [167].

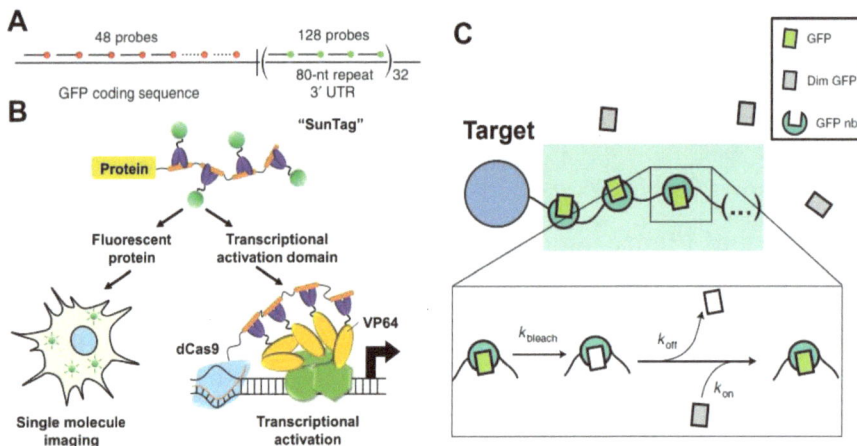

Fig. (20). Imaging target mRNA using multiple-labeling strategies. (**A**) 48 linear fluorescent probes were used to tag an mRNA for imaging. Reprinted from [164] with the permission by Springer Nature. (**B**) SunTag. Adapted from [166]. (**C**) Fluorogenic arrays. Reprinted from [167] with the permission by Springer Nature.

Ligation-based PCR Assay

In the above two methods, signal amplification is achieved without using any enzymes. In nucleic acid detection, a number of enzymatic reactions have been widely used to increase the target signals, including ligation chain reaction [168,

169], ligation with rolling-circle amplification [170], and loop-mediated isot-hermal amplification [171]. In these approaches, the amplified signal comes indirectly from the target hybridization-triggered enzymatic reaction products (for example, ligated linear probes [169], ligated padlock probes [170], or extended loop-formation primers [171]) rather than directly from the amplification of target binding signal. For instance, the LigAmp assay [169] is based on ligation chain reaction [168] in which the two adjacently hybridized oligonucleotides are ligated, amplified by PCR, and detected by a TaqMan probe (Fig. **21**). As only the perfect matched sequences at the nick site enable ligation, LigAmp is particularly useful for single-nucleotide polymorphism detection.

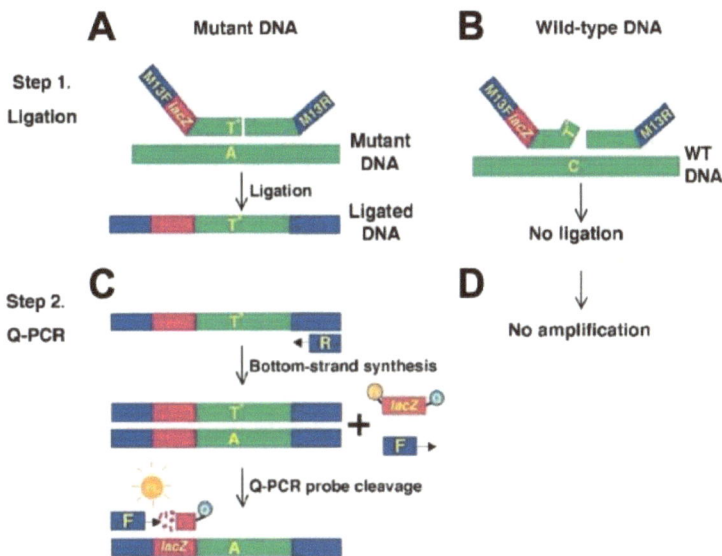

Fig. (21). Schematic diagram of the LigAmp assay. Two DNAs are ligated (A, B) and the ligated DNAs are detected by quantitative PCR (C, D). Reprinted from [169] with the permission by Springer Nature.

Proximity Probes

There is no PCR analogous target-based amplification method for proteins. One indirect way to convert protein amplification into DNA amplification is immuno-PCR [172, 173]. Mirkin's group designed a protein sensor based on the immuno-PCR concept, but it required magnetic-bead separation and chip-based detection [174]. To bypass the need for separation, Landegren's group developed a proximity probe for protein detection that takes advantage of proximal binding of a target protein by two DNA aptamers, which promotes ligation of oligonucleotides linked to each aptamer (Fig. **22A**) [175]. The ligated products can then be amplified by PCR. Similar idea has been applied to detect protein complexes, where the ligated products are amplified by rolling circle amplification (RCA, Fig. **22B**) [176]. Taking advantage of nucleic acid ampli-fication, proximity probes are a highly specific and sensitive way for protein detection *in vitro*.

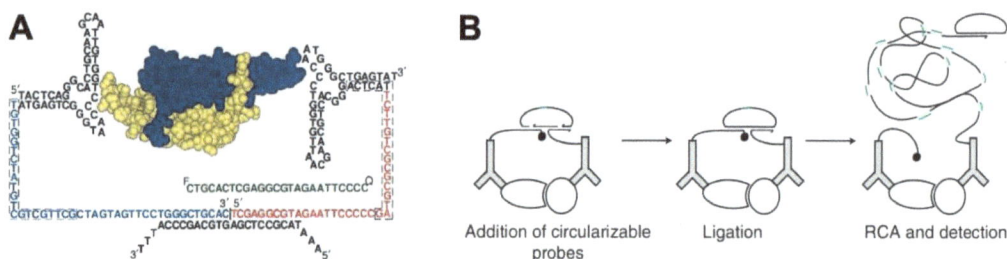

Fig. (22). Schematic diagram of proximity probes. (**A**) Two DNA probes are linked to two aptamers against a target protein. Proximal binding, thus, promotes ligation of the DNA probes. The ligated products can be amplified by PCR. Reprinted from [175] with the permission by Springer Nature. (**B**) Similarly, the proximity probes can be two antibodies that are against a protein complex, where the circular ligation products are amplified by RCA. Reprinted from [176] with the permission by Springer Nature.

REQUIREMENTS FOR USING FLUORESCENCE SENSORS IN BIOMEDICAL IMAGING

Here, the characteristics of successful fluorescence sensors in biomedical detection and imaging are described. Satisfying all of the criteria is desirable, but difficult in many situations. Hence, trade-offs have to be made for different applications under different detection/imaging conditions.

Wavelength

The ideal spectral window for both excitation and emission of a fluorophore in tissues is within the 650-900 nm range, which encompasses the deep red to the near-infrared light (Fig. **23**). Blue to green excitation light (488-532 nm) has a shallow tissue penetration depth, which is only used for superficial imaging of the tissue samples. Yellow to red light (561-600 nm) causes excessive autofluorescence due to the excitation of hemoglobin and other endogenous fluorophores. Excitation in the UV range leads to tissue damage, whereas excitation beyond 900 nm causes tissue heating due to water absorption. At the 650-900 nm window, both hemoglobin autofluorescence and water absorption are relatively low, resulting in a deep excitation penetration depth. As silicon-based detectors have a low quantum efficiency in the near-infrared range, special detectors, such as an InGaAs camera (900-1,700 nm range), could be needed for some fluorescence sensor imaging applications in tissues. One advantage of tunable fluorescence sensors is that they enable ratiometric imaging *in vivo*, such as SNARF dyes, for pH sensing [113]. Compared with the single-channel intensity measurements, ratiometric imaging is less sensitive to the variations in optical path length, excitation intensity, and sensor concentration in tissue imaging.

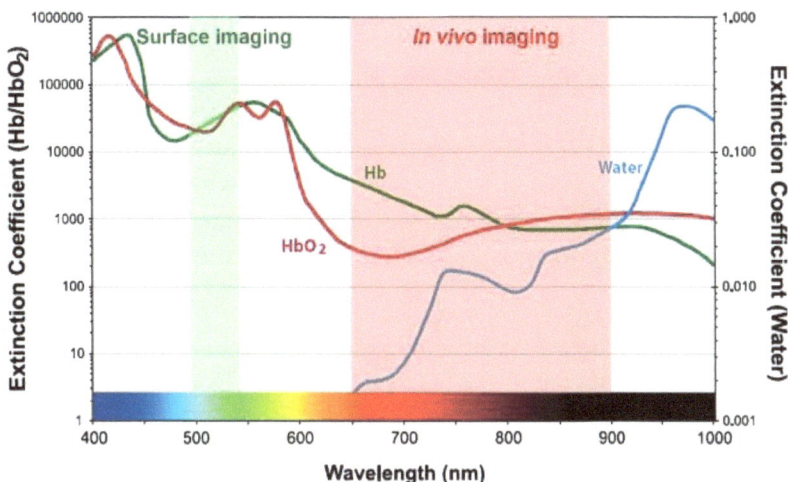

Fig. (23). Extinction coefficient value of water and oxyhemoglobin and deoxyhemoglobin in the range between visible and near-infrared wavelength. Reprinted from [4] with permission by the American Chemical Society.

Brightness

Although fluorescence sensors provide a higher signal-to-noise ratio in detection, they often come at the cost of larger sensor sizes. One example is the polymer-dot (pdot) sensors that Chiu developed for the *in-vivo* monitoring of small molecules [177, 178]. While being very bright, the size of a typical pdot is around 5-10 nm [179]. Another example is the semiconductor quantum dots that often have the size in the 15-20 nm range after functionalization. Other than the size issue, commercial QDs also have the cytotoxicity issue due to their heavy metal core/shell materials, cadmium, and selenium. Despite the toxicity issue, a few reports use QDs as contrast agents for multiphoton imaging in tissues [180].

Stability

Photostability is an issue for all organic dyes and fluorescent proteins. For *in-vitro* studies, oxygen scavenger systems [181] and antifading agents (*e.g.* Vectashield) [57] can be used to reduce photobleaching. While these methods are generally not live-cell compatible and mainly used in *in-vitro* studies, some reports suggested a reduced amount of oxygen scavenger system can still maintain cell health [182]. Recently Kusumi's group reported a method of combining low concentrations of dissolved oxygen with a reducing-plus-oxidizing system (ROXS) to achieve super-long observation (~ 7 minutes) of single-fluorescent molecules in live cells [183]. Other than the photostability issue, the chemical stability of fluorophores is also a problem for intracellular studies. Once in lysosomes, organic dyes, such as fluorescein, Bodipy, and cyanine derivatives, lose their fluorescence within several days [184]. Only rhodamine derivatives maintain their fluorescence for more than a week. Rather than repeated injection of fluorophores to achieve long-term observation of activities in live cells, Liphardt's group recently achieved temporally unlimited tracking of single molecules using a fluorogenic protein-nanobody array system and a stochastic binder exchange scheme [167]. Combining brightness, fluorogenicity, and fluorescence replenishment, these fluorogenic arrays open new avenues for imaging single molecules in live cells.

Pharmacokinetics and Biodistribution

Organic dyes or nanocrystals can alter the pharmacokinetics of target molecules to which they are conjugated. The situation is even worse when multiple fluorophores bind with a single target [185]. For nanoparticle-based sensors, particle size, shape, and surface charge dictate pharmacokinetics and biodistribution among the different organs, including the lungs, liver, spleen, and kidneys [186]. Highly cationic nanoparticles are more rapidly cleared from circulation, as compared with highly anionic nanoparticles [187]. In contrast, neutral nanoparticles, as well as slightly negatively charged particles, show significantly prolonged circulating half-lives. Longer circulation improves accumulation in tumors, which has led to recent research efforts aimed at creating functionalizing nanoparticles with zwitterionic surfaces [188]. For organic dye-based imaging probes, such as Cy5.5 and rhodamine X, rapid liver accumulation before successful targeting was reported [189]. Pharmacokinetics, target tissue uptake, and biodistribution are all factors that need to be considered when designing fluorescence biosensors for the *in-vivo* use.

CONCLUDING REMARKS

In the past thirty years, we have witnessed the development of many important fluorescence biosensors that change the way we study complex biological and chemical systems. In this chapter, we have discussed the design principles, functions, and limitations of several key fluorescence biosensors that are widely used in quantitative biology, analytical chemistry, and clinical medicine. Despite the rich arsenal of fluorophores and fluorescence techniques available today, researchers are still searching for smaller, cheaper, brighter, and more stable fluorophores whose fluorescence can be modulated by an entirely new physical or chemical means. With new capabilities given by new sensors, researchers may unveil more "dark matter" in live cells or tissues and solve unanswered questions.

CONSENT FOR PUBLICATION

Not applicable.

CONFLICT OF INTEREST

The authors confirm that this chapter contents have no conflict of interest.

ACKNOWLEDGEMENTS

The authors thank the financial support from the Texas 4000 Foundation, Welch Foundation (F-1833), National Science Foundation (1611451), and National Institutes of Health (GM129617).

REFERENCES

[1]   Lakowicz JR, Ed. Principles of fluorescence spectroscopy. 3rd ed., Boston: Springer 2006.
        [http://dx.doi.org/10.1007/978-0-387-46312-4]

[2]   Zander C, Enderlein J, Keller RA, Eds. Single molecule detection in solution: Methods and applications. Berlin: Wiley-VCH 2002.
        [http://dx.doi.org/10.1002/3527600809]

[3]   Eisenstein M. Helping cells to tell a colorful tale. Nat Methods 2006; 3(8): 647-55.
        [http://dx.doi.org/10.1038/nmeth0806-647] [PMID: 16892526]

[4]   Kobayashi H, Ogawa M, Alford R, Choyke PL, Urano Y. New strategies for fluorescent probe design in medical diagnostic imaging. Chem Rev 2010; 110(5): 2620-40.
        [http://dx.doi.org/10.1021/cr900263j] [PMID: 20000749]

[5]   Schultz J. Design of fibre-optic biosensors based on bioreceptors. New York: Oxford University Press 1987; pp. 638-54.

[6]   Tyagi S, Kramer FR. Molecular beacons: probes that fluoresce upon hybridization. Nat Biotechnol 1996; 14(3): 303-8.
        [http://dx.doi.org/10.1038/nbt0396-303] [PMID: 9630890]

[7]   Tyagi S, Bratu DP, Kramer FR. Multicolor molecular beacons for allele discrimination. Nat Biotechnol 1998; 16(1): 49-53.
        [http://dx.doi.org/10.1038/nbt0198-49] [PMID: 9447593]

[8]   Holland PM, Abramson RD, Watson R, Gelfand DH. Detection of specific polymerase chain reaction product by utilizing the 5′----3′ exonuclease activity of Thermus aquaticus DNA polymerase. Proc Natl Acad Sci USA 1991; 88(16): 7276-80.
        [http://dx.doi.org/10.1073/pnas.88.16.7276] [PMID: 1871133]

[9]   Lee LG, Connell CR, Bloch W. Allelic discrimination by nick-translation PCR with fluorogenic probes. Nucleic Acids Res 1993; 21(16): 3761-6.
        [http://dx.doi.org/10.1093/nar/21.16.3761] [PMID: 8367293]

[10]   Heid CA, Stevens J, Livak KJ, Williams PM. Real time quantitative PCR. Genome Res 1996; 6(10): 986-94.
        [http://dx.doi.org/10.1101/gr.6.10.986] [PMID: 8908518]

[11]   Miyawaki A, Llopis J, Heim R, *et al.* Fluorescent indicators for Ca2+ based on green fluorescent

proteins and calmodulin. Nature 1997; 388(6645): 882-7.
[http://dx.doi.org/10.1038/42264] [PMID: 9278050]

[12]   Medintz IL, Clapp AR, Mattoussi H, Goldman ER, Fisher B, Mauro JM. Self-assembled nanoscale biosensors based on quantum dot FRET donors. Nat Mater 2003; 2(9): 630-8.
[http://dx.doi.org/10.1038/nmat961] [PMID: 12942071]

[13]   Zhang CY, Yeh HC, Kuroki MT, Wang TH. Single-quantum-dot-based DNA nanosensor. Nat Mater 2005; 4(11): 826-31.
[http://dx.doi.org/10.1038/nmat1508] [PMID: 16379073]

[14]   Kamiya M, Kobayashi H, Hama Y, *et al.* An enzymatically activated fluorescence probe for targeted tumor imaging. J Am Chem Soc 2007; 129(13): 3918-29.
[http://dx.doi.org/10.1021/ja067710a] [PMID: 17352471]

[15]   Urano Y, Asanuma D, Hama Y, *et al.* Selective molecular imaging of viable cancer cells with pH-activatable fluorescence probes. Nat Med 2009; 15(1): 104-9.
[http://dx.doi.org/10.1038/nm.1854] [PMID: 19029979]

[16]   Cabantous S, Terwilliger TC, Waldo GS. Protein tagging and detection with engineered self-assembling fragments of green fluorescent protein. Nat Biotechnol 2005; 23(1): 102-7.
[http://dx.doi.org/10.1038/nbt1044] [PMID: 15580262]

[17]   Cabantous S, Waldo GS. *In vivo* and *in vitro* protein solubility assays using split GFP. Nat Methods 2006; 3(10): 845-54.
[http://dx.doi.org/10.1038/nmeth932] [PMID: 16990817]

[18]   Feinberg EH, Vanhoven MK, Bendesky A, *et al.* GFP Reconstitution Across Synaptic Partners (GRASP) defines cell contacts and synapses in living nervous systems. Neuron 2008; 57(3): 353-63.
[http://dx.doi.org/10.1016/j.neuron.2007.11.030] [PMID: 18255029]

[19]   Nakai J, Ohkura M, Imoto K. A high signal-to-noise Ca(2+) probe composed of a single green fluorescent protein. Nat Biotechnol 2001; 19(2): 137-41.
[http://dx.doi.org/10.1038/84397] [PMID: 11175727]

[20]   Wang Q, Shui B, Kotlikoff MI, Sondermann H. Structural basis for calcium sensing by GCaMP2. Structure 2008; 16(12): 1817-27.
[http://dx.doi.org/10.1016/j.str.2008.10.008] [PMID: 19081058]

[21]   Guo ZV, Hart AC, Ramanathan S. Optical interrogation of neural circuits in Caenorhabditis elegans. Nat Methods 2009; 6(12): 891-6.
[http://dx.doi.org/10.1038/nmeth.1397] [PMID: 19898486]

[22]   Chen Q, Cichon J, Wang W, *et al.* Imaging neural activity using Thy1-GCaMP transgenic mice. Neuron 2012; 76(2): 297-308.
[http://dx.doi.org/10.1016/j.neuron.2012.07.011] [PMID: 23083733]

[23]   Conley NR, Pomerantz AK, Wang H, Twieg RJ, Moerner WE. Bulk and single-molecule characterization of an improved molecular beacon utilizing H-dimer excitonic behavior. J Phys Chem B 2007; 111(28): 7929-31.
[http://dx.doi.org/10.1021/jp073310d] [PMID: 17583944]

[24]   Ogawa M, Kosaka N, Choyke PL, Kobayashi H. H-type dimer formation of fluorophores: a mechanism for activatable, *in vivo* optical molecular imaging. ACS Chem Biol 2009; 4(7): 535-46.
[http://dx.doi.org/10.1021/cb900089j] [PMID: 19480464]

[25]   Nesterova IV, Erdem SS, Pakhomov S, Hammer RP, Soper SA. Phthalocyanine dimerization-based molecular beacons using near-IR fluorescence. J Am Chem Soc 2009; 131(7): 2432-3.
[http://dx.doi.org/10.1021/ja8088247] [PMID: 19191492]

[26]   Julia LB, Yuri LS, Ihor DP, Alexander PD. Fluorescent j-aggregates of cyanine dyes: Basic research and applications review. Methods Appl Fluoresc 2018; 6(1)012001
[PMID: 30457122]

[27]   Cannon BL, Patten LK, Kellis DL, *et al.* Large davydov splitting and strong fluorescence suppression: An investigation of exciton delocalization in DNA-templated holliday junction dye aggregates. J Phys Chem A 2018; 122(8): 2086-95.
[http://dx.doi.org/10.1021/acs.jpca.7b12668] [PMID: 29420037]

[28]   Knemeyer JP, Marmé N, Sauer M. Probes for detection of specific DNA sequences at the single-molecule level. Anal Chem 2000; 72(16): 3717-24.
[http://dx.doi.org/10.1021/ac000024o] [PMID: 10959954]

[29]   Tanaka K, Miura T, Umezawa N, *et al.* Rational design of fluorescein-based fluorescence probes. Mechanism-based design of a maximum fluorescence probe for singlet oxygen. J Am Chem Soc 2001; 123(11): 2530-6.
[http://dx.doi.org/10.1021/ja0035708] [PMID: 11456921]

[30]   Miura T, Urano Y, Tanaka K, Nagano T, Ohkubo K, Fukuzumi S. Rational design principle for modulating fluorescence properties of fluorescein-based probes by photoinduced electron transfer. J Am Chem Soc 2003; 125(28): 8666-71.
[http://dx.doi.org/10.1021/ja035282s] [PMID: 12848574]

[31]   Urano Y, Kamiya M, Kanda K, Ueno T, Hirose K, Nagano T. Evolution of fluorescein as a platform for finely tunable fluorescence probes. J Am Chem Soc 2005; 127(13): 4888-94.
[http://dx.doi.org/10.1021/ja043919h] [PMID: 15796553]

[32]   Lerman LS. Structural considerations in the interaction of DNA and acridines. J Mol Biol 1961; 3(1): 18-30.
[http://dx.doi.org/10.1016/S0022-2836(61)80004-1] [PMID: 13761054]

[33]   Glazer AN, Peck K, Mathies RA. A stable double-stranded DNA-ethidium homodimer complex: application to picogram fluorescence detection of DNA in agarose gels. Proc Natl Acad Sci USA 1990; 87(10): 3851-5.
[http://dx.doi.org/10.1073/pnas.87.10.3851] [PMID: 2339125]

[34]   Glazer AN, Rye HS. Stable dye-DNA intercalation complexes as reagents for high-sensitivity fluorescence detection. Nature 1992; 359(6398): 859-61.
[http://dx.doi.org/10.1038/359859a0] [PMID: 1436062]

[35]   Rye HS, Yue S, Wemmer DE, *et al.* Stable fluorescent complexes of double-stranded DNA with bis-intercalating asymmetric cyanine dyes: properties and applications. Nucleic Acids Res 1992; 20(11): 2803-12.
[http://dx.doi.org/10.1093/nar/20.11.2803] [PMID: 1614866]

[36]   Spielmann HP, Wemmer DE, Jacobsen JP. Solution structure of a DNA complex with the fluorescent bis-intercalator TOTO determined by NMR spectroscopy. Biochemistry 1995; 34(27): 8542-53.
[http://dx.doi.org/10.1021/bi00027a004] [PMID: 7612596]

[37]   Kapuscinski J. DAPI: a DNA-specific fluorescent probe. Biotech Histochem 1995; 70(5): 220-33.
[http://dx.doi.org/10.3109/10520299509108199] [PMID: 8580206]

[38]   Sanchez-Galvez A, Hunt P, Robb MA, *et al.* Ultrafast radiationless deactivation of organic dyes: Evidence for a two-state two-mode pathway in polymethine cyanines. J Am Chem Soc 2000; 122(12): 2911-24.
[http://dx.doi.org/10.1021/ja993985x]

[39]   Silva GL, Ediz V, Yaron D, Armitage BA. Experimental and computational investigation of unsymmetrical cyanine dyes: understanding torsionally responsive fluorogenic dyes. J Am Chem Soc 2007; 129(17): 5710-8.
[http://dx.doi.org/10.1021/ja070025z] [PMID: 17411048]

[40]   Dragan AI, Pavlovic R, McGivney JB, *et al.* SYBR Green I: fluorescence properties and interaction with DNA. J Fluoresc 2012; 22(4): 1189-99.
[http://dx.doi.org/10.1007/s10895-012-1059-8] [PMID: 22534954]

[41]   Griffin BA, Adams SR, Tsien RY. Specific covalent labeling of recombinant protein molecules inside live cells. Science 1998; 281(5374): 269-72.
[http://dx.doi.org/10.1126/science.281.5374.269] [PMID: 9657724]

[42]   Adams SR, Campbell RE, Gross LA, *et al.* New biarsenical ligands and tetracysteine motifs for protein labeling *in vitro* and *in vivo*: synthesis and biological applications. J Am Chem Soc 2002; 124(21): 6063-76.
[http://dx.doi.org/10.1021/ja017687n] [PMID: 12022841]

[43]   Tuerk C, Gold L. Systematic evolution of ligands by exponential enrichment: RNA ligands to bacteriophage T4 DNA polymerase. Science 1990; 249(4968): 505-10.
[http://dx.doi.org/10.1126/science.2200121] [PMID: 2200121]

[44]   Hermann T, Patel DJ. Adaptive recognition by nucleic acid aptamers. Science 2000; 287(5454): 820-5.
[http://dx.doi.org/10.1126/science.287.5454.820] [PMID: 10657289]

[45]   Babendure JR, Adams SR, Tsien RY. Aptamers switch on fluorescence of triphenylmethane dyes. J Am Chem Soc 2003; 125(48): 14716-7.
[http://dx.doi.org/10.1021/ja037994o] [PMID: 14640641]

[46]   Paige JS, Wu KY, Jaffrey SR. RNA mimics of green fluorescent protein. Science 2011; 333(6042): 642-6.
[http://dx.doi.org/10.1126/science.1207339] [PMID: 21798953]

[47]   Filonov GS, Moon JD, Svensen N, Jaffrey SR. Broccoli: rapid selection of an RNA mimic of green fluorescent protein by fluorescence-based selection and directed evolution. J Am Chem Soc 2014; 136(46): 16299-308.
[http://dx.doi.org/10.1021/ja508478x] [PMID: 25337688]

[48]   Dolgosheina EV, Jeng SC, Panchapakesan SS, *et al.* RNA mango aptamer-fluorophore: a bright, high-affinity complex for RNA labeling and tracking. ACS Chem Biol 2014; 9(10): 2412-20.
[http://dx.doi.org/10.1021/cb500499x] [PMID: 25101481]

[49]   Jepsen MDE, Sparvath SM, Nielsen TB, *et al.* Development of a genetically encodable FRET system using fluorescent RNA aptamers. Nat Commun 2018; 9(1): 18.
[http://dx.doi.org/10.1038/s41467-017-02435-x] [PMID: 29295996]

[50]   Yeh H-C, Sharma J, Han JJ, Martinez JS, Werner JHA. A DNA--silver nanocluster probe that fluoresces upon hybridization. Nano Lett 2010; 10(8): 3106-10.
[http://dx.doi.org/10.1021/nl101773c] [PMID: 20698624]

[51]   Yeh H-C, Sharma J, Han JJ, Martinez JS, Werner JH. A beacon of light. IEEE Nanotechnol Mag 2011; 5(2): 28-33.
[http://dx.doi.org/10.1109/MNANO.2011.940951]

[52]   Yeh H-C, Sharma J, Shih IeM, Vu DM, Martinez JS, Werner JH. A fluorescence light-up Ag nanocluster probe that discriminates single-nucleotide variants by emission color. J Am Chem Soc 2012; 134(28): 11550-8.
[http://dx.doi.org/10.1021/ja3024737] [PMID: 22775452]

[53]   Obliosca JM, Liu C, Yeh H-C. Fluorescent silver nanoclusters as DNA probes. Nanoscale 2013; 5(18): 8443-61.
[http://dx.doi.org/10.1039/c3nr01601c] [PMID: 23828021]

[54]   Obliosca JM, Liu C, Batson RA, Babin MC, Werner JH, Yeh HC. DNA/RNA detection using DNA-templated few-atom silver nanoclusters. Biosensors (Basel) 2013; 3(2): 185-200.
[http://dx.doi.org/10.3390/bios3020185] [PMID: 25586126]

[55]   Obliosca JM, Babin MC, Liu C, *et al.* A complementary palette of nanocluster beacons. ACS Nano 2014; 8(10): 10150-60.
[http://dx.doi.org/10.1021/nn505338e] [PMID: 25299363]

[56] Chen Y-A, Obliosca JM, Liu Y-L, Liu C, Gwozdz ML, Yeh HC. NanoCluster Beacons enable detection of a single n 6-methyladenine. J Am Chem Soc 2015; 137(33): 10476-9.
[http://dx.doi.org/10.1021/jacs.5b06038] [PMID: 26261877]

[57] Juul S, Obliosca JM, Liu C, *et al.* NanoCluster Beacons as reporter probes in rolling circle enhanced enzyme activity detection. Nanoscale 2015; 7(18): 8332-7.
[http://dx.doi.org/10.1039/C5NR01705J] [PMID: 25901841]

[58] Chen YA, Vu HT, Liu YL, *et al.* Improving NanoCluster Beacon performance by blocking the unlabeled NC probes. Chem Commun (Camb) 2019; 55(4): 462-5.
[http://dx.doi.org/10.1039/C8CC08291J] [PMID: 30547174]

[59] Heller DA, Jeng ES, Yeung TK, *et al.* Optical detection of DNA conformational polymorphism on single-walled carbon nanotubes. Science 2006; 311(5760): 508-11.
[http://dx.doi.org/10.1126/science.1120792] [PMID: 16439657]

[60] Sorokina M, Koh H-R, Patel SS, Ha T. Fluorescent lifetime trajectories of a single fluorophore reveal reaction intermediates during transcription initiation. J Am Chem Soc 2009; 131(28): 9630-1.
[http://dx.doi.org/10.1021/ja902861f] [PMID: 19552410]

[61] Yeh HC, Puleo CM, Ho YP, *et al.* Tunable blinking kinetics of cy5 for precise DNA quantification and single-nucleotide difference detection. Biophys J 2008; 95(2): 729-37.
[http://dx.doi.org/10.1529/biophysj.107.127530] [PMID: 18424494]

[62] Tyagi S, Marras SA, Kramer FR. Wavelength-shifting molecular beacons. Nat Biotechnol 2000; 18(11): 1191-6.
[http://dx.doi.org/10.1038/81192] [PMID: 11062440]

[63] Zhao Q, Lv Q, Wang H. Aptamer fluorescence anisotropy sensors for adenosine triphosphate by comprehensive screening tetramethylrhodamine labeled nucleotides. Biosens Bioelectron 2015; 70: 188-93.
[http://dx.doi.org/10.1016/j.bios.2015.03.031] [PMID: 25814408]

[64] Gokulrangan G, Unruh JR, Holub DF, Ingram B, Johnson CK, Wilson GS. DNA aptamer-based bioanalysis of IgE by fluorescence anisotropy. Anal Chem 2005; 77(7): 1963-70.
[http://dx.doi.org/10.1021/ac0483926] [PMID: 15801725]

[65] Yeh H-C, Puleo CM, Lim TC, *et al.* A microfluidic-fcs platform for investigation on the dissociation of sp1-DNA complex by doxorubicin. Nucleic Acids Research 2006; 34(21): e144-.
[http://dx.doi.org/10.1093/nar/gkl787]

[66] Kinjo M, Rigler R. Ultrasensitive hybridization analysis using fluorescence correlation spectroscopy. Nucleic Acids Res 1995; 23(10): 1795-9.
[http://dx.doi.org/10.1093/nar/23.10.1795] [PMID: 7784185]

[67] Elghanian R, Storhoff JJ, Mucic RC, Letsinger RL, Mirkin CA. Selective colorimetric detection of polynucleotides based on the distance-dependent optical properties of gold nanoparticles. Science 1997; 277(5329): 1078-81.
[http://dx.doi.org/10.1126/science.277.5329.1078] [PMID: 9262471]

[68] Sapsford KE, Algar WR, Berti L, *et al.* Functionalizing nanoparticles with biological molecules: developing chemistries that facilitate nanotechnology. Chem Rev 2013; 113(3): 1904-2074.
[http://dx.doi.org/10.1021/cr300143v] [PMID: 23432378]

[69] Magde D, Elson E, Webb WW. Thermodynamic fluctuations in a reacting system—measurement by fluorescence correlation spectroscopy. Phys Rev Lett 1972; 29(11): 705.
[http://dx.doi.org/10.1103/PhysRevLett.29.705]

[70] Rigler R, Elson ES. Fluorescence correlation spectroscopy: Theory and applications. Springer Science & Business Media 2012.

[71] Chan WC, Nie S. Quantum dot bioconjugates for ultrasensitive nonisotopic detection. Science 1998;

281(5385): 2016-8.
[http://dx.doi.org/10.1126/science.281.5385.2016] [PMID: 9748158]

[72] Bruchez M, Moronne M, Gin P, Weiss S, Alivisatos AP. Semiconductor nanocrystals as fluorescent biological labels. science 1998; 281(5385): 2013-6.

[73] Petty JT, Zheng J, Hud NV, Dickson RM. DNA-templated Ag nanocluster formation. J Am Chem Soc 2004; 126(16): 5207-12.
[http://dx.doi.org/10.1021/ja031931o] [PMID: 15099104]

[74] Zheng J, Nicovich PR, Dickson RM. Highly fluorescent noble-metal quantum dots. Annu Rev Phys Chem 2007; 58: 409-31.
[http://dx.doi.org/10.1146/annurev.physchem.58.032806.104546] [PMID: 17105412]

[75] Hink MA, Griep RA, Borst JW, *et al.* Structural dynamics of green fluorescent protein alone and fused with a single chain Fv protein. J Biol Chem 2000; 275(23): 17556-60.
[http://dx.doi.org/10.1074/jbc.M001348200] [PMID: 10748019]

[76] Yu WW, Qu L, Guo W, Peng X. Experimental determination of the extinction coefficient of cdte, cdse, and cds nanocrystals. Chem Mater 2003; 15(14): 2854-60.
[http://dx.doi.org/10.1021/cm034081k]

[77] Levy M, Cater SF, Ellington AD. Quantum-dot aptamer beacons for the detection of proteins. ChemBioChem 2005; 6(12): 2163-6.
[http://dx.doi.org/10.1002/cbic.200500218] [PMID: 16254932]

[78] Santangelo PJ, Nix B, Tsourkas A, Bao G. Dual FRET molecular beacons for mRNA detection in living cells. Nucleic Acids Res 2004; 32(6)e57
[http://dx.doi.org/10.1093/nar/gnh062] [PMID: 15084672]

[79] Zhang M, Li M, Zhang W, Han Y, Zhang Y-H. Simple and efficient delivery of cell-impermeable organic fluorescent probes into live cells for live-cell superresolution imaging. Light Sci Appl 2019; 8(1): 73.
[http://dx.doi.org/10.1038/s41377-019-0188-0] [PMID: 31666945]

[80] Pan D, Hu Z, Qiu F, *et al.* A general strategy for developing cell-permeable photo-modulatable organic fluorescent probes for live-cell super-resolution imaging. Nat Commun 2014; 5(1): 5573.
[http://dx.doi.org/10.1038/ncomms6573] [PMID: 25410769]

[81] Verkman AS, Sellers MC, Chao AC, Leung T, Ketcham R. Synthesis and characterization of improved chloride-sensitive fluorescent indicators for biological applications. Anal Biochem 1989; 178(2): 355-61.
[http://dx.doi.org/10.1016/0003-2697(89)90652-0] [PMID: 2751097]

[82] Verkman AS. Development and biological applications of chloride-sensitive fluorescent indicators. Am J Physiol 1990; 259(3 Pt 1): C375-88.
[http://dx.doi.org/10.1152/ajpcell.1990.259.3.C375] [PMID: 2205105]

[83] Chojnacki J, Eggeling C, Caesar I, *et al.* Advances in super-resolution microscopy. Advances in Super-resolution Microscopy 2018; p. 348.

[84] Zhang J, Campbell RE, Ting AY, Tsien RY. Creating new fluorescent probes for cell biology. Nat Rev Mol Cell Biol 2002; 3(12): 906-18.
[http://dx.doi.org/10.1038/nrm976] [PMID: 12461557]

[85] Kitamura Y, Ihara T, Tsujimura Y, Osawa Y, Tazaki M, Jyo A. Colorimetric allele typing through cooperative binding of DNA probes carrying a metal chelator for luminescent lanthanide ions. Anal Biochem 2006; 359(2): 259-61.
[http://dx.doi.org/10.1016/j.ab.2006.09.009] [PMID: 17055995]

[86] Kitamura Y, Ihara T, Tsujimura Y, *et al.* Template-directed formation of luminescent lanthanide complexes: versatile tools for colorimetric identification of single nucleotide polymorphism. J Inorg Biochem 2008; 102(10): 1921-31.

[http://dx.doi.org/10.1016/j.jinorgbio.2008.06.016] [PMID: 18707760]

[87] Grossmann TN, Seitz O. DNA-catalyzed transfer of a reporter group. J Am Chem Soc 2006; 128(49): 15596-7.
[http://dx.doi.org/10.1021/ja0670097] [PMID: 17147362]

[88] Grossmann TN, Seitz O. Nucleic acid templated reactions: consequences of probe reactivity and readout strategy for amplified signaling and sequence selectivity. Chemistry 2009; 15(27): 6723-30.
[http://dx.doi.org/10.1002/chem.200900025] [PMID: 19496097]

[89] Mergny JL, Boutorine AS, Garestier T, *et al.* Fluorescence energy transfer as a probe for nucleic acid structures and sequences. Nucleic Acids Res 1994; 22(6): 920-8.
[http://dx.doi.org/10.1093/nar/22.6.920] [PMID: 8152922]

[90] Cardullo RA, Agrawal S, Flores C, Zamecnik PC, Wolf DE. Detection of nucleic acid hybridization by nonradiative fluorescence resonance energy transfer. Proc Natl Acad Sci USA 1988; 85(23): 8790-4.
[http://dx.doi.org/10.1073/pnas.85.23.8790] [PMID: 3194390]

[91] Kolpashchikov DM. Binary probes for nucleic acid analysis. Chem Rev 2010; 110(8): 4709-23.
[http://dx.doi.org/10.1021/cr900323b] [PMID: 20583806]

[92] Vendrell M, Zhai D, Er JC, Chang Y-T. Combinatorial strategies in fluorescent probe development. Chem Rev 2012; 112(8): 4391-420.
[http://dx.doi.org/10.1021/cr200355j] [PMID: 22616565]

[93] Teo YN, Kool ET. DNA-multichromophore systems. Chem Rev 2012; 112(7): 4221-45.
[http://dx.doi.org/10.1021/cr100351g] [PMID: 22424059]

[94] Yang Y, Zhao Q, Feng W, Li F. Luminescent chemodosimeters for bioimaging. Chem Rev 2013; 113(1): 192-270.
[http://dx.doi.org/10.1021/cr2004103] [PMID: 22702347]

[95] Ranasinghe RT, Brown T. Ultrasensitive fluorescence-based methods for nucleic acid detection: towards amplification-free genetic analysis. Chem Commun (Camb) 2011; 47(13): 3717-35.
[http://dx.doi.org/10.1039/c0cc04215c] [PMID: 21283891]

[96] Ihara T, Kitamura Y. Photochemically relevant DNA-based molecular systems enabling chemical and signal transductions and their analytical applications. J Photochem Photobiol Photochem Rev 2012; 13: 148-67.
[http://dx.doi.org/10.1016/j.jphotochemrev.2012.03.002]

[97] Miyawaki A. Visualization of the spatial and temporal dynamics of intracellular signaling. Dev Cell 2003; 4(3): 295-305.
[http://dx.doi.org/10.1016/S1534-5807(03)00060-1] [PMID: 12636912]

[98] Hoffmann A, Nettels D, Clark J, *et al.* Quantifying heterogeneity and conformational dynamics from single molecule FRET of diffusing molecules: recurrence analysis of single particles (RASP). Phys Chem Chem Phys 2011; 13(5): 1857-71.
[http://dx.doi.org/10.1039/c0cp01911a] [PMID: 21218223]

[99] Nazarenko IA, Bhatnagar SK, Hohman RJ. A closed tube format for amplification and detection of DNA based on energy transfer. Nucleic Acids Res 1997; 25(12): 2516-21.
[http://dx.doi.org/10.1093/nar/25.12.2516] [PMID: 9171107]

[100] Whitcombe D, Theaker J, Guy SP, Brown T, Little S. Detection of PCR products using self-probing amplicons and fluorescence. Nat Biotechnol 1999; 17(8): 804-7.
[http://dx.doi.org/10.1038/11751] [PMID: 10429248]

[101] Saiki RK, Gelfand DH, Stoffel S, *et al.* Primer-directed enzymatic amplification of DNA with a thermostable DNA polymerase. Science 1988; 239(4839): 487-91.
[http://dx.doi.org/10.1126/science.239.4839.487] [PMID: 2448875]

[102] Whitcombe D, Brownie J, Gillard HL, *et al.* A homogeneous fluorescence assay for PCR amplicons:

its application to real-time, single-tube genotyping. Clin Chem 1998; 44(5): 918-23.
[http://dx.doi.org/10.1093/clinchem/44.5.918] [PMID: 9590362]

[103] Johansson MK. Choosing reporter-quencher pairs for efficient quenching through formation of intramolecular dimers Fluorescent energy transfer nucleic acid probes. Springer 2006; pp. 17-29.
[http://dx.doi.org/10.1385/1-59745-069-3:17]

[104] Marras SA, Kramer FR, Tyagi S. Efficiencies of fluorescence resonance energy transfer and contact☐mediated quenching in oligonucleotide probes. Nucleic acids research 2002; 30(21): e122-.
[http://dx.doi.org/10.1093/nar/gnf121]

[105] Wang K, Tang Z, Yang CJ, *et al.* Molecular engineering of DNA: molecular beacons. Angew Chem Int Ed Engl 2009; 48(5): 856-70.
[http://dx.doi.org/10.1002/anie.200800370] [PMID: 19065690]

[106] Ginzinger DG. Gene quantification using real-time quantitative PCR: an emerging technology hits the mainstream. Exp Hematol 2002; 30(6): 503-12.
[http://dx.doi.org/10.1016/S0301-472X(02)00806-8] [PMID: 12063017]

[107] Wang DG, Fan J-B, Siao C-J, *et al.* Large-scale identification, mapping, and genotyping of single-nucleotide polymorphisms in the human genome. Science 1998; 280(5366): 1077-82.
[http://dx.doi.org/10.1126/science.280.5366.1077] [PMID: 9582121]

[108] Walia A, Waadt R, Jones AM. Genetically encoded biosensors in plants: Pathways to discovery. Annu Rev Plant Biol 2018; 69(1): 497-524.
[http://dx.doi.org/10.1146/annurev-arplant-042817-040104] [PMID: 29719164]

[109] Joiner ML, Koval OM, Li J, *et al.* CaMKII determines mitochondrial stress responses in heart. Nature 2012; 491(7423): 269-73.
[http://dx.doi.org/10.1038/nature11444] [PMID: 23051746]

[110] Miyawaki A, Griesbeck O, Heim R, Tsien RY. Dynamic and quantitative Ca2+ measurements using improved cameleons. Proc Natl Acad Sci USA 1999; 96(5): 2135-40.
[http://dx.doi.org/10.1073/pnas.96.5.2135] [PMID: 10051607]

[111] Kerr R, Lev-Ram V, Baird G, Vincent P, Tsien RY, Schafer WR. Optical imaging of calcium transients in neurons and pharyngeal muscle of C. elegans. Neuron 2000; 26(3): 583-94.
[http://dx.doi.org/10.1016/S0896-6273(00)81196-4] [PMID: 10896155]

[112] Suzuki H, Thiele TR, Faumont S, Ezcurra M, Lockery SR, Schafer WR. Functional asymmetry in Caenorhabditis elegans taste neurons and its computational role in chemotaxis. Nature 2008; 454(7200): 114-7.
[http://dx.doi.org/10.1038/nature06927] [PMID: 18596810]

[113] Haugland RP. Handbook of fluorescent probes and research products. Molecular Probes 2002.

[114] Stosiek C, Garaschuk O, Holthoff K, Konnerth A. *In vivo* two-photon calcium imaging of neuronal networks. Proc Natl Acad Sci USA 2003; 100(12): 7319-24.
[http://dx.doi.org/10.1073/pnas.1232232100] [PMID: 12777621]

[115] Kuner T, Augustine GJ. A genetically encoded ratiometric indicator for chloride: capturing chloride transients in cultured hippocampal neurons. Neuron 2000; 27(3): 447-59.
[http://dx.doi.org/10.1016/S0896-6273(00)00056-8] [PMID: 11055428]

[116] Esposito A, Gralle M, Dani MAC, Lange D, Wouters FS. pHlameleons: a family of FRET-based protein sensors for quantitative pH imaging. Biochemistry 2008; 47(49): 13115-26.
[http://dx.doi.org/10.1021/bi8009482] [PMID: 19007185]

[117] Surdo NC, Berrera M, Koschinski A, *et al.* FRET biosensor uncovers cAMP nano-domains at β-adrenergic targets that dictate precise tuning of cardiac contractility. Nat Commun 2017; 8: 15031.
[http://dx.doi.org/10.1038/ncomms15031] [PMID: 28425435]

[118] Xu X, Gerard AL, Huang BC, Anderson DC, Payan DG, Luo Y. Detection of programmed cell death

using fluorescence energy transfer. Nucleic Acids Res 1998; 26(8): 2034-5.
[http://dx.doi.org/10.1093/nar/26.8.2034] [PMID: 9518501]

[119]   Kardash E, Bandemer J, Raz E. Imaging protein activity in live embryos using fluorescence resonance energy transfer biosensors. Nat Protoc 2011; 6(12): 1835-46.
[http://dx.doi.org/10.1038/nprot.2011.395] [PMID: 22051797]

[120]   Aoki K, Matsuda M. Visualization of small GTPase activity with fluorescence resonance energy transfer-based biosensors. Nat Protoc 2009; 4(11): 1623-31.
[http://dx.doi.org/10.1038/nprot.2009.175] [PMID: 19834477]

[121]   Itoh RE, Kurokawa K, Ohba Y, Yoshizaki H, Mochizuki N, Matsuda M. Activation of rac and cdc42 video imaged by fluorescent resonance energy transfer-based single-molecule probes in the membrane of living cells. Mol Cell Biol 2002; 22(18): 6582-91.
[http://dx.doi.org/10.1128/MCB.22.18.6582-6591.2002] [PMID: 12192056]

[122]   Mochizuki N, Yamashita S, Kurokawa K, *et al.* Spatio-temporal images of growth-factor-induced activation of Ras and Rap1. Nature 2001; 411(6841): 1065-8.
[http://dx.doi.org/10.1038/35082594] [PMID: 11429608]

[123]   Zhang J, Ma Y, Taylor SS, Tsien RY. Genetically encoded reporters of protein kinase A activity reveal impact of substrate tethering. Proc Natl Acad Sci USA 2001; 98(26): 14997-5002.
[http://dx.doi.org/10.1073/pnas.211566798] [PMID: 11752448]

[124]   Ting AY, Kain KH, Klemke RL, Tsien RY. Genetically encoded fluorescent reporters of protein tyrosine kinase activities in living cells. Proc Natl Acad Sci USA 2001; 98(26): 15003-8.
[http://dx.doi.org/10.1073/pnas.211564598] [PMID: 11752449]

[125]   Wang Y, Botvinick EL, Zhao Y, *et al.* Visualizing the mechanical activation of Src. Nature 2005; 434(7036): 1040-5.
[http://dx.doi.org/10.1038/nature03469] [PMID: 15846350]

[126]   Pertz O, Hodgson L, Klemke RL, Hahn KM. Spatiotemporal dynamics of RhoA activity in migrating cells. Nature 2006; 440(7087): 1069-72.
[http://dx.doi.org/10.1038/nature04665] [PMID: 16547516]

[127]   Fosbrink M, Aye-Han N-N, Cheong R, Levchenko A, Zhang J. Visualization of JNK activity dynamics with a genetically encoded fluorescent biosensor. Proc Natl Acad Sci USA 2010; 107(12): 5459-64.
[http://dx.doi.org/10.1073/pnas.0909671107] [PMID: 20212108]

[128]   Bermejo C, Haerizadeh F, Takanaga H, Chermak D, Frommer WB. Optical sensors for measuring dynamic changes of cytosolic metabolite levels in yeast. Nat Protoc 2011; 6(11): 1806-17.
[http://dx.doi.org/10.1038/nprot.2011.391] [PMID: 22036883]

[129]   Hudson DA, Caplan JL, Thorpe C. Designing flavoprotein-gfp fusion probes for analyte-specific ratiometric fluorescence imaging. Biochemistry 2018; 57(7): 1178-89.
[http://dx.doi.org/10.1021/acs.biochem.7b01132] [PMID: 29341594]

[130]   Hama Y, Urano Y, Koyama Y, *et al.* A target cell-specific activatable fluorescence probe for *in vivo* molecular imaging of cancer based on a self-quenched avidin-rhodamine conjugate. Cancer Res 2007; 67(6): 2791-9.
[http://dx.doi.org/10.1158/0008-5472.CAN-06-3315] [PMID: 17363601]

[131]   Hama Y, Urano Y, Koyama Y, Gunn AJ, Choyke PL, Kobayashi H. A self-quenched galactosamine-serum albumin-rhodamineX conjugate: a "smart" fluorescent molecular imaging probe synthesized with clinically applicable material for detecting peritoneal ovarian cancer metastases. Clin Cancer Res 2007; 13(21): 6335-43.
[http://dx.doi.org/10.1158/1078-0432.CCR-07-1004] [PMID: 17975145]

[132]   Tyagi S. Splitting or stacking fluorescent proteins to visualize mRNA in living cells. Nat Methods 2007; 4(5): 391-2.

[http://dx.doi.org/10.1038/nmeth0507-391] [PMID: 17464293]

[133] Rossi F, Charlton CA, Blau HM. Monitoring protein-protein interactions in intact eukaryotic cells by beta-galactosidase complementation. Proc Natl Acad Sci USA 1997; 94(16): 8405-10.
[http://dx.doi.org/10.1073/pnas.94.16.8405] [PMID: 9237989]

[134] Johnsson N, Varshavsky A. Split ubiquitin as a sensor of protein interactions *in vivo*. Proc Natl Acad Sci USA 1994; 91(22): 10340-4.
[http://dx.doi.org/10.1073/pnas.91.22.10340] [PMID: 7937952]

[135] Pelletier JN, Campbell-Valois FX, Michnick SW. Oligomerization domain-directed reassembly of active dihydrofolate reductase from rationally designed fragments. Proc Natl Acad Sci USA 1998; 95(21): 12141-6.
[http://dx.doi.org/10.1073/pnas.95.21.12141] [PMID: 9770453]

[136] Blakely BT, Rossi FMV, Tillotson B, Palmer M, Estelles A, Blau HM. Epidermal growth factor receptor dimerization monitored in live cells. Nat Biotechnol 2000; 18(2): 218-22.
[http://dx.doi.org/10.1038/72686] [PMID: 10657132]

[137] Ghosh I, Hamilton AD, Regan L. Antiparallel leucine zipper-directed protein reassembly: Application to the green fluorescent protein. J Am Chem Soc 2000; 122(23): 5658-9.
[http://dx.doi.org/10.1021/ja994421w]

[138] Lindenburg L, Merkx M. Engineering genetically encoded FRET sensors. Sensors (Basel) 2014; 14(7): 11691-713.
[http://dx.doi.org/10.3390/s140711691] [PMID: 24991940]

[139] Mank M, Griesbeck O. Genetically encoded calcium indicators. Chem Rev 2008; 108(5): 1550-64.
[http://dx.doi.org/10.1021/cr078213v] [PMID: 18447377]

[140] Last NB, Rhoades E, Miranker AD. Islet amyloid polypeptide demonstrates a persistent capacity to disrupt membrane integrity. Proc Natl Acad Sci USA 2011; 108(23): 9460-5.
[http://dx.doi.org/10.1073/pnas.1102356108] [PMID: 21606325]

[141] Kotlikoff MI. Genetically encoded Ca2+ indicators: using genetics and molecular design to understand complex physiology. J Physiol 2007; 578(Pt 1): 55-67.
[http://dx.doi.org/10.1113/jphysiol.2006.120212] [PMID: 17038427]

[142] Svanvik N, Westman G, Wang D, Kubista M. Light-up probes: thiazole orange-conjugated peptide nucleic acid for detection of target nucleic acid in homogeneous solution. Anal Biochem 2000; 281(1): 26-35.
[http://dx.doi.org/10.1006/abio.2000.4534] [PMID: 10847607]

[143] Bethge L, Jarikote DV, Seitz O. New cyanine dyes as base surrogates in PNA: forced intercalation probes (FIT-probes) for homogeneous SNP detection. Bioorg Med Chem 2008; 16(1): 114-25.
[http://dx.doi.org/10.1016/j.bmc.2006.12.044] [PMID: 17981472]

[144] Holzhauser C, Wagenknecht H-A. DNA and RNA "traffic lights": synthetic wavelength-shifting fluorescent probes based on nucleic acid base substitutes for molecular imaging. J Org Chem 2013; 78(15): 7373-9.
[http://dx.doi.org/10.1021/jo4010102] [PMID: 23796243]

[145] Carreon JR, Stewart KM, Mahon KP Jr, Shin S, Kelley SO. Cyanine dye conjugates as probes for live cell imaging. Bioorg Med Chem Lett 2007; 17(18): 5182-5.
[http://dx.doi.org/10.1016/j.bmcl.2007.06.097] [PMID: 17646099]

[146] Sha X-L, Niu J-Y, Sun R, Xu Y-J, Ge J-F. Synthesis and optical properties of cyanine dyes with an aromatic azonia skeleton. Org Chem Front 2018; 5(4): 555-60.
[http://dx.doi.org/10.1039/C7QO00889A]

[147] Manders EM, Kimura H, Cook PR. Direct imaging of DNA in living cells reveals the dynamics of chromosome formation. J Cell Biol 1999; 144(5): 813-21.
[http://dx.doi.org/10.1083/jcb.144.5.813] [PMID: 10085283]

[148] Halstead JM, Lionnet T, Wilbertz JH, *et al.* Translation. An RNA biosensor for imaging the first round of translation from single cells to living animals. Science 2015; 347(6228): 1367-671.
[http://dx.doi.org/10.1126/science.aaa3380] [PMID: 25792328]

[149] Fusco D, Accornero N, Lavoie B, *et al.* Single mRNA molecules demonstrate probabilistic movement in living mammalian cells. Curr Biol 2003; 13(2): 161-7.
[http://dx.doi.org/10.1016/S0960-9822(02)01436-7] [PMID: 12546792]

[150] Bertrand E, Chartrand P, Schaefer M, Shenoy SM, Singer RH, Long RM. Localization of ASH1 mRNA particles in living yeast. Mol Cell 1998; 2(4): 437-45.
[http://dx.doi.org/10.1016/S1097-2765(00)80143-4] [PMID: 9809065]

[151] Paige JS, Nguyen-Duc T, Song W, Jaffrey SR. Fluorescence imaging of cellular metabolites with RNA. Science 2012; 335(6073): 1194.
[http://dx.doi.org/10.1126/science.1218298] [PMID: 22403384]

[152] Strack RL, Song W, Jaffrey SR. Using Spinach-based sensors for fluorescence imaging of intracellular metabolites and proteins in living bacteria. Nat Protoc 2014; 9(1): 146-55.
[http://dx.doi.org/10.1038/nprot.2014.001] [PMID: 24356773]

[153] Gwinn E, Schultz D, Copp SM, Swasey S. DNA-protected silver clusters for nanophotonics. Nanomaterials (Basel) 2015; 5(1): 180-207.
[http://dx.doi.org/10.3390/nano5010180] [PMID: 28347005]

[154] Zheng J, Zhang C, Dickson RM. Highly fluorescent, water-soluble, size-tunable gold quantum dots. Phys Rev Lett 2004; 93(7)077402
[http://dx.doi.org/10.1103/PhysRevLett.93.077402] [PMID: 15324277]

[155] Petty JT, Ganguly M, Yunus AI, *et al.* A DNA-encapsulated silver cluster and the roles of its nucleobase ligands. J Phys Chem C 2018; 122(49): 28382-92.
[http://dx.doi.org/10.1021/acs.jpcc.8b09414]

[156] Torimura M, Kurata S, Yamada K, *et al.* Fluorescence-quenching phenomenon by photoinduced electron transfer between a fluorescent dye and a nucleotide base. Anal Sci 2001; 17(1): 155-60.
[http://dx.doi.org/10.2116/analsci.17.155] [PMID: 11993654]

[157] Huard DJ, Demissie A, Kim D, *et al.* Atomic structure of a fluorescent ag8 cluster templated by a multistranded DNA scaffold. J Am Chem Soc 2018.
[PMID: 30562465]

[158] Jung C, Ellington AD. Diagnostic applications of nucleic acid circuits. Acc Chem Res 2014; 47(6): 1825-35.
[http://dx.doi.org/10.1021/ar500059c] [PMID: 24828239]

[159] Dirks RM, Pierce NA. Triggered amplification by hybridization chain reaction. Proc Natl Acad Sci USA 2004; 101(43): 15275-8.
[http://dx.doi.org/10.1073/pnas.0407024101] [PMID: 15492210]

[160] Choi HM, Chang JY, Trinh A, Padilla JE, Fraser SE, Pierce NA. Programmable in situ amplification for multiplexed imaging of mRNA expression. Nat Biotechnol 2010; 28(11): 1208-12.
[http://dx.doi.org/10.1038/nbt.1692] [PMID: 21037591]

[161] Wang F, Elbaz J, Orbach R, Magen N, Willner I. Amplified analysis of DNA by the autonomous assembly of polymers consisting of DNAzyme wires. J Am Chem Soc 2011; 133(43): 17149-51.
[http://dx.doi.org/10.1021/ja2076789] [PMID: 21954996]

[162] Chen X, Briggs N, McLain JR, Ellington AD. Stacking nonenzymatic circuits for high signal gain. Proc Natl Acad Sci USA 2013; 110(14): 5386-91.
[http://dx.doi.org/10.1073/pnas.1222807110] [PMID: 23509255]

[163] Vargas DY, Raj A, Marras SA, Kramer FR, Tyagi S. Mechanism of mRNA transport in the nucleus. Proc Natl Acad Sci USA 2005; 102(47): 17008-13.

[http://dx.doi.org/10.1073/pnas.0505580102] [PMID: 16284251]

[164] Raj A, van den Bogaard P, Rifkin SA, van Oudenaarden A, Tyagi S. Imaging individual mRNA molecules using multiple singly labeled probes. Nat Methods 2008; 5(10): 877-9.
[http://dx.doi.org/10.1038/nmeth.1253] [PMID: 18806792]

[165] Tyagi S. Imaging intracellular RNA distribution and dynamics in living cells. Nat Methods 2009; 6(5): 331-8.
[http://dx.doi.org/10.1038/nmeth.1321] [PMID: 19404252]

[166] Tanenbaum ME, Gilbert LA, Qi LS, Weissman JS, Vale RD. A protein-tagging system for signal amplification in gene expression and fluorescence imaging. Cell 2014; 159(3): 635-46.
[http://dx.doi.org/10.1016/j.cell.2014.09.039] [PMID: 25307933]

[167] Ghosh RP, Franklin JM, Draper WE, *et al.* A fluorogenic array for temporally unlimited single-molecule tracking. Nat Chem Biol 2019; 15(4): 401-9.
[http://dx.doi.org/10.1038/s41589-019-0241-6] [PMID: 30858596]

[168] Barany F. Genetic disease detection and DNA amplification using cloned thermostable ligase. Proc Natl Acad Sci USA 1991; 88(1): 189-93.
[http://dx.doi.org/10.1073/pnas.88.1.189] [PMID: 1986365]

[169] Shi C, Eshleman SH, Jones D, *et al.* LigAmp for sensitive detection of single-nucleotide differences. Nat Methods 2004; 1(2): 141-7.
[http://dx.doi.org/10.1038/nmeth713] [PMID: 15782177]

[170] Larsson C, Koch J, Nygren A, *et al.* In situ genotyping individual DNA molecules by target-primed rolling-circle amplification of padlock probes. Nat Methods 2004; 1(3): 227-32.
[http://dx.doi.org/10.1038/nmeth723] [PMID: 15782198]

[171] Notomi T, Okayama H, Masubuchi H, *et al.* Loop-mediated isothermal amplification of DNA. Nucleic Acids Res 2000; 28(12): e63-.
[http://dx.doi.org/10.1093/nar/28.12.e63]

[172] Sano T, Smith CL, Cantor CR. Immuno-PCR: very sensitive antigen detection by means of specific antibody-DNA conjugates. Science 1992; 258(5079): 120-2.
[http://dx.doi.org/10.1126/science.1439758] [PMID: 1439758]

[173] Giljohann DA, Mirkin CA. Drivers of biodiagnostic development. Nature 2009; 462(7272): 461-4.
[http://dx.doi.org/10.1038/nature08605] [PMID: 19940916]

[174] Nam J-M, Thaxton CS, Mirkin CA. Nanoparticle-based bio-barcodes for the ultrasensitive detection of proteins. science 2003; 301(5641): 1884-6.

[175] Fredriksson S, Gullberg M, Jarvius J, *et al.* Protein detection using proximity-dependent DNA ligation assays. Nat Biotechnol 2002; 20(5): 473-7.
[http://dx.doi.org/10.1038/nbt0502-473] [PMID: 11981560]

[176] Söderberg O, Gullberg M, Jarvius M, *et al.* Direct observation of individual endogenous protein complexes in situ by proximity ligation. Nat Methods 2006; 3(12): 995-1000.
[http://dx.doi.org/10.1038/nmeth947] [PMID: 17072308]

[177] Wu L, Wu I-C, DuFort CC, *et al.* Photostable ratiometric pdot probe for *in vitro* and *in vivo* imaging of hypochlorous acid. J Am Chem Soc 2017; 139(20): 6911-8.
[http://dx.doi.org/10.1021/jacs.7b01545] [PMID: 28459559]

[178] Sun K, Tang Y, Li Q, *et al. In vivo* dynamic monitoring of small molecules with implantable polymer-dot transducer. ACS Nano 2016; 10(7): 6769-81.
[http://dx.doi.org/10.1021/acsnano.6b02386] [PMID: 27303785]

[179] Wu C, Chiu DT. Highly fluorescent semiconducting polymer dots for biology and medicine. Angew Chem Int Ed Engl 2013; 52(11): 3086-109.
[http://dx.doi.org/10.1002/anie.201205133] [PMID: 23307291]

[180]   Larson DR, Zipfel WR, Williams RM, *et al*. Water-soluble quantum dots for multiphoton fluorescence imaging *in vivo*. Science 2003; 300(5624): 1434-6.
[http://dx.doi.org/10.1126/science.1083780] [PMID: 12775841]

[181]   Aitken CE, Marshall RA, Puglisi JD. An oxygen scavenging system for improvement of dye stability in single-molecule fluorescence experiments. Biophys J 2008; 94(5): 1826-35.
[http://dx.doi.org/10.1529/biophysj.107.117689] [PMID: 17921203]

[182]   Jones SA, Shim S-H, He J, Zhuang X. Fast, three-dimensional super-resolution imaging of live cells. Nat Methods 2011; 8(6): 499-508.
[http://dx.doi.org/10.1038/nmeth.1605] [PMID: 21552254]

[183]   Tsunoyama TA, Watanabe Y, Goto J, *et al*. Super-long single-molecule tracking reveals dynamic-anchorage-induced integrin function. Nat Chem Biol 2018; 14(5): 497-506.
[http://dx.doi.org/10.1038/s41589-018-0032-5] [PMID: 29610485]

[184]   Hama Y, Urano Y, Koyama Y, Bernardo M, Choyke PL, Kobayashi H. A comparison of the emission efficiency of four common green fluorescence dyes after internalization into cancer cells. Bioconjug Chem 2006; 17(6): 1426-31.
[http://dx.doi.org/10.1021/bc0601626] [PMID: 17105220]

[185]   Kobayashi H, Choyke PL. Target-cancer-cell-specific activatable fluorescence imaging probes: rational design and *in vivo* applications. Acc Chem Res 2011; 44(2): 83-90.
[http://dx.doi.org/10.1021/ar1000633] [PMID: 21062101]

[186]   Blanco E, Shen H, Ferrari M. Principles of nanoparticle design for overcoming biological barriers to drug delivery. Nat Biotechnol 2015; 33(9): 941-51.
[http://dx.doi.org/10.1038/nbt.3330] [PMID: 26348965]

[187]   Arvizo RR, Miranda OR, Moyano DF, *et al*. Modulating pharmacokinetics, tumor uptake and biodistribution by engineered nanoparticles. PLoS One 2011; 6(9)e24374
[http://dx.doi.org/10.1371/journal.pone.0024374] [PMID: 21931696]

[188]   Yao C, Wang P, Zhou L, *et al*. Highly biocompatible zwitterionic phospholipids coated upconversion nanoparticles for efficient bioimaging. Anal Chem 2014; 86(19): 9749-57.
[http://dx.doi.org/10.1021/ac5023259] [PMID: 25075628]

[189]   Ogawa M, Regino CA, Choyke PL, Kobayashi H. *In vivo* target-specific activatable near-infrared optical labeling of humanized monoclonal antibodies. Mol Cancer Ther 2009; 8(1): 232-9.
[http://dx.doi.org/10.1158/1535-7163.MCT-08-0862] [PMID: 19139133]

CHAPTER 6

Plasmonic Label-Free Optical Biosensors

Wonju Lee[1], Seongmin Im[2] and Donghyun Kim[2,*]

[1] *Korea Electrotechnology Research Institute, 111 Hanggaul-ro, Ansan, Gyeonggi-do, Republic of Korea*

[2] *School of Electrical and Electronic Engineering, Yonsei University, 50 Yonsei-ro, Seodaemun-gu, Seoul, Republic of Korea*

Abstract: Plasmonics has provided one of the commercially proven label-free biosensing platforms to date. Traditional surface plasmon resonance (SPR) sensors, however, suffer from moderate sensitivity because of the label-free nature. In this chapter, we review various recent approaches that have attempted to produce improved detection characteristics with unique strengths and weaknesses. We first explore plasmonic field localization for self-aligned overlap or colocalization between localized near-fields and target molecules developed for dramatically enhanced detection performance. Localized SPR sensors based on metallic nanoparticles for amplification of plasmonic optical signatures measured by target molecular interactions have also been reviewed. Phase-sensitive SPR configurations based on optical path difference as well as temporal difference control have been explored for sensitivity improvement compared with conventional intensity-based SPR sensors with measurement of angular and frequency characteristics. Relatively new analytical methods based on whispering gallery mode sensors coupled to nanostructures that support localized surface plasmon to achieve ultrahigh sensitivity that may enable single molecular detection were also described. We have also included the use of SPR imaging for high-throughput label-free detection. Finally, surface-enhanced Raman spectroscopy using plasmonic near-field enhancement was discussed for the amplification of molecular signals. This chapter highlights many exciting research directions that have been unraveled to develop high-performance optical label-free biosensors based on diverse plasmonic platforms.

Keywords: Field enhancement, Label-free optical biosensor, Plasmonic localization, Phase-sensitive measurement, Surface plasmon resonance, Surface-enhanced Raman spectroscopy.

INTRODUCTION

In the last several decades, numerous studies have been conducted to develop tec-

* **Corresponding author Donghyun Kim:** School of Electrical and Electronic Engineering, Yonsei University; E-mail: kimd@yonsei.ac.kr

Han-Sheng Chuang & Yi-Ping Ho (Eds.)

hniques for label-free optical detection of target interaction that measure signals without binding labels such as fluorophores. In comparison with those required labels, label-free sensing provides several advantages, for example, the technical simplicity and rapid detection. Label-free sensing is typically based on the measurement of optical signatures that are directly or indirectly sensitive to changes in the refractive index as a result of target molecular binding interactions. The capability of real-time monitoring molecular interactions, therefore, allows a detailed understanding of reaction kinetics without the interference from labels.

Surface plasmon resonance (SPR) based biosensors have been widely investigated for the label-free detection of molecular interactions, since its introduction into a commercial setting in the 1980s [1, 2]. Despite being widely successful, traditional SPR sensing suffers from many limitations, particularly the moderate detection sensitivity due to the very label-free nature of the technique. The strict control of experimental conditions has significantly reduced the molecular weight that can be detected by SPR sensing, thus improved the detection sensitivity, over the years. Yet, the prospect of single-molecule detection remains very far, if notunimaginable. For this reason, many diverse approaches have been attempted with varying degrees of success.

In this chapter, we intend to detail these approaches that have recently been attempted based on the excitation of surface plasmon (SP). The theoretical background of SP is discussed, followed by the history of SPR sensing and traditional applications over the last few decades. We have classified the efforts to improve traditional SPR sensors into sections of: (1) enhancement of detection sensitivity by spatial overlapping (*i.e.*, colocalization) between fields and analytical molecules, (2) amplification by nanoparticles (NPs), (3) measurement of phase associated with a target interaction, (4) combination with other modalities, especially whispering gallery mode sensors, (5) improved capability of imaging, and (6) LSP-based surface-enhanced Raman spectroscopy (SERS). The summary and outlooks are discussed in the concluding remarks at the end. We acknowledge that this chapter is far from being comprehensive of what has happened in the area since new developments may have been reported even while we were writing this chapter. Nonetheless, we hope that this chapter would serve as one of the reviews helping readers understand what has happened, and more importantly what will happen, in plasmonic biosensing technology with more clarity.

BACKGROUNDS OF PLASMONIC BIOSENSING

Theory

The term "surface plasmon" (SP) is collectively referred to as resonant oscillations of conducting electrons that occur in the optical geometry of a metal-dielectric interface. Theoretically, *p*-polarized light excites SP when the real part of metal permittivity is negative with its magnitude larger than that of the dielectric permittivity for momentum-matching. The dispersion relation of SP can be obtained from Maxwell's equations as given below [1]:

$$Re\{k_{SP}\} = \frac{\omega}{c} Re\{\sqrt{\frac{\varepsilon_m \varepsilon_d}{\varepsilon_m + \varepsilon_d}}\} = k_0 n_s sin\theta_{SP} \qquad (1)$$

k_{SP} is the wavenumber of SPs. ω, c, ε_m, and ε_d represent the angular frequency of the incident light, speed of light, metal permittivity, and dielectric permittivity, respectively. k_0, n_s, and θ_{SP} on the right-hand side are the wave number in the free space, the refractive index of a substrate, and the incident angle at resonance. As mentioned above, for excitation of SP with metal such as gold or silver, the condition of $|Re(\varepsilon_m)| \gg |Im(\varepsilon_m)|$ should be satisfied so that $sin\theta \approx \sqrt{\varepsilon_m \varepsilon_d/(\varepsilon_m + \varepsilon_d)}/n_s$ at the resonance angle. The resonance condition as well as the near-fields associated with the excitation of SP is sensitive to biomolecular interactions that take place on the dielectric surface. The interaction can be quantitatively detected in real-time by measuring changes in the resonance condition. In Equation (1), the change of ε_d before and after biomolecular interactions is the quantity that gives rise to the shift in SPR. Electronic dipoles associated with SP create electromagnetic near-fields localized within 200 nm from the metal surface. In other words, electromagnetic fields are highly enhanced by axial localization under the SPR condition. The phenomenon of coupling of SP waves to photon propagating along the surface is well-known as SP polariton (SPP), conceptually illustrated in Fig. (**1**). Various approaches by which momentum-matching between photon and SP is fulfilled and SPP wave is supported, for example, using Otto and Kretschmann configuration and also by way of grating-based excitation, have been widely explored for traditional SPR biosensors, as presented in Fig. (**2**).

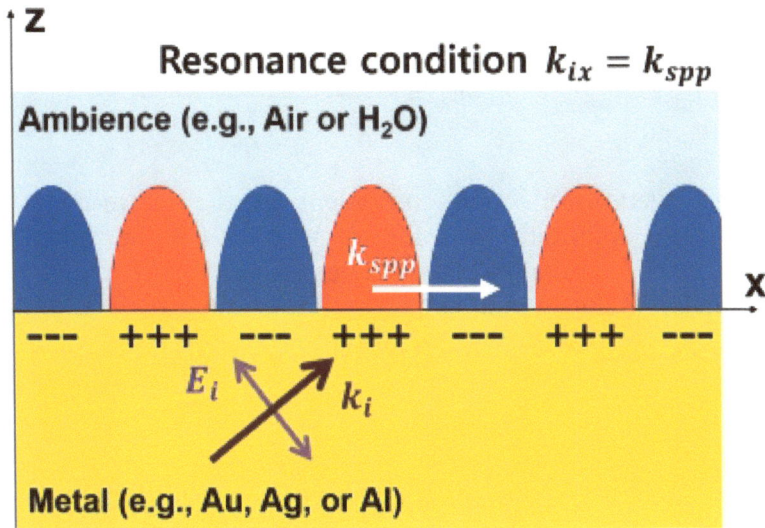

Fig. (1). Conceptual illustration of SPPs at metal-dielectric interface under the SPR condition. x and z represent the direction of SPP propagation and the depth axis away from the metal surface.

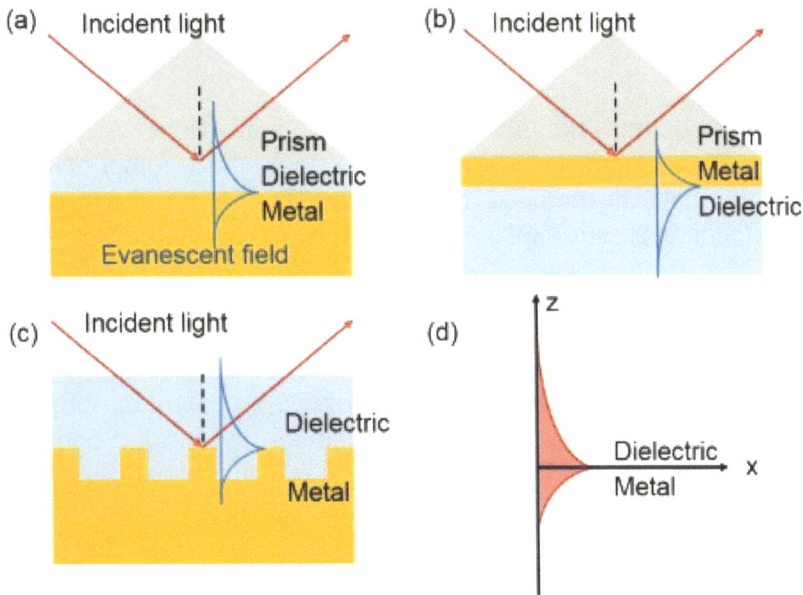

Fig. (2). Schematics of various approaches for SPP excitation: **(a)** Otto and **(b)** Kretschmann configuration. **(c)** Grating-based excitation. **(d)** Typical amplitude distribution along the depth (z) axis.

On the other hand, we can express the amplitude and phase of reflected p-polarized light upon prism-metal-dielectric interfaces from the Fresnel equation, as shown below [3]:

$$r_{pmd} = |r_{pmd}|\, exp(i\phi) = \frac{r_{pm} + r_{md}\, exp(2ik_{my}d)}{1 + r_{pm}r_{md}\, exp(2ik_{my}d)} \tag{2}$$

with r_{pmd} is the overall reflection coefficient of the prism-metal-dielectric structure. $|r_{pmd}|$ is the amplitude, ϕ is the phase, and d is the metal thickness. Reflection coefficient r_{jl} at the interface between layer j and l, where j and l can either be p, m, or d for prism substrate, metal and dielectric layer, and wavenumber k_{jz} of the propagating waves in medium j along the axial z-direction are represented as:

$$r_{jl} = \frac{\epsilon_l k_{jy} - \epsilon_j k_{ly}}{\epsilon_l k_{jy} + \epsilon_j k_{ly}} \tag{3}$$

$$k_{jz} = \sqrt{\left(\frac{\omega}{c}\right)^2 \epsilon_j - k_x^2} \tag{4}$$

In Equation (4), x denotes the propagation direction of SP waves and z is an axial coordinate orthogonal to the x-direction (Fig. 1). k_x is the x-component of incident light waves momentum-matched to SPP. Equations (2)-(4) can be used to calculate SPR characteristics in the far-field.

Note that the geometrical specifications of metal structures affect the propagation and distribution of SP waves traveling along the interface. Subwavelength metallic structures including NPs and surface relief nanopatterns smaller in size than the wavelength of incident light localize SP, which is aptly termed as localized SP (LSP). LSP may be accompanied by strong confinement of plasmonic fields near the surface and be the basis to overcome the limitations of thin film-based conventional SPR sensing. Subwavelength nanopatterns can modulate the near-field distribution at the surface and amplify localized fields, which directly affects the performance of biomolecular sensing. In other words, highly enhanced LSP can be employed to improve the sensitivity of SPR biosensors using well-defined plasmonic nanostructures. For this reason, some parts of Chapter 6 address LSP excitation by various nanostructures and associated near-field enhancement, which can lead to amplification of the signature produced by biomolecular interactions.

Brief History and Traditional Applications

Plasmonics have been utilized for more than 1700 years. A well-known example of plasmonic materials is the famous "Lycurgus Cup" made in the fourth century AD. It consists of Au-Ag alloys of NPs, which give rise to a different appearance in color depending on the transmission or reflection of light. Another ancient plasmonic phenomenon is the stained-glass windows of gothic cathedrals in medieval Europe. Plasmonic resonance of colloidal NPs in stained glasses is affected by the optical properties of material constituents, which determines different colors. For instance, gold NPs (AuNPs) give a characteristic of a brilliant red color. Modern understanding of SPR was first presented by R. M. Wood in 1902 and then by Lord Rayleigh in 1907 [4, 5]. The potential of SPR for thin-film characterization was first recognized in the 1970s [6]. Since the 1980s, numerous investigations of SPR have been carried out as one of the representative technologies for biosensing. In this regard, several influential reviews of SPR biosensors have been reported [7 - 11].

SPR sensors have been widely used for fundamental biological studies and an extensive list of bioengineering applications such as in the clinical diagnosis, drug evaluation, environmental monitoring, and food safety. The wide applicability of SPR sensors is credited with its capability of detecting biomolecular interactions both in qualitative and quantitative manner without any labeling procedure and in real-time. It is also possible to extract kinetic coefficients of interaction without much difficulty. SPR biosensing technology has attracted diverse instrumental developments: commercialization was first completed by Biacore AB (now part of GE Healthcare, Uppsala, Sweden) in the early 1990s and remains one of the most commercially successful biosensor technologies to date [12, 13].

Commercial SPR biosensors are mostly based on the measurement of reflectivity with respect to angle and spectral interrogation of the incident light. Despite the simplicity offered by the measurement of reflected intensity, however, the sensitivity of such conventional SPR sensors is relatively low on the order of 1 pg/mm^2, which corresponds to $10^{-5} \sim 10^{-6}$ RIU (refractive index unit). The challenge in the sensitivity has prompted an array of approaches to attain ultra-high sensitivity with the ultimate goal of detecting single molecules, for example, using plasmonic nanotechnology and a combination of complementary detection modalities. Many studies of SPR have also been conducted to develop multi-analysis and low-cost miniaturized systems.

PLASMON ENHANCEMENT BASED LABEL-FREE OPTICAL BIOSENSOR

In this section, we explore various studies that have been attempted to enhance the sensitivity of plasmonic biosensors. We focus on applications of LSPs excited at surface-relief nanostructures including nanometer-scale gratings, periodic nanoholes and post structures, and arrays of nanogaps. In the second half, NP-based plasmonic field amplification, phase-sensitive SPR measurement, combinatorial approaches of plasmonic sensing with whispering gallery modes, and finally sensitivity enhancement in SERS by highly localized plasmonic fields are addressed.

Plasmonic Colocalization

This section is focused on a technique for overlapping the distribution of target molecules and localized light fields, which is termed colocalization. In the near-field regime, electromagnetic waves are localized at one side of the ridge of the plasmonic nanostructure. If target molecules are made to bind only at the ridge, the interaction may become self-aligned for colocalization with the electromagnetic fields and therefore maximize the use of light fields available for the detection. In other words, the detection sensitivity, which may be evaluated by an overlap integral between target distribution and near-fields, can be maximized if target molecules are spatially colocalized with the localized fields [14 - 16]. While there may be diverse approaches to produce a nanoscale gap structure for light-matter colocalization, for example, the one utilizing plasmonic lithography [17], the discussion herein mainly constrains on oblique or angled evaporation on subwavelength plasmonic nanostructures.

Oblique evaporation as a fabrication technique *per se* has been investigated to make nanogaps of molecular electronic devices [18, 19], or to produce optically enhanced hot spots for SERS platforms [20, 21]. The directionality of an evaporation process can be utilized for target colocalization in LSPR biosensing. Fig. (**3**) presents a three-dimensional schematic diagram of an obliquely evaporated nanograting structure. In other words, a small opening can be formed as a result of the angled deposition of SiO_2 (SiO_2 used as a mask layer) at one ridge of grating, which corresponds to the light volume of localized fields. Furthermore, the SiO_2 dielectric layer prevents target molecules such as antibody linkers or DNA strands from being immobilized to the top. Only the gap opening beside grating ridges provides access to the underlying metal and becomes available for molecular immobilization [22, 23]. By modifying the chemistry, for example, by thiolation in this particular case, probe molecules of interaction may be made to prefer binding to the gap, thereby, colocalization between an interaction and light fields was achieved. For example, single-stranded DNA (ssDNA) molecules can be immobilized or hybridized to the complementary strands at the opening for colocalized binding, as shown in Fig. (**3**). The size of a nanogap or opening length can be approximated by the angle of oblique evaporation θ_{eva} in the following simple relation.

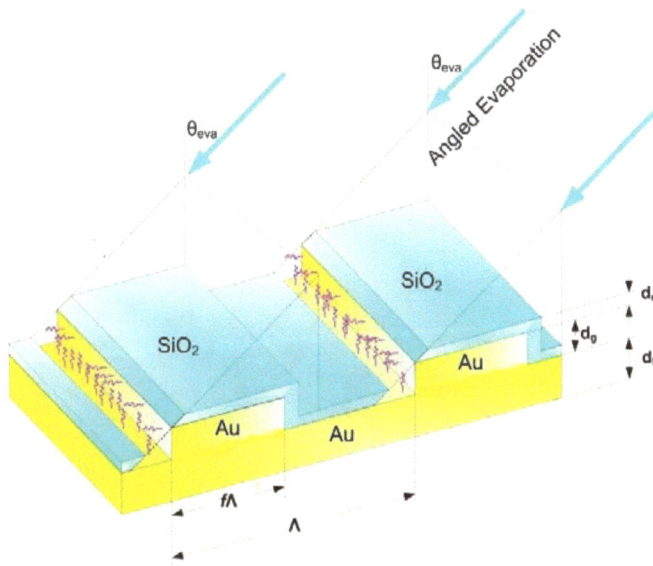

Fig. (3). Schematic of oblique evaporation for colocalization using a nanograting structure. Various design parameters are shown. The thick blue arrows represent the direction of oblique evaporation of SiO_2. The schematic also shows DNA oligomer probe molecules immobilized in the dielectric opening (reprinted with permission from [15]; copyright 2010 the Institute of Electrical and Electronic Engineers).

$$tan(90° - \theta_{eva}) = \frac{d_g}{L} \qquad (5)$$

In Equation (5), d_g is the height or depth of nanograting ridge and L is the opening length or gap size for colocalization. For example, the opening length is estimated as $L = 11.6$ nm using a nanograting with $d_g = 20$ nm. Grating ridge wall is also open for interaction, therefore the total opening size becomes $L + d_g = 31.6$ nm. Other geometrical parameters including nanograting array period (Λ), fill factor of grating (f), and film thickness of gold (d_f) and SiO_2 deposition mask layer (d_m) affect the way that light fields are localized in the near field.

The overall processes to fabricate the linear nanograting structure in Fig. (3) are presented in Fig. (4). Grating arrays were defined by electron beam lithography using polymethylmethacrylate (PMMA) photoresist on an SF10 glass substrate. This was followed by the evaporation of the 40-nm-thick gold and 2-nm-thick chromium adhesion layer. Metallic nanograting arrays could then be implemented after a lift-off process. The fabricated nanograting arrays are shown in an SEM image of Fig. (**5a**). To form the opening for colocalization, SiO_2 was deposited as a dielectric mask layer with a design thickness (d_m) at an angle θ_{eva}. In this particular example, θ_{eva} was fixed at 30°. From Fig. (**5b**), the gap opening formed by angled evaporation of the SiO_2 dielectric layer could be visually confirmed.

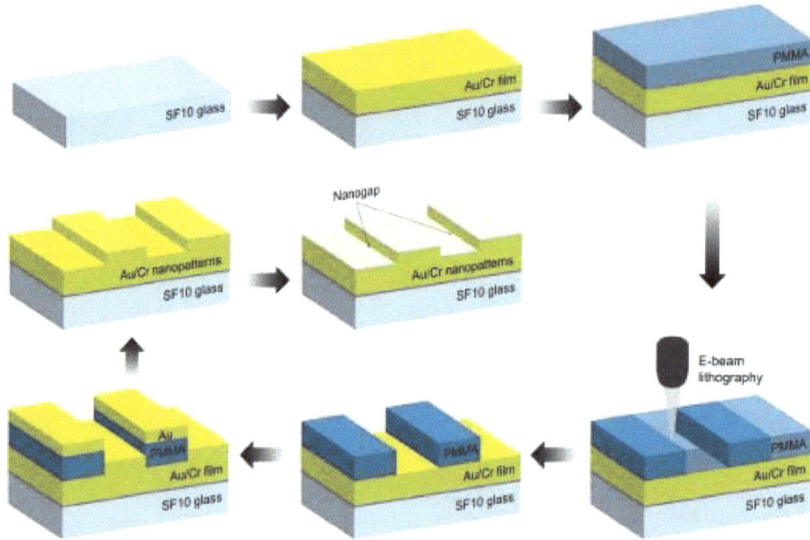

Fig. (4). Processes to fabricate 2D nanogaps based on linear grating. Self-aligned colocalization between electromagnetic near-fields and molecular interaction (DNA hybridization in this case) is achieved by electron-beam lithography followed by oblique evaporation of a mask layer (reprinted with permission from [24]; copyright 2014 Elsevier).

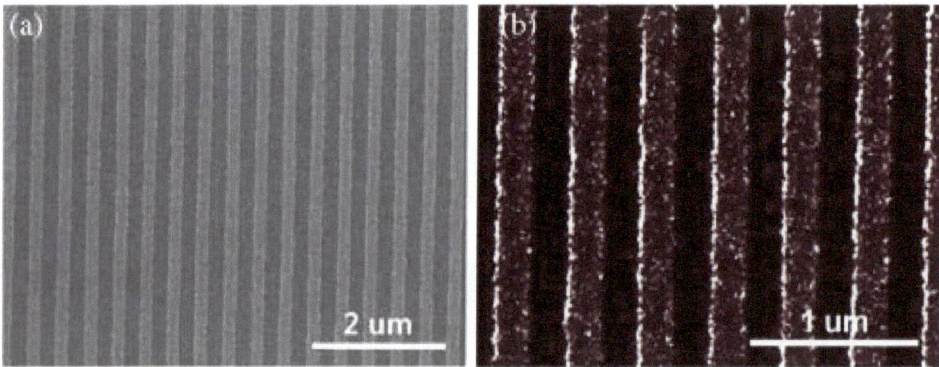

Fig. (5). (a) SEM image of a nanogap sample formed by oblique evaporation. **(b)** Magnified image of the nanogap confirms gap opening as a result of oblique evaporation (reprinted with permission from [15]; copyright 2010 the Institute of Electrical and Electronics Engineers).

Oftentimes, insights can be gained from the dispersion relation of light waves in a medium. The dispersion relation can be revised for LSP-based nanostructures as shown in the following [28 - 30]:

$$k_{SP} = \frac{\omega}{c}\sqrt{\frac{\varepsilon_m \varepsilon_{eff}}{\varepsilon_m + \varepsilon_{eff}}} = k_0 n_s sin\theta_{SP} \tag{6}$$

The main distinction between Equation (6) from Equation (1) is that the permittivity for dielectric ambience is replaced by ε_{eff}, which is the effective permittivity reflecting the combined effect of biomolecular interactions and plasmonic nanostructures in ambience. The use of effective indices tends to homogenize local field irregularities, therefore, Equation (6) should only be treated as an approximation. Since linear nanograting arrays are a 2D nanostructure considering axial variation, effective medium based on the Rytov effective medium theory (EMT) may be used to express the optical properties of a nanograting layer [28, 29], *i.e.*, an overall effective medium that consists of surface nanograting and an ambient medium may be estimated as

$$\varepsilon_{eff} = \varepsilon_{eff,TM}^{(0)} + \frac{\pi^2}{3}\varepsilon_{eff,TE}^{(0)}(\varepsilon_{eff,TM}^{(0)})^3 \cdot f^2(1-f)^2 \times \left(\frac{1}{\varepsilon_m} - \frac{1}{\varepsilon_d}\right)^2 \left(\frac{\Lambda}{\lambda}\right)^2 \tag{7}$$

$$\varepsilon_{eff,TE}^{(0)} = f\varepsilon_m + (1-f)\varepsilon_d \quad and \quad \frac{1}{\varepsilon_{eff,TM}^{(0)}} = \frac{f}{\varepsilon_m} + \frac{1-f}{\varepsilon_d} \tag{8}$$

where $\varepsilon_{eff}^{(0)}$ is the zeroth-order effective dielectric constant for TE and TM polarization and λ is a wavelength of the incident light. The validity of an effective medium has been studied phenomenologically and the approximation of subwavelength nanostructures was used in analyses based on the Fresnel coefficients [22, 31, 32].

With regard to improving the detection sensitivity in LSP-based sensing, sensitivity enhancement by plasmonic nanostructures can be evaluated with a number of quantitative metrics. A very simple measure of the enhancement is the sensitivity enhancement factor (SEF), which is a ratio of resonance shifts after molecular target binding with LSPR to those with conventional SPR. Therefore, SEF based on the resonance angle scanning can be expressed as below:

$$SEF = \frac{\Delta\theta_{LSP}}{\Delta\theta_{con}} = \frac{[\theta(analyte) - \theta(no\ analyte)]_{LSP}}{[\theta(analyte) - \theta(no\ analyte)]_{con}} \qquad (9)$$

Here, $\Delta\theta_{LSP}$ and $\Delta\theta_{con}$ denote the resonance shift detected by LSP-based nanostructures and film-based conventional SPR sensing. For the evaluation of a target localized SPR biosensor, a SEF needs to be defined per-unit-target volume (SEF_{UTV}) as a ratio of resonance shifts per-unit-target volume because SEF_{UTV} is more relevant to the evaluation of the detection sensitivity since the sensing area is changed by the process to produce target colocalization. SEF_{UTV} for 2D nanograting structures may be simply expressed as the SEF per-unit-target cross section, *i.e.*,

$$SEF_{UTV} \approx \frac{\Delta\theta_{LSP}/(d_g + d_g\tan\theta_{eva})}{\Delta\theta_{con}/\Lambda} =$$
$$SEF\frac{\Lambda}{d_g(1 + \tan\theta_{eva})} \qquad (10)$$

Recently, Oh *et al.* reported that ultra-high detection sensitivity can be achieved in LSPR biosensors based on self-aligned target colocalization using three-dimensional (3D) nanogap arrays [24]. The study was motivated by the fact that 3D arrays of nanopatterns such as nanohole apertures may produce a colocalization area that is far smaller than the case of using 2D nanograting patterns, as illustrated in Fig. (6), which shows 3D plasmonic nanogap arrays formed by periodic nanohole arrays for colocalized detection of hybridization between ssDNAs. A smaller nanogap area for colocalization suggests the feasibility of detecting much smaller amount of molecules that participate in an interaction. Colocalization area formed by 3D nanoaperture arrays can be estimated in a manner similar to Equation (5). For example, the nanogap area defined by a triangular aperture can be calculated as

$$Ld_g \times \left[(1 + \tan\theta_{eva}) + \frac{d_g\tan\theta_{eva}}{\sqrt{3}L}(2 - \tan\theta_{eva})\right] \qquad (11)$$

Here, L denotes the side length of triangular nanoapertures. Evaporation angle θ_{eva} is presented in Fig. (6b).

The fabrication processes to create 3D nanogap arrays are presented in Fig. (7). A 40-nm gold film was first evaporated on a SF10 glass substrate with a 2-nm chromium adhesion layer. Nanoapertures with circular and triangular shapes were periodically defined by electron beam lithography with a 2-μm array period and an aperture size at 600 nm. 20-nm-thick holes were formed after gold deposition and an ensuing lift-off process of e-beam resist. ITO mask was obliquely evaporated as a 5-nm dielectric layer to form 3D nanogap arrays with an evaporation angle θ_{eva} = 30°, 45°, and 60°. The angle was adjusted to vary the gap area.

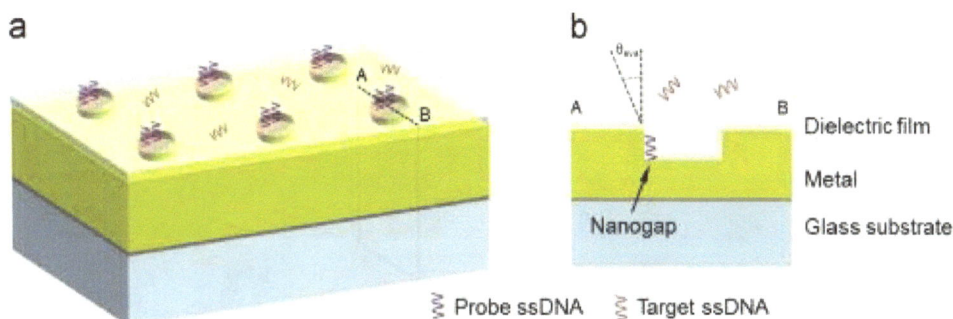

Fig. (6). (a) Schematic illustration of 3D nanogap-based colocalization of DNA hybridization. (b) Cross-section corresponding to the dashed line A-B in (a) (reprinted with permission from [24]; copyright 2014 Elsevier).

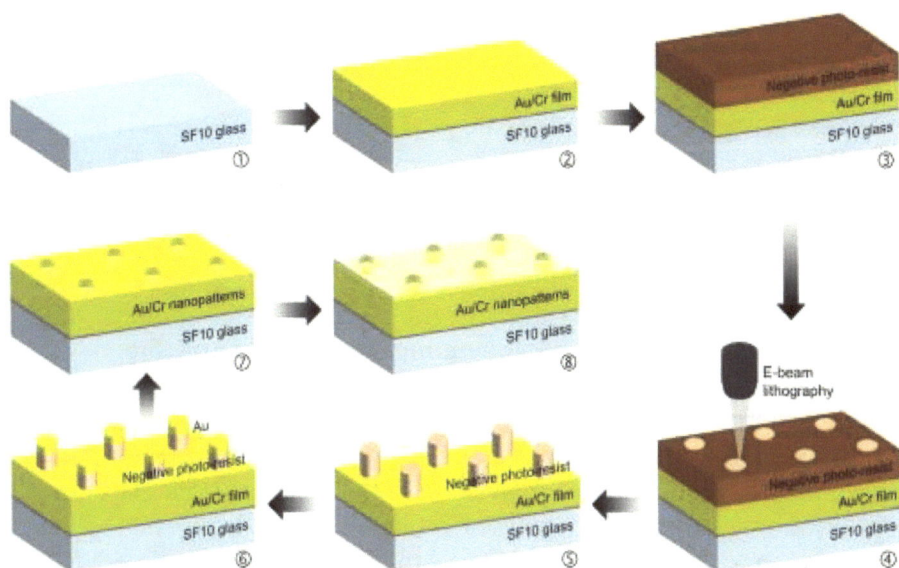

Fig. (7). Fabrication steps for 3D arrays of nanogaps based on circular and triangular nanopatterns. The procedure employed electron-beam lithography and oblique evaporation for self-aligned colocalization of electromagnetic near-fields and DNA hybridization (reprinted with permission from [24]; copyright 2014 Elsevier).

SEM images of the fabricated 3D nanogap structure formed on circular and triangular aperture arrays are shown in Fig. (**8**). The existence of nanogap can be visually confirmed at the ridge of nanoaperture. The binding mainly takes place on the bottom area of a nanogap, the area of which was estimated to be 24.6 ± 7 μm^2 and 19.3 ± 5 μm^2 for a real aperture presented in Fig. (**8**) without considering the sidewall. Electromagnetic field distribution at the nanogap was numerically calculated by rigorous coupled wave analysis and indeed confirmed that the fields are highly localized at the opening region of a nanogap, as shown in Fig. (**9**).

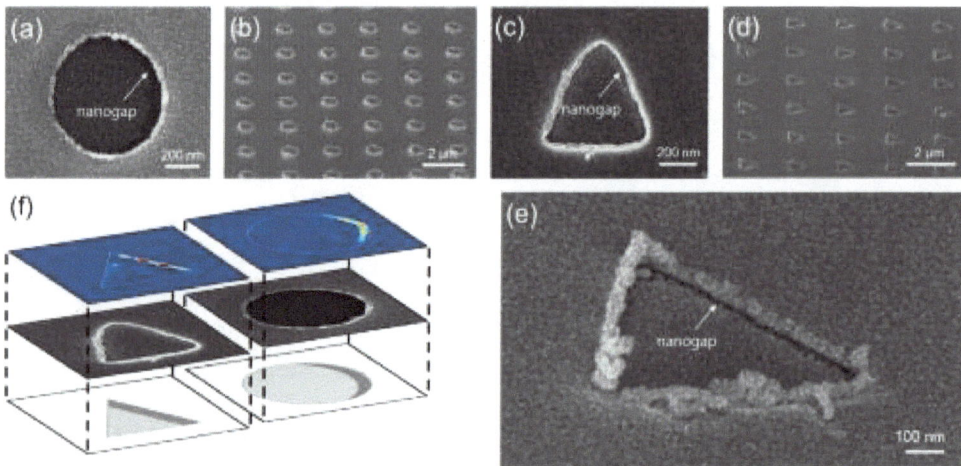

Fig. (8). SEM image: **(a)** a circular nanoaperture and **(b)** arrays. **(c)** A triangular aperture and **(d)** arrays. **(e)** A slanted image of a triangular nanoaperture. Both circular and triangular patterns were fabricated at $\theta_{eva} = 60°$ and $\Lambda = 2$ μm. **(f)** Near-field distribution (top) formed by circular and triangular nanoapertures overlaid with SEM images (middle). Schematics of the nanoapertures are also shown (bottom) (reprinted with permission from [24]; copyright 2014 Elsevier).

Fig. (**10**) shows experimental results to validate SPR shifts obtained with 3D nanopattern arrays as well as linear nanogratings for DNA hybridization. Circular and triangular nanoapertures as well as nanogratings were first employed to generate the plasmonic nanogap structures for colocalization. Resonance angle shifts due to the biomolecular interaction occurred at the nanogap were measured compared to the conventional detection without the nanogap. Fig. (**10a**) presents measured SPR angle shifts $\Delta\theta_{SPR}$. In case of non-colocalized detection, resonance angle shifts by nanostructures were measured to be larger than that in the thin film because the total region where DNA hybridization occurs is increased by existence of nanostructures. Since the whole nanogap region by nanogratings is relatively larger than that of 3D nanopattern arrays, colocalized detection by nanogratings induced larger resonance shifts due to more targets hybridized on nanogratings rather than 3D nanogaps. In order to consider the number of molecules that may contribute to the measured optical signals, it was assumed that the amount is proportional to the total area of nanogap to which target molecules can bind and a new parameter was defined by normalization: relative angle shift $(RAS) = \Delta\theta_{SPR}/A$ (A: nanogap area). Fig. (**10b**) shows RAS measured at each case in Fig. (**10a**). Compared with RAS by non-colocalization, RAS_{3D} by colocalization using 3D nanogaps produced at the circular and triangular nanopatterns was increased more than two orders of magnitude. RAS_{2D} was increased by one order of magnitude in case of using 2D nanogaps by nanograting arrays. The maximum RAS_{3D} at $\theta_{eva} = 60°$ colocalized by triangular nanoaperture-based 3D nanogaps was 460 times larger than non-colocalized RAS_{2D} at the thin film. Efficient localization of SPs at triangular nanopatterns was previously reported [33, 34]. Resonance characteristics for nanogap-based colocalization (Insets C and D in Fig. (**10b**)) as well as non-colocalization (Insets A and B in Fig. (**10a**)) were presented in the insets of Fig. (**10**). In particular, little broadening in the SPR curve shown in the inset C is to be noted for low plasmonic damping caused by long array period and relatively small amount of target molecules.

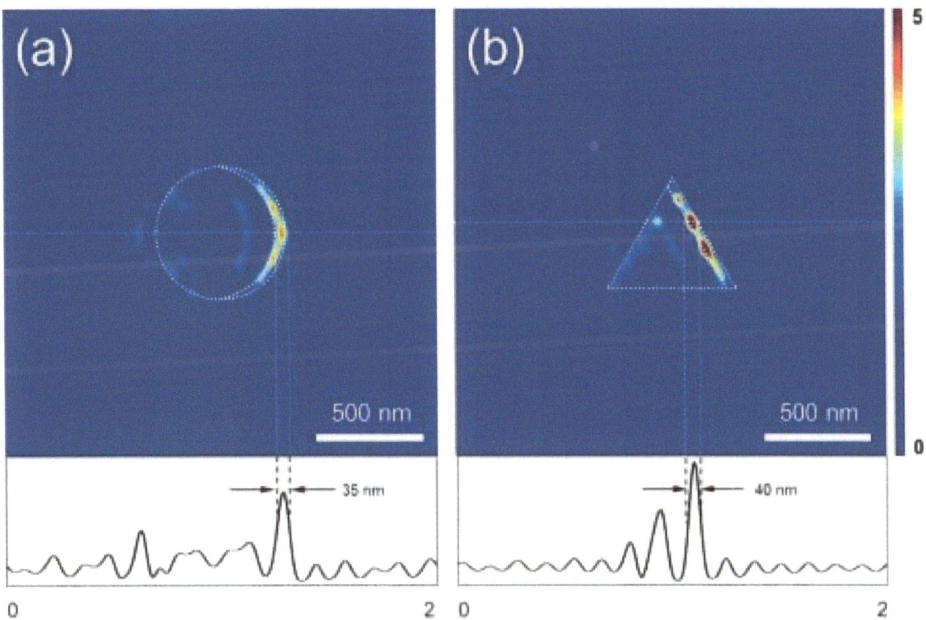

Fig. (9). Near-field distribution that is formed by **(a)** circular and **(b)** triangular nanoaperture (period $\Lambda = 2$ µm). Lateral unit in µm. Fluorescent intensity in arbitrary unit (color bar) (reprinted with permission from [24]; copyright 2014 Elsevier).

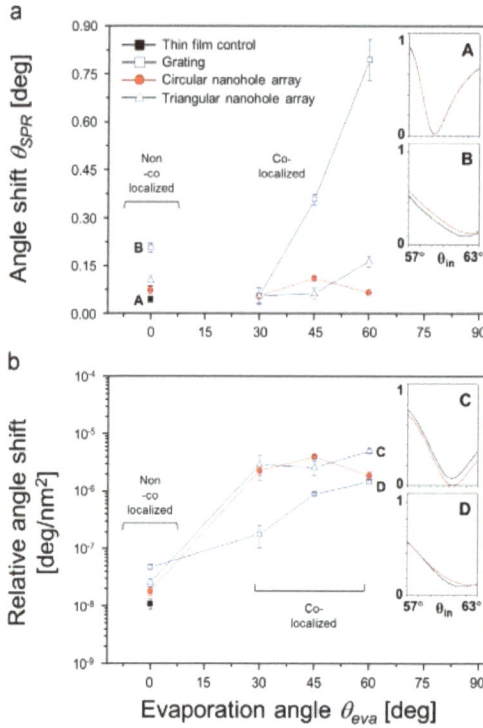

Fig. (10). SPR shifts measured with circular and triangular arrays of nanopatterns compared with 2D grating. The evaporation angle θ_{eva} is varied. SPR shifts ($\Delta\theta_{SPR}$): **(a)** before and **(b)** after being normalized by the nanogap surface area (RAS). $\Delta\theta_{SPR}$ ($\theta_{eva} = 0°$) corresponds to the case of no colocalization without a mask layer. The nanogap area, which is proportionate to the number of probe molecules increases with θ_{eva}. Reflectance curves near resonance (immobilization of p-DNAs in black solid lines and hybridization with t-DNAs in red solid lines) are provided in the insets. θ_{in}: angle of incidence. A: conventional SPR detection using thin films, B: $\theta_{eva} = 0°$ with 2D linear gratings, and colocalized detection with $\theta_{eva} = 60°$: C with 3D triangular nanoarrays and D with 2D linear gratings (reprinted with permission from [24]; copyright 2014 Elsevier).

Plasmonic Localization Using NPs

NPs have been actively explored to enhance localized electromagnetic fields and to boost optical signals and ultimately detection capabilities that may be obtained from SPR sensors. When light is incident on metallic NPs, plasmonic hybridization of electrons leads to high localization of electromagnetic fields near the surface and field intensity can be greatly enhanced under the resonance condition. As a result, metallic NPs can amplify optical signals of SPR sensors [35, 36]. Resonance wavelength and field intensity of induced LSPR can be adjusted by changing geometrical parameters such as size, shape, and surrounding environment [37, 38]. Gold and silver NPs are often used. However, AuNPs have been widely adopted for LSPR studies due to good biocompatibility. Furthermore, it is easy to control the surface condition through conjugation of antibody or biomarker molecules since the surface area/volume ratio of AuNPs is high. Variations of surrounding environment near NP surface cause a change in the resonance wavelength, which is measurable by taking light absorption or scattering spectra [39]. Furthermore, the shift of SPR wavelengths from visible to near-infrared waveband tends to be accompanied by improved sensitivity. In consequence, SPR biosensing with AuNPs has been investigated in numerous applications for biological and chemical detection.

One such example is a recent study of SPR sensors using aptamer-based AuNPs for label-free and real-time detection of subnanomolar thrombin [40]. Aptamers, which refer to oligonucleotide or peptide molecules, recognize and bind to the specific molecules by changing their structures [41]. In this study, a SPR sensor was based on AuNPs coupled with thrombin-specific aptamers to explore recognition of thrombin and to determine its concentration by enhanced near-fields. The possibility of precise detection of thrombin concentration has long attracted attention since thrombin is one of the key enzymes of blood clotting [42]. While thrombin converts fibrinogen to fibrin which clots the wound, the thrombin concentration changes from nM to µM by the coagulation of blood [43]. For this purpose, an aptamer/thrombin/aptamer-AuNPs sandwich assay was investigated on the surface of a SPR aptasensor [40]. In this work, two thrombin aptamers were used: TBA29 was thiol-modified and fixed by Au-S bonding and biotinylated TBA15 was fixed by biotin-streptavidin interaction on the surface of streptavidin attached to a gold film. By thrombin, TBA15 and TBA29 change their structures from coil-like to suitable G-quadruplex conformer for binding to the fibrinogen-recognition exosite of thrombin. Consequently, injection of highly concentrated thrombin can increase the quantity of thrombin captured on the sensor chip, which directly induces the enhancement of SPR signals. Furthermore, TBA29-AuNPs improved the SPR detection sensitivity based on the excitation of highly enhanced plasmonic fields when thrombin bound to AuNPs.

Another study shows the amplification of resonance wavelength shifts by LSPR bioassays using AuNPs, which were conjugated to antibodies [44]. The ability of these AuNPs for enhancement of LSPR sensor response to observe antibody-antigen binding was demonstrated using biotin-terminated ligands functionalized on silver nanoprism arrays (Fig. 11). These silver nanoprism structures shaped like a pyramidal feature with edge lengths of 100 nm and heights of 20 nm were fabricated on a glass substrate by using nanosphere lithography. A carboxylic acid-terminated self-assembled monolayer was formed on the silver nanoprism arrays to stabilize the biotin-functionalized surface and NPs. Finally, the extinction spectrum of LSPR was measured after an incubation process of NP-conjugated antibiotin antibodies binding to biotin-functionalized nanoprism arrays. LSPR enhanced resonance wavelength shift with antibiotin-labeled NPs in comparison to an identical experiment substituting unlabeled anti-biotin, as presented in Fig. (**11b** and **c**), respectively. In cased of LSPR sensing using NP-antibiotin, the resonance wavelength shift of $\Delta\lambda_{NP\text{-}Ab}$ was measured to be 42.7 nm whereas the shift $\Delta\lambda_{Ab}$ was 11 nm for native antibiotin. In other words, this value obtained by the NP-based LSPR biosensor represented the sensitivity improvement by more than 400% over the performance of conventional LSPR sensing without NPs.

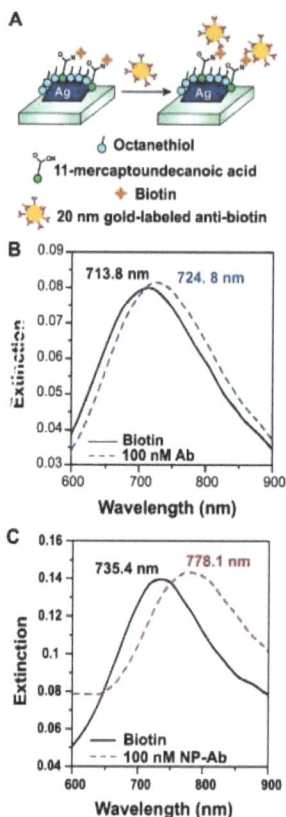

Fig. (11). Schematic and experimental LSPR spectra. **(A)** With biotin covalently linked to the NPs, AuNPs labeled with antibiotin are exposed to the surface. **(B)** LSPR spectra acquired before (solid black) and after binding of native antibiotin (dashed blue). The resonance shift was measured to be 11 nm. **(C)** LSPR spectra before (solid black) and after binding of NPs labeled with antibiotin (dashed red). The resonance shift was 42.7 nm (reprinted with permission from [44]; copyright 2011 American Chemical Society).

Enhancement of resonance wavelength shifts by NPs occurs due to additional extinction shifts by LSPs of NP-coupling to plasmonic substrates as well as the shift induced by an increase of refractive index. Several papers have reported the detection of single molecule or single DNA hybridization event by AuNP labels [45, 46], since plasmonic coupling can dramatically change the observed resonance depending on the distance between NPs [47 - 50]. A diffractive grating-based long-range SPR sensor was also described to detect bacterial pathogens with much enhanced sensitivity using magnetic NPs [51]. Here, the employment of magnetic NPs increased the sensor response by amplification of refractive index changes as target analytes were delivered fast to the sensor surface. This amplification strategy using magnetic NPs to implement an enhanced long-range SPR sensor can be applied to detecting numerous analytes that diffuse slowly at the sensor surface. The feasibility of the approach was verified by detecting *Escherichia coli* at concentration as low as 50 cfu/mL, about 4 times improvement over the detection limit of existing grating-coupled SPR sensors.

Phase-sensitive Surface Plasmon Resonance Sensing

In this section, we describe phase-sensitive SPR biosensing which achieves improved resonance characteristics by measuring phase difference of light induced after a molecular interaction. When SP is excited under the resonance condition, phase of the reflected light may change sharply compared to the change observed in the reflected intensity dip (Fig. **12**). For this reason, phase-sensitive SPR biosensor has produced extremely high detection sensitivity ($<10^{-7}$ RIU) compared to a typical intensity-based SPR measurement ($10^{-5} \sim 10^{-6}$ RIU). The fundamental principle of phase measurement is to control temporal or optical path difference for the phase detection. Three approaches are described to measure the phase of light waves upon SPR.

The first example of phase-sensitive SPR sensing is to take advantage of heterodyne detection to measure reflected light phase. Heterodyne detection is a well-known technique in wireless communications to transform frequency of an electromagnetic wave using "beat phenomenon" which occurs between two waves having slightly different frequencies. An optical heterodyne technique can detect temporal modulation of light. Suppose that an electromagnetic wave propagates in vacuum along the *x* direction [53]:

$$E = E_0 e^{\{j(\omega t - kx + \phi_1)\}} = E_0 e^{j(2\pi f t - 2\pi f x/c + \phi_1)} \tag{12}$$

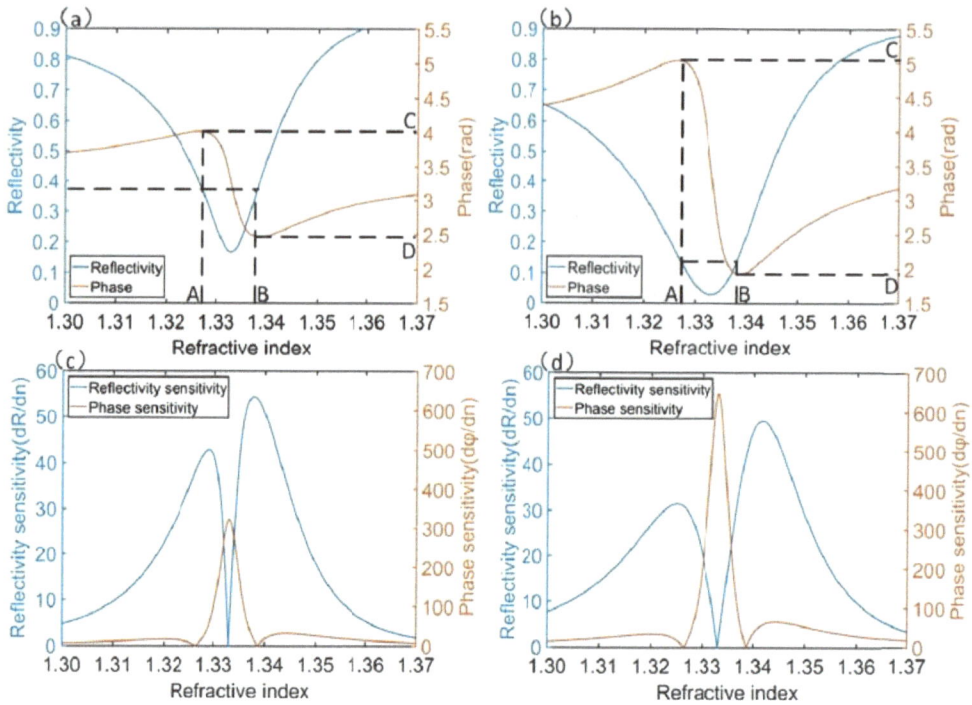

Fig. (12). Relationship between reflectivity and phase observed in phase-sensitive SPR biosensing with **(a)** traditional intensity-based two-beam interferometry and **(b)** self-mixing interference (SMI). Reflectivity sensitivity *vs.* phase sensitivity: **(c)** traditional two-beam interferometry and **(d)** SMI (reprinted with permission from [52]; copyright 2018 Optical Society).

E_0 is the electric field amplitude, f is the linear optical wave frequency ($f = \omega/2\pi$), wave number k = $2\pi/\lambda$ and ϕ_1 is the initial phase. Visible wave band oscillates with extremely high frequency components on the order of 10^{14} Hz, which is too fast to resolve directly by a photodetector. For this reason, a photodetector detects only the average intensity $I = E.E^* = E_0^2$, where * denotes conjugate operation and thus loses phase information. If E_r is used as a heterodyne reference in a form,

$$E_r = E_0' e^{j[2\pi(f+\Delta f)+2\pi(f+\Delta f)x/c+\phi_2]}$$ (13)

where E_0' and ϕ_2 are the electric field amplitude and the phase of the reference wave. The frequency is similar to that of the original wave as $f + \Delta f$. The intensity of light interference between E and Er is expressed by the superposition:

$$I = (E + E_r) \cdot (E + E_r)^* = E_0^2 + E_0'^2 + 2E_0E_0' \cos\left(2\pi\Delta ft - \frac{2\pi\Delta fx}{c} + \Delta\phi\right) \quad (14)$$

$\Delta\phi$ denotes the phase difference between the two waves. The result is the fluctuation with beat frequency Δf. A photodetector can observe a time-varying intensity when the response frequency of a photodetector is higher than the frequency difference Δf. If we record a time-varying intensity whose frequency matches the beat frequency Δf, the initial phase difference $\Delta\phi$ can be extracted by post-processing the intensity data.

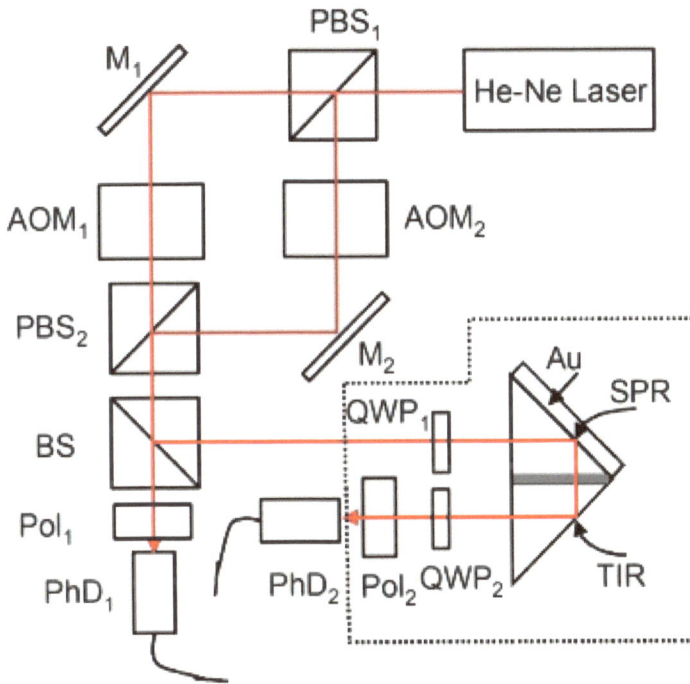

Fig. (13). A schematic diagram of phase-sensitive SPR biosensing based on optical heterodyne detection (PBS: polarizing beam splitter, AOM: acousto-optic modulator, BS: beam splitter, QWP: quarter-wave plate, Pol: polarizer, PhD: photodetector, Au: gold, SPR, surface plasmon resonance, TIR: total internal reflection, and M: mirror) (reprinted with permission from [54]; copyright 2004 Optical Society).

Nelson *et al.* reported a SPR biosensor based on optical heterodyne scheme using an acousto-optic modulators (AOM) to generate heterodyne light sources with a beat frequency $\Delta f \sim$ 10 kHz [56]. It was reported that the highest resolution of an AOM-based phase-sensitive SPR biosensor was estimated to be 5×10^{-7} RIU with an optimized set-up. Wu *et al.* also used two AOMs to generate a beat frequency of 60 kHz using a set-up shown in Fig. (**13**) [54, 57]. The refractive index resolution as a measure of detection sensitivity was improved to be 2×10^{-7} RIU. Instead of using an optical modulator to achieve optical heterodyne detection, Shen *et al.* employed a frequency-stabilized Zeeman laser as an optical heterodyne light source to implement a phase-sensitive SPR system [58]. A Zeeman laser provides two orthogonally polarized light waves at a frequency difference $\Delta f = 60$ kHz with good stability without any optical modulator, as shown in Fig. (**14**). Similarly, Xinglong *et al.* reported an SPR immunosensor based on optical heterodyne phase measurement using a commercial Zeeman laser with excellent frequency stability for a frequency difference of 33.2 kHz [59].

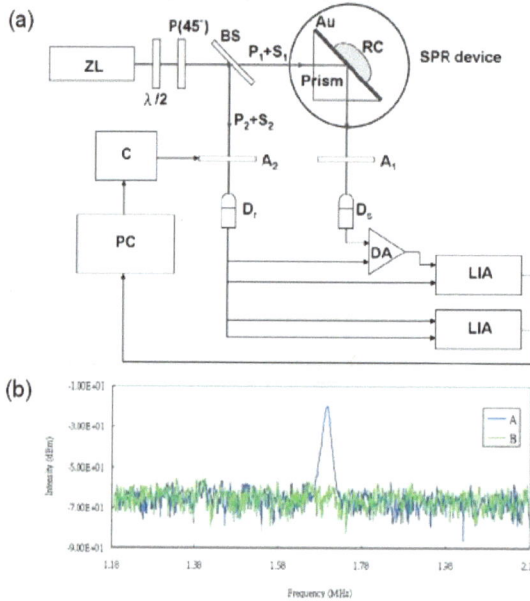

Fig. (**14**). (**a**) Schematic set-up of the differential-phase SPR biosensor (ZL: Zeeman laser, $\lambda/2$: half-wave plate, P: polarizer, BS: beam splitter, RC: reaction chamber, D_p, D_s: photodetectors, A: analyzers, DA: differential amplifier, LIA: lock-in amplifier, C: controller, PC: personal computer). (**b**) Power spectrum of the output signal from the DA. Curve A: noise floor of the detected heterodyne signal at tridistilled water. Curve B: electronic noise level when the laser beam was totally blocked in the measurement (reprinted with permission from [55]; copyright 2008 American Chemical Society).

Second phase measurement technique is the use of polarimetry which measures the changes of polarization states upon reflection or transmission of optical waves and is very similar to ellipsometry. Polarimetry investigates the interference of two orthogonally polarized components of light after passing through a polarizer. Consider two orthogonally polarized light waves with amplitude E_p and E_s propagating along the x direction and the phase difference between the two waves as $\Delta\phi$. A polarizer with the principal axis oriented at an angle θ from p-polarized waves is used to create interference of the two waves at a photodetector. The interference pattern shows the phase difference between *p*- and *s*-polarized waves. The intensity can be expressed by classical interference formula [60]:

$$I = E_p^2 \cos^2 \theta + E_s^2 \sin^2 \theta + E_p E_s \sin 2\theta \cos(\Delta\phi) \qquad (15)$$

The interference intensity is a function of θ and the phase difference $\Delta\phi$. Therefore, we can measure a series of interference patterns by rotating a polarizer, *i.e.*, modulating the oriented angle θ, or using phase retarders for determining accurate phases difference $\Delta\phi$.

Compared with the optical heterodyne detection, polarimetry allows phase measurement with time-invariant intensity. By modulating phase or polarization, various intensity data with phase information can be conveniently obtained from the reflected light wave. In return, the use of polarimetry often needs to build complex optical set-up for accurate phase measurement with additional optical components such as wave plates or polarizers and to generate enough intensity patterns for signal processing.

In 1976, Abeles first confirmed the possibility of investigating surface interaction by using ellipsometry to measure phase difference of surface wave [61]. In 1990s, Herminghaus *et al.* used polarimetry to characterize thin films [62]. Since 1998, many research groups have reported polarimetry-based SPR systems to improve sensitivity and image performance of SPR sensors. For example, Nikitin and co-workers proposed application of polarimetry to phase-sensitive SPR measurement while scanning incident angles [63 - 65]. Westphal *et al.* used a commercially available ellipsometer to combine with a SPR sensor for measuring immobilization of antibodies and DNA hybridization [66]. The results showed the sensitivity on the order of 10^{-5} RIU. On the other hand, Naraoka *et al.* proposed phase measurement based on a rotating analyzer with a sensitivity of 10^{-7} RIU [67]. Recently, Hooper *et al.* applied various optical components, such as Faraday rotator [68] and liquid crystal polarization modulator [69, 70], to build high performance phase-sensitive SPR biosensors, in which the sensitivity of the phase detection reached $\sim 2 \times 10^{-7}$ RIU. More recently, polarimetry has been combined with photo-elastic modulation (PEM). Ho and co-workers have reported various polarimetry configurations based on PEM for measurement of phase information [71 - 73]. Kabashin and co-workers have used pumping beams whose phase can be modulated spatially and temporally to extract two-dimensional phase distribution in the Fourier domain [74 - 78]. An experimental set-up and the results are shown in Figs. (**15** and **16**). Phase difference can be simply obtained by subtracting the phase map successively.

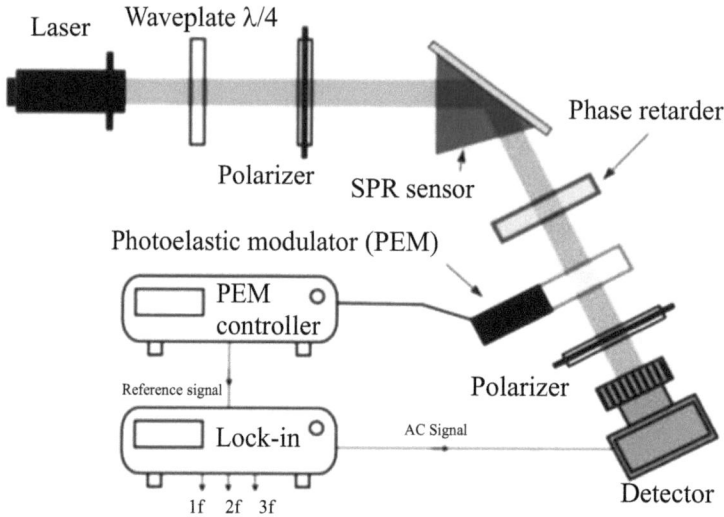

Fig. (15). Experimental set-up for the polarimetry-based phase-sensitive SPR biosensor (PEM: photo-elastic modulator) (reprinted with permission from [75]; copyright 2007 Optical Society).

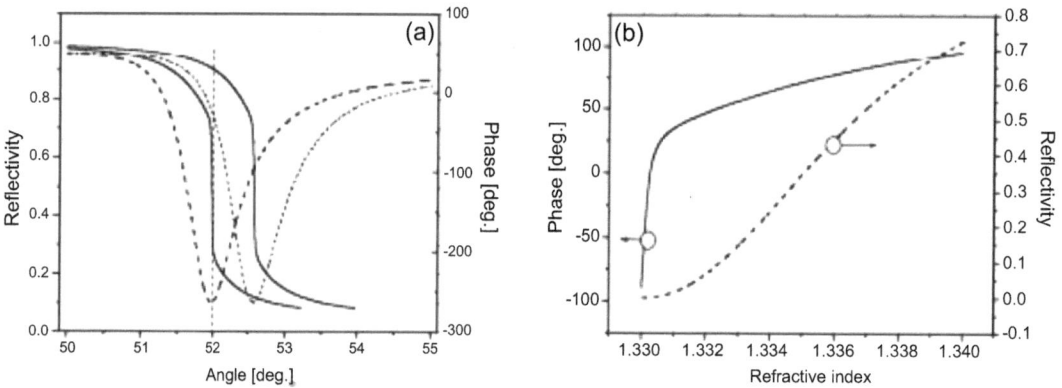

Fig. (16). Phase (solid line) and intensity (dotted) measured of reflected light under SPR condition using the polarimetry-based phase-sensitive SPR biosensor (schematic in Fig. (**15**)) (reprinted with permission from [75]; copyright 2007 Optical Society).

The third technique used for phase-sensitive SPR systems is based on interferometry which is well-known to provide a way to extract phase information of light from interference of known reference and unknown object beam. Suppose that two waves with an identical frequency f propagate in different directions [53]:

$$E_1 = E_0 e^{j(\omega t - \boldsymbol{k_1} \cdot \boldsymbol{r} + \phi_1)} \tag{16}$$

$$E_2 = E_0' e^{j(\omega t - \boldsymbol{k_2} \cdot \boldsymbol{r} + \phi_2)} \tag{17}$$

The interference intensity can be obtained from the superposition of Equations (16) and (17) and expressed as

$$I = (E_1 + E_2) \cdot (E_1 + E_2)^* = E_0^2 + E_0'^2 + 2E_0 E_0' cos(\Delta \boldsymbol{k} \cdot \boldsymbol{r} + \Delta \phi) \tag{18}$$

with $\Delta \boldsymbol{k} = \boldsymbol{k_2} - \boldsymbol{k_1}$ and $\Delta \phi = \phi_2 - \phi_1$ as the difference in the wave vector and the initial phase. The intensity expression of Equation (18) shows a steady-state interference pattern in the spatial domain, out of which a phase difference $\Delta \phi$ can be extracted based on various phase modulation methods. For example, a simple Mach-Zehnder interferometer was used to implement a SPR biosensor [79, 80], in which an incident beam was divided into a signal and a reference part by a beam splitter. The reference arm was directed to the image plane by a mirror system without phase changes, while the p-polarized signal propagates to the sample and carries a phase change upon reflection. The two beams are reunited by another beam splitter and made interference fringe patterns in the image plane induced by the phase difference. An ultrasensitive detection limit on the order of 4×10^{-8} RIU in gas exchange experiments was reported based on an assumption of $0.01°$ phase resolution. Also proposed was a small angle interferometer which uses a birefringence crystal to separate a convergent beam to p and s-polarization component [81]. This technique is similar to the case of polarimetry-based phase-sensitive SPR sensing in the sense that interference patterns are formed due to the optical path difference between two orthogonal waves. Furthermore, Notcovich *et al.* proposed SPR phase imaging based on Mach-Zehnder interferometry using only p-polarization [82]. In addition, Ho and co-workers conducted SPR phase detection based on white-light spectral interferometry, as shown in Fig. (**17**) [83, 84], where a half wave plate was used to rotate the polarization direction for interference, instead of using polarizers and/or birefringent crystals, along with a piezoelectric transducer for driving linear time-variant phase and detecting spatial shifts in the interference patterns. The experimental results showed detection sensitivity of 5.5×10^{-8} RIU with a $0.01°$ phase resolution.

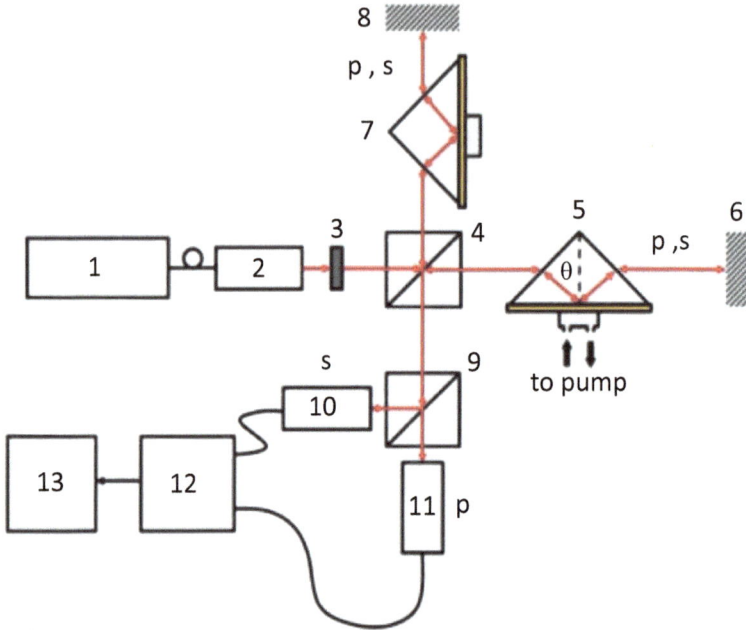

Fig. (17). Block diagram of the white-light SPR spectral interferometer for differential phase measurement. 1: white light emitting diode (LED), 2: collimator, 3: broadband linear polarizer, 4: broadband non-polarizing beam splitter, 5: SPR probe cell attached to the peristaltic pump; 6/8: high precision mirrors, 7: SPR reference cell filled with distilled water, 9: broadband polarizing beam splitter which divides the two polarization components into different paths, 10/11: collimators that collect the interference fringes, 12: dual channel spectrometer, 13: personal computer for analysis (reprinted with permission from [84]; copyright 2011 Optical Society).

Plasmon-enhanced Whispering Gallery Mode Sensing

There have been many attempts of combining SPR sensing with various modalities to achieve desired sensor characteristics. Here, we focus on the efforts to take advantage of the strengths of whispering gallery modes (WGMs) for SPR sensors. A WGM has been widely investigated as one of the well-defined optical methods for label-free detection of biomolecular recognition and interactions. High-Q resonant modes are generated when incoming light is trapped inside the surface of a microsphere or disk cavity due to total internal reflection at the air-dielectric interface. The resonant mode is called a WGM [85, 86]. In 2002, the utility of a microcavity was validated as a WGM resonator by guiding and trapping incident photons in a silica microsphere of ~100 μm radius [87]. Recirculation of photon in the microsphere provides a mechanism for improving detection sensitivity [88]. A WGM is established when incident light guided in the microcavity is driven coherently by satisfying the constructive interference condition, *i.e.,* forming an integer number of wavelengths in one circumnavigation. A resonance dip in wavelength (λ_r) can be measured in the transmission spectrum coupled to an optical fiber. Binding interactions of biomolecules that occur on the cavity surface can be detected by measurement of resonance wavelength shifts [89]. Molecular binding increases the optical path length of light inside the microcavity, leading to a red shift in the resonance wavelength, where the resonance can be compensated by increasing the light wavelength by resonance shift, $\Delta\lambda_r$. This enables subtle changes of the microsphere radius R and refractive index on the surface n to be observed by detecting fractional shifts of the resonance wavelength, *i.e.,* $\Delta\lambda_r/\lambda_r = \Delta R/R + \Delta n/n$. WGM biosensors have been well known for ultra-high sensitivity to the degree of detecting single virus [90] and even single molecular interactions with field enhancement [91 - 94].

Now, we introduce plasmon-enhanced WGM biosensors using various metal nanostructures such as NPs. A fractional shift of resonance frequency in WGM, $\delta\omega$, is presented below in accordance with Refs [88, 89]:

$$\frac{\delta\omega}{\omega} \cong \frac{-(\alpha/\varepsilon_0)|E(r_t)|^2}{2\int \varepsilon_r(r)|E(r)|^2 dV} \tag{19}$$

where α is the real part of molecular polarizability in the surrounding medium, ε_r is the permittivity of dielectric cavity, r_t is the molecular binding site, E is the electric field of WGM. Resonance wavelength shifts increase proportionally to the electric field intensity, $|E(r_t)|^2$, locally amplified at biomolecular binding sites. In other words, the detection sensitivity can be enhanced by local amplification of an electric field without significantly degrading of the WGM Q-factor. Thus, plasmonic nanostructures may be used to localize fields with highly amplified intensities, which can induce enhancement of WGM detection sensitivity. For more convenient plasmonic field localization, metal NP structures have been widely used to create local field enhancement in WGM sensors [95 - 99]. On the other hand, WGM biosensors based on metallic nanostructures on a planar platform can enlarge the effect of plasmon field localization, which can be controlled precisely between the surface of nanostructure and WGM [100 - 105].

For example, NP-based WGM biosensors were studied for the detection of protein binding [95]. A platform of plasmonic AuNPs was used for nonspecific absorption of Bovine Serum Albumin (BSA) proteins. High-Q resonance shifts were observed by evanescent coupling of a microcavity resonator to NPs. For experimentally verification, the AuNPs were prepared, as shown in Fig. (**18a**), following the Lee and Meisel's method after modification [106]. AuNPs were mixed with BSA and a solution of AuNPs-BSA was formed after incubation. AAO membranes with a hole diameter of ~100 nm were saturated in a solution of polyethyleneinimide to enhance adhesion of the NP-layer to the AAO membrane, which was subsequently were washed and dried under vacuum. Fig. (**18b**) presents SEM images of the AAO substrate and the AuNPs captured on the AAO. Fig. (**18**)(c) shows a concept illustration of the microsphere cavity coupled to the AuNp-layer captured on the AAO membrane. The WGM spectrum before and after coupling to NPs are presented in Fig. (**18(d)**), showing two resonance dips and frequency shifts centered around ~633.014 nm (peak 1) and ~633.016 nm (peak 2) wavelengths. Theoretical calculations were performed based on the Mie theory to investigate detailed interactions of WGM with LSP of the AuNPs as well. Through approximation to the first-order perturbation [89], fractional shifts in wavelength were found to be directly proportional to the magnitude of E-field intensity at the molecular site, $|E(r_s)|^2$, whereas inversely proportional to the integrated energy density in the entire volume, *i.e.*, Higher sensitivity enhancement of the WGM-NP sensor is associated with stronger localization of fields created in the microsphere-NP structure, where protein molecules were accessible. For instance, simulation results show difference in resonance wavelength shifts between conventional and the NP-coupled WGM method. When a single BSA molecule was adsorbed in the evanescent field formed at the nanosphere surface with a 3.4 nm radius, no detectable resonance shift of WGM was measured at $\lambda = \sim 580$ nm. However, a significant resonance shift of $\Delta\lambda = \sim 1.06 \times 10^{-4}$ nm was detected when a BSA molecule was located in a hot spot region created in the NP-coupled WGM structure.

$$\frac{\Delta\lambda_r}{\lambda_r} \cong \frac{\alpha/\varepsilon_0 |E(r_t)|^2}{2\int_V \varepsilon_r(r)|E(r)|^2 dV} \tag{20}$$

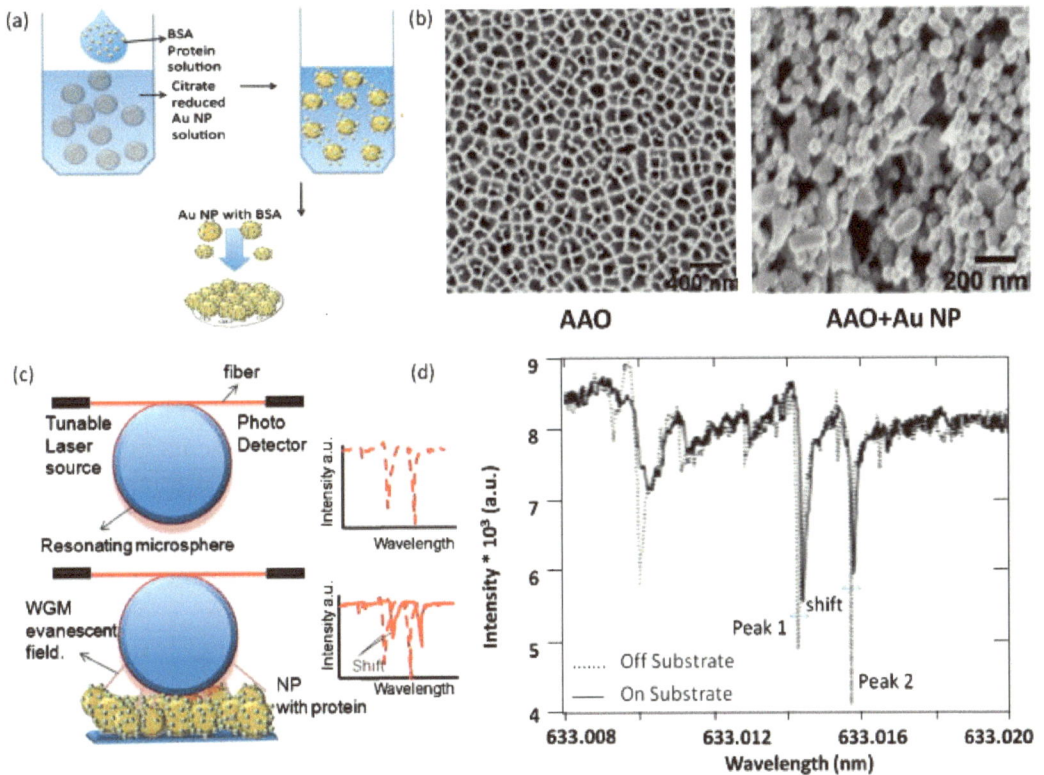

Fig. (18). (a) Preparation of AuNPs. AuNPs mixed with BSA are incubated to form BSA-AuNP complexes. AAO membranes were soaked in polyethyleneinimide for enhanced adhesion between AuNPs and AAO membrane. AAO membranes were washed with pure water and dried under vacuum. **(b)** Electron microscopy images of bare AAO and AAO-AuNPs. **(c)** Schematic diagram of the optical set-up to couple WGM to the AuNP layer. WGM transmission spectrum: (top) for the microsphere in air and (bottom) for microsphere in contact with NPs. The coupling induces a WGM wavelength shift. **(d)** Example spectrum of WGP in air (dotted line) and after evanescent coupling to a BSA-NP layer (solid line) (reprinted with permission from [95]; copyright 2011 American Institute of Physics).

Another study reported plasmonic coupling of LSP-based nanodisk structures to a WGM microsphere cavity for sensitivity enhancement in various applications of sensing, for example, biomolecular interactions, protein-protein folding, and single molecular detection [107]. Authors investigated energy fraction of WGM coupled to plasmonic nanodisks depending on the polarization of light. WGM resonance shifts in wavelength was observed for only *p*-polarized light incidence. Theoretical calculation of near-field distributions between a microsphere cavity and nanodisk arrays showed highly localized energy fraction of WGM fields. A detailed comparison of plasmonic coupling in case of using a single nanodisk vs. double was performed experimentally based on simulation results. The localized distribution and intensity of the near-fields formed at a microcavity-nanostructure interface change by plasmonic characteristics based on the inter-relation between nanostructure geometry and light fields and influence the wavelength shifts of WGM resonance.

Fig. (**19**) presents the concept of coupling a plasmonic nanodisk to a WGM sensor and also SEM images of fabricated nanodisk arrays. WGM resonance wavelength perturbations ($\Delta\lambda/\lambda$) are directly affected by energy fractions ($\Delta E/E$) when a microsphere cavity is coupled to the plasmonic structure, *i.e.*, $\Delta\lambda/\lambda \approx (\Delta E/E)^2$. Here, a microcavity with 200-μm diameter was repetitively coupled to a 50-nm-height single nanodisk fabricated on gold thin film. WGM resonance shifts in wavelength were then measured in the range of ~ 1300-nm wavelength. By plasmonic coupling of a WGM shown in Fig. (**20a**), red shift was observed with TM polarized light as shown in Fig. (**20b**), whereas Fig. (**20c**) presents no visible red shift for TE-polarization since electromagnetic fields between a microsphere and the nanodisk are not locally enhanced in this case.

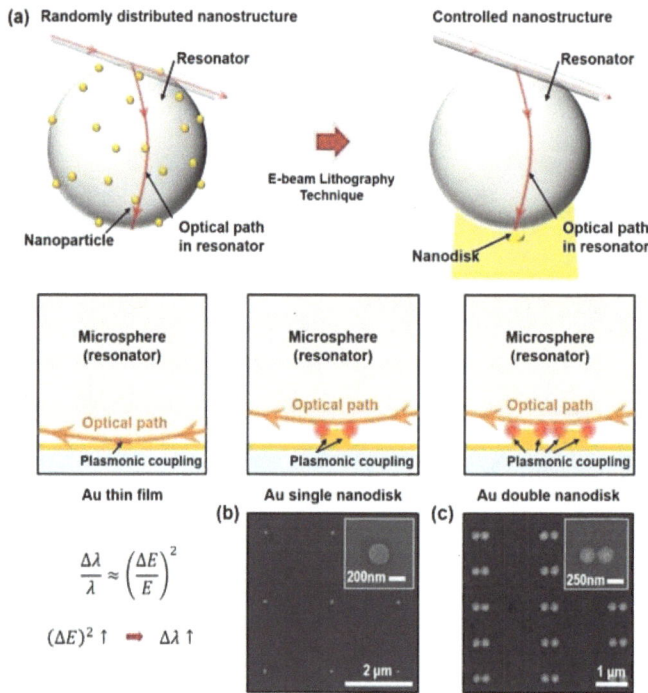

Fig. (19). (a) Schematic illustration of nanodisk-coupled WGM sensor. Electron-beam lithography can be used to fabricate nanodisks. The position of the microsphere with respect to the nanodisk array may be controlled by piezoelectric actuators. **(b and c)** SEM images of an array of single and double nanodisks. The diameter and the thickness of each nanodisk were chosen to be 300 and 50 nm (reprinted with permission from [107]; copyright 2017 Scientific Reports).

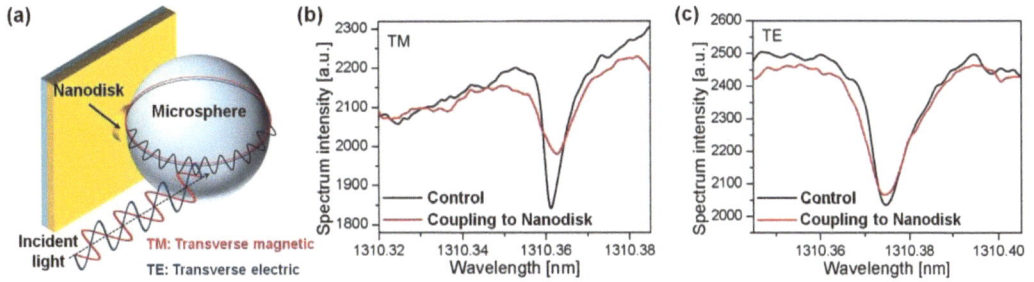

Fig. (20). (a) Schematic illustration of WGM based on microsphere cavity that is coupled to a single nanodisk for light incidence in TM and TE polarization. A photodetector connected to an optical fiber records the transmission spectrum in real-time. The spectrum intensity of WGM resonance with **(b)** TM and **(c)** TE polarized light incidence (reprinted with permission from [107]; copyright 2017 Scientific Reports). (https://creativecommons.org/license/by/4.0).

In order to investigate the difference in degrees of plasmon-coupled energy fraction between single and double nanodisk structure, spectral characteristics of WGMs were theoretically and experimentally analyzed as shown in Figs. (**21** and **22**), respectively. Highly localized near-fields were created at edges of a nanodisk ridge within the evanescent region from the microsphere surface. From theoretical calculation, much stronger field localization was observed with a double nanodisk structure, which induced a larger wavelength shift: $(\Delta\lambda/\lambda)_{double} = 3.4 \times 10^{-4}$, compared with the wavelength shift of $(\Delta\lambda/\lambda)_{single} = 1.7 \times 10^{-4}$ with a single nanodisk (see the results in Fig. (**21**)). Much more energy fraction being available by a double nanodisk structure was in good agreement with experimental results presented in Fig. (**22**). The fractional wavelength shift of a double nanodisk structure was experimentally determined to be $(\Delta\lambda/\lambda)_{double} = 1.76 \times 10^{-5}$ in an incident wavelength range of 1310 nm, while $(\Delta\lambda/\lambda)_{single} = 4.58 \times 10^{-6}$ was measured.

For plasmonic label-free optical biosensors, highly amplified field localization has allowed dramatically enhanced sensitivity [15, 108]. Good spatial overlap between highly localized near-fields and molecules in WGM sensing can improve the detection sensitivity (equal to $\Delta\lambda/\lambda$) to a sufficient degree for single molecule detection, compared with bare WGM systems. By combination, plasmon-coupled WGM biosensors can capitalize on the strengths of plasmonic sensing such as detection stability and specificity while it can further enhance the sensitivity by the efficient spatial overlap between fields and analytes. Plasmonic localization in WGM biosensors has the potential for new approaches by optimizing colocalization efficiency and localized energy fraction. Further increases in WGM sensitivity can be tailored by introducing more optimized nanostructure designs, for example, bowties [109], nanopyramids [110], or concentric necklace nanolenses [111].

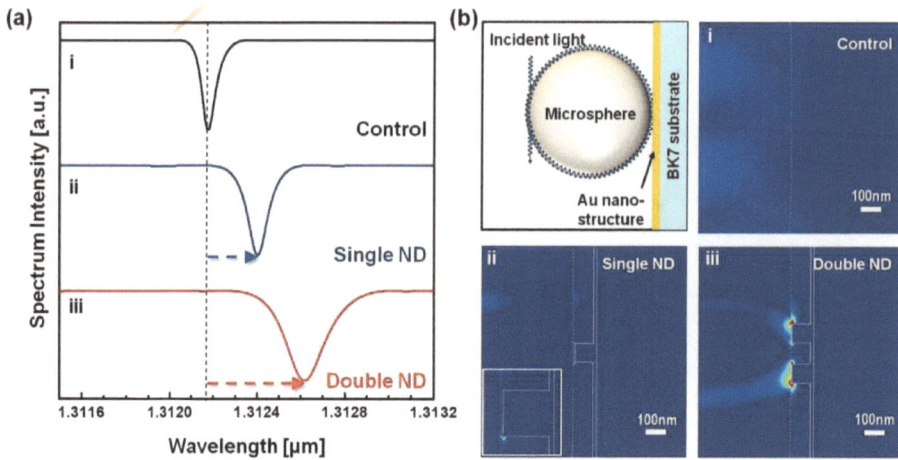

Fig. (21). Numerically simulated plasmonic coupling of WGM sensor to the single and double metallic nanodisks. **(a)** The WGM spectrum intensity of light in microsphere on thin film and single and double nanodisk shows resonance when incident light is TM polarized. **(b)** Electric field intensity distribution near (i) thin film, (ii) single nanodisk, and (iii) double nanodisk (reprinted with permission from [107]; copyright 2017 Scientific Reports).

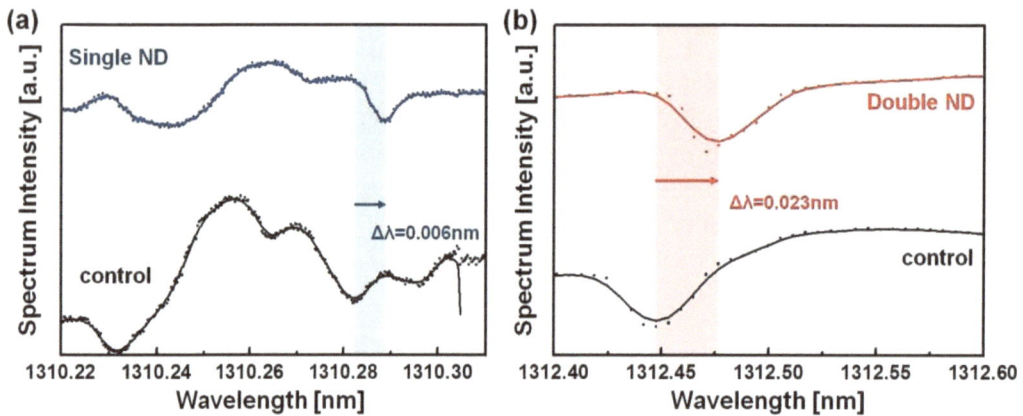

Fig. (22). Wavelength shift $\Delta\lambda$ presented in the spectrum of WGM sensor based on metallic nanodisk arrays: **(a)** single and **(b)** double nanodisk (reprinted with permission from [107]; copyright 2017 Scientific Reports). (https://creativecommons.org/license/by/4.0).

Localized Surface Plasmon Resonance Imaging

Conventional SPR sensing is a point measurement technique and typically not employed for image acquisition. However, with an imaging detector, *e.g.*, charge coupled device (CCD), SPR sensing can be used to provide spatial distribution of target molecules [112] or multiplexed sensing of identical or various molecules simultaneously [113]. The technique is usually terms as SPR imaging or imaging

SPR, which refers to multiplexed SPR sensing for high-throughput measurement. In SPR imaging, reflected light intensity is measured instead of interrogating resonance shift in wavelength or incident angle [114, 115].

The set-up for SPR imaging can also be extended to microscopy applications, thus SP microscopy (SPM) or sometimes SPR microscopy (SPRM), in which cell/substrate contacts of living cells can be imaged by the interference between cells and evanescent waves without fluorescent labels [116]. The distance of cells membrane from the substrate is estimated by the correlation with reflectance. Furthermore, SPM was employed for label-free imaging of H1N1 influenza A virus as well as silica NPs with spatial location data, in which scattering patterns were shown to depend on the size and mass of particle [117]. The calibration of SPR intensity with particle volume enables the mass estimation of virus and particle. SPM was constructed on an inverted microscope with a high numerical aperture objective lens (NA > 1.4) and a 633-nm He-Ne laser. Using a linear motorized stage, the laser beam focused by a convex lens on the back focal plane of an objective was moved toward off-axis and obliquely incident to substrate. In order to obtain the reflected intensity distribution from an objective and to avoid interference effects, a pellicle beam splitter was employed. V shaped diffraction patterns were observed due to the scattering of propagating SP wave. Evanescent waves on the plasmonic metal surface were scattered by the attachment of a NP. As shown in Fig. (**23**), the pattern was found not to depend on the NP or virus size and the full-width-at-half-maximum of the patterns along the x direction was ~ 0.5 μm, which corresponds to the diffraction limit, as shown in Fig. (**23b**), and falls with a decay length of ~ 3 μm (Fig. (**23c**)). The diffraction pattern was determined by the formation condition of SPP, such as laser wavelength, metal, and angle of incidence. This was confirmed by the results of finite element method (FEM) numerical simulation shown in the insets of Fig. (**23a**). The changes of the detection signal depending on specific and non-specific binding were studied with different surface modification. Influenza viruses adsorb onto bare gold irreversibly and nonspecifically. Fig. (**24a**) shows snapshots of virus attachment to gold surface in time and indicates that the adsorbed viruses do not leave the surface. As shown in Fig. (**24b**), the irreversible links were also found by averaged intensity change of the squared area (red rectangles in Fig. (**24a**) numbered as 1, 2, and 3). Once viruses attach themselves to gold, SPR intensity rises sharply and is maintained.

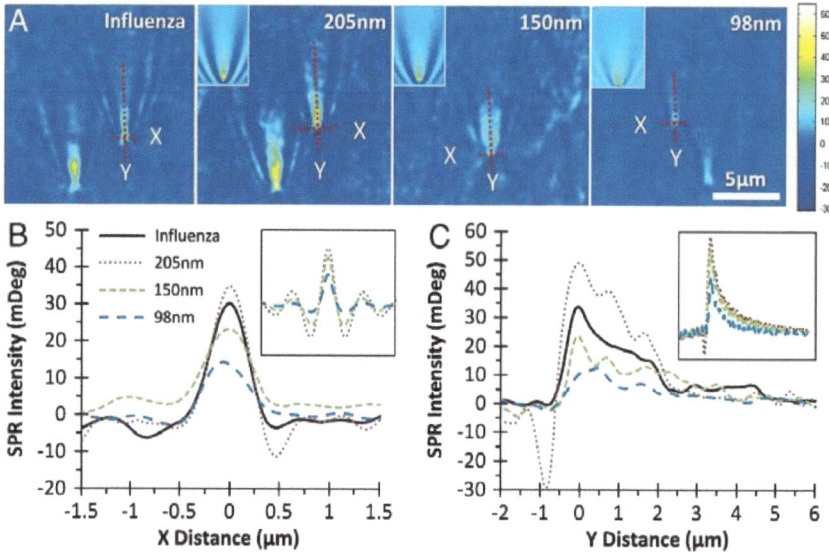

Fig. (23). (a) SPM images of H1N1 influenza A virus and silica NPs of three different sizes (in PBS buffer). Insets are the images of a NP produced by numerical simulation. **(b and c)** SPR intensity profiles of NPs along the *x* and *y* axis. The axis is defined by dashed lines in the SPM images of **(a)**. Inset profiles represent those from simulated images (reprinted with permission from [117]; copyright 2017 National Academy of Sciences).

In contrast, individual viruses show transient movement on PEG-coated surface, in which the V diffraction patterns are blinking due to Brownian motion of particle near the surface. Because PEG is used for blocking non-specific binding, the virus adsorption to the surface was prevented. Moreover, specific binding of influenza virus on antibody-coated surface was tested. More than 2-fold SPR intensity increase was observed with influenza on antibody-coated surface compared to influenza of PEG-coated surface or other viruses on antibody coated surface. For the quantitative analysis, histograms of SPR intensity with respect to the particle size were presented in Fig. (**25a**). The histogram fits well to Gaussian distribution and strong correlation between the particle size and SPR intensity was found. The small peaks that do not follow the distribution (marked with black arrow) are expected to be due to dimerization. Fig. (**25b**) shows the plot of the center SPR intensity which was obtained in the histograms of Fig. (**25a**) with respect to the particle volume. The particle volume overlapping with the evanescent wave is estimated to be proportional to the SPR intensity. The fitting curve corresponds well with the measured value and can be used for calibration for detecting the volume of unknown particle. The size of influenza was found to be 109 ± 13 nm which agrees with its literature value, around 90-110 nm [89]. The same procedure was done with human cytomegalovirus to confirm reliability.

Its size was found to be 218 ± 10 nm which is in line with the literature [118]. Mass of the particle can also be obtained from estimated volume from calibration curve and additional mass density of the particle.

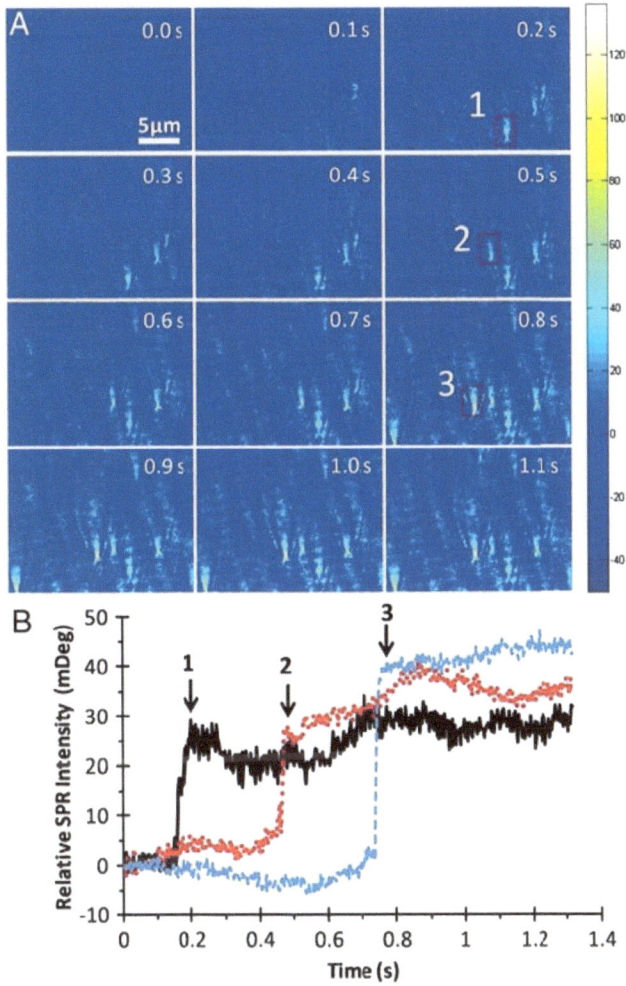

Fig. (24). (a) Time-lapse sequence of SPM image sequence of influenza A virus on bare gold. Color map: relative SPR image intensity in mDeg. (b) Temporal changes of SPR intensity in the regions indicated by rectangles in (a) where individual virus particles are adsorbed onto the gold surface (reprinted with permission from [117]; copyright 2017 National Academy of Sciences).

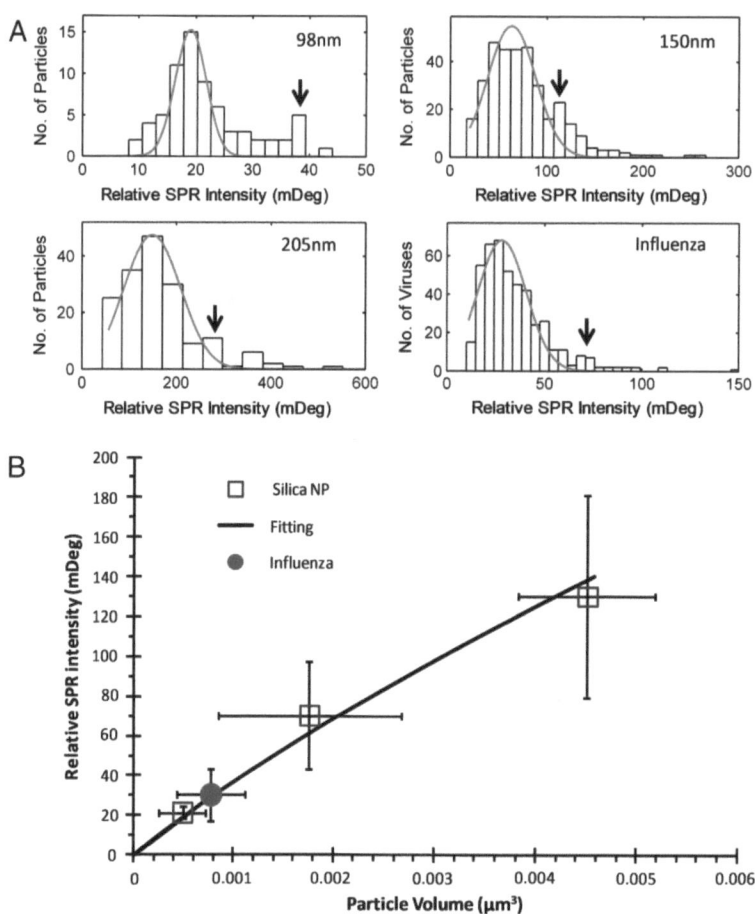

Fig. (25). (a) Relative SPR intensity distributions of individual silica NPs and influenza virus particles in histograms. The distributions are Gaussian-fitted (solid lines). Arrows represent peaks likely due to the formation of dimmers. **(b)** Calibration curve of SPR intensity *vs.* particle volumes provides the average volume of an influenza particle and the average SPR intensity in the histogram (reprinted with permission from [117]; copyright 2017 National Academy of Sciences).

In general, conventional SPM suffers from low image resolution due to severe SP scattering. Many studies have been performed to alleviate the effects of scattering. For example, surface nanoaperture arrays were confirmed to reduce the propagation length of SP scattering by more than 3 times, although the enhancement depends on the type of nanoapertures [119]. More recently, switching of light incidence, combined with minimum filtering, was shown to achieve significantly improved image resolution, one almost diffraction-limited in SPM [120]. The approach can be interpreted as an application of structured illumination to label-free SPM.

Biosensing Based on Surface-enhanced Raman Spectroscopy

SERS is one of the most studied surface-sensitive biosensing techniques based on unique Raman scattering signatures of molecules [121 - 123]. In recent decades, SERS has attracted much attention in chemical sensing and biomedical applications as an analytical technique because of high sensitivity, unique spectral characteristics of analytes with narrow bandwidth, simple sample preparation procedure, and non-invasive nature that allows multiple high-throughput detection and point-of-care analysis [124 - 132]. Several studies reported high SERS enhancement that is achieved by extreme localization of SP [133 - 135]. Raman scattering is known to be dramatically amplified with an enhancement factor up to 10^{10} and 10^{11} using metallic rough surfaces or artificial nanostructures, which has permitted the practical application of Raman scattering to be possible with high sensitivity to the degree of single molecular detection [136, 137].

In SERS, chemical enhancement originates from charge transfer between energy levels of metal nanostructures and the adsorbate molecules based on metal-molecule interactions. On the other hand, locally amplified near-fields created at the surface of plasmonic metal nanostructures induce electromagnetic field enhancement. Recent studies suggested that electromagnetic enhancement should make a dominant contribution to SERS in terms of the enhancement factor by about 10^3 to 10^8 times more than chemical enhancement [138, 139]. For the electromagnetic enhancement, high localization of light field can be produced in nanoscale LSP structures, such as gaps, holes, ridges, or sharp features of metal materials. In other words, understanding interactions between analyte molecules and plasmonic "hot spot" is a key component for SERS biosensors. Metal NPs can also amplify SERS signals. Geometrical shape and size in case of using metal NPs strongly influence the enhancement of SERS signals at absorption and scattering events. An ideal SERS substrate must possess high field enhancement with excellent uniformity. Reproducible and robust structures that strongly enhance the electromagnetic field are desirable. Such substrates can be fabricated on a wafer scale. Label-free super-resolution microscopy was also demonstrated using the fluctuation of SERS signal with such high-performance plasmonic metasurfaces [140].

Fig. (26) shows a schematic illustration of the SERS sensor based on plasmonic nanostructures coupled to metallic nanoarrays for ultrasensitive detection of hepatitis B virus (HBV) DNA [129]. SERS signals can be further enhanced by excitation of highly localized light fields when two plasmonic NPs are located closely for the strong coupling of LSP fields. NP-like sandwich structures of Ag nanorice@Raman label@SiO$_2$ coupled to Au triangle nanoarrays *via* DNA linkers were developed and resulted in spatially enhanced electromagnetic fields, which enabled ultrasensitive SERS with a discrimination capacity of single-base mutant of DNA. Here, Ag nanorice as a form of the sandwich NP was synthesized by a polyol process [141]. Au triangle nanoarray chips were fabricated using nanosphere lithography on a Si wafer [142, 143] and DNA hybridization occurred between nanorice structures and the Au chip. Raman spectrum of malachite green isothiocyanate as a Raman label was measured on the NP/DNA/chip structure, where the number of NPs proportional to DNA concentration affected the Raman intensity. The SERS signal on the NP/DNA/triangle nanoarray chip was highly enhanced until very low limit of detection of 50 aM was reached, compared with that of the NP/DNA/planar film chip. The results confirmed that SERS signals were significantly amplified by electromagnetic enhancement on the plasmonic NP/DNA/chip structure. SERS amplification by the electromagnetic enhancement of plasmonic nanostructures was also numerically confirmed. Fig. (**27**) presents the 3D FDTD calculation results of electromagnetic field enhancement at various plasmonic nanostructures. First of all, the electromagnetic field intensity of the Ag nanorice was locally amplified by about 50 times. Since SERS enhancement is approximately proportional to the fourth power of the field ($|E|^4$), Ag nanorice structure induces SERS enhancement by ~ 2,500 in Fig. (**27a**). In regard to the Au chip consisting of triangular nanoarrays, the largest field enhancement was observed to be ~ 14 and consequently SERS enhancement to be on the order of ~ 200, as shown in Fig. (**27b**). When nanodimers of two nanorices were placed on the arrayed nanotriangle, the degree of enhancement associated with LSP varies depending on the orientation of coupled nanostructure.

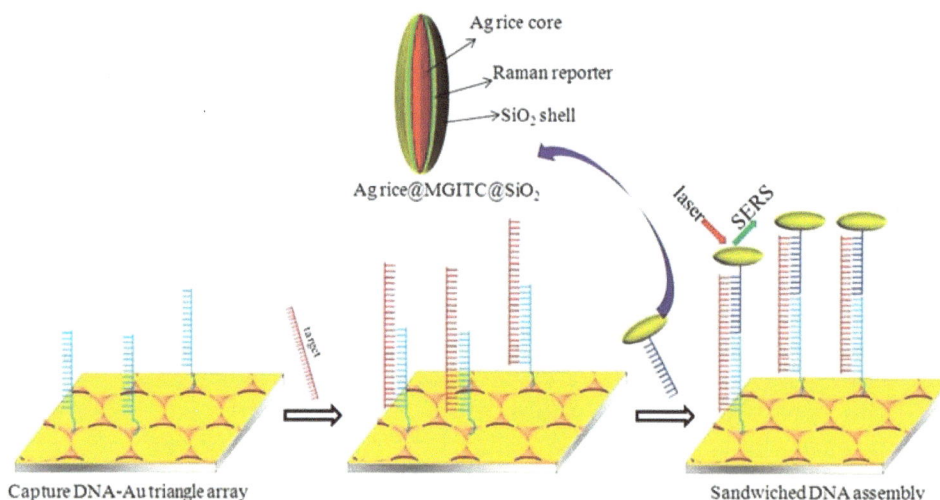

Fig. (26). Sandwiched structure of Ag nanorice@Raman label@SiO$_2$ used for DNA-Au triangle array in the SERS sensor that aims HBV DNA detection (reprinted with permission from [129]; copyright 2013 American Chemical Society).

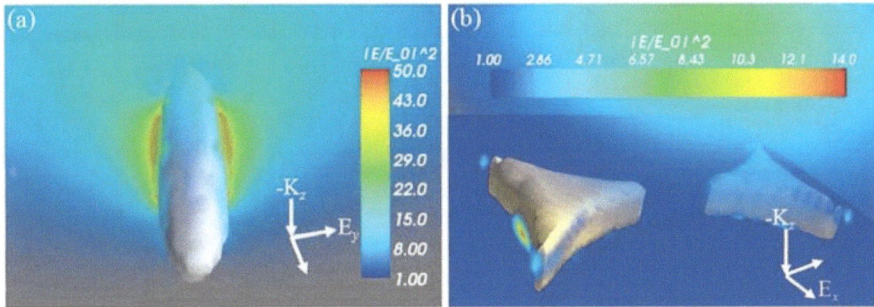

Fig. (27). 3D Electromagnetic field distribution (FDTD) produced by **(a)** Ag nanorice, **(b)** Au triangle nanoarrays after normalization by $|E/E_0|^2$. Wavelength $\lambda = 785$ nm with normal light incidence to the surface (K_z: incident wavevector, and E_x or E_y: electric field polarization) (reprinted with permission from [129]; copyright 2013 American Chemical Society).

CONCLUDING REMARKS AND OUTLOOK

In this chapter, we have explored various plasmonic techniques for improved detection characteristics. Among various approaches to attain enhanced detection sensitivity, particular emphasis has been placed upon plasmonic localization using nanostructures. Plasmonic colocalization based on the self-aligned overlap between localized near-fields and target molecules has been developed for dramatically enhanced detection performance of SPR sensing. LSPR using metal NPs has been investigated to amplify plasmonic optical signatures induced by molecular interactions. Aside from the traditional measurement based on angular and spectral interrogation, phase-sensitive SPR configurations based on optical path difference as well as temporal difference control have also been described for sensitivity improvement compared with conventional SPR detection. Relatively new LSPR-based analytical approaches based on the coupling of WGM with LSP modes using metallic nanostructures for ultrahigh sensitivity that may lead to single molecular detection have also been discussed. Label-free SPR imaging is considered as a way to achieve both improved sensitivity and high-throughput imaging capability. Finally, we have presented Raman spectroscopy enhanced by LSP to amplify signals that are unique for each molecule. These approaches have been actively pursued as an analytical tool with ultrahigh sensitivity for the measurement of molecules and binding kinetics and/or detection of structural changes of analytes.

Despite the incredible development that has taken place for the past decade, there are still limitations to address, to name a few, more practical implementation and further improvement of sensitivity. The development of nanofabrication techniques and the integration with other complementary sensing methods, *e.g.*, WGM resonators, have been one of the driving forces for plasmonic label-free biosensors in the future. Would it attain to a degree of single molecule detection?

The answer would have been no many years ago. However, it now becomes more and more likely than ever.

CONSENT FOR PUBLICATION

Not applicable.

CONFLICT OF INTEREST

The authors confirm that this chapter contents have no conflict of interest.

ACKNOWLEDGEMENTS

This work was supported by the National Research Foundation (NRF) grants funded by the Korean Government (NRF-2019R1A4A1025958, 2019R1F1A1063602, and 2019K2A9A2A08000198).

REFERENCES

[1] Raether H. Surface plasmons on smooth and rough surfaces and on gratings. Berlin, Germany: Springer-Verlag Berlin Heidelberg 1988.
[http://dx.doi.org/10.1007/BFb0048317]

[2] Zhang D, Men L, Chen Q. Microfabrication and applications of opto-microfluidic sensors. Sensors (Basel) 2011; 11(5): 5360-82.
[http://dx.doi.org/10.3390/s110505360] [PMID: 22163904]

[3] Hecht E. Optics. 4th International edition., San Francisco, United States: Addison-Wesley 2002.

[4] Wood RW. On a remarkable case of uneven distribution of light in a diffraction grating spectrum. Philos Mag 1902; 4: 396-402.
[http://dx.doi.org/10.1080/14786440209462857]

[5] Strutt JW. On the dynamical theory of gratings. Proc R Soc Lond, A Contain Pap Math Phys Character 1907; 79: 399-416.
[http://dx.doi.org/10.1098/rspa.1907.0051]

[6] Pockrand I, Swalen JD, Gordon JG, Philpott MR. Surface plasmon spectroscopy of organic monolayer assemblies. Surf Sci 1978; 74: 237-44.
[http://dx.doi.org/10.1016/0039-6028(78)90283-2]

[7] Homola J. Surface plasmon resonance sensors for detection of chemical and biological species. Chem Rev 2008; 108(2): 462-93.
[http://dx.doi.org/10.1021/cr068107d] [PMID: 18229953]

[8] Homola J, Yee SS, Gauglitz G. Surface plasmon resonance sensors. Sens Actuators B Chem 1999; 54: 3-15.
[http://dx.doi.org/10.1016/S0925-4005(98)00321-9]

[9] Homola J, Ed. Surface plasmon resonance based sensors. 2006.
[http://dx.doi.org/10.1007/b100321]

[10] Hoa XD, Kirk AG, Tabrizian M. Towards integrated and sensitive surface plasmon resonance biosensors: a review of recent progress. Biosens Bioelectron 2007; 23(2): 151-60.
[http://dx.doi.org/10.1016/j.bios.2007.07.001] [PMID: 17716889]

[11] Brolo AG. Plasmonics for future biosensors. Nat Photonics 2012; 6: 709-13.

[http://dx.doi.org/10.1038/nphoton.2012.266]

[12]   Jönsson U, Fägerstam L, Ivarsson B, *et al.* Real-time biospecific interaction analysis using surface plasmon resonance and a sensor chip technology. Biotechniques 1991; 11(5): 620-7.
       [PMID: 1804254]

[13]   Liedberg B, Lundström I, Stenberg E. Principles of biosensing with an extended coupling matrix and surface plasmon resonance. Sens Actuators B Chem 1993; 11(1-3): 63-72.
       [http://dx.doi.org/10.1016/0925-4005(93)85239-7]

[14]   Yoon SJ, Kim D. Target dependence of the sensitivity in periodic nanowire-based localized surface plasmon resonance biosensors. J Opt Soc Am A Opt Image Sci Vis 2008; 25(3): 725-35.
       [http://dx.doi.org/10.1364/JOSAA.25.000725] [PMID: 18311243]

[15]   Ma K, Kim DJ, Kim K, Moon S, Kim D. Target-localized nanograting-based surface plasmon resonance detection toward label-free molecular biosensing. IEEE J Sel Top Quantum Electron 2010; 16: 1004-14.
       [http://dx.doi.org/10.1109/JSTQE.2009.2034123]

[16]   Kim Y, Chung K, Lee W, Kim DH, Kim D. Nanogap-based dielectric-specific colocalization for highly sensitive surface plasmon resonance detection of biotin-streptavidin interactions. Appl Phys Lett 2012; 101233701
       [http://dx.doi.org/10.1063/1.4769108]

[17]   Kim K, Lee W, Chung K, *et al.* Molecular overlap with optical near-fields based on plasmonic nanolithography for ultrasensitive label-free detection by light-matter colocalization. Biosens Bioelectron 2017; 96: 89-98.
       [http://dx.doi.org/10.1016/j.bios.2017.04.046] [PMID: 28463741]

[18]   Kubatkin S, Danilov A, Hjort M, *et al.* Single-electron transistor of a single organic molecule with access to several redox states. Nature 2003; 425(6959): 698-701.
       [http://dx.doi.org/10.1038/nature02010] [PMID: 14562098]

[19]   Kumagai S, Yoshii S, Matsukawa N, Nishio K, Tsukamoto R, Yamashita I. Self-aligned placement of biologically synthesized Coulomb islands within nanogap electrodes for single electron transistor. Appl Phys Lett 2009; 94083103
       [http://dx.doi.org/10.1063/1.3085767]

[20]   Theiss J, Pavaskar P, Echternach PM, Muller RE, Cronin SB. Plasmonic nanoparticle arrays with nanometer separation for high-performance SERS substrates. Nano Lett 2010; 10(8): 2749-54.
       [http://dx.doi.org/10.1021/nl904170g] [PMID: 20698586]

[21]   Siegfried T, Ekinci Y, Solak HH, Martin OJF, Sigg H. Fabrication of sub-10 nm gap arrays over large areas for plasmonic sensors. Appl Phys Lett 2011; 99263302
       [http://dx.doi.org/10.1063/1.3672045]

[22]   Hermanson GT. Bioconjugate Techniques. London, UK: Academic Press 1996.

[23]   Fixe F, Branz HM, Louro N, Chu V, Prazeres DMF, Conde JP. Immobilization and hybridization by single sub-millisecond electric field pulses, for pixel-addressed DNA microarrays. Biosens Bioelectron 2004; 19(12): 1591-7.
       [http://dx.doi.org/10.1016/j.bios.2003.12.012] [PMID: 15142592]

[24]   Oh Y, Lee W, Kim Y, Kim D. Self-aligned colocalization of 3D plasmonic nanogap arrays for ultra-sensitive surface plasmon resonance detection. Biosens Bioelectron 2014; 51: 401-7.
       [http://dx.doi.org/10.1016/j.bios.2013.08.008] [PMID: 24012773]

[25]   Kim D, Yoon SJ. Effective medium-based analysis of nanowire-mediated localized surface plasmon resonance. Appl Opt 2007; 46(6): 872-80.
       [http://dx.doi.org/10.1364/AO.46.000872] [PMID: 17279132]

[26]   Kim D. Effect of resonant localized plasmon coupling on the sensitivity enhancement of nanowire-based surface plasmon resonance biosensors. J Opt Soc Am A Opt Image Sci Vis 2006; 23(9): 2307-

14.
[http://dx.doi.org/10.1364/JOSAA.23.002307] [PMID: 16912758]

[27]　Kim D. Nanostructure-based localized surface plasmon resonance biosensors.Optical Guided-Wave Chemical and Biosensors, Springer Series on Chemical Sensors and Biosensors. New York: Springer 2010.
[http://dx.doi.org/10.1007/978-3-540-88242-8_7]

[28]　Rytov SM. Electromagnetic properties of a finely stratified medium. Sov Phys JETP 1956; 2: 466-75.

[29]　Lalanne P, Lemercier-Lalanne D. On the effective medium theory of subwavelength periodic structures. J Mod Opt 1996; 43: 2063-85.
[http://dx.doi.org/10.1080/09500349608232871]

[30]　Lalanne P, Hutley M. The optical properties of artificial media structured at a subwavelength scale.Encyclopedia of Optical Engineering. New York: Marcel Dekker 2003; pp. 62-71.

[31]　Moon S, Kim D. Fitting-based determination of an effective medium of a metallic periodic structure and application to photonic crystals. J Opt Soc Am A Opt Image Sci Vis 2006; 23(1): 199-207.
[http://dx.doi.org/10.1364/JOSAA.23.000199] [PMID: 16478078]

[32]　Kang K, Kim D. Effective optical properties of nanoparticle-mediated surface plasmon resonance sensors. Opt Express 2019; 27(3): 3091-100.
[http://dx.doi.org/10.1364/OE.27.003091] [PMID: 30732335]

[33]　Fromm DP, Sundaramurthy A, Schuck PJ, Kino G, Moerner WE. Gap-dependent optical coupling of single "bowtie" nanoantennas resonant in the visible. Nano Lett 2004; 4: 957-61.
[http://dx.doi.org/10.1021/nl049951r]

[34]　Haes AJ, Zou S, Schatz GC, Van Duyne RP. Nanoscale optical biosensor: short range distance dependence of the localized surface plasmon resonance of noble metal nanoparticles. J Phys Chem B 2004; 108: 6961-8.
[http://dx.doi.org/10.1021/jp036261n]

[35]　He L, Musick MD, Nicewarner SR, *et al.* Colloidal Au-enhanced surface plasmon resonance for ultrasensitive detection of DNA hybridization. J Am Chem Soc 2000; 122: 9071-7.
[http://dx.doi.org/10.1021/ja001215b]

[36]　Moon S, Kim DJ, Kim K, *et al.* Surface-enhanced plasmon resonance detection of nanoparticle-conjugated DNA hybridization. Appl Opt 2010; 49(3): 484-91.
[http://dx.doi.org/10.1364/AO.49.000484] [PMID: 20090815]

[37]　Liz-Marzán LM. Tailoring surface plasmons through the morphology and assembly of metal nanoparticles. Langmuir 2006; 22(1): 32-41.
[http://dx.doi.org/10.1021/la0513353] [PMID: 16378396]

[38]　Lee KS, El-Sayed MA. Gold and silver nanoparticles in sensing and imaging: sensitivity of plasmon response to size, shape, and metal composition. J Phys Chem B 2006; 110(39): 19220-5.
[http://dx.doi.org/10.1021/jp062536y] [PMID: 17004772]

[39]　Jans H, Huo Q. Gold nanoparticle-enabled biological and chemical detection and analysis. Chem Soc Rev 2012; 41(7): 2849-66.
[http://dx.doi.org/10.1039/C1CS15280G] [PMID: 22182959]

[40]　Bai Y, Feng F, Zhao L, *et al.* Aptamer/thrombin/aptamer-AuNPs sandwich enhanced surface plasmon resonance sensor for the detection of subnanomolar thrombin. Biosens Bioelectron 2013; 47: 265-70.
[http://dx.doi.org/10.1016/j.bios.2013.02.004] [PMID: 23584389]

[41]　Ellington AD, Szostak JW. In vitro selection of RNA molecules that bind specific ligands. Nature 1990; 346(6287): 818-22.
[http://dx.doi.org/10.1038/346818a0] [PMID: 1697402]

[42]　Coughlin SR. Thrombin signalling and protease-activated receptors. Nature 2000; 407(6801): 258-64.

[http://dx.doi.org/10.1038/35025229] [PMID: 11001069]

[43]   Arai T, Miklossy J, Klegeris A, Guo JP, McGeer PL. Thrombin and prothrombin are expressed by neurons and glial cells and accumulate in neurofibrillary tangles in Alzheimer disease brain. J Neuropathol Exp Neurol 2006; 65(1): 19-25.
[http://dx.doi.org/10.1097/01.jnen.0000196133.74087.cb] [PMID: 16410745]

[44]   Hall WP, Ngatia SN, Van Duyne RP. LSPR biosensor signal enhancement using nanoparticle-antibody conjugates. J Phys Chem C Nanomater Interfaces 2011; 115(5): 1410-4.
[http://dx.doi.org/10.1021/jp106912p] [PMID: 21660207]

[45]   Reinhard BM, Sheikholeslami S, Mastroianni A, Alivisatos AP, Liphardt J. Use of plasmon coupling to reveal the dynamics of DNA bending and cleavage by single EcoRV restriction enzymes. Proc Natl Acad Sci USA 2007; 104(8): 2667-72.
[http://dx.doi.org/10.1073/pnas.0607826104] [PMID: 17307879]

[46]   Sannomiya T, Hafner C, Voros J. In situ sensing of single binding events by localized surface plasmon resonance. Nano Lett 2008; 8(10): 3450-5.
[http://dx.doi.org/10.1021/nl802317d] [PMID: 18767880]

[47]   Su KH, Wei QH, Zhang X, Mock JJ, Smith DR, Schultz S. Interparticle coupling effects on plasmon resonances of nanogold particles. Nano Lett 2003; 3: 1087-90.
[http://dx.doi.org/10.1021/nl034197f]

[48]   Gunnarsson L, Rindzevicius T, Prikulis J, *et al.* Confined plasmons in nanofabricated single silver particle pairs: experimental observations of strong interparticle interactions. J Phys Chem B 2005; 109(3): 1079-87.
[http://dx.doi.org/10.1021/jp049084e] [PMID: 16851063]

[49]   Jain PK, Huang WY, El-Sayed MA. On the universal scaling behavior of the distance decay of plasmon coupling in metal nanoparticle pairs: a plasmon ruler equation. Nano Lett 2007; 7: 2080-8.
[http://dx.doi.org/10.1021/nl071008a]

[50]   Ross BM, Waldeisen JR, Wang T, Lee LP. Strategies for nanoplasmonic core-satellite biomolecular sensors: Theory-based Design. Appl Phys Lett 2009; 95(19): 193112-4.
[http://dx.doi.org/10.1063/1.3254756] [PMID: 19997582]

[51]   Wang Y, Knoll W, Dostalek J. Bacterial pathogen surface plasmon resonance biosensor advanced by long range surface plasmons and magnetic nanoparticle assays. Anal Chem 2012; 84(19): 8345-50.
[http://dx.doi.org/10.1021/ac301904x] [PMID: 22931462]

[52]   Qi P, Zhou B, Zhang Z, Li S, Li Y, Zhong J. Phase-sensitivity-doubled surface plasmon resonance sensing *via* self-mixing interference. Opt Lett 2018; 43(16): 4001-4.
[http://dx.doi.org/10.1364/OL.43.004001] [PMID: 30106937]

[53]   Huang YH, Ho HP, Kong SK, Kabashin AV. Phase-sensitive surface plasmon resonance biosensors: methodology, instrumentation and applications. Ann Phys 2012; 524: 637-62.
[http://dx.doi.org/10.1002/andp.201200203]

[54]   Wu CM, Pao MC. Sensitivity-tunable optical sensors based on surface plasmon resonance and phase detection. Opt Express 2004; 12(15): 3509-14.
[http://dx.doi.org/10.1364/OPEX.12.003509] [PMID: 19483879]

[55]   Li YC, Chang YF, Su LC, Chou C. Differential-phase surface plasmon resonance biosensor. Anal Chem 2008; 80(14): 5590-5.
[http://dx.doi.org/10.1021/ac800598c] [PMID: 18507400]

[56]   Nelson SG, Johnston KS, Yee SS. High sensitivity surface plasmon resonance sensor based on phase detection. Sens Actuators B Chem 1996; 35: 187-91.
[http://dx.doi.org/10.1016/S0925-4005(97)80052-4]

[57]   Wu CM, Jian ZC, Joe SF, Chang LB. High-sensitivity sensor based on surface plasmon resonance and heterodyne interferometry. Sens Actuators B Chem 2003; 92: 133-6.

[http://dx.doi.org/10.1016/S0925-4005(03)00157-6]

[58]   Shen S, Liu T, Guo J. Optical phase-shift detection of surface plasmon resonance. Appl Opt 1998; 37(10): 1747-51.
[http://dx.doi.org/10.1364/AO.37.001747] [PMID: 18273083]

[59]   Xinglong Y, Lequn Z, Hong J, Haojuan W, Chunyong Y, Shenggeng Z. Immunosensor based on optical heterodyne phase detection. Sens Actuators B Chem 2001; 76: 199-202.
[http://dx.doi.org/10.1016/S0925-4005(01)00636-0]

[60]   Born M, Wolf E. Principles of Optics. 1st ed. Cambridge: Cambridge University Press 1999; pp. 752-8.
[http://dx.doi.org/10.1017/CBO9781139644181]

[61]   Abeles F. Surface electromagnetic waves ellipsometry. Surf Sci 1976; 56: 237-51.
[http://dx.doi.org/10.1016/0039-6028(76)90450-7]

[62]   Herminghaus S, Bechinger C, Petersen W, Leiderer P. Phase contrast surface mode resonance microscopy. Opt Commun 1994; 112: 16-20.
[http://dx.doi.org/10.1016/0030-4018(94)90072-8]

[63]   Kabashin AV, Kochergin VE, Beloglazov AA, Nikitin PI. Phase-polarisation contrast for surface plasmon resonance biosensors. Biosens Bioelectron 1998; 13(12): 1263-9.
[http://dx.doi.org/10.1016/S0956-5663(98)00088-8] [PMID: 9883560]

[64]   Kabashin AV, Kochergin VE, Nikitin PI. Surface plasmon resonance bio-and chemical sensors with phase-polarisation contrast. Sens Actuators B Chem 1999; 54: 51-6.
[http://dx.doi.org/10.1016/S0925-4005(98)00326-8]

[65]   Kochergin VE, Valeiko MV, Beloglazov AA, Ksenevich TI, Nikitin PI. Visualisation of the angular dependence of the reflected-radiation phase under conditions of a surface-plasmon resonance and its sensor applications. Quantum Electron 1998; 28: 835.
[http://dx.doi.org/10.1070/QE1998v028n09ABEH001338]

[66]   Westphal P, Bornmann A. Biomolecular detection by surface plasmon enhanced ellipsometry. Sens Actuators B Chem 2002; 84: 278-82.
[http://dx.doi.org/10.1016/S0925-4005(02)00037-0]

[67]   Naraoka R, Kajikawa K. Phase detection of surface plasmon resonance using rotating analyzer method. Sens Actuators B Chem 2005; 107: 952-6.
[http://dx.doi.org/10.1016/j.snb.2004.12.044]

[68]   Hooper IR, Sambles JR. Sensing using differential surface plasmon ellipsometry. J Appl Phys 2004; 96: 3004-11.
[http://dx.doi.org/10.1063/1.1778218]

[69]   Hooper IR, Sambles JR. Differential ellipsometric surface plasmon resonance sensors with liquid crystal polarization modulators. Appl Phys Lett 2004; 85: 3017-9.
[http://dx.doi.org/10.1063/1.1806273]

[70]   Hooper IR, Sambles JR, Pitter MC, Somekh MG. Phase sensitive array detection with polarisation modulated differential sensing. Sens Actuators B Chem 2006; 119: 651-5.
[http://dx.doi.org/10.1016/j.snb.2006.01.022]

[71]   Peng HJ, Wong SP, Lai YW, Liu XH, Ho HP, Zhao S. Simplified system based on photoelastic modulation technique for low-level birefringence measurement. Rev Sci Instrum 2003; 74: 745-4749.
[http://dx.doi.org/10.1063/1.1614875]

[72]   Ho HP, Law WC, Wu SY, *et al.* Phase-sensitive surface plasmon resonance biosensor using the photoelastic modulation technique. Sens Actuators B Chem 2006; 114: 80-4.
[http://dx.doi.org/10.1016/j.snb.2005.04.007]

[73]   Wu SY, Ho HP. Single-beam self-referenced phase-sensitive surface plasmon resonance sensor with

high detection resolution. Chin Opt Lett 2008; 6: 176-8.
[http://dx.doi.org/10.3788/COL20080603.0176]

[74]   Patskovsky S, Jacquemart R, Meunier M, De Crescenzo G, Kabashin AV. Phase-sensitive spatially-modulated surface plasmon resonance polarimetry for detection of biomolecular interactions. Sens Actuators B Chem 2008; 133: 628-31.
[http://dx.doi.org/10.1016/j.snb.2008.03.044]

[75]   Markowicz PP, Law WC, Baev A, Prasad PN, Patskovsky S, Kabashin A. Phase-sensitive time-modulated surface plasmon resonance polarimetry for wide dynamic range biosensing. Opt Express 2007; 15(4): 1745-54.
[http://dx.doi.org/10.1364/OE.15.001745] [PMID: 19532412]

[76]   Patskovsky S, Meunier M, Kabashin AV. Surface plasmon resonance polarizer for biosensing and imaging. Opt Commun 2008; 281: 5492-6.
[http://dx.doi.org/10.1016/j.optcom.2008.07.061]

[77]   Patskovsky S, Vallieres M, Maisonneuve M, Song IH, Meunier M, Kabashin AV. Designing efficient zero calibration point for phase-sensitive surface plasmon resonance biosensing. Opt Express 2009; 17(4): 2255-63.
[http://dx.doi.org/10.1364/OE.17.002255] [PMID: 19219129]

[78]   Patskovsky S, Meunier M, Prasad PN, Kabashin AV. Self-noise-filtering phase-sensitive surface plasmon resonance biosensing. Opt Express 2010; 18(14): 14353-8.
[http://dx.doi.org/10.1364/OE.18.014353] [PMID: 20639919]

[79]   Kabashin AV, Nikitin PI. Interferometer based on a surface-plasmon resonance for sensor applications. Quantum Electron 1997; 27: 653.
[http://dx.doi.org/10.1070/QE1997v027n07ABEH001013]

[80]   Kabashin AV, Nikitin PI. Surface plasmon resonance interferometer for bio-and chemical-sensors. Opt Commun 1998; 150: 5-8.
[http://dx.doi.org/10.1016/S0030-4018(97)00726-8]

[81]   Kochergin VE, Beloglazov AA, Valeiko MV, Nikitin PI. Phase properties of a surface-plasmon resonance from the viewpoint of sensor applications. Quantum Electron 1998; 28: 444.
[http://dx.doi.org/10.1070/QE1998v028n05ABEH001245]

[82]   Notcovich AG, Zhuk V, Lipson SG. Surface plasmon resonance phase imaging. Appl Phys Lett 2000; 76: 1665-7.
[http://dx.doi.org/10.1063/1.126129]

[83]   Wu SY, Ho HP, Law WC, Lin C, Kong SK. Highly sensitive differential phase-sensitive surface plasmon resonance biosensor based on the Mach-Zehnder configuration. Opt Lett 2004; 29(20): 2378-80.
[http://dx.doi.org/10.1364/OL.29.002378] [PMID: 15532273]

[84]   Ng SP, Wu CML, Wu SY, Ho HP. White-light spectral interferometry for surface plasmon resonance sensing applications. Opt Express 2011; 19(5): 4521-7.
[http://dx.doi.org/10.1364/OE.19.004521] [PMID: 21369283]

[85]   Foreman MR, Swaim JD, Vollmer F. Whispering gallery mode sensors. Adv Opt Photonics 2015; 7(2): 168-240.
[http://dx.doi.org/10.1364/AOP.7.000168] [PMID: 26973759]

[86]   Righini GC, Dumeige Y, Féron P, *et al.* Whispering gallery mode microresonators: Fundamentals and applications. Riv Nuovo Cim 2011; 37: 435-88.

[87]   Vollmer F, Braun D, Libchaber A. Protein detection by optical shift of a resonant microcavity. Appl Phys Lett 2002; 80: 4057-9.
[http://dx.doi.org/10.1063/1.1482797]

[88]   Arnold S, Khoshsima M, Teraoka I, Holler S, Vollmer F. Shift of whispering-gallery modes in

microspheres by protein adsorption. Opt Lett 2003; 28(4): 272-4.
[http://dx.doi.org/10.1364/OL.28.000272] [PMID: 12653369]

[89]   Vollmer F, Arnold S, Keng D. Single virus detection from the reactive shift of a whispering-gallery mode. Proc Natl Acad Sci USA 2008; 105(52): 20701-4.
[http://dx.doi.org/10.1073/pnas.0808988106] [PMID: 19075225]

[90]   Vollmer F, Arnold S. Whispering-gallery-mode biosensing: label-free detection down to single molecules. Nat Methods 2008; 5(7): 591-6.
[http://dx.doi.org/10.1038/nmeth.1221] [PMID: 18587317]

[91]   Dantham VR, Holler S, Kolchenko V, Wan Z, Arnold S. Taking whispering gallery-mode single virus detection and sizing to the limit. Appl Phys Lett 2012; 101043704
[http://dx.doi.org/10.1063/1.4739473]

[92]   Shopova SI, Blackledge CW, Rosenberger AT. Enhanced evanescent coupling to whispering-gallery modes due to gold nanorods grown on the microresonator surface. Appl Phys B 2008; 93: 183-7.
[http://dx.doi.org/10.1007/s00340-008-3180-6]

[93]   Shopova SI, Rajmangal R, Holler S, Arnold S. Plasmonic enhancement of a whispering-gallery-mode biosensor for single nanoparticle detection. Appl Phys Lett 2011; 98243104
[http://dx.doi.org/10.1063/1.3599584]

[94]   Swaim JD, Knittel J, Bowen WP. Detection limits in whispering gallery biosensors with plasmonic enhancement. Appl Phys Lett 2011; 99243109
[http://dx.doi.org/10.1063/1.3669398]

[95]   Santiago-Cordoba MA, Boriskina SV, Vollmer F, Demirel MC. Nanoparticle-based protein detection by optical shift of a resonant microcavity. Appl Phys Lett 2011; 99073701
[http://dx.doi.org/10.1063/1.3599706]

[96]   Santiago-Cordoba MA, Cetinkaya M, Boriskina SV, Vollmer F, Demirel MC. Ultrasensitive detection of a protein by optical trapping in a photonic-plasmonic microcavity. J Biophotonics 2012; 5(8-9): 629-38.
[http://dx.doi.org/10.1002/jbio.201200040] [PMID: 22707455]

[97]   Baaske MD, Vollmer F. Optical observation of single atomic ions interacting with plasmonic nanorods in aqueous solution. Nat Photonics 2016; 10: 733-9.
[http://dx.doi.org/10.1038/nphoton.2016.177]

[98]   Arnold S, Dantham VR, Barbre C, Garetz BA, Fan X. Periodic plasmonic enhancing epitopes on a whispering gallery mode biosensor. Opt Express 2012; 20(24): 26147-59.
[http://dx.doi.org/10.1364/OE.20.026147] [PMID: 23187470]

[99]   Ahn W, Boriskina SV, Hong Y, Reinhard BM. Photonic-plasmonic mode coupling in on-chip integrated optoplasmonic molecules. ACS Nano 2012; 6(1): 951-60.
[http://dx.doi.org/10.1021/nn204577v] [PMID: 22148502]

[100] Kim SA, Byun KM, Kim K, *et al.* Surface-enhanced localized surface plasmon resonance biosensing of avian influenza DNA hybridization using subwavelength metallic nanoarrays. Nanotechnology 2010; 21(35)355503
[http://dx.doi.org/10.1088/0957-4484/21/35/355503] [PMID: 20693616]

[101] Kim K, Choi JW, Ma K, *et al.* Nanoisland-based random activation of fluorescence for visualizing endocytotic internalization of adenovirus. Small 2010; 6(12): 1293-9.
[http://dx.doi.org/10.1002/smll.201000058] [PMID: 20517876]

[102] Kim K, Yajima J, Oh Y, *et al.* Nanoscale localization sampling based on nanoantenna arrays for super-resolution imaging of fluorescent monomers on sliding microtubules. Small 2012; 8(6): 892-900, 786.
[http://dx.doi.org/10.1002/smll.201101840] [PMID: 22170849]

[103] Zhu S, Li H, Yang M, Pang SW. High sensitivity plasmonic biosensor based on nanoimprinted quasi

3D nanosquares for cell detection. Nanotechnology 2016; 27(29)295101
[http://dx.doi.org/10.1088/0957-4484/27/29/295101] [PMID: 27275952]

[104]   Choi JR, Kim K, Oh Y, *et al.* Extraordinary transmission□based plasmonic nanoarrays for axially
        super□resolved cell imaging. Adv Opt Mater 2014; 2: 48-55.
        [http://dx.doi.org/10.1002/adom.201300330]

[105]   Otte MA, Estévez MC, Carrascosa LG, González-Guerrero AB, Lechuga LM, Sepúlveda B. Improved
        biosensing capability with novel suspended nanodisks. J Phys Chem 2011; 115: 5344-51.

[106]   Cryankiewicz M, Kruszewski T, Kruszewski S. Study of SERS efficiency of metallic colloidal
        systems. J Phys Conf Ser 2007; 79012013
        [http://dx.doi.org/10.1088/1742-6596/79/1/012013]

[107]   Kang TY, Lee W, Ahn H, *et al.* Plasmon-coupled whispering gallery modes on nanodisk arrays for
        signal enhancements. Sci Rep 2017; 7(1): 11737.
        [http://dx.doi.org/10.1038/s41598-017-12053-8] [PMID: 28916835]

[108]   Oh Y, Lee W, Kim D. Colocalization of gold nanoparticle-conjugated DNA hybridization for
        enhanced surface plasmon detection using nanograting antennas. Opt Lett 2011; 36(8): 1353-5.
        [http://dx.doi.org/10.1364/OL.36.001353] [PMID: 21499354]

[109]   Kinkhabwala A, Yu Z, Fan S, Avlasevich Y, Mullen K, Moerner WE. Large single-molecule
        fluorescence enhancements produced by a bowtie nanoantenna. Nat Photonics 2009; 3: 654-7.
        [http://dx.doi.org/10.1038/nphoton.2009.187]

[110]   Jin M, Pully V, Otto C, van den Berg A, Carlen ET. High-density periodic arrays of self-aligned
        subwavelength nanopyramids for surface-enhanced Raman spectroscopy. J Phys Chem C 2010; 114:
        21953-9.
        [http://dx.doi.org/10.1021/jp106245a]

[111]   Pasquale AJ, Reinhard BM, Dal Negro L. Concentric necklace nanolenses for optical near-field
        focusing and enhancement. ACS Nano 2012; 6(5): 4341-8.
        [http://dx.doi.org/10.1021/nn301000u] [PMID: 22537221]

[112]   Huang B, Yu F, Zare RN. Surface plasmon resonance imaging using a high numerical aperture
        microscope objective. Anal Chem 2007; 79(7): 2979-83.
        [http://dx.doi.org/10.1021/ac062284x] [PMID: 17309232]

[113]   Steiner G. Surface plasmon resonance imaging. Anal Bioanal Chem 2004; 379(3): 328-31.
        [http://dx.doi.org/10.1007/s00216-004-2636-8] [PMID: 15127177]

[114]   Lee HJ, Wark AW, Corn RM. Microarray methods for protein biomarker detection. Analyst (Lond)
        2008; 133(8): 975-83.
        [http://dx.doi.org/10.1039/b717527b] [PMID: 18645635]

[115]   Halpern AR, Chen Y, Corn RM, Kim D. Surface plasmon resonance phase imaging measurements of
        patterned monolayers and DNA adsorption onto microarrays. Anal Chem 2011; 83(7): 2801-6.
        [http://dx.doi.org/10.1021/ac200157p] [PMID: 21355546]

[116]   Giebel K, Bechinger C, Herminghaus S, *et al.* Imaging of cell/substrate contacts of living cells with
        surface plasmon resonance microscopy. Biophys J 1999; 76(1 Pt 1): 509-16.
        [http://dx.doi.org/10.1016/S0006-3495(99)77219-X] [PMID: 9876164]

[117]   Wang S, Shan X, Patel U, *et al.* Label-free imaging, detection, and mass measurement of single
        viruses by surface plasmon resonance. Proc Natl Acad Sci USA 2010; 107(37): 16028-32.
        [http://dx.doi.org/10.1073/pnas.1005264107] [PMID: 20798340]

[118]   Jin YL, Chen JY, Xu L, Wang PN. Refractive index measurement for biomaterial samples by total
        internal reflection. Phys Med Biol 2006; 51(20): N371-9.
        [http://dx.doi.org/10.1088/0031-9155/51/20/N02] [PMID: 17019025]

[119]   Kim DJ, Kim D. Subwavelength grating-based nanoplasmonic modulation for surface plasmon

resonance imaging with enhanced resolution. J Opt Soc Am B 2010; 27: 1252-9.
[http://dx.doi.org/10.1364/JOSAB.27.001252]

[120] Son T, Lee C, Seo J, Choi I-H, Kim D. Surface plasmon microscopy by spatial light switching for label-free imaging with enhanced resolution. Opt Lett 2018; 43(4): 959-62.
[http://dx.doi.org/10.1364/OL.43.000959] [PMID: 29444037]

[121] Raman CV. A new radiation. Indian J Phys 1928; 2: 387-98.

[122] Kohlrausch KGF. Der Smekal-Raman-Effekt. Berlin, Germany: Verlag von Julius Springer 1931.
[http://dx.doi.org/10.1007/978-3-642-90744-9]

[123] Singh RCV. Raman and the discovery of the Raman effect. Phys Perspect 2002; 4: 399-420.
[http://dx.doi.org/10.1007/s000160200002]

[124] Sha MY, Xu H, Penn SG, Cromer R. SERS nanoparticles: a new optical detection modality for cancer diagnosis. Nanomedicine (Lond) 2007; 2(5): 725-34.
[http://dx.doi.org/10.2217/17435889.2.5.725] [PMID: 17976033]

[125] Hudson SD, Chumanov G. Bioanalytical applications of SERS (surface-enhanced Raman spectroscopy). Anal Bioanal Chem 2009; 394(3): 679-86.
[http://dx.doi.org/10.1007/s00216-009-2756-2] [PMID: 19343331]

[126] Li M, Zhang J, Suri S, Sooter LJ, Ma D, Wu N. Detection of adenosine triphosphate with an aptamer biosensor based on surface-enhanced Raman scattering. Anal Chem 2012; 84(6): 2837-42.
[http://dx.doi.org/10.1021/ac203325z] [PMID: 22380526]

[127] Li M, Cushing SK, Zhang J, *et al.* Shape-dependent surface-enhanced Raman scattering in gold-Raman probe-silica sandwiched nanoparticles for biocompatible applications. Nanotechnology 2012; 23(11)115501
[http://dx.doi.org/10.1088/0957-4484/23/11/115501] [PMID: 22383452]

[128] Wang Y, Yan B, Chen L. SERS tags: novel optical nanoprobes for bioanalysis. Chem Rev 2013; 113(3): 1391-428.
[http://dx.doi.org/10.1021/cr300120g] [PMID: 23273312]

[129] Li M, Cushing SK, Liang H, Suri S, Ma D, Wu N. Plasmonic nanorice antenna on triangle nanoarray for surface-enhanced Raman scattering detection of hepatitis B virus DNA. Anal Chem 2013; 85(4): 2072-8.
[http://dx.doi.org/10.1021/ac303387a] [PMID: 23320458]

[130] Zong S, Wang Z, Chen H, Yang J, Cui Y. Surface enhanced Raman scattering traceable and glutathione responsive nanocarrier for the intracellular drug delivery. Anal Chem 2013; 85(4): 2223-30.
[http://dx.doi.org/10.1021/ac303028v] [PMID: 23327663]

[131] Li M, Cushing SK, Zhang J, *et al.* Three-dimensional hierarchical plasmonic nano-architecture enhanced surface-enhanced Raman scattering immunosensor for cancer biomarker detection in blood plasma. ACS Nano 2013; 7(6): 4967-76.
[http://dx.doi.org/10.1021/nn4018284] [PMID: 23659430]

[132] Yang J, Palla M, Bosco FG, *et al.* Surface-enhanced Raman spectroscopy based quantitative bioassay on aptamer-functionalized nanopillars using large-area Raman mapping. ACS Nano 2013; 7(6): 5350-9.
[http://dx.doi.org/10.1021/nn401199k] [PMID: 23713574]

[133] Wang H, Li H, Xu S, Zhao B, Xu W. Integrated plasmon-enhanced Raman scattering (iPERS) spectroscopy. Sci Rep 2017; 7(1): 14630.
[http://dx.doi.org/10.1038/s41598-017-15111-3] [PMID: 29116139]

[134] Lin KQ, Yi J, Zhong JH, *et al.* Plasmonic photoluminescence for recovering native chemical information from surface-enhanced Raman scattering. Nat Commun 2017; 8: 14891.
[http://dx.doi.org/10.1038/ncomms14891] [PMID: 28348368]

[135] Li ZY. Mesoscopic and Microscopic Strategies for Engineering Plasmon□Enhanced Raman Scattering. Adv Opt Mater 2018; 61701097
[http://dx.doi.org/10.1002/adom.201701097]

[136] Nie S, Emory SR. Probing single molecules and single nanoparticles by surface-enhanced Raman scattering. Science 1997; 275(5303): 1102-6.
[http://dx.doi.org/10.1126/science.275.5303.1102] [PMID: 9027306]

[137] Le Ru EC, Meyer M, Etchegoin PG. Proof of single-molecule sensitivity in surface enhanced Raman scattering (SERS) by means of a two-analyte technique. J Phys Chem B 2006; 110(4): 1944-8.
[http://dx.doi.org/10.1021/jp054732v] [PMID: 16471765]

[138] Kanipe KN, Chidester PP, Stucky GD, Moskovits M. Large format surface-enhanced Raman spectroscopy substrate optimized for enhancement and uniformity. ACS Nano 2016; 10(8): 7566-71.
[http://dx.doi.org/10.1021/acsnano.6b02564] [PMID: 27482725]

[139] Sharma B, Cardinal MF, Ross MB, et al. Aluminum film-over-nanosphere substrates for deep-UV surface-enhanced resonance Raman spectroscopy. Nano Lett 2016; 16(12): 7968-73.
[http://dx.doi.org/10.1021/acs.nanolett.6b04296] [PMID: 27960451]

[140] Ayas S, Cinar G, Ozkan AD, et al. Label-free nanometer-resolution imaging of biological architectures through surface enhanced Raman scattering. Sci Rep 2013; 3: 2624.
[http://dx.doi.org/10.1038/srep02624] [PMID: 24022059]

[141] Liang H, Zhao H, Rossouw D, et al. Silver nanorice structures: oriented attachment-dominated growth, high environmental sensitivity, and real-space visualization of multipolar resonances. Chem Mater 2012; 24: 2339-46.
[http://dx.doi.org/10.1021/cm3006875]

[142] Li H, Low J, Brown KS, Wu N. Large-area well-ordered nanodot array pattern fabricated with self-assembled nanosphere template. IEEE Sens J 2008; 8: 880-4.
[http://dx.doi.org/10.1109/JSEN.2008.923266]

[143] Li H, Wu N. A large-area nanoscale gold hemisphere pattern as a nanoelectrode array. Nanotechnology 2008; 19(27)275301
[http://dx.doi.org/10.1088/0957-4484/19/27/275301] [PMID: 21828697]

CHAPTER 7

Micro/Nano-fluidics Based Biosensors

Eunseop Yeom[*]

School of Mechanical Engineering, Pusan National University, Busan, South Korea

Abstract: Integrated microfluidic sensors have been developed with the understanding of fundamental laws of blood flow and its non-Newtonian properties and the advent of microfluidic technology to diagnose various diseases. Lab-on-a-chip platforms based on hemodynamics allow the highly accurate detection of the pathological changes in the behaviors of blood (*i.e.*, red blood cells, white blood cells, and platelets) and cells. Hemorheology depends on the complex interactions of immune response and cardiovascular and other diseases. The nanofluidic systems initiated by flow characteristics remain insufficient, but the ongoing development of microfluidic and nanofluidic systems and the identification of key players and risk factors enable the study of disease onset and progression, thereby leading to a spectrum of clinically relevant findings.

Keywords: Blood flow, Cell deformation, Drag force, ESR (erythrocyte sedimentation rate), Image processing, Lab-on-a-chip, Microfluidics, Pressure, RBC aggregation, Shear stress, Platelet activation, PIV (particle image velocimetry), Viscosity.

INTRODUCTION

The cardiovascular system is vital for the transport of fluids and molecules in and out of cells for humans and living animals. Blood vessels, which are composed of three tunicae, namely, intima, media, and adventitia, have wide diameters (5 μm–4 mm) in an adult human depending on their functions and locations. The vascular system is exposed to mechanical forces induced by pressure and shear forces. According to previous studies, extremely low shear forces acting on endothelial cells may lead to an increased risk of atherosclerosis characterized by the thickening of plaques. The accumulation of plaque in the arteries leads to the blockage of blood flow and eventually plaque rupture. Hemodynamic and hemorheological features have been suggested to be closely related to the cause, progression, and prognosis of atherosclerosis because the wall shear stress (WSS)

[*] **Corresponding author Eunseop Yeom:** School of Mechanical Engineering, Pusan National University, Busan, South Korea; E-mail: esyeom@pusan.ac.kr

Han-Sheng Chuang & Yi-Ping Ho (Eds.)

intensity, exposure time, and turbidity affect the structure and function of the endothelium [1 - 3]. Low and oscillating WSS, which is affected by disturbed flow, may result in endothelial cell dysfunction, thereby leading to atherogenesis and thrombosis [4]. For a long time, many researchers have tried to understand the cardiovascular system, including the nature and properties of the blood vessels, hemodynamic and hemorheological behaviors, and blood components.

Microfluidic-based biosensors are composed of the manipulation (such as transportation, mixing, and separation) and analysis of fluids within micrometer-sized channels (1 μm = 10^{-6} m). In order to provide diagnostic results for various cardiovascular diseases, most micro biosensors are based on the detection of biomolecules such as proteins [5, 6], peptides [7, 8], enzymes [9 - 11] and DNA [12]. In addition to the detection of cellular activity, electrical activity, and physical and chemical signals transmitted by the cells, microfluidic devices that mimic blood vessels or induce sudden flow disturbances have been proposed for biosensing. New devices and systems for biological and medical research especially nanofluidics have been developed due to the size of biological molecules (*i.e.*, nucleic acids, amino acids, and proteins) and implemented to determine the unique properties of nanomaterials. Nanofluidics manipulate nanometer-sized fluids (typically 1–100 nm, 1 nm = 10^{-9} m) [13].

Several studies have provided a summary of microfluidic devices for the measurement of blood viscosity, blood viscoelasticity, red blood cell (RBC) aggregation, RBC deformability, and platelet (PLT) activation [14 - 17], but comprehensive information on fluidic biosensors remains insufficient due to the various biophysical properties of blood. In this chapter, the discussion is focused on the basic mechanism of some biosensors initiated by flow characteristics.

MICROFLUIDIC DEVICES BASED ON HEMODYNAMICS

Measurement of Cell Deformation

RBC Deformability

RBCs are the major carriers of oxygen and carbon dioxide in the circulatory system. Particularly, RBCs experience shear stress in microvessels and capillaries that have a diameter of 3 μm [18]. RBCs are highly deformable biconcave disks that have a diameter and thickness of 8 and 2 μm, respectively. A hemoglobin-rich cytoplasm in RBC is enclosed by a molecularly thin membrane consisting of a lipid bilayer, membrane skeleton network, and transmembrane proteins. Complex dynamics, such as tumbling, tank-treading (the membrane rotates around the cell body), and swinging of RBCs, are observed under steady-shear flow conditions [19]. During the flow in capillaries, RBCs can be deformed due to the interplay of bending and stretching forces of the RBC membrane and the lubrication forces of the fluid passing in the narrow gap between the RBC membrane and the capillary walls. Although the main features during flow in the capillary are parachute-like cells, nonaxisymmetric slipper-like cells can be observed depending on the capillary radius and apparent fluid viscosity [20 - 22]. When the capillary radius is reduced to become comparable to the maximum diameter of the RBC, a single RBC temporarily blocks the channel. This blockage increases the pressure drop (ΔP) in the capillary, and the cell is squeezed and gradually deformed. When the hydrodynamic force reaches a certain threshold, the RBC pushes through the capillary into a veinlet [23]. Under this deformation, RBCs can release chemicals, such as adenosine triphosphate (ATP), to participate in vascular signaling and control systemic circulation [24].

RBC deformability can be pathologically varied due to inherited genetic disorders, such as sickle cell, noninfectious [25] and infectious diseases [26] because RBC deformability can contribute to the variations in cytoskeleton composition, network structure, and protein density. Healthy RBCs have high deformability under relatively small ΔP. By contrast, unhealthy RBCs are stiff and require a high ΔP to move across the capillary. Therefore, the reduced deformability of RBCs can result in serious vascular complications, and the measurement of RBC deformability can be used as a marker to identify pathological changes [27, 28].

A micropipette aspiration technology monitor is widely used to measure the mechanical properties of the RBC membrane under static conditions [29]. The elastic modulus of the cell membrane can be extracted from the suction pressure and the length of the membrane aspirated into the pipette. Similarly, the mechanical deformation of a single cell can be measured using experimental tools, such as atomic force microscopy and optical and magnetic tweezers. However, these quantitative single-cell measurements are generally labor- and skill-intensive [15].

The measurement of the biophysical properties of cells by using microfluidic technologies has several advantages, such as small sample volume, integration capability, and fast response. Thus, several microchannel devices have been proposed to provide information for the clinical diagnosis and therapy of blood diseases [15, 23, 30 - 38]. RBCs are mostly studied in the majority of existing constriction channel-based devices to induce the human capillary-like environment. The shear rate ($\dot{\gamma}$) of a flow in the rectangular microchannel is approximately estimated using the following equation. The flow is assumed to be a simple Poiseuille flow [39].

$$\dot{\gamma} = \frac{12Q}{WH^2} \qquad (1)$$

where W and H denote the width and height, respectively, of a rectangular channel. As the size of the rectangular channel is reduced, high shear flow can be induced in the microfluidic device. Most of the proposed microfluidic devices to estimate RBC deformability focus on this high-shear effect. The first malaria diagnosis based on RBC deformability by using microfluidic devices was reported in 2003 [40]. In this study, constriction channels with various channel widths were used to determine the deformability changes depending on the malaria stage (*i.e.*, early ring stage, early trophozoite, late trophozoite, and schizont). The deformability of malaria-infected RBCs is reduced as the parasite progresses from the early ring stage to the schizont, whereas healthy RBCs are deformable to travel through the constriction channels. Similar to this study, microcontractions (due to velocity transition) and bifurcations (around the apex region and small branch) have been adopted to induce a high shear flow in the device. The deformation of RBCs can be quantified through high-speed imaging as a deformation index (DI) or stretch ratio [30, 41 - 43]. Forsyth and coworkers have reported that three different types of motion, namely, stretching, tumbling, and recoiling, are induced as the $\dot{\gamma}$ in the microfluidic channel increases [41]. A micronetwork with converging–diverging flow sections and decreasing width (reduced to 10 μm) is proposed by mimicking the human microcirculation network [43]. The hydrodynamic force can deform RBCs with respect to the biconcave rest configuration (parachute-like shape). The degree of RBC deformation is defined as DI, which is the aspect ratio of a cell rectangular bounding box. As expected, DI tends to increase with an increase in *P* and cell velocity.

The conception of conventional pipette aspiration is adopted in the microfluidic characterization of cells. A single RBC is infused into a microfluidic channel and deformed through funnel-shaped constrictions (Fig. **1**). RBC deformation can be estimated through electrical and mechanical characterization by using impedance spectroscopy [44]. Two Ag/AgCl electrodes are inserted into the inlet and the outlet ports of the device. As a single RBC passes through the constriction channel, the RBC perturbs the electric field in the channel, generating a current impulse. The sealing resistance between the RBC membrane and the channel walls can be estimated by sensing the current change in the circuit loop *via* input impedance. From the optical and electrical information, the multiple parameters quantified as mechanical and electrical signatures include transit time, impedance amplitude ratio, and impedance phase increase. These parameters reveal different biophysical properties across samples and between the adult and the neonatal

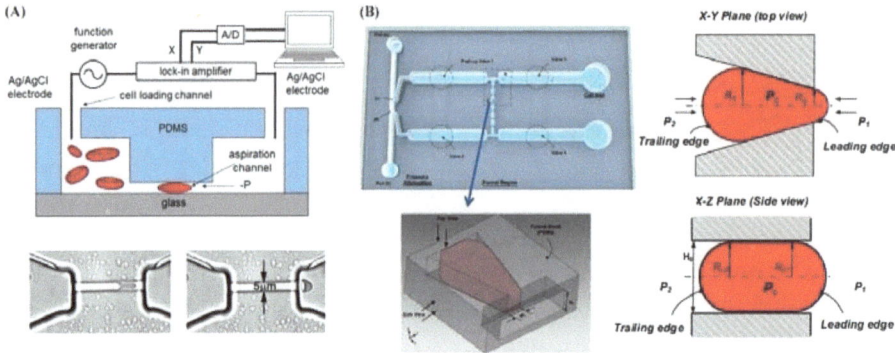

Fig. (1). (A) Schematic of the microfluidic system for electrical and mechanical characterization of RBCs. Measurements are made when an RBC passes through the constriction channel [44]. Copyright 2012 The Royal Society of Chemistry. **(B)** Microchannel with a funnel constriction. Geometric representations of both RBCs and the relevant funnel constrictions. Top and side view illustrations of a single RBC [45]. Copyright 2014 Elsevier.

RBC populations. In addition to impedance, the cortical tension (T_C) of RBC in passing funnel constriction with a 30° contraction angle is estimated on the basis of the Laplace law to assess cell deformability [45]. The threshold pressure ($P_{threshold}$) for RBC transit through a constriction can be estimated as follows:

$$P_{threshold} = T_C \left(\frac{1}{R_a} - \frac{1}{R_b} \right) \tag{2}$$

where R_a and R_b are the widths of the RBC and the funnel pore, respectively. In Eq. 2, the T_C of an RBC membrane, which contributes to the RBC deformability, is used. The T_C of RBC can be estimated by measuring the pressure and used to distinguish the biological variation in RBC deformability.

The shape of RBCs flowing through small capillaries is dependent on various factors, such as flow rate, the initial position relative to the central line of the capillary, and the diameter of the capillary [20]. Thus, RBCs need to be centered in the microchannel for the consistent measurement of RBC deformation. Hydrodynamic focusing is used to position the RBCs close to the central line of the microchannel [46]. In addition to positioning the RBC in the central line, the usage of hydrodynamic focusing can apply forces to cells for deformation measurement. As shown in Fig. (**2**), hydrodynamic focusing centers the cell, and the RBC in the central channel (8 μm × 8 μm) is folded into a parachute-like shape. In the recovery region with a cross-sectional area of 200 μm × 8 μm, shear stress is released, and the RBC gradually recovers its original shape. Difference of DI, which is defined as DI = L/D, before the RBC exits the central channel and enters the recovery region, is used to quantify the deformation behavior of RBCs. To monitor the variation in RBC deformability during blood storage, the collected blood samples are suspended in saline–adenine–glucose mannitol solution (110 ml) and stored in a blood bank refrigerator (4 °C) after the separation of plasma and buffy coat. During blood storage, the morphological change from the biconcave RBC to the spherical RBC is observed. Circularity, which is defined as circularity = 4π × area/perimeter^2, is used to depict the morphology of each stored RBC. The time constant (t_c) of each RBC is determined by fitting its DI values over time to an exponential function to characterize the recovery rate of the RBC. t_c and DI decrease as circularity increases, indicating that the morphological changes of RBCs cause changes in RBC deformability during blood storage. The average t_c is reduced as the RBCs are stored longer. The low t_c may be attributed to ATP depletion. ATP alteration results in the stiffening and recovery of the RBC structure. Fresh and stored blood samples can be distinguished on the basis of multiple parameters by using high-speed imaging system and automated image processing. Similar to the focusing flow, an extensional flow at the intersection of four channels is proposed to study the polymer extensional hysteresis [47]. In a microfluidic cross-slot channel with four channels, the extensional flow is induced by providing inflows through two opposite channels and draining outflows through two perpendicular channels. The RBC deformation under extensional flow is simulated in a cross-slot microchannel based on the basis of a finite-difference flow solver and the front-tracking method [48]. RBC is deformed along the major axis when entering near the centerline. RBCs that enter further away from the centerline have asymmetrical shapes due to the shear in the channel arm, and their maximally deformed shape results from a combination of shear and extension. This simulation differentiating healthy and diseased RBCs has provided information about the experimental conditions and design of the channel.

However, the overall throughput for the measurement of single cell is relatively low compared to bulk assay methods [15]. Bulk microfiltration techniques have been used for several decades to investigate microcirculatory diseases by measuring the variations in the pressure or the flow rate of RBC solutions when the fluid is passed through micropore filters. By adopting the conception of the capillary network, Shevkoplyas and coworkers have proposed a microchannel network with width of 6–70 μm and depth of 6 μm [31]. The proposed device is compared with conventional filtration with pore of 5 μm (Fig. **3A**). The microchannel can be easily plugged by RBCs as the concentration of glutaraldehyde increases because the glutaraldehyde treatment reduces the RBC deformability. Conventional filtration measures the filtration time (FT), which is the time required for a fixed volume (50 µl) of the sample to pass through the

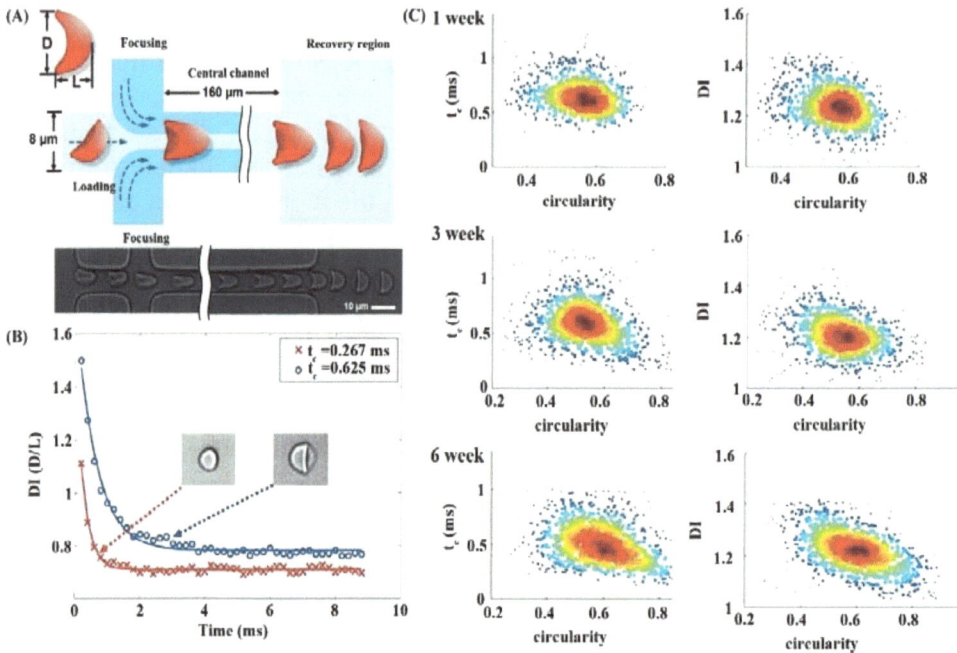

Fig. (2). (A) Schematic of the microfluidic device showing the centering, orienting, folding, and shape recovering of an RBC. **(B)** Shape recovery of a RBC stored for 1 week and RBC stored for 6 weeks. Fitting lines to an exponential model were inserted. **(C)** The scatter plots showing comparisons between t_c and circularity, and between DI and circularity depending on blood storage [46]. Copyright 2014 The Royal Society of Chemistry.

filter, to quantify the RBC deformability. However, the FT is only weakly dependent on glutaraldehyde treatment. At a glutaraldehyde concentration of 0.08%, the filter is completely plugged. In contrast to the filtration method, RBC velocity passing the microchannel network under given pressure drop (ΔP) decreased quasi-linearly with increasing concentration of glutaraldehyde.

Besides the high shear flow in the microchannel, the microstructure in the device can be applied to measure the RBC deformation [34, 36, 45, 49, 50]. The structure of deterministic lateral displacement (DLD) makes the asymmetric flow pattern around obstacles. Beech and coworkers have observed the different behaviors of RBCs depending on RBC shape (*i.e.*, discocyte, echinocyte, and stomatocyte) [51]. This work indicates great potential in the use of microstructures, like DLD devices, to estimate cellular properties. Bow and coworkers have proposed a flow cytometer with periodically spaced triangle-shaped pillars by adopting an oblique angle with slits to avoid the clogging problem observed in the filters [52]. The constrictions of pillars in parallel across the width of the channel ensure higher throughput, and the constrictions of pillars in series along the length of the channel ensure repeatability. An inverse correlation exists between the degree of artificial stiffening and the velocity of the RBCs through the channels. As shown in Fig. (**3B**), the noninfected RBC moves about twice as far as each infected RBC in 8.3 s. Triangle-shaped pillars can have different tendency of constriction by rotating as much as 180° (diverging and converging channels). In the regime of the laminar flow with low Reynolds number, the forward and backward fluid velocities and resistances are identical [53]. When the confounding effects caused by temperature, cell age, buffer conditions, pressure, and device variability are obviated, the difference in the velocity of cells moving in the two channels with 180° rotation, results from cell deformation. From the velocity difference, the difference in deformability between the noninfected and the ring stage-infected RBCs can be quantitatively and statistically distinguished. Recently, the complexity of cell traversal in the DLD device with geometric obstacles (from circle to diamond) is investigated through hydrodynamic simulations for the development of novel DLD devices [54].

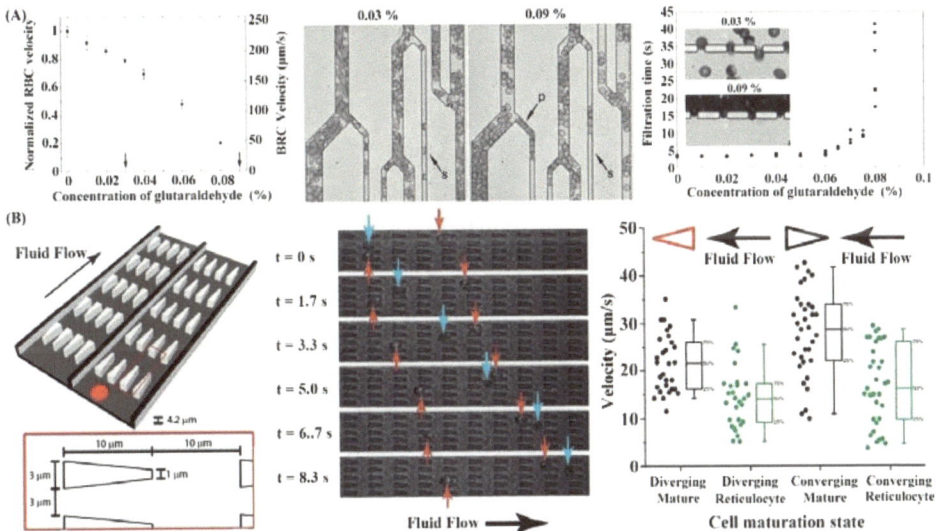

Fig. (3). (A) (Top left) Dependence of the average RBC velocity in the input channel on the concentration of glutaraldehyde. Typical blood flow patterns within the network corresponding to treatment with 0.03% and 0.09% glutaraldehyde. (Top right) Filtration time according to the glutaraldehyde concentration. Images of RBC filterability for the glutaraldehyde concentration (0.03 and 0.09 %). Sample with 1% hematocrit pass through 5 μm polycarbonate filter [31]. Copyright 2006 The Royal Society of Chemistry. (B) (Bottom left) Illustration of the device design; each channel of the actual device is 10 pores wide and 200 pores long. (Bottom center) Experimental images of ring stage P. falciparum-infected (red arrows) and uninfected (blue arrows) RBCs at a pressure gradient of 0.24 Pa μm⁻¹. (Bottom right) Variation of velocity depending on cell maturation state and flow direction [52]. Copyright 2011 The Royal Society of Chemistry.

In case of Plasmodium falciparum malaria, the ring stage-infected RBCs are observed in the circulation, whereas later stage-infected RBCs are either removed by the spleen or adhere to the vascular endothelium. The filtering capacity of the spleen is inherently related to the blood passage through the reticular meshwork of the red pulp. As depicted in Fig. (**4**), 90% of the blood circulates through the closed-fast microcirculation and directly bypasses the spleen's filtration capacity. The remaining 10% of the blood circulates through the open-slow microcirculation with the filtration beds of the cords, where the hematocrit is significantly augmented, facilitating the recognition and the destruction of unhealthy RBCs [55]. Before reaching the venous system, 10% of the blood in the open-slow microcirculation of sinusal spleens must pass through the interendothelial slits (IES) of the splenic sinusoids. This passage is the second stringent test for the functionality of RBCs. Specifically, less deformable unhealthy cells cannot traverse the IES [56]. Some microfluidic devices are proposed by mimicking the spleen's circulation [36, 50]. Rigat-Brugarolas and coworkers have designed the microfluidic device with the closed-fast and the open-slow microcirculations to provide a physiological flow division. In the open-slow channel, the hematocrit is augmented by passing through a pillar matrix that resembles the reticular mesh. At the end of the slow flow channel, physically constrained RBCs are distinguished by parallel 2 μm micro-constrictions that resemble the IES. Cell deformability is estimated by measuring the elongation of blood cells as follows:

$$D_{M\%} = \frac{L_S - L_{RM}}{L_{RM}} \times 100 \tag{3}$$

In Eq. 3, L_S and L_{RM} are the lengths in microns of a single cell in the slit and in the pillar matrix zone, respectively. A statistically significant difference is observed between the deformation percentages of fresh and aged human RBCs due to the reduced RBC deformability of old RBCs. The deformation percentage of RBCs from mice with *Plasmodium yoelii,* which are known to increase membrane rigidity and reduce RBCs deformability, are highly significantly different with that of noninfected RBCs. Picot *et al.* have proposed a microfluidic device with width of 2–5 μm by monitoring IES. Infected RBCs are perfused to the device to determine their differential retention. Infected RBCs have a cell suspension of 0.1% hematocrit containing three different RBC populations: 5% blue-labeled ring-infected RBCs, 5% green-labeled trophozoite-infected RBCs, and 90% noninfected unlabeled control RBCs. The infected RBCs (blue- and green-labeled RBCs) are easily plugged in the slits compared with the noninfected control RBCs (unlabeled). The spleen-like microfluidic device successfully discriminates infected RBCs from noninfected RBCs and the newly infected RBCs from the late

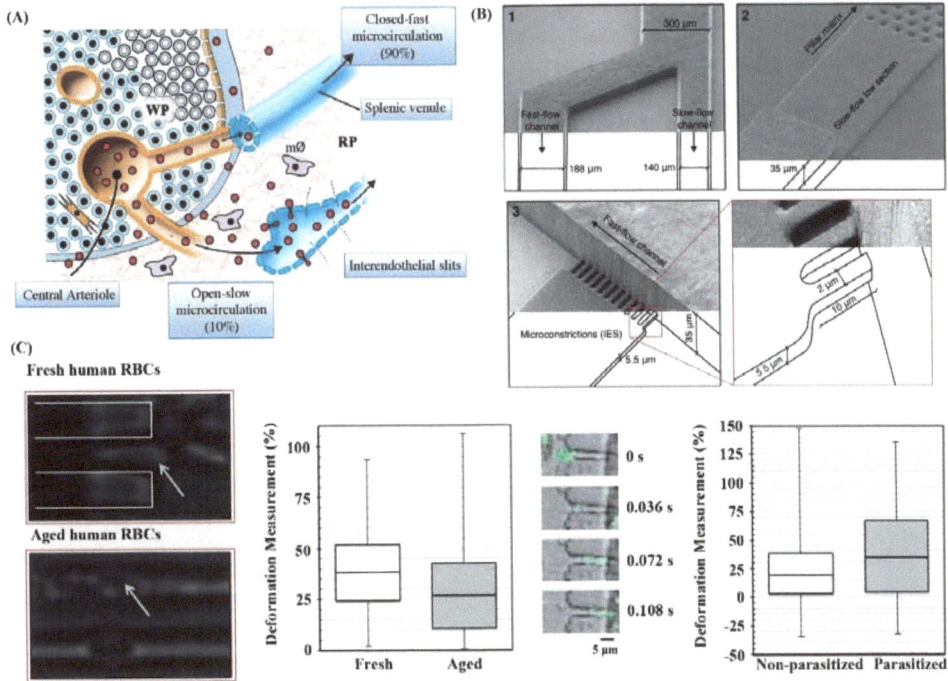

Fig. (4). (A) Diagram of the human splenon showing the closed-fast and open-slow microcirculations as well as the interendothelial slits (IES). **(B)** Details of the slow-flow channel. (1) Flow division zone; (2) Slow-flow low section and the pillar matrix; (3) Microconstrictions representing the IES. **(C)** Deformability of fresh and aged RBCs inside the slow-flow channel. Median and the quartiles of the deformation percentage of fresh and aged RBC populations. Time lapse-series showing the passage of one infected reticulocyte (green) going through a microconstriction [36]. Copyright 2014 The Royal Society of Chemistry.

infected RBCs by measuring the number of cells trapped in the slits.

On the basis of RBC deformability, the clinical device was proposed by sorting *P. falciparum*-infected RBCs (Fig. **5**) [57]. The device consists of a constriction matrix (35 rows and 630 columns of tapered constrictions), which has a thickness of 4.5 μm and is used to sort RBCs. The pore size decreases every four rows from bottom to top. The fluid flow in the constriction matrix is controlled by the upward filtration flow and the downward declogging flow. More deformable cells, such as noninfected RBCs, travel further up the matrix of funnel constrictions than less deformable cells, such as *P. falciparum*-infected RBCs at the late (trophozoite and schizont) stages of infection, which are blocked midway and separated from the main population.

Recently, the high-throughput analysis of RBC deformability with single-cell resolution is proposed through an image processing-based program [58]. By using this method, the RBC deformability of

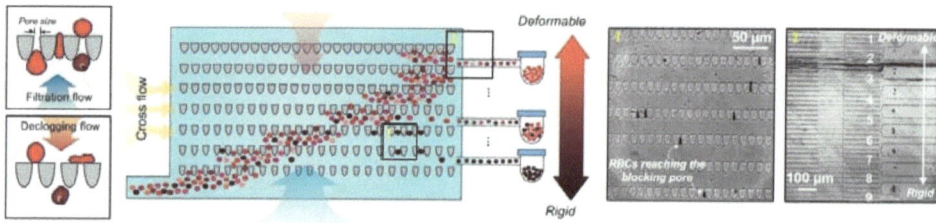

Fig. (5). Design of the ratchet-sorting device. Tapered funnel constriction allowing unidirectional flow of cells under oscillation excitation which consists of upward filtration flow, downward de-clogging flow, and cell sorting using a matrix of funnel constrictions. RBCs are introduced through the inlet, (1) transit the sorting matrix until reaching the blocking pore sizes, where (2) they proceed horizontally towards the appropriate outlet [57]. Copyright 2016 The Royal Society of Chemistry.

patients with sickle cell disease and healthy volunteers are monitored. In addition, the deformability and size of stored and packed RBCs are monitored to investigate the effects of blood storage.

Deformability of other Cells

The mechanical properties of cells have emerged as compelling biomarkers for estimating cell state and various disease processes [59]. The variation in cell deformability of invasive cancer cells compared with that of normal cells of the same origin are reported [60]. The changes in the cytoskeletal and the nuclear organizations accompanying differentiation, activation, pluripotency, or malignancy result in measurable changes in the mechanical properties of cells [28]. By adopting the conception of the aforementioned methods, the different deformability of living cells can be distinguished for the diagnosis of diseases. The increased rigidity of neutrophils is related to increased capillary retention, resulting in tissue ischemia seen in sepsis and acute respiratory distress syndrome [61]. A microdevice that is geometrically similar to capillary networks is proposed to measure the deformability of leucocytes [62]. The transit time passing through microchannels is measured by image processing. Results show that the leukostasis-symptomatic sample with low deformability have nine times higher transit time than the leukostasis-asymptomatic samples. The inflammatory mediators involved in sepsis are observed to significantly affect the magnitude of the neutrophil transit time. The deformability of individual normal and cancerous oral epithelial cells is serially investigated using microfluidic optical stretchers [63]. In this device, a dual-beam laser trap deforms single cells in the suspension by two counterpropagating laser beams. The cancer cells rapidly deform upon stress application, and the extension reaches a plateau after about 0.2 s. The normal cells exhibit a retarded behavior. The cancer cells are 2.5 times more deformable and can be clearly distinguished from the normal cells due to the relatively low deformation resistance of cancer cells compared with that of normal cells. The increase in deformability is likely caused by the decrease in filamentous actin, which is reduced by 30% in cancerous keratinocytes compared with that in normal keratinocytes.

Di Carlo's group has proposed a hydropipetting method based on the extensional flow [27]. This method has relatively high throughput of approximately 2000 cells s^{-1}. In this method, hydrodynamic forces are used to align and apply stress to the cells in flow. In a curved channel, the cells are focused to the channel centerline by a combination of inertial lift forces and secondary flows in a series of asymmetric curving channels. The cells in a straight channel are tightly focused to the channel centerline, thereby mitigating offsets due to secondary flows. Moreover, the microchannel branches with the main channel with focused cells and two side branches with cell-free fluid. The two-branch flows are subsequently returned to the main stream with cell suspension to apply extensional flow to the central channel. The focused cells are deformed by the rejoining cell-free "sheath" fluid that increases flow velocity by narrowing the width of the branches [33]. This deformation is regulated by several hydrodynamic forces. The opposite directed pressure gradients induced by the incident sheath fluid is estimated by a pressure drag (F_D) expressed as follows:

$$F_D = 0.5\rho U^2 C_D A_P \tag{4}$$

In this equation, ρ is fluid density, U is average transverse fluid velocity from the branch flow, C_D is the drag coefficient of a sphere, and A_p is the cross-sectional area of a sphere. The viscous force from the fast-moving sheath fluid leads to a net stretching force in the cell. The viscous stress is estimated as $\tau \sim \mu \dot{\gamma}$. By the combination of hydrodynamic forces, travelling cells are forced through a 2D fluid orifice formed at this interface that is conceptually analogous to a micropipette orifice. As shown in Fig. (**6A**), Jurkat leukemia cells and HeLa cervical cancer cells reveal separate deformability profiles, showing an inverse relationship between size and deformability. Based on the hydropipetting device, circulating tumor cells with increased size and deformability are distinguished from healthy blood and isolated in patients with cancer [64]. Otto and coworkers have proposed real-time deformability cytometry to improve the measurement rates for the diagnostic analysis [65]. The flow inside a microfluidic channel constriction can induce the deformation of cells without contact by shear stress and pressure gradient. As shown in Fig. (**6B**), the tangential (shear) and normal (pressure) stresses over a spherical cell's surface lead to the cell deformation from a spherical shape into a bullet-like shape. Given that the deformation is dependent

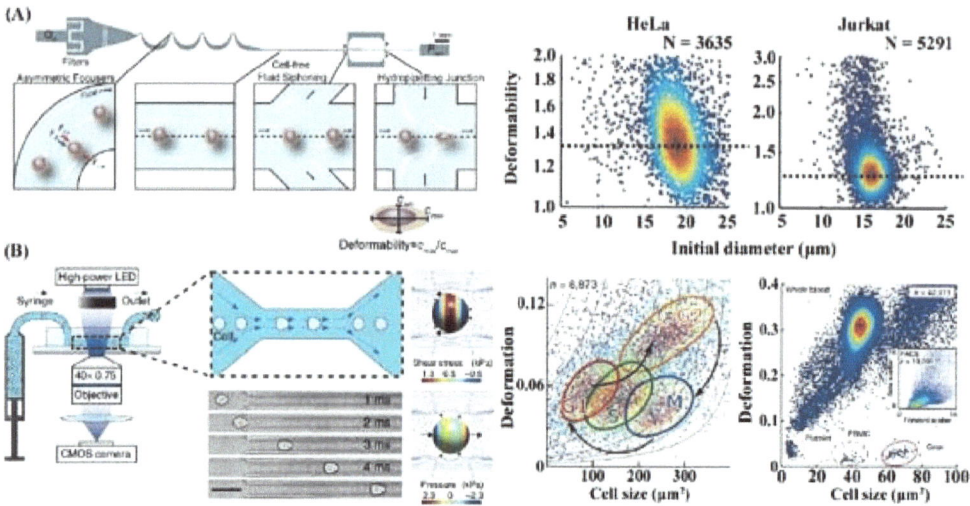

Fig. (6). (A) Method of hydropipetting. Cells are positioned in flow centerline by a combination of drag from the secondary flow, F_D, present in curving microchannels and inertial lift forces, $F_{L,s}$ and $F_{L,w}$. In the hydropipetting junction, the cell-free fluid incident on the focused cell suspension. HeLa cervical cancer cell deformability and Jurkat leukemia cell deformability [33]. Copyright 2013 The Royal Society of Chemistry. **(B)** Setup and measurement principle (inset shows top view of constriction). Time series of a cell deformed through constriction. Scale bar, 50 µm. Shear stress and pressure on the cell surface inside the constriction. 50%-density contour plots and measurement data of human leukemic (HL60) cells chemically synchronized in G1, S, G2 and M phases of the cell cycle. scatter plot of whole blood (diluted 1:50 in PBS containing 0.5% methylcellulose). Three distinct subpopulations are circled with red dotted (platelets), dashed (peripheral blood mononucleated cells, PBMC) and solid lines (granulocytes, gran) [65]. Copyright 2015 Nature Publishing.

on cell size, deformation ($D = 1 - $ circularity) and size (cross-sectional area) are displayed as a scatter plot to quantify the cell deformation. The proposed method can distinguish human leukemic (HL60) cells that are chemically synchronized in different cell cycle stages. As the reference, the expected deformations of an isotropic linearly elastic sphere with given elastic modulus (E_0) have overlapped with the results. The changes in the actin cytoskeleton may contribute to the difference between the G2 and the M phase cells. The distinction of the G2 and the M phases with considerable decrease in deformation distributions becomes possible by using this method. In addition, HL60 cells are differentiated into granulocytes, monocytes, and macrophages. Finally, the cells in a mixed population, *i.e.*, whole blood, is assessed to have a rate of 40 000 blood cells in 85 s. Results show that abundant RBCs are clearly separated from the other cells by large deformation. The shift of the RBCs away from the other blood cells is helpful to identify the remaining populations as PLTs, peripheral blood mononucleated cells, and granulocytes.

Measurement of RBC Aggregation

RBCs are the most important component of the blood because they occupy approximately 45% of the physiological volume concentration (hematocrit). In plasma, RBCs are prone to form rouleaux (RBC aggregates) and 3D networks as a reversible process. The extent of RBC aggregation is affected by force balance. An aggregating force is induced by the presence of macromolecules, and disaggregating forces include the negative surface charge and shear force developed in blood flows [66]. The shear dependence of viscosity is attributed to RBC aggregation, which is of interest in hemorheology. Specifically, a large formation of RBC aggregates under low-shear conditions lead to the elevation of blood viscosity. Moreover, the RBC aggregation is affected by the presence and concentrations of macromolecules in the plasma (fibrinogen or dextran). The hyperaggregation of RBCs significantly impedes blood flow in blood vessels and increase vascular flow resistance [67, 68]. In addition, the increase in RBC aggregation is somewhat correlated with various CVDs [69, 70] and diabetes mellitus [71, 72]. The two hypotheses (bridging and depletion) are proposed to explain RBC aggregation [73]. The bridge model insists that the RBCs are aggregated due to the attractive forces caused by the adsorption of the macromolecules on the cell surfaces. The depletion model insists that the osmotic force in the vicinity of RBCs leads to RBC aggregation when the macromolecule concentration near the cell surface is low [68].

In terms of data acquisition, several assessment techniques for the RBC aggregation can be classified into direct [74 - 76], and indirect measurements. Indirect measurement techniques include erythrocyte sedimentation rate (ESR) [77, 78], ultrasonic [79 - 81], electrorheological [82], and light transmission or reflection methods [83]. The aforementioned techniques have merits and demerits in terms of complexity and practicality [84].

Various phenomena related to RBC aggregation have been directly investigated using microscopy [75, 85]. For example, the alteration in RBC aggregation changes the thickness of a cell-free layer by modifying the lateral migration of RBCs [86, 87]. The formation and disaggregation of RBC aggregates in rectangular channels have been observed using time-resolved scanning confocal microscopy [88]. The plasma gaps in the captured blood images are detected on the basis of digital image processing techniques to directly evaluate the degree of RBC aggregation [74, 89] The size and the flow velocity of RBC aggregates in the microchannel are simultaneously measured by adopting the image processing method and the microparticle image velocimetry technique [90, 91]. The direct assessment techniques can monitor the size and dynamic motions of rouleaux, but the hematocrit of blood samples should be adjusted to less than 10% for the accurate quantification of RBC aggregation [76, 92].

Therefore, the degree of RBC aggregation has been measured mostly indirectly under various physiological conditions. The ESR method is first described by Westergren in 1921 [93]. The sedimentation rate in $mm·h^{-1}$ is determined by measuring the distance from the meniscus to the top of the column of sedimented RBCs in a 200 mm glass tube with a diameter of 2.5 mm for 1 h. The ESR measurement with minor modifications has been widely used clinically as a nonspecific indicator of inflammation in the diagnosis of chronic diseases [94, 95]. When the ESR values are higher than 30 $mm·h^{-1}$, further clinical investigation is required [73]. The ESR value highly depends on physiological conditions, such as plasma protein and hematocrit. The ESR value increases by 0.85 $mm·h^{-1}$ for each 5-year increase the in age-elevated levels of fibrinogen or high occult disease prevalence in the elderly. Particularly, the ESR value significantly reflects the degree of RBC aggregation [77]. Based on Stokes' Law, the settling velocity of a spherical particle in a medium is dependent on its size [96].

$$V_{Settling} = \frac{2g}{9} \frac{(\rho_{particle} - \rho_{medium})}{\mu} r^2 \tag{5}$$

$V_{settling}$ is the particle settling velocity, ρ is density, g is gravitational acceleration constant, μ is the medium dynamic viscosity, and r is the particle radius. Eq. 5 indicates that the $V_{settling}$ of a particle is dependent on its size. Thus, the large aggregates of RBCs have high $V_{settling}$ However, the conventional ESR method only provides a mean ESR value for each blood sample. Yeom and coworkers have proposed an index representing the degree of ESR [97]. The images of a blood sample in the syringe are acquired during RBC sedimentation. Through image processing, the boundaries between the sedimented RBCs and the RBC-depleted plasma are detected (Fig. 7). The volume of the sedimented RBCs (V_{RBC}) is gradually decreased with the lapse of time. The degree of RBC aggregation is controlled by changing the plasma dextran concentrations ($C_{Dextran}$) because the dextran treatment promotes the formation and propagation of RBC aggregates under a defined hemodynamic condition. As expected, V_{RBC} decreases as $C_{Dextran}$ increases. V_{RBC}/V_{Total} is approximately modeled as follows to quantify the variation in ESR in accordance with the physiological conditions.

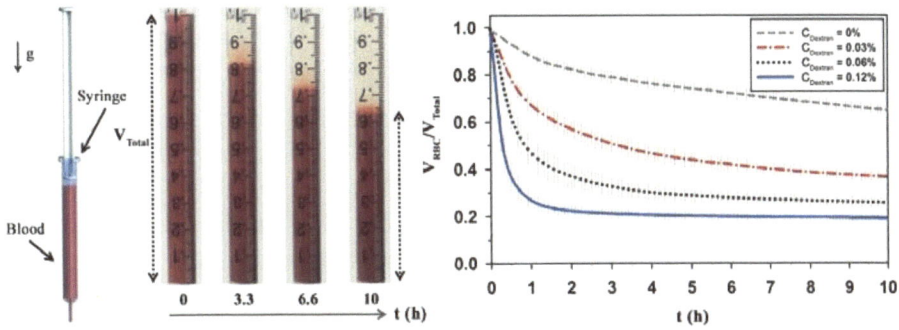

Fig. (7). Modified ESR method to measure erythrocyte aggregation. After loading a blood sample in the disposable syringe (1 ml), the syringe is vertically disposed at an inverted position. Typical images showing the sedimentation of RBCs in a blood sample with a total volume of 1ml with respect to time (*t*). Temporal variations of V_{RBC}/V_{Total} with respect to dextran concentration ($C_{Dextran}$) at hematocrit of 20% [97].

$$\frac{V_{RBC}}{V_{Total}} = \alpha + \beta \cdot e^{(-t \cdot \lambda)} \tag{6}$$

Three fitting parameters, namely, initial value (α), fitting constant (β) and characteristic time (λ_{ESR}), can be determined through regression analysis. Among the fitting parameters, λ_{ESR} decreases as the $C_{Dextran}$ increases. Low λ_{ESR} value can indicate the fast completion of the RBC sedimentation in a disposable syringe. By using λ_{ESR}, the diabetic blood (1.10 ± 0.41) can be distinguished from the normal blood (4.08 ± 0.34). However, the ESR method requires a long measurement time (h), and its measurement accuracy is influenced by several factors, including the installation angle and the surface condition of the specimen tubes.

The electrical properties of blood change depending on the hemorheological condition. As such, the electrical property has been monitored to obtain information about the degree and the time course of RBC aggregation [98, 99]. However, the electrical property cannot solely reflect the aggregation process. The light intensity (LI) analysis, which utilizes either transmitted or backscattered light through RBCs under a specific condition, has been widely used [100]. Prior to the measurement of RBC aggregation, the rouleaux completely disaggregate into separate RBCs under high-shear conditions. The LI is then recorded after a sudden decrement in $\dot{\gamma}$. On the basis of the measurement of light transmittance or reflectance, several commercially available instruments exist, in which cone-plate or rotational Couette shearing systems are used to adjust $\dot{\gamma}$ conditions [83, 101]. However, these rotational flows are somewhat different from real blood flow in blood vessels. In addition, the rotational shearing systems are expensive and require cleaning after each measurement.

Various microfluidic devices have been developed because microfluidic platforms have great potential for sensing and diagnostics when the rapid analysis of samples with low volumes is needed [97, 102 - 107]. Shin's group has estimated the degree of RBC aggregation by using a pressure-driven microfluidic aggregometer [102, 103, 105 - 107]. The LI of a laser beam scattered or transmitted by RBCs in the microchannel is measured under the pulse flow controlled by the vacuum generator. In light-backscattering aggregometry, the light scattered by the RBCs is captured by photodiodes. When a high pressure difference is initially applied, a strong shear flow starts to disaggregate the RBC aggregates with increased LI. Disaggregated RBCs reaggregate, and the corresponding LI decreases as $\dot{\gamma}$ decreases. In contrast to light-backscattering aggregometer, the transmitted aggregometer measures the transmitted LI, and LI increases with decreasing $\dot{\gamma}$. Thus, the decrease in shear flow induces the reduction of scattered LI due to RBC aggregation. The aggregation index, which is the ratio of the area above the syllectogram to the total area over the measurement time period, has been proposed to quantify RBC aggregation. The aggregation exhibits strong shear-dependent characteristics. The degree of RBC aggregation for heated RBCs is somewhat lower than that for normal RBCs due to the reduction of deformability. The critical shear stress is proposed to depict the RBC aggregability. As the reduced shear stress is applied to the microchannel flow, the aggregated RBCs start to disaggregate. When the microchannel flow is significantly decreased, the aggregated RBCs can resist the disaggregative shear flow. Thus, RBCs tend to aggregate, and the corresponding LI starts to decrease. The maximum LI over the running indicates the critical time, and the shear stress at the critical time is the critical shear stress. These indices can distinguish the difference caused by physiological variation, but measuring the pressure and LI separately is required to monitor the hemodynamic information accurately.

Similar to the pressure-driven microfluidic aggregometer, a micro-ESR with a solenoid pinch valve, a light-emitting diode, and photodetector is proposed [108]. The solenoid pinch valve disaggregates the RBCs after sample loading in the PMMA (polymethyl methacrylate) chip by inducing the back and forth motion of the blood. After finishing the operation of the pinch valve, the RBCs start to reaggregate. The LI of the transmitted optical signal increases until the RBCs completely aggregate. Three sedimentation indices from the transmitted LI are compared. The first index is calculated by taking the ratio of the area under the signal curve to the total area of the signal (120 s). The second index is the maximum amplitude of the LI, and the third index is the time when the intensity reaches half of the maximum value. Results show that the second index is suitable due to its almost linear increase with $C_{Dextran}$.

However, the LI transmitted through the channel does not accurately depict the degree of RBC aggregation [97]. Similar to the aforementioned method, the flow rate of the blood supplied in the straight channel is rapidly reduced to induce the formation of RBC aggregates after disaggregating.

As shown in Fig. (8), the optical images of blood flow darken as the hematocrit increases, and the formation of RBC aggregates caused by the decrease in flow rate creates speckle patterns with increasing intensity. Instead of LI, the normalized autocovariance function in the image plane is calculated to estimate the average speckle size from blood images. The average speckle area ($A_{Speckle}$) can be calculated by multiplying the horizontal and the vertical speckle sizes. As the flow rate decreases from 1 ml·h^{-1} to 0 ml·h^{-1}, the $A_{Speckle}$ gradually increases with time. The two fitting parameters, namely, the initial value (A_0) and the characteristic time ($\lambda_{Speckle}$), are obtained using the following fitting equation to quantify the increasing trend of $A_{Speckle}$.

$$A_{Speckle} = A_0 + e^{[(t-60)/\lambda_{Speckle}]} \tag{7}$$

where t is the measurement time. As $C_{Dextran}$ increases, $\lambda_{Speckle}$ is reduced, and A_0 increases. These results indicate that the high $C_{Dextran}$ create clear speckle patterns in a short time. From these results, $\lambda_{Speckle}$ can be used to reasonably estimate the

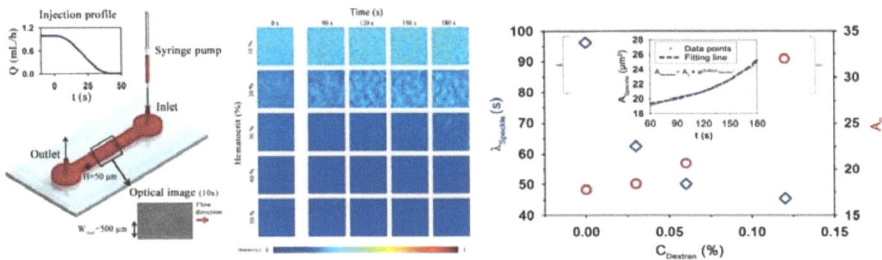

Fig. (8). Blood is supplied into the straight channel with a width of 1000μm and a depth of 50μm using a programmable syringe pump with decreasing flow rate from 1 to 0 mL/h. Speckle images of blood samples with respect to hematocrit level and elapsed time. The size of each image is 150 pixels, corresponding to 303.6μm in physical dimension. Quantitative evaluations of the characteristic time ($\lambda_{Speckle}$) and A_0 according to $C_{Dextran}$. Data points ($C_{Dextran}$ = 0.03%) and its fitting curve are included [97]. Copyright 2015 American Institute of Physics.

extent of RBC aggregation under various physiological conditions. The diabetic blood (54.8 ± 9.3 s) can be distinguished from the normal blood (96.1 ± 3.8 s) by using $\lambda_{Speckle}$. In addition to the diabetes, the degree of sepsis can be determined using this method by detecting the increase in RBC aggregation [109].

Measurement of Blood Viscosity

The shear viscosity of blood decreases with increasing $\dot{\gamma}$. Considering the relationship between blood viscosity and biological systems, the measurement of the blood viscosity is important for biological and medical applications. Several conventional viscometers, including a capillary type [110], rotating (cone-an--plate and Couette) [111, 112], and falling ball [113], viscometers, are widely used but suffer from some drawbacks [114]. In the case of capillary viscometers, the flow rate and pressure in a capillary tube should be measured, and regular calibrations are necessary to verify their credibility. In addition, conventional viscometers consume large sample quantities as a result of repetitive tests and inefficient time-consuming procedures [114]. In the last decade, microfluidic viscometers have emerged as alternative tools that can address the abovementioned limitations of conventional viscometers [16, 115, 116]. Depending on the basic principle underlying each viscometer, its methodology and representative results are described.

Surface Tension Viscometers

Surface tension viscometers are dependent on the capillary pressure (ΔP_C) and the wetting properties of surfaces to passively draw samples into the channels [110, 117]. ΔP_C is given by:

$$\Delta P_C = 2\sigma cos\theta \left(\frac{1}{H} + \frac{1}{W}\right) \tag{8}$$

where θ is the contact angle, and σ is the surface tension of the liquid. For Newtonian fluids, the viscosity is determined using the following equation when the flow is assumed as the Hagen–Poiseuille flow.

$$\mu = \frac{H^2}{S}\frac{\Delta P_C}{V(t)L(t)} \tag{9}$$

where $V(t)$ is the time-dependent velocity, $L(t)$ is the instantaneous length of the liquid column in the channel, and S is a constant specific to channel geometry. In case of a non-Newtonian liquid, the viscosity, which is a function of $\dot{\gamma}$, may either increase (shear thickening) or decrease (shear thinning) with increasing $\dot{\gamma}$ values. A simple empirical model called the power law expression is widely used to describe the non-Newtonian behavior.

$$\mu(\dot{\gamma}) = m\dot{\gamma}^{n-1} \tag{10}$$

where m is a constant depicting the fluid, and n is the power law exponent. Depending on the n value, the fluid can be considered as Newtonian ($n = 1$), shear-thinning ($n < 1$), or shear-thickening ($n > 1$) liquid. Based on the above equations and assumption ($H \ll W$), Srivastava and Burns have estimated a range of viscosities in accordance with the $\dot{\gamma}$ from a single experiment because the velocity of liquid interface varies with time in surface tension viscometers [110].

$$\mu(\dot{\gamma}) = \frac{H^2}{S} \frac{1}{\left(\frac{2}{3}+\frac{1}{3n}\right)} \frac{\Delta P}{V(t)L(t)} \tag{11}$$

Microfluidic surface tension viscometers, which consist of a long microchannel, have relatively simple operation without active or moving parts. The viscosity can be estimated by measuring the dynamic velocity and the length of a traveling liquid column. However, the device material is an important parameter because it dictates the wettability of the fluid. In this method, two parameters, namely, the geometric factor H^2/S and the driving ΔP, are critical for viscosity measurement. Two sealed and two open chambers are fabricated on the chip to obtain these parameters. The geometric factor is obtained by observing the velocity of the calibrating fluid (*e.g.*, water) in the open channel. The ΔP_C for the test fluid can be obtained by placing a drop at the inlet of the sealed chamber. The rheology of complex fluids, such as blood plasma, polyethylene oxide (PEO)–xanthan gum solutions, and polyacrylamide solutions, can be measured through robust self-calibration. The major advantages of the surface tension viscometer are extremely low consumption of sample (~0.6 µl), simple operation, and quick readout times (< 1 min) [117]. The limitations of this method are wetting defects, inability to access very high $\dot{\gamma}$, and complex flow issues caused by entrance effects.

Pressure-sensing Viscometers

The second instrument is microfluidic viscometers based on pressure sensing. By measuring the ΔP across a microchannel, viscosity can be estimated using the Hagen–Poiseuille equation for a one-dimensional flow as follows:

$$\mu(\dot{\gamma}) = \frac{WH\Delta P}{2l_0(W+H)}\frac{1}{\dot{\gamma}} \tag{12}$$

where l_0 is distance between the pressure sensors, and H denotes the width and height of a rectangular channel. As shown in Fig. (**9**), the embedded flush-mounted pressure transducers measure pressure in the microchannels with widths between 2 and 3 mm and depths lower than 100 μm for the validity of Eq. 13 based on low aspect ratios (<< 1) [118]. The pressure sensor array is mounted at a sufficient distance downstream of the inlet to neglect any entrance effects. In addition to the pressure sensor array [119], the pressure in microfluidic channels can be estimated through sideways tapping into the microchannel [120]. Another distinct approach to measure the pressure in the channel is by using pump-mounted pressure transducers [121]. However, such off-chip pressure transduction requires careful design and analysis considerations because the sensor is located away from the main microchannel, and some errors caused by the connection of channel and the entrance effects are considered in the overall ΔP.

The shear-thinning behavior of xanthan gum solution (blood analog fluid) and PEO and the worm-like micellar solution of cetylpyridinium chloride/sodium salicylate (CpCl/NaSal) in sodium chloride brine is clearly measured using the flush-mounted pressure transducers (Fig. 9). Over a wide range of $\dot{\gamma}$ values (20–1,000 s⁻¹), the shear-thinning viscosity of embryonic avian blood is measured using a microviscometer based on flush-mounted pressure sensors [122]. The viscosity of saliva is also estimated on the basis of this approach [123].

Considering the simplicity of pressure-sensing viscometers, the viscosity of complex fluids can be measured using a small sample volume (> 20 μl) with high $\dot{\gamma}$ (0.5–1,400,000 s⁻¹). However, the devices with the on-chip pressure sensor are not disposable. Given the active contact of the fluid and the pressure sensor, the devices should be washed after measurement especially if biofluids are used. Depending on the sensitivity of the pressure sensor, the measurement error can be involved in the results at the lowest $\dot{\gamma}$ values [16].

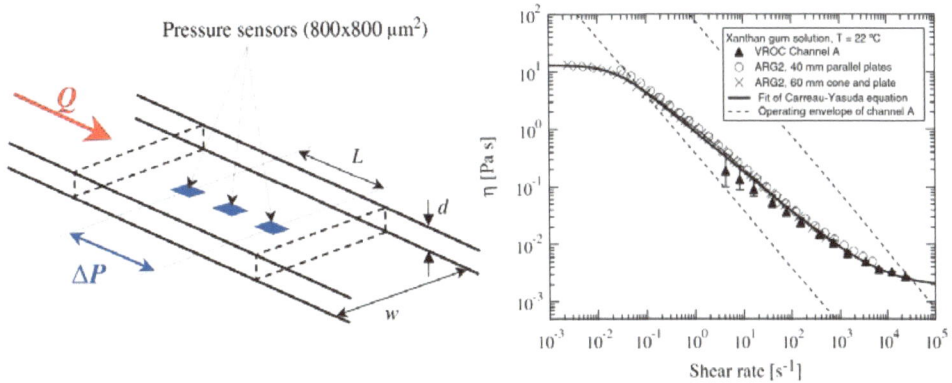

Fig. (9). Pressure sensing microfluidic viscometer with flush mounted pressure sensors. Variation of viscosity as a function of shear rate for aqueous xanthan gum solution (10^{-3}-10^4) [118]. Copyright 2008 Springer.

Flow Rate-sensing Viscometers

Similar to the working principle of pressure-sensing microfluidic viscometers, the viscosity can be determined by inserting the flow rate into Eq. 12 instead of measuring ΔP. The microcapillary rheometer, which is a miniature capillary viscometer, is combined with an in-line commercially available flowmeter to measure flow rate [124]. Hudson *et al.* have demonstrated that this device can measure the viscosity of antibody solutions (0.7–10 mPa·s) over a wide range of $\dot{\gamma}$ values over three decades (10–10,000 s_{-1}). Results are compared with those measured using a commercial device of m-VROC rheometer and are in good agreement. In addition, the total volume of samples consumed for each measurement are low (10 µl).

As an alternative to flow rate-sensing viscometers, the iCapillary is proposed by Solomon *et al.* (Fig. **10**) [125]. Under fixed-pressure conditions, the flow rate is estimated by detecting the interface between the air and the sample in a glass capillary attached with the microchannel based on the small assumption effects of the Laplace pressure (< 5%) across a relatively large diameter capillary. A smartphone camera is used to record the interface motion. The iCapillary viscometer can measure the viscosity of PEO solutions over a wide range of $\dot{\gamma}$ values (10–10,000 s^{-1}). The parallel analysis of bovine serum albumin (BSA) solutions (5–250 mg·ml^{-1}) is conducted using multiple capillaries.

The flow rate-sensing viscometers are adaptable to the parallel analysis of samples, but achieving viscosity data at extremely high $\dot{\gamma}$ values (> 10,000 s^{-1}) is difficult due to the limitation of flow rate sensors. Another limitation is that these

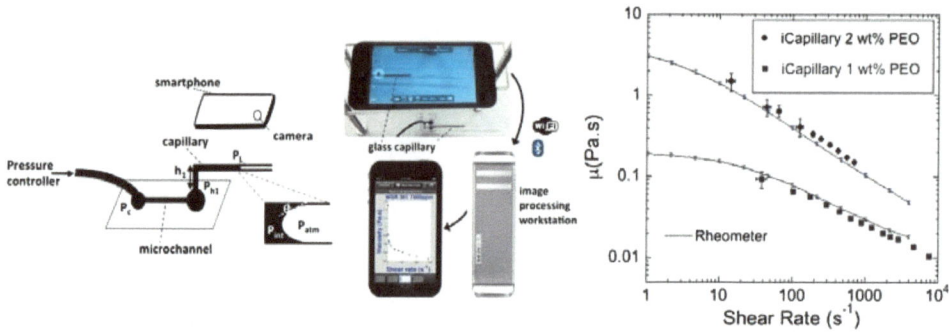

Fig. (10). An i capillary viscometer setup and operation. Viscosity values of 2 wt% (circles) and 1 wt% (squares) concentrations of PEO solution [125]. Copyright 2016 Springer.

viscometers require pressure controllers to impose fixed-pressure conditions, thereby requiring additional instrumentation compared with other simpler techniques.

Co-flowing Stream Viscometers

Microfluidic devices that use co-flowing laminar streams have been proposed [126 - 128]. In this method, two fluids, one with well-known viscosity (reference fluid) and the other with unknown viscosity (test sample), are delivered through each inlet and form an interface between the two streams in the confluence region [129, 130]. The geometry of devices is either a T- [127] or Y-junction [109, 131] or a cross-channel [132]. The interface between two co-flowing laminar streams in the confluence region is described by the inlet flow rates and viscosity to determine the viscosity of the test sample.

$$\frac{P_{Sample}}{P_{Reference}} = \frac{\mu_{Sample}}{\mu_{Reference}}\frac{Q_{Sample}}{Q_{Reference}} = f\left(\frac{W_{Reference}}{W}, \frac{H}{W}\right) \tag{13}$$

where the subscripts Sample and Reference indicate the properties of the sample and the reference fluids, respectively. The pressure ratio is a function of the relative width of the reference flows and the channel aspect ratio (H/W). f, a complex function, is simply dependent on the width ratio when the microchannel is a thin slit or the flow is one dimensional [133]. The mean flow rate (Q_{Sample}) of the test sample is evaluated by integrating the flow velocity along y, z transverse directions to the flow. In the case of a low aspect ratio or thin-slit channel, the mean $\dot{\gamma}$ can be expressed as:

$$\dot{\gamma}_{Sample} = \frac{3Q_{Sample}}{H^2 W_{Sample}} \qquad (14)$$

The viscosity of the test sample can be measured by experimentally measuring the width ratio and the injection flow rate. The first main method for co-flowing stream viscometry is the interface compensation method. Fig. (**11A**) shows the microfluidic device that can measure the viscosity of sample by manually matching the pressures of the reference and the blood streams [134]. The pressure difference between the reference and the sample streams can generate a flow passing through the bridge channel, which connects two identical side channels. When both pressures are the same (a hydrodynamic balancing [HB] state), no flow is observed in the bridge channel, as depicted in right inset (IV) of Fig. (**11A**). The viscosity of the test sample can be measured using Eq. 14.

$$\mu_{Sample} = \mu_{Reference} \frac{Q_{Reference}^{HB}}{Q_{Sample}^{HB}} \qquad (15)$$

The shear-thinning behavior of the blood sample under low-shear conditions can be measured using this device. Yeom *et al.* can distinguish the diabetic blood from the normal blood [135]. Choi and Park have measured the viscosity of BSA solutions depending on temperature [136].

The other approach is the interface displacement method. Under the given flow rates, the interface is allowed to freely form in the downstream of the channel (Fig. **11B**). Prior to the viscosity measurement, the relationship between the pressure and the width ratios $f(W_{Reference}/W)$ should be defined. The viscosity can be evaluated by measuring the width ratio and the following expression

$$\mu_{Sample} = \mu_{Reference} \, f\left(\frac{W_{Reference}}{W}\right) \frac{Q_{Reference}}{Q_{Sample}} \qquad (16)$$

On the basis of the increase in blood viscosity, the degree of sepsis is estimated using the co-flowing stream viscometers [109]. In addition to sepsis, malaria-infected RBCs have been distinguished on the basis of the ring, trophozoite, and schizont stages by Kang and coworkers [137]. Hong and coworkers have developed a 3D-printed microfluidic viscometer and validated their device by clinically comparing patients with diabetes and healthy volunteers [138].

In contrast to other viscometers, co-flowing stream viscometers are well suited for fluids with very low viscosity and can measure the viscosity of biofluids over almost one decade of $\dot{\gamma}$ variation (1-1000 s^{-1}) with relatively small sample volume (~0.1–1.0 ml). In addition, the implementation of this flow comparator-based technique is simple because pressure sensors are not required. The microfluidic geometry design is simple, and effect of surface tension can be negligible. However, a potential drawback is that the diffusion across the interface may preclude the accurate estimation of viscosity under extremely low-shear conditions. In addition, repetitive tests by using the same sample are difficult to due to mixing between the reference fluid and the test sample. Hydrodynamic instabilities can be observed in the comparator region at very high $\dot{\gamma}$ values [133].

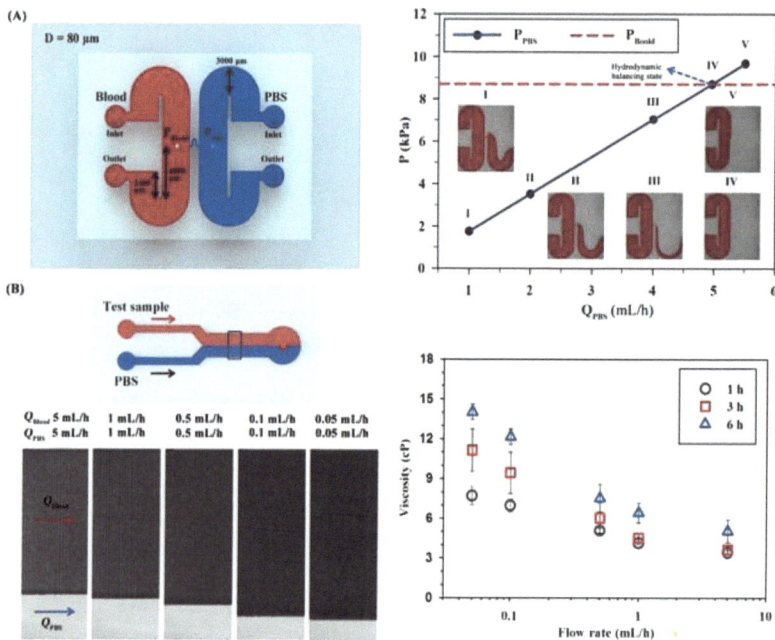

Fig. (11). (A) A microfluidic device with two identical side channels and a connecting bridge channel. The width and height of the channels are 3000 and 80 μm, respectively. Variation of pressure at the right side end of the bridge channel (P$_{PBS}$) according to the flow rate of PBS solution (Q$_{PBS}$). Pressure at the left side end of the bridge channel (P$_{Blood}$) is constant, because the blood flow rate is fixed at 1 mL/h [134]. Copyright 2015 Nature Publishing. **(B)** Measurement of variation in viscosity based on interfacial width between the test sample and PBS solution. The channel downstream has a width (W) of 3000 μm and a height (H) of 50 μm. Variations in blood viscosity according to flow rate and lapsed time after LPS injection [109]. Copyright 2017 Nature Publishing.

Measurement of Platelet Aggregation

PLTs, or thrombocytes, are anuclear cells with a discoid shape in inactive state (diameter of 2-4 μm). Although platelet are more abundant than WBCs, they constitute merely ~0.1% of the blood volume due to their small size. PLTs play an important role in wound healing; however, their influence on hemorheology is negligible. In their activated state, chemical signaling leads to plug formation and the induction of primary coagulation [139]. A multistep adhesion process between PLT membrane receptors and adhesive ligands efficiently enables adhesion under dynamic blood flows. Subendothelial matrix proteins [140], biochemical activators [141, 142] and hemodynamic features [143 - 145] contribute to cell adhesion mechanism. Among them high shear stress, induced by arterial narrowing, establish a potentially hazardous cycle of further PLT activation and thrombus growth [146]. In addition, the PLT activation plays a critical role in cardiovascular diseases including arteriosclerosis, stroke, and diabetes mellitus [139, 147, 148].

The mechanisms underlying PLT aggregation and thrombus formation are different depending on shear rate conditions to some extent. Under a relatively low shear condition (0 - 1,000 s^{-1}), PLT aggregation is primarily regulated by soluble fibrinogen [149, 150]. Fibrinogen support both adhesion and aggregation of PLTs by binding to glycoprotein (GP) IIb/IIIa receptor and integrin $\alpha_{IIb}\beta_3$ [142]. Under progressively high shear conditions, the fibrinogen plays a supportive role and von Willebrand factor (vWF) is more prominent [149]. The GPIb on the PLT engages in vWF [151]. When the shear rate is over 10,000 s^{-1}, the aggregation mechanism becomes exclusively influenced by the vWF engagement of GPIb [152].

Several devices were proposed to measure PLT functions [17, 145, 153 - 156]. A light transmission aggregometry (LTA) uses PLT-rich plasma (PRP) for testing PLT functions [153, 157]. However, LTA is time-consuming and difficult to standardize the PLT function. Given these reasons, alternative methods such as impedance aggregometry, rapid PLT function analyzer (RPFA), PLT function analyzer 100 (PFA-100, Siemens, Germany), 96-well plate aggregometry, and flow cytometry were developed to estimate PLT aggregation in PRP or whole blood [155, 158]. Although impedance aggregometry estimates the extent of PLT aggregation by measuring variations in electrical resistance [159, 160], relatively much sample volume is required and the analysis is time-consuming and expensive. The RPFA developed as a point-of-care instrument is based on monitoring integrin $\alpha_{IIb}\beta_3$ (GPIIb/IIIa) [161]. However, the measurement performance of this aggregometry is improved by the presence of fibrinogen-coated beads. The PFA-100 is composed of a sample reservoir, a capillary, and a biologically active membrane with a central aperture (collagen-epinephrine-coated or collagen-ADP-coated). A test sample is delivered from the reservoir through the capillary and the aperture under high shear rate conditions (5,000-6,000 s^{-1}). For quantification of PLT aggregation, the time which is necessary for a PLT plug to occlude the aperture is observed [162]. However, this method has limitation of sensitivity and specificity [155, 163]. Although the PLT aggregation can be measured using 96-well plate reader with relatively low sample volume [164], preparation of PRP sample is required for measurement. A flow cytometry assay was used to assess the PLT function from small volume of blood with low PLT numbers [165, 166]. However, this is quite an elaborate technique because blood sample should be divided into two parts by labeling PLTs with different biomarkers, washing away the excess of antibodies, and then reconstituting cells in a buffer solution with plasma prior to the actual assessment [158, 167].

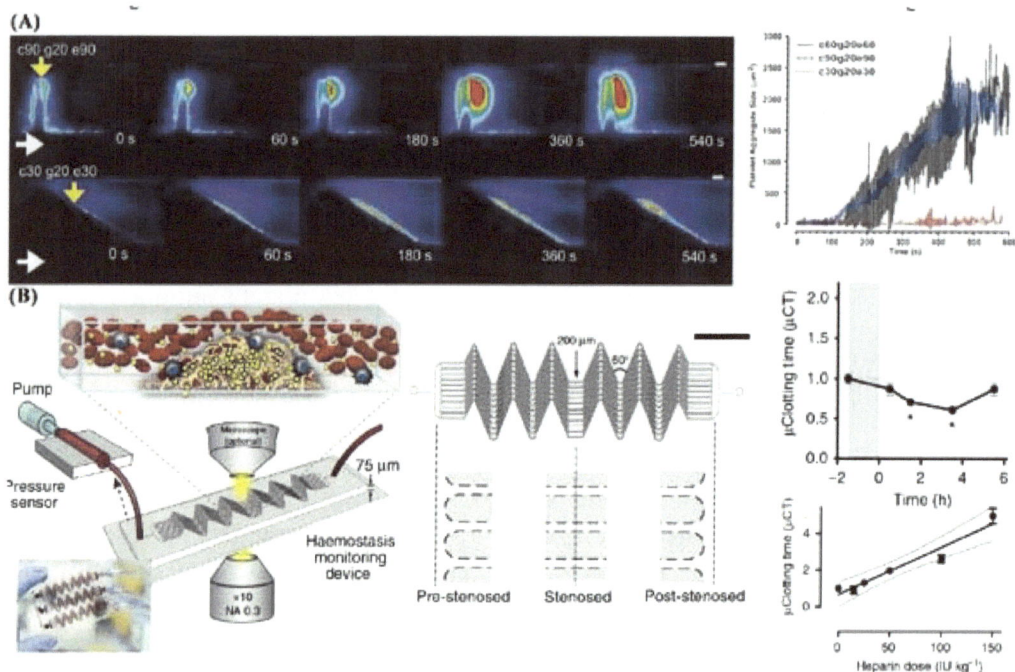

Fig. (12). (A) Representative epi-fluorescence image sequences of blood perfusion through the c90g20e90 and c30g20c30 microchannel cases (c [contraction angle], g [gap distance], e [expansion angle]); the yellow arrows denote the points of initial aggregation [t = 0 s], the white arrows designate the direction of blood flow (scale bar= 15 μm) [144]. Copyright 2010 The Royal Society of Chemistry. **(B)** Schematic of the haemostasis monitor device and method. Photograph of three haemostasis monitoring devices formed in a single piece of PDMS mould on top of a standard glass slide. The central stenosed region contains 12 parallel lanes of 200-μm-wide and 75-μm-high channels that repeatedly turn 60° a few times in each channel (scale bar, 500 μm). crofluidic clotting time (μCT) calculated using the microfluidic device attached to the femoral vein of a pig *via* a trilumen catheter. Heparin therapy model μCT (black circles) measured using the microfluidic haemostasis monitor [173]. Copyright 2016 Nature Publishing.

Microfluidic devices can measure the functions of PLTs in whole blood with or without using biomarkers [168, 169]. Especially, it is demonstrated that the microfluidic system can provide diagnostic information related to hemostatics [155]. For these reasons, several microfluidic systems have been developed by using small sample volume [143, 144, 167, 170 - 172]. The development of more complex microfluidic platforms with functionalized surfaces (endothelial cell; EC or collagen layer)c allows researchers to study the shear-mediated progression of PLTs activation [173 - 175]. Tovar-Lopez *et al.* checked formation of PLT aggregate depending on the degree of stenosis under *in vivo* condition and systematically investigated the effect of high shear gradients generated by vascular constrictions mimicking the stenosis on PLT aggregation *in vitro* [144]. As shown in Fig. (**12A**), different constriction geometries were designed ranging from gradual to immediate constriction, thereby generating a variety of shear gradients. The geometric properties of vessel constrictions establish distinct shear flows, inducing different aggregate formation and stabilization. However, the dynamics and mechanisms of PLT aggregation around stenosed vessels remain poorly understood. Shear-dependent PLT adhesion onto flow-modulating geometries precoated with vWF at physiological and pathological flows could show clinically relevant diagnosis of the disease.

The development of stenosis models for the use of clinical samples under physiological and pathological flows generated more sensitive readouts. Jain *et al.* mimicked as closely as possible stenosis in arterioles using a bifurcating channel system consisting of accelerating (prestenotic), constant (stenotic), and decelerating (poststenotic) sections [173]. This method uses clotting time as a marker of hemostasis levels in blood. Similar to clotting times in patients with bleeding disorders, clotting time control was shear-dependent at pathological flow rates. *Ex vivo* coagulation monitoring of a living pig can be possible by using this device (Fig. **12B**). It can provide great potential for real-time patient surveillance in a clinical setting. In addition, platelet function analysis with clotting time were monitored for healthy donors and patients with bleeding disorders taking aspirin and Plavix [173]. By measuring occlusion times and thrombus detachment in the device with stenosis coated by collagen, effects of antiplatelet therapy were clinically investigated [176]. To eliminate the need for lab-based evaluation of collected blood samples, correlation mapping method was applied to flow images to distinguish adhered platelets from flowing blood [177]. Each image was divided into small tiles ($m \times n$), and the 2D correlation coefficient (R) of two tiles is calculated. After labeling the centroid of the tile with R squared, the labeling process is repeated for all captured images. Application of the correlation mapping allows constant monitoring of biophysical markers of cardiovascular disease (diabetes and sepsis models) under *ex vivo* conditions without labelling [109, 135].

Besides to the bifurcating channel with the stenosed channel, DLD arrays in the microfluidic devices offer continuous-flow separation of particles suspended in a fluid (Fig. 13A). By using this flow disturbance around DLD arrays, the formation of blood clots were investigated under various biophysical conditions [178]. To quantify the blood clots, they used labelled WBCs because activated PLTs can be adhered with PLTs and WBCs. As shown in Fig. (13A), different clogging pattern expressed by labelled WBCs was observed depending on the DLD arrays. As the gap was reduced, it was observed that more clogging immediately after the beginning of the array, with short transportation of WBCs. Instead of flow disturbance induced by the obstacles in the microchannel, the rotating stirrer or rotors of the peristaltic pump was adopted to induce PLT aggregation (Fig. 13B) [145, 179]. Considering that high shear force can initiate PLT aggregation, this kind of collision in the microfluidic device can induce PLT aggregation. By measuring migration distance or area of correlation map, the function of PLTs can be easily estimated. Different biophysical parameters (PLTs and blood viscosity) can be distinguished in normal and diabetic rats [179].

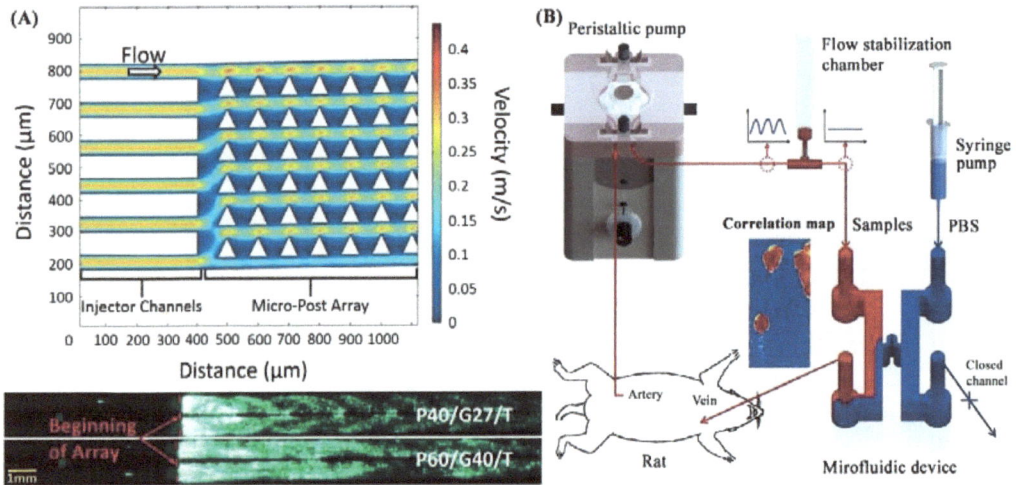

Fig. (13). (A) Color contour plot of the magnitude of the flow velocity in the injector channels and beginning of the DLD array. Injector channels are 40 μm wide, and the micro-post array is composed of 60 μm right isosceles triangles with 40 μm gaps. Fluorescent image of stained WBCs in whole blood entering two micro-post arrays (40 μm triangles with gap of 27 μm, and 60 μm triangles with gap of 40 μm) [178]. Copyright 2015 The Royal Society of Chemistry. (B) Schematic of the measurement system composed of a peristaltic pump, a flow stabilization chamber, and a microfluidic device. A correlation map depicting adhered PLTs of the microfluidic device is inserted. The outlet of the PBS flow is closed to induce an interfacial line between the PBS solution and blood sample. Blood is supplied by a rat extracorporeal loop. The blood and PBS solution mixture is returned to the jugular vein of the rat model [179]. Copyright 2016 Nature Publishing.

Nanofluidic Biosensors

Although various nanofluidic biosensors have been developed to detect organic components, such as enzymes, antibodies, DNA and amino acids *et al.*, most of them are many flower-shaped inorganic nanomaterials based on chemical reaction or electrical detection [5, 180]. There are few nanofluidic biosensors initiated by the flow characteristic. Diffusion viscometers can measure viscosity by using diffusive motion of nano-scale tracer particles. Particles suspended in a Newtonian fluid can be used to quantify its viscosity using the Stokes-Einstei--Sutherland relation [181].

$$\mu = \frac{kT}{3\pi d_p D} \tag{17}$$

where k is the Boltzmann constant, T is the temperature, d_p is the nanoparticle diameter, and D is diffusion coefficient of the nanoparticles. Diffusion viscometers offer distinct advantages. They are a convenient means to measure viscosity in the "absence of shear," with the benefits of small sample volumes, parallel analysis and high sensitivity in measurement. They offer a novel way to depict viscosity under local variations of temperature, pH, and so on. However, the limitations of diffusion viscometers are unstable in measuring rheology depending on particle size and chemistry, and unwanted interactions with the material [16].

CONCLUDING REMARKS

Throughout a fundamental understanding of hemorheology and blood flow and the advent of microfluidics technology, various microfluidic platforms precisely mimic blood systems to diagnose various diseases (Table 1). Microfluidic platforms based on hemodynamics mainly assess the pathophysiological behavior of cells by measuring membrane deformability; A disease marker and indicator of severity in malaria, sickle cell diseases, and cancer cell. Alternative detection methods for RBC aggregation and blood viscosity have emerged in recent years. Though these devices, variations in the hemorheology caused by the diabetes, the sepsis and malaria were detected. Besides hemorheological features, PLTs are involved in complex interactions of immune response and cardiovascular and other diseases. Functionalization of microchannel surfaces with ECs and associated proteins enables replication of complex diseases such as thrombosis. Microfluidic platforms with from simple laminar flow assays to complex model vasculatures distinguish different PLT dynamics and functions induced by cardiovascular diseases. Nanofluidic systems initiated by the flow characteristic are insufficient until now.

Table 1. Summary of microfluidic biosensors.

		Properties	Target Samples	Comment	Ref.
RBC Deformability		Capillary blockage	Malaria-infected RBC	Constriction channel Various channel width High shear flow	40
		RBC Velocity(cm/s)	Healthy valunteer RBC Hardend RBC	Mimicking Human microcirculation Kelvin-Voight model	43,34, 36,45, 49,50
		RBC Velocity(μm/s)	Malaria-infected RBC	Dissipative particle dynamics Triangle-shaped pillars High throghput	52
		RBC transit(Impedance change(cells/s))	Healthy adult and neonatal RBC	High throughoutput	44
		Pressure(Bar)	Hemolytic anemia	Funnel constriction	45
		Deformation index(L/D)	Degradation of store RBC	Centered RBC Parchute-like shape Focusing Flow	46
		Elasticity(μN/m)	Malaria-infected RBC	Extensional flow Cross-slot channel Wilcoxon rank-sum test	48
		Filtration time(s)	Hardend RBC with Glutaraldehyde	Filtraration channel	31
		Percentage of RBCs in each sorting outlet (%)	Malaria-infected RBC Hardended RBC	Constriction matrix Soarting infected RBC	57
		Single cell deformability index (μm/s)	Sickle cell disease & Storage monitoring	Single-cell resolution High throughput Automated image processing	58
		Other cells Deformability	Transit time(s)	Leukostasis Image processing	62
		Fraction of cells(%)	OSCC(Cancer cell)	Mechanical phenotyping Cancer cells	63
		CTCs in whool blood (mL)	CTCs	Circulating tumor cells Vortex-mediated deformability cytometry	64

(Table 1) cont.....

RBC Deformability	Deformation(1-circularity) and size(cross-section)	Leukostasis	Chemically synchronized in different cell-cycle stages	65
RBC Aggregation	Sedimentation rate(%)	Aggregated RBC with dextran	Image processing	97
	Light intensity (LI)	Hardened RBC	Light-backscattering aggregometer	100, 102,103, 105-107
Blood viscosity	Pressure drop(Pa)	Xanthan gum solution and PEO	Pressure-sensing Flush-mounted pressure transducer	118
	Flow rate(mL/s)	PEO	Flow rate-sensing	125
	Width ratio(%)	Diabetes RBC of rat	Co-flowing stream	135-138
Platelet aggregation	PLT aggregation size(μm^2)	Stenosis on PLT aggregation *in vitro*	Shear-dependent PLT adhesion	144
	Clotting time(s)	Bleeding disorders	Hemostasis level	173
	Brightness(a.u.)	Healthy valunteer whole blood	Micro-post array Rare cell capture.	178
	Platelet adhesion index ($mm^2 \cdot s$)	Diabetic rats	Rotating stirrer or rotors	179

As summarized in Table **2**, commercialized products for the clinical measurement of haemorheological properties were focused on a single property rather than multiple properties. To effectively diagnose haematological diseases, comprehensive analysis of haemorheological properties should be considered. Thus, a microfluidic platform, which can simultaneous measurements of haemorheological properties from a blood sample with a small volume, needs to be developed. In addition, most techniques require bulk-sized instruments, including a microscope and a high-speed camera to visualize inside of chips, and the pump. In the near future, a miniaturised device will be employed to diagnose haematological disorders and to screen effective treatment methods for curing them.

Table 2. Summary of commercial products for measurement of haemorheological properties.

Measurement Properties	Commercial products
Viscosity	Hemathix Blood Analyzer (Health Onvector, USA) EMS-1000S (Kyoto electronics, Japan) Viscore (Nano Biz, Korea)

Measurement Properties	Commercial products
RBC Deformability & RBC aggregation	LORRCA (RR Mechatronics, netherlands) Rheodyne SSD (Myrenne GmbH,. Germany) RheoScan(RheoMeditech, Korea)
ESR	ESR 2010(labONE, India) Starrsed ST (RR Mechatronics, netherlands)

The ongoing development of microfluidic and nanofluidic systems may result in a new analytical methodology based on a microfluidic platform with miniature instruments for clinical application and point-of-care diagnostics and identify new disease markers in the near future.

CONSENT FOR PUBLICATION

Not applicable.

CONFLICT OF INTEREST

The authors confirm that this chapter contents have no conflict of interest.

ACKNOWLEDGEMENTS

Hyeonji Hong and Suhwan Lee were acknowledged for searching and summarizing the articles in this chapter. This work was supported by the National Research Foundation of Korea(NRF) grant funded by the Korea government(MSIT) (No. NRF-2018R1A5A2023879).

REFERENCES

[1]   Fisher AB, Chien S, Barakat AI, Nerem RM. Endothelial cellular response to altered shear stress. Am J Physiol Lung Cell Mol Physiol 2001; 281(3): L529-33.
[http://dx.doi.org/10.1152/ajplung.2001.281.3.L529] [PMID: 11504676]

[2]   Dolan JM, Kolega J, Meng H. High wall shear stress and spatial gradients in vascular pathology: a review. Ann Biomed Eng 2013; 41(7): 1411-27.
[http://dx.doi.org/10.1007/s10439-012-0695-0] [PMID: 23229281]

[3]   Samady H, Eshtehardi P, McDaniel MC, et al. Coronary artery wall shear stress is associated with progression and transformation of atherosclerotic plaque and arterial remodeling in patients with coronary artery disease. Circulation 2011; 124(7): 779-88.
[http://dx.doi.org/10.1161/CIRCULATIONAHA.111.021824] [PMID: 21788584]

[4]   Chiu J-J, Chien S. Effects of disturbed flow on vascular endothelium: pathophysiological basis and clinical perspectives. Physiol Rev 2011; 91(1): 327-87.
[http://dx.doi.org/10.1152/physrev.00047.2009] [PMID: 21248169]

[5]   Esteves-Villanueva JO, Trzeciakiewicz H, Martic S. A protein-based electrochemical biosensor for detection of tau protein, a neurodegenerative disease biomarker. Analyst (Lond) 2014; 139(11): 2823-31.
[http://dx.doi.org/10.1039/C4AN00204K] [PMID: 24740472]

[6]   Vistas CR, Soares SS, Rodrigues RM, Chu V, Conde JP, Ferreira GN. An amorphous silicon photodiode microfluidic chip to detect nanomolar quantities of HIV-1 virion infectivity factor. Analyst (Lond) 2014; 139(15): 3709-13.
[http://dx.doi.org/10.1039/C4AN00695J] [PMID: 24922601]

[7]   Zhang M, Yin BC, Wang XF, Ye BC. Interaction of peptides with graphene oxide and its application for real-time monitoring of protease activity. Chem Commun (Camb) 2011; 47(8): 2399-401.
[http://dx.doi.org/10.1039/C0CC04887A] [PMID: 21305066]

[8]   Das G, Chirumamilla M, Toma A, *et al.* Plasmon based biosensor for distinguishing different peptides mutation states. Sci Rep 2013; 3: 1792.
[http://dx.doi.org/10.1038/srep01792] [PMID: 23652645]

[9]   Mishra GK, Sharma A, Deshpande K, Bhand S. Flow injection analysis biosensor for urea analysis in urine using enzyme thermistor. Appl Biochem Biotechnol 2014; 174(3): 998-1009.
[http://dx.doi.org/10.1007/s12010-014-0985-0] [PMID: 24907044]

[10]   Jing-Juan X, Hong-Yuan C. Amperometric glucose sensor based on coimmobilization of glucose oxidase and Poly(p-phenylenediamine) at a platinum microdisk electrode. Anal Biochem 2000; 280(2): 221-6.
[http://dx.doi.org/10.1006/abio.2000.4502] [PMID: 10790304]

[11]   Huang X, Leduc C, Ravussin Y, *et al.* A differential dielectric affinity glucose sensor. Lab Chip 2014; 14(2): 294-301.
[http://dx.doi.org/10.1039/C3LC51026C] [PMID: 24220675]

[12]   de-Carvalho J, Rodrigues RM, Tomé B, *et al.* Conformational and mechanical changes of DNA upon transcription factor binding detected by a QCM and transmission line model. Analyst (Lond) 2014; 139(8): 1847-55.
[http://dx.doi.org/10.1039/C3AN01682J] [PMID: 24352369]

[13]   Song Y, Zhang J, Li D. Microfluidic and nanofluidic resistive pulse sensing: A review. Micromachines (Basel) 2017; 8(7): 204.
[http://dx.doi.org/10.3390/mi8070204] [PMID: 30400393]

[14]   Kang YJ, Lee SJ. *In vitro* and ex vivo measurement of the biophysical properties of blood using microfluidic platforms and animal models. Analyst (Lond) 2018; 143(12): 2723-49.
[http://dx.doi.org/10.1039/C8AN00231B] [PMID: 29740642]

[15]   Zheng Y, Nguyen J, Wei Y, Sun Y. Recent advances in microfluidic techniques for single-cell biophysical characterization. Lab Chip 2013; 13(13): 2464-83.
[http://dx.doi.org/10.1039/c3lc50355k] [PMID: 23681312]

[16]   Gupta S, Wang WS, Vanapalli SA. Microfluidic viscometers for shear rheology of complex fluids and biofluids. Biomicrofluidics 2016; 10(4)043402
[http://dx.doi.org/10.1063/1.4955123] [PMID: 27478521]

[17]   Combariza ME, Yu X, Nesbitt WS, Mitchell A, Tovar-Lopez FJ. Nonlinear dynamic modelling of platelet aggregation via microfluidic devices. IEEE Trans Biomed Eng 2015; 62(7): 1718-27.
[http://dx.doi.org/10.1109/TBME.2015.2403266] [PMID: 25706500]

[18]   Schmid-Schönbein GW, Shih YY, Chien S. Morphometry of human leukocytes. Blood 1980; 56(5): 866-75.
[http://dx.doi.org/10.1182/blood.V56.5.866.866] [PMID: 6775712]

[19]   Fischer TM, Stöhr-Lissen M, Schmid-Schönbein H. The red cell as a fluid droplet: tank tread-like motion of the human erythrocyte membrane in shear flow. Science 1978; 202(4370): 894-6.
[http://dx.doi.org/10.1126/science.715448] [PMID: 715448]

[20]   Abkarian M, Faivre M, Horton R, Smistrup K, Best-Popescu CA, Stone HA. Cellular-scale hydrodynamics. Biomed Mater 2008; 3(3)034011
[http://dx.doi.org/10.1088/1748-6041/3/3/034011] [PMID: 18765900]

[21]   Wan J, Forsyth AM, Stone HA. Red blood cell dynamics: from cell deformation to ATP release. Integr Biol 2011; 3(10): 972-81.
[http://dx.doi.org/10.1039/c1ib00044f] [PMID: 21935538]

[22]   Pozrikidis C. Axisymmetric motion of a file of red blood cells through capillaries. Phys Fluids 2005; 17031503
[http://dx.doi.org/10.1063/1.1830484]

[23]   Chen YC, Chen GY, Lin YC, *et al*. A lab-on-a-chip capillary network for red blood cell hydrodynamics. Microfluid Nanofluidics 2010; 9: 585-91.
[http://dx.doi.org/10.1007/s10404-010-0591-6]

[24]   Sprague RS, Stephenson AH, Ellsworth ML. Red not dead: signaling in and from erythrocytes. Trends Endocrinol Metab 2007; 18(9): 350-5.
[http://dx.doi.org/10.1016/j.tem.2007.08.008] [PMID: 17959385]

[25]   McMillan DE, Utterback NG, La Puma J. Reduced erythrocyte deformability in diabetes. Diabetes 1978; 27(9): 895-901.
[http://dx.doi.org/10.2337/diab.27.9.895] [PMID: 689301]

[26]   Cranston HA, Boylan CW, Carroll GL, *et al*. Plasmodium falciparum maturation abolishes physiologic red cell deformability. Science 1984; 223(4634): 400-3.
[http://dx.doi.org/10.1126/science.6362007] [PMID: 6362007]

[27]   Gossett DR, Tse HT, Lee SA, *et al*. Hydrodynamic stretching of single cells for large population mechanical phenotyping. Proc Natl Acad Sci USA 2012; 109(20): 7630-5.
[http://dx.doi.org/10.1073/pnas.1200107109] [PMID: 22547795]

[28]   Cross SE, Jin YS, Rao J, Gimzewski JK. Nanomechanical analysis of cells from cancer patients. Nat Nanotechnol 2007; 2(12): 780-3.
[http://dx.doi.org/10.1038/nnano.2007.388] [PMID: 18654431]

[29]   Rand RP, Burton AC. Mechanical properties of the red cell membrane. I. Membrane stiffness and intracellular pressure. Biophys J 1964; 4: 115-35.
[http://dx.doi.org/10.1016/S0006-3495(64)86773-4] [PMID: 14130437]

[30]   Tsukada K, Sekizuka E, Oshio C, Minamitani H. Direct measurement of erythrocyte deformability in diabetes mellitus with a transparent microchannel capillary model and high-speed video camera system. Microvasc Res 2001; 61(3): 231-9.
[http://dx.doi.org/10.1006/mvre.2001.2307] [PMID: 11336534]

[31]   Shevkoplyas SS, Yoshida T, Gifford SC, Bitensky MW. Direct measurement of the impact of impaired erythrocyte deformability on microvascular network perfusion in a microfluidic device. Lab Chip 2006; 6(7): 914-20.
[http://dx.doi.org/10.1039/b601554a] [PMID: 16804596]

[32]   Wan J, Ristenpart WD, Stone HA. Dynamics of shear-induced ATP release from red blood cells. Proc Natl Acad Sci USA 2008; 105(43): 16432-7.
[http://dx.doi.org/10.1073/pnas.0805779105] [PMID: 18922780]

[33]   Dudani JS, Gossett DR, Tse HT, Di Carlo D. Pinched-flow hydrodynamic stretching of single-cells. Lab Chip 2013; 13(18): 3728-34.
[http://dx.doi.org/10.1039/c3lc50649e] [PMID: 23884381]

[34]   Huang S, Undisz A, Diez-Silva M, Bow H, Dao M, Han J. Dynamic deformability of Plasmodium falciparum-infected erythrocytes exposed to artesunate in vitro. Integr Biol 2013; 5(2): 414-22.
[http://dx.doi.org/10.1039/C2IB20161E] [PMID: 23254624]

[35]   Yaginuma T, Oliveira MS, Lima R, Ishikawa T, Yamaguchi T. Human red blood cell behavior under homogeneous extensional flow in a hyperbolic-shaped microchannel. Biomicrofluidics 2013; 7(5): 54110.
[http://dx.doi.org/10.1063/1.4820414] [PMID: 24404073]

[36] Rigat-Brugarolas LG, Elizalde-Torrent A, Bernabeu M, *et al.* A functional microengineered model of the human splenon-on-a-chip. Lab Chip 2014; 14(10): 1715-24.
[http://dx.doi.org/10.1039/C3LC51449H] [PMID: 24663955]

[37] Sakuma S, Kuroda K, Tsai CH, Fukui W, Arai F, Kaneko M. Red blood cell fatigue evaluation based on the close-encountering point between extensibility and recoverability. Lab Chip 2014; 14(6): 1135-41.
[http://dx.doi.org/10.1039/c3lc51003d] [PMID: 24463842]

[38] Zhao Y, Chen D, Luo Y, *et al.* Simultaneous characterization of instantaneous Young's modulus and specific membrane capacitance of single cells using a microfluidic system. Sensors (Basel) 2015; 15(2): 2763-73.
[http://dx.doi.org/10.3390/s150202763] [PMID: 25633598]

[39] Lu H, Koo LY, Wang WM, Lauffenburger DA, Griffith LG, Jensen KF. Microfluidic shear devices for quantitative analysis of cell adhesion. Anal Chem 2004; 76(18): 5257-64.
[http://dx.doi.org/10.1021/ac049837t] [PMID: 15362881]

[40] Shelby JP, White J, Ganesan K, Rathod PK, Chiu DT. A microfluidic model for single-cell capillary obstruction by Plasmodium falciparum-infected erythrocytes. Proc Natl Acad Sci USA 2003; 100(25): 14618-22.
[http://dx.doi.org/10.1073/pnas.2433968100] [PMID: 14638939]

[41] Forsyth AM, Wan J, Ristenpart WD, Stone HA. The dynamic behavior of chemically "stiffened" red blood cells in microchannel flows. Microvasc Res 2010; 80(1): 37-43.
[http://dx.doi.org/10.1016/j.mvr.2010.03.008] [PMID: 20303993]

[42] Lee SS, Yim Y, Ahn KH, Lee SJ. Extensional flow-based assessment of red blood cell deformability using hyperbolic converging microchannel. Biomed Microdevices 2009; 11(5): 1021-7.
[http://dx.doi.org/10.1007/s10544-009-9319-3] [PMID: 19434498]

[43] Tomaiuolo G, Barra M, Preziosi V, Cassinese A, Rotoli B, Guido S. Microfluidics analysis of red blood cell membrane viscoelasticity. Lab Chip 2011; 11(3): 449-54.
[http://dx.doi.org/10.1039/C0LC00348D] [PMID: 21076756]

[44] Zheng Y, Shojaei-Baghini E, Azad A, Wang C, Sun Y. High-throughput biophysical measurement of human red blood cells. Lab Chip 2012; 12(14): 2560-7.
[http://dx.doi.org/10.1039/c2lc21210b] [PMID: 22581052]

[45] Guo Q, Duffy SP, Matthews K, Santoso AT, Scott MD, Ma H. Microfluidic analysis of red blood cell deformability. J Biomech 2014; 47(8): 1767-76.
[http://dx.doi.org/10.1016/j.jbiomech.2014.03.038] [PMID: 24767871]

[46] Zheng Y, Chen J, Cui T, Shehata N, Wang C, Sun Y. Characterization of red blood cell deformability change during blood storage. Lab Chip 2014; 14(3): 577-83.
[http://dx.doi.org/10.1039/C3LC51151K] [PMID: 24296983]

[47] Schroeder CM, Babcock HP, Shaqfeh ES, Chu S. Observation of polymer conformation hysteresis in extensional flow. Science 2003; 301(5639): 1515-9.
[http://dx.doi.org/10.1126/science.1086070] [PMID: 12970560]

[48] Henon Y, Sheard GJ, Fouras A. Erythrocyte deformation in a microfluidic cross-slot channel. RSC Advances 2014; 4: 36079-88.
[http://dx.doi.org/10.1039/C4RA04229H]

[49] Preira P, Grandné V, Forel JM, Gabriele S, Camara M, Theodoly O. Passive circulating cell sorting by deformability using a microfluidic gradual filter. Lab Chip 2013; 13(1): 161-70.
[http://dx.doi.org/10.1039/C2LC40847C] [PMID: 23147069]

[50] Picot J, Ndour PA, Lefevre SD, *et al.* A biomimetic microfluidic chip to study the circulation and mechanical retention of red blood cells in the spleen. Am J Hematol 2015; 90(4): 339-45.
[http://dx.doi.org/10.1002/ajh.23941] [PMID: 25641515]

[51] Beech JP, Holm SH, Adolfsson K, Tegenfeldt JO. Sorting cells by size, shape and deformability. Lab Chip 2012; 12(6): 1048-51.
[http://dx.doi.org/10.1039/c2lc21083e] [PMID: 22327631]

[52] Bow H, Pivkin IV, Diez-Silva M, *et al.* A microfabricated deformability-based flow cytometer with application to malaria. Lab Chip 2011; 11(6): 1065-73.
[http://dx.doi.org/10.1039/c0lc00472c] [PMID: 21293801]

[53] Deen WM. Analysis of Transport Phenomena, Topics in Chemical Engineering. New York: Oxford University Press 1998; Vol. 3.

[54] Zhang ZM, Chien W, Henry E, *et al.* Sharp-edged geometric obstacles in microfluidics promote deformability-based sorting of cells. Phys Rev Fluids 2019; 4024201
[http://dx.doi.org/10.1103/PhysRevFluids.4.024201]

[55] Bowdler AJ. The complete spleen: structure, function, and clinical disorders. Springer Science & Business Media 2001.

[56] Mohandas N, Gallagher PG. Red cell membrane: past, present, and future. Blood 2008; 112(10): 3939-48.
[http://dx.doi.org/10.1182/blood-2008-07-161166] [PMID: 18988878]

[57] Guo Q, Duffy SP, Matthews K, *et al.* Deformability based sorting of red blood cells improves diagnostic sensitivity for malaria caused by *Plasmodium falciparum*. Lab Chip 2016; 16(4): 645-54.
[http://dx.doi.org/10.1039/C5LC01248A] [PMID: 26768227]

[58] Guruprasad P, Mannino RG, Caruso C, *et al.* Integrated automated particle tracking microfluidic enables high-throughput cell deformability cytometry for red cell disorders. Am J Hematol 2019; 94(2): 189-99.
[http://dx.doi.org/10.1002/ajh.25345] [PMID: 30417938]

[59] Di Carlo D. A mechanical biomarker of cell state in medicine. J Lab Autom 2012; 17(1): 32-42.
[http://dx.doi.org/10.1177/2211068211431630] [PMID: 22357606]

[60] Suresh S. Biomechanics and biophysics of cancer cells. Acta Biomater 2007; 3(4): 413-38.
[http://dx.doi.org/10.1016/j.actbio.2007.04.002] [PMID: 17540628]

[61] Skoutelis AT, Kaleridis V, Athanassiou GM, Kokkinis KI, Missirlis YF, Bassaris HP. Neutrophil deformability in patients with sepsis, septic shock, and adult respiratory distress syndrome. Crit Care Med 2000; 28(7): 2355-9.
[http://dx.doi.org/10.1097/00003246-200007000-00029] [PMID: 10921564]

[62] Rosenbluth MJ, Lam WA, Fletcher DA. Analyzing cell mechanics in hematologic diseases with microfluidic biophysical flow cytometry. Lab Chip 2008; 8(7): 1062-70.
[http://dx.doi.org/10.1039/b802931h] [PMID: 18584080]

[63] Remmerbach TW, Wottawah F, Dietrich J, Lincoln B, Wittekind C, Guck J. Oral cancer diagnosis by mechanical phenotyping. Cancer Res 2009; 69(5): 1728-32.
[http://dx.doi.org/10.1158/0008-5472.CAN-08-4073] [PMID: 19223529]

[64] Che J, Yu V, Garon EB, Goldman JW, Di Carlo D. Biophysical isolation and identification of circulating tumor cells. Lab Chip 2017; 17(8): 1452-61.
[http://dx.doi.org/10.1039/C7LC00038C] [PMID: 28352869]

[65] Otto O, Rosendahl P, Mietke A, *et al.* Real-time deformability cytometry: on-the-fly cell mechanical phenotyping. Nat Methods 2015; 12: 199-202, 4 p following 02.
[http://dx.doi.org/10.1038/nmeth.3281]

[66] Paeng DG, Nam KH. Ultrasonic visualization of dynamic behavior of red blood cells in flowing blood. J Vis 2009; 12: 295-306.
[http://dx.doi.org/10.1007/BF03181874]

[67] Ong PK, Namgung B, Johnson PC, Kim S. Effect of erythrocyte aggregation and flow rate on cell-free

layer formation in arterioles. Am J Physiol Heart Circ Physiol 2010; 298(6): H1870-8.
[http://dx.doi.org/10.1152/ajpheart.01182.2009] [PMID: 20348228]

[68]   Bishop JJ, Popel AS, Intaglietta M, Johnson PC. Rheological effects of red blood cell aggregation in the venous network: a review of recent studies. Biorheology 2001; 38(2-3): 263-74.
[PMID: 11381180]

[69]   Rainer C, Kawanishi DT, Chandraratna PA, *et al.* Changes in blood rheology in patients with stable angina pectoris as a result of coronary artery disease. Circulation 1987; 76(1): 15-20.
[http://dx.doi.org/10.1161/01.CIR.76.1.15] [PMID: 3594763]

[70]   Justo D, Mashav N, Arbel Y, *et al.* Increased erythrocyte aggregation in men with coronary artery disease and erectile dysfunction. Int J Impot Res 2009; 21(3): 192-7.
[http://dx.doi.org/10.1038/ijir.2009.6] [PMID: 19242480]

[71]   Le Devehat C, Khodabandehlou T, Vimeux M. Impaired hemorheological properties in diabetic patients with lower limb arterial ischaemia. Clin Hemorheol Microcirc 2001; 25(2): 43-8.
[PMID: 11790869]

[72]   Cloutier G, Zimmer A, Yu FT, Chiasson JL. Increased shear rate resistance and fastest kinetics of erythrocyte aggregation in diabetes measured with ultrasound. Diabetes Care 2008; 31(7): 1400-2.
[http://dx.doi.org/10.2337/dc07-1802] [PMID: 18375419]

[73]   Baskurt O, Neu B, Meiselman HJ. Red blood cell aggregation. CRC Press 2011.
[http://dx.doi.org/10.1201/b11221]

[74]   Kaliviotis E, Ivanov I, Antonova N, Yianneskis M. Erythrocyte aggregation at non-steady flow conditions: a comparison of characteristics measured with electrorheology and image analysis. Clin Hemorheol Microcirc 2010; 44(1): 43-54.
[http://dx.doi.org/10.3233/CH-2009-1251] [PMID: 20134092]

[75]   Barshtein G, Wajnblum D, Yedgar S. Kinetics of linear rouleaux formation studied by visual monitoring of red cell dynamic organization. Biophys J 2000; 78(5): 2470-4.
[http://dx.doi.org/10.1016/S0006-3495(00)76791-9] [PMID: 10777743]

[76]   Chen S, Barshtein G, Gavish B, *et al.* Monitoring of red blood cell aggregability in a flow-chamber by computerized image analysis. Clin Hemorheol Microcirc 1994; 14: 497-508.
[http://dx.doi.org/10.3233/CH-1994-14405]

[77]   Olshaker JS, Jerrard DA. The erythrocyte sedimentation rate. J Emerg Med 1997; 15(6): 869-74.
[http://dx.doi.org/10.1016/S0736-4679(97)00197-2] [PMID: 9404806]

[78]   Kang YJ, Ha YR, Lee SJ. Microfluidic-based measurement of erythrocyte sedimentation rate for biophysical assessment of blood in an *in vivo* malaria-infected mouse. Biomicrofluidics 2014; 8(4)044114
[http://dx.doi.org/10.1063/1.4892037] [PMID: 25379099]

[79]   Qin Z, Durand LG, Cloutier G. Kinetics of the "black hole" phenomenon in ultrasound backscattering measurements with red blood cell aggregation. Ultrasound Med Biol 1998; 24(2): 245-56.
[http://dx.doi.org/10.1016/S0301-5629(97)00273-1] [PMID: 9550183]

[80]   Nam KH, Yeom E, Ha H, Lee SJ. Simultaneous measurement of red blood cell aggregation and whole blood coagulation using high-frequency ultrasound. Ultrasound Med Biol 2012; 38(3): 468-75.
[http://dx.doi.org/10.1016/j.ultrasmedbio.2011.11.013] [PMID: 22264408]

[81]   Paeng DG, Nam KH, Choi MJ, Shung KK. Three-dimensional reconstruction of the "bright ring" echogenicity from porcine blood upstream in a stenosed tube. IEEE Trans Ultrason Ferroelectr Freq Control 2009; 56(4): 880-5.
[http://dx.doi.org/10.1109/TUFFC.2009.1113] [PMID: 19406719]

[82]   Pribush A, Meiselman HJ, Meyerstein D, Meyerstein N. Dielectric approach to the investigation of erythrocyte aggregation: I. Experimental basis of the method. Biorheology 1999; 36(5-6): 411-23.
[PMID: 10818639]

[83]   Hardeman MR, Goedhart PT, Dobbe JGG, *et al.* Laser-assisted optical rotational cell analyser
        (L.O.R.C.A.); I. A new instrument for measurement of various structural hemorheological parameters.
        Clin Hemorheol Microcirc 1994; 14: 605-18.
        [http://dx.doi.org/10.3233/CH-1994-14416]

[84]   Rampling MW, Whittingstall P. A comparison of five methods for estimating red cell aggregation.
        Klin Wochenschr 1986; 64(20): 1084-8.
        [PMID: 3784460]

[85]   Bishop JJ, Nance PR, Popel AS, Intaglietta M, Johnson PC. Effect of erythrocyte aggregation on
        velocity profiles in venules. Am J Physiol Heart Circ Physiol 2001; 280(1): H222-36.
        [http://dx.doi.org/10.1152/ajpheart.2001.280.1.H222] [PMID: 11123237]

[86]   Sherwood JM, Dusting J, Kaliviotis E, Balabani S. The effect of red blood cell aggregation on velocity
        and cell-depleted layer characteristics of blood in a bifurcating microchannel. Biomicrofluidics 2012;
        6(2): 24119.
        [http://dx.doi.org/10.1063/1.4717755] [PMID: 23667411]

[87]   Kim S, Kong RL, Popel AS, Intaglietta M, Johnson PC. Temporal and spatial variations of cell-free
        layer width in arterioles. Am J Physiol Heart Circ Physiol 2007; 293(3): H1526-35.
        [http://dx.doi.org/10.1152/ajpheart.01090.2006] [PMID: 17526647]

[88]   Patrick MJ, Chen CY, Frakes DH, *et al.* Cellular-level near-wall unsteadiness of high-hematocrit
        erythrocyte flow using confocal μPIV. Exp Fluids 2011; 50: 887-904.
        [http://dx.doi.org/10.1007/s00348-010-0943-8]

[89]   Kaliviotis E, Yianneskis M. Fast response characteristics of red blood cell aggregation. Biorheology
        2008; 45(6): 639-49.
        [http://dx.doi.org/10.3233/BIR-2008-0514] [PMID: 19065011]

[90]   Mehri R, Mavriplis C, Fenech M. Design of a microfluidic system for red blood cell aggregation
        investigation. J Biomech Eng 2014; 136(6)064501
        [http://dx.doi.org/10.1115/1.4027351] [PMID: 24700377]

[91]   Mehri R, Laplante J, Mavriplis C, *et al.* Investigation of Blood Flow Analysis and Red Blood Cell
        Aggregation. J Med Biol Eng 2014; 34: 469-74.
        [http://dx.doi.org/10.5405/jmbe.1695]

[92]   Berliner S, Ben-Ami R, Samocha-Bonet D, *et al.* The degree of red blood cell aggregation on
        peripheral blood glass slides corresponds to inter-erythrocyte cohesive forces in laminar flow. Thromb
        Res 2004; 114(1): 37-44.
        [http://dx.doi.org/10.1016/j.thromres.2004.04.009] [PMID: 15262483]

[93]   Westergren ALF. Studies of the suspension stability of the blood in pulmonary tuberculosis. Acta Med
        Scand 1921; 54: 247-82.
        [http://dx.doi.org/10.1111/j.0954-6820.1921.tb15179.x]

[94]   Jou JM, Lewis SM, Briggs C, Lee SH, De La Salle B, McFadden S. ICSH review of the measurement
        of the erythrocyte sedimentation rate. Int J Lab Hematol 2011; 33(2): 125-32.
        [http://dx.doi.org/10.1111/j.1751-553X.2011.01302.x] [PMID: 21352508]

[95]   Bull BS, Caswell M, Ernst E, *et al.* ICSH recommendations for measurement of erythrocyte
        sedimentation rate. J Clin Pathol 1993; 46(3): 198-203.
        [http://dx.doi.org/10.1136/jcp.46.3.198] [PMID: 8463411]

[96]   Stokes GG. On the effect of the internal friction of fluids on the motion of pendulums. Pitt Press
        Cambridge 1851; Vol. 9.

[97]   Yeom E, Lee SJ. Microfluidic-based speckle analysis for sensitive measurement of erythrocyte
        aggregation: A comparison of four methods for detection of elevated erythrocyte aggregation in
        diabetic rat blood. Biomicrofluidics 2015; 9(2)024110
        [http://dx.doi.org/10.1063/1.4917023] [PMID: 25945136]

[98]   Antonova N, Riha P, Ivanov I. Time dependent variation of human blood conductivity as a method for an estimation of RBC aggregation. Clin Hemorheol Microcirc 2008; 39(1-4): 69-78.
[http://dx.doi.org/10.3233/CH-2008-1114] [PMID: 18503112]

[99]   Balan C, Balut C, Gheorghe L, Gheorghe C, Gheorghiu E, Ursu G. Experimental determination of blood permittivity and conductivity in simple shear flow. Clin Hemorheol Microcirc 2004; 30(3-4): 359-64.
[PMID: 15258367]

[100]   Baskurt OK, Meiselman HJ, Kayar E. Measurement of red blood cell aggregation in a "plate-plate" shearing system by analysis of light transmission. Clin Hemorheol Microcirc 1998; 19(4): 307-14.
[PMID: 9972668]

[101]   Klose HJ, Volger E, Brechtelsbauer H, Heinich L, Schmid-Schönbein H. Microrheology and light transmission of blood. I. The photometric effects of red cell aggregation and red cell orientation. Pflugers Arch 1972; 333(2): 126-39.
[http://dx.doi.org/10.1007/BF00586912] [PMID: 4538028]

[102]   Lee BK, Ko JY, Lim HJ, Nam JH, Shin S. Investigation of critical shear stress with simultaneous measurement of electrical impedance, capacitance and light backscattering. Clin Hemorheol Microcirc 2012; 51(3): 203-12.
[http://dx.doi.org/10.3233/CH-2011-1526] [PMID: 22240385]

[103]   Shin S, Yang Y, Suh JS. Measurement of erythrocyte aggregation in a microchip stirring system by light transmission. Clin Hemorheol Microcirc 2009; 41(3): 197-207.
[http://dx.doi.org/10.3233/CH-2009-1172] [PMID: 19276517]

[104]   Kaliviotis E, Dusting J, Sherwood JM, Balabani S. Quantifying local characteristics of velocity, aggregation and hematocrit of human erythrocytes in a microchannel flow. Clin Hemorheol Microcirc 2015; 63(2): 123-48.
[http://dx.doi.org/10.3233/CH-151980] [PMID: 26444611]

[105]   Nam JH, Xue S, Lim H, Shin S. Study of erythrocyte aggregation at pulsatile flow conditions with backscattering analysis. Clin Hemorheol Microcirc 2012; 50(4): 257-66.
[http://dx.doi.org/10.3233/CH-2011-1434] [PMID: 22240363]

[106]   Shin S, Park MS, Ku YH, Suh JS. Shear-dependent aggregation characteristics of red blood cells in a pressure-driven microfluidic channel. Clin Hemorheol Microcirc 2006; 34(1-2): 353-61.
[PMID: 16543657]

[107]   Shin S, Nam JH, Hou JX, Suh JS. A transient, microfluidic approach to the investigation of erythrocyte aggregation: the threshold shear-stress for erythrocyte disaggregation. Clin Hemorheol Microcirc 2009; 42(2): 117-25.
[http://dx.doi.org/10.3233/CH-2009-1191] [PMID: 19433885]

[108]   Isiksacan Z, Asghari M, Elbuken C. A microfluidic erythrocyte sedimentation rate analyzer using rouleaux formation kinetics. Microfluid Nanofluidics 2017; 21: 44.
[http://dx.doi.org/10.1007/s10404-017-1878-7]

[109]   Yeom E, Kim HM, Park JH, Choi W, Doh J, Lee SJ. Microfluidic system for monitoring temporal variations of hemorheological properties and platelet adhesion in LPS-injected rats. Sci Rep 2017; 7(1): 1801.
[http://dx.doi.org/10.1038/s41598-017-01985-w] [PMID: 28496179]

[110]   Srivastava N, Burns MA. Analysis of non-Newtonian liquids using a microfluidic capillary viscometer. Anal Chem 2006; 78(5): 1690-6.
[http://dx.doi.org/10.1021/ac0518046] [PMID: 16503624]

[111]   Krieger IM. Shear rate in the Couette viscometer. Trans Soc Rheol 1968; 12: 5-11.
[http://dx.doi.org/10.1122/1.549097]

[112]   Gent AN. Theory of the parallel plate viscometer. Br J Appl Phys 1960; 11: 85.

[http://dx.doi.org/10.1088/0508-3443/11/2/310]

[113] Cho YI, Hartnett JP, Lee WY. Non-Newtonian viscosity measurements in the intermediate shear rate range with the falling-ball viscometer. J Non-Newt Fluid Mech 1984; 15: 61-74.
[http://dx.doi.org/10.1016/0377-0257(84)80028-2]

[114] Kim H, Cho YI, Lee DH, *et al.* Analytical performance evaluation of the scanning capillary tube viscometer for measurement of whole blood viscosity. Clin Biochem 2013; 46(1-2): 139-42.
[http://dx.doi.org/10.1016/j.clinbiochem.2012.10.015] [PMID: 23099199]

[115] Liu M, Xie S, Ge J, *et al.* Microfluidic assessment of frying oil degradation. Sci Rep 2016; 6: 27970.
[http://dx.doi.org/10.1038/srep27970] [PMID: 27312884]

[116] Allmendinger A, Dieu LH, Fischer S, Mueller R, Mahler HC, Huwyler J. High-throughput viscosity measurement using capillary electrophoresis instrumentation and its application to protein formulation. J Pharm Biomed Anal 2014; 99: 51-8.
[http://dx.doi.org/10.1016/j.jpba.2014.07.005] [PMID: 25077704]

[117] Srivastava N, Davenport RD, Burns MA. Nanoliter viscometer for analyzing blood plasma and other liquid samples. Anal Chem 2005; 77(2): 383-92.
[http://dx.doi.org/10.1021/ac0494681] [PMID: 15649032]

[118] Pipe CJ, Majmudar TS, McKinley GH. High shear rate viscometry. Rheol Acta 2008; 47: 621-42.
[http://dx.doi.org/10.1007/s00397-008-0268-1]

[119] Pan LC, Arratia PE. A high-shear, low Reynolds number microfluidic rheometer. Microfluid Nanofluidics 2013; 14: 885-94.
[http://dx.doi.org/10.1007/s10404-012-1124-2]

[120] Chevalier J, Ayela F. Microfluidic on chip viscometers. Rev Sci Instrum 2008; 79(7)076102
[http://dx.doi.org/10.1063/1.2940219] [PMID: 18681739]

[121] Kang K, Lee LJ, Koelling KW. High shear microfluidics and its application in rheological measurement. Exp Fluids 2005; 38: 222-32.
[http://dx.doi.org/10.1007/s00348-004-0901-4]

[122] Al-Roubaie S, Jahnsen ED, Mohammed M, Henderson-Toth C, Jones EA. Rheology of embryonic avian blood. Am J Physiol Heart Circ Physiol 2011; 301(6): H2473-81.
[http://dx.doi.org/10.1152/ajpheart.00475.2011] [PMID: 21963831]

[123] Haward SJ, Odell JA, Berry M, *et al.* Extensional rheology of human saliva. Rheol Acta 2011; 50: 869-79.
[http://dx.doi.org/10.1007/s00397-010-0494-1]

[124] Hudson SD, Sarangapani P, Pathak JA, Migler KB. A microliter capillary rheometer for characterization of protein solutions. J Pharm Sci 2015; 104(2): 678-85.
[http://dx.doi.org/10.1002/jps.24201] [PMID: 25308758]

[125] Solomon DE, Abdel-Raziq A, Vanapalli SA. A stress-controlled microfluidic shear viscometer based on smartphone imaging. Rheol Acta 2016; 55: 727-38.
[http://dx.doi.org/10.1007/s00397-016-0940-9]

[126] Galambos P, Forster F. An optical micro-fluidic viscometer. ASME Int Mech Eng Cong Exp. Anaheim, CA. 1998; pp. 187-91.

[127] Guillot P, Panizza P, Salmon JB, *et al.* Viscosimeter on a microfluidic chip. Langmuir 2006; 22(14): 6438-45.
[http://dx.doi.org/10.1021/la060131z] [PMID: 16800711]

[128] Kang YJ, Yoon SY, Lee KH, Yang S. A highly accurate and consistent microfluidic viscometer for continuous blood viscosity measurement. Artif Organs 2010; 34(11): 944-9.
[http://dx.doi.org/10.1111/j.1525-1594.2010.01078.x] [PMID: 20946281]

[129] Vanapalli SA, van den Ende D, Duits MHG, *et al.* Scaling of interface displacement in a microfluidic

comparator. Appl Phys Lett 2007; 90114109
[http://dx.doi.org/10.1063/1.2713800]

[130] Groisman A, Enzelberger M, Quake SR. Microfluidic memory and control devices. Science 2003;
       300(5621): 955-8.
       [http://dx.doi.org/10.1126/science.1083694] [PMID: 12738857]

[131] Kim S, Kim KC, Yeom E. Microfluidic method for measuring viscosity using images from
       smartphone. Opt Lasers Eng 2018; 104: 237-43.
       [http://dx.doi.org/10.1016/j.optlaseng.2017.05.016]

[132] Nguyen NT, Yap YF, Sumargo A. Microfluidic rheometer based on hydrodynamic focusing. Meas Sci
       Technol 2008; 19085405
       [http://dx.doi.org/10.1088/0957-0233/19/8/085405]

[133] Solomon DE, Vanapalli SA. Multiplexed microfluidic viscometer for high-throughput complex fluid
       rheology. Microfluid Nanofluidics 2014; 16: 677-90.
       [http://dx.doi.org/10.1007/s10404-013-1261-2]

[134] Yeom E, Jun Kang Y, Lee SJ. Hybrid system for *ex vivo* hemorheological and hemodynamic analysis:
       A feasibility study. Sci Rep 2015; 5: 11064.
       [http://dx.doi.org/10.1038/srep11064] [PMID: 26090816]

[135] Yeom E, Byeon H, Lee SJ. Effect of diabetic duration on hemorheological properties and platelet
       aggregation in streptozotocin-induced diabetic rats. Sci Rep 2016; 6: 21913.
       [http://dx.doi.org/10.1038/srep21913] [PMID: 26898237]

[136] Choi S, Park JK. Microfluidic rheometer for characterization of protein unfolding and aggregation in
       microflows. Small 2010; 6(12): 1306-10.
       [http://dx.doi.org/10.1002/smll.201000210] [PMID: 20461729]

[137] Kang YJ, Ha YR, Lee SJ. High-throughput and label-free blood-on-a-chip for malaria diagnosis. Anal
       Chem 2016; 88(5): 2912-22.
       [http://dx.doi.org/10.1021/acs.analchem.5b04874] [PMID: 26845250]

[138] Hong H, Song JM, Yeom E. 3D printed microfluidic viscometer based on the co-flowing stream.
       Biomicrofluidics 2019; 13(1)014104
       [http://dx.doi.org/10.1063/1.5063425] [PMID: 30867875]

[139] Massberg S, Brand K, Grüner S, *et al.* A critical role of platelet adhesion in the initiation of
       atherosclerotic lesion formation. J Exp Med 2002; 196(7): 887-96.
       [http://dx.doi.org/10.1084/jem.20012044] [PMID: 12370251]

[140] Hansen RR, Tipnis AA, White-Adams TC, Di Paola JA, Neeves KB. Characterization of collagen thin
       films for von Willebrand factor binding and platelet adhesion. Langmuir 2011; 27(22): 13648-58.
       [http://dx.doi.org/10.1021/la2023727] [PMID: 21967679]

[141] Fabre JE, Nguyen M, Latour A, *et al.* Decreased platelet aggregation, increased bleeding time and
       resistance to thromboembolism in P2Y1-deficient mice. Nat Med 1999; 5(10): 1199-202.
       [http://dx.doi.org/10.1038/13522] [PMID: 10502826]

[142] Gogstad GO, Brosstad F, Krutnes MB, Hagen I, Solum NO. Fibrinogen-binding properties of the
       human platelet glycoprotein IIb-=IIIa complex: a study using crossed-radioimmunoelectrophoresis.
       Blood 1982; 60(3): 663-71.
       [http://dx.doi.org/10.1182/blood.V60.3.663.663] [PMID: 6286013]

[143] Nesbitt WS, Westein E, Tovar-Lopez FJ, *et al.* A shear gradient-dependent platelet aggregation
       mechanism drives thrombus formation. Nat Med 2009; 15(6): 665-73.
       [http://dx.doi.org/10.1038/nm.1955] [PMID: 19465929]

[144] Tovar-Lopez FJ, Rosengarten G, Westein E, *et al.* A microfluidics device to monitor platelet
       aggregation dynamics in response to strain rate micro-gradients in flowing blood. Lab Chip 2010;
       10(3): 291-302.

[http://dx.doi.org/10.1039/B916757A] [PMID: 20091000]

[145] Song SH, Lim CS, Shin S. Migration distance-based platelet function analysis in a microfluidic system. Biomicrofluidics 2013; 7(6): 64101.
[http://dx.doi.org/10.1063/1.4829095] [PMID: 24396535]

[146] Kroll MH, Hellums JD, McIntire LV, Schafer AI, Moake JL. Platelets and shear stress. Blood 1996; 88(5): 1525-41.
[http://dx.doi.org/10.1182/blood.V88.5.1525.1525] [PMID: 8781407]

[147] Ruggeri ZM. Platelets in atherothrombosis. Nat Med 2002; 8(11): 1227-34.
[http://dx.doi.org/10.1038/nm1102-1227] [PMID: 12411949]

[148] Colwell JA, Halushka PV, Sarji K, Levine J, Sagel J, Nair RM. Altered platelet function in diabetes mellitus. Diabetes 1976; 25(2 SUPPL): 826-31.
[PMID: 823064]

[149] Savage B, Saldívar E, Ruggeri ZM. Initiation of platelet adhesion by arrest onto fibrinogen or translocation on von Willebrand factor. Cell 1996; 84(2): 289-97.
[http://dx.doi.org/10.1016/S0092-8674(00)80983-6] [PMID: 8565074]

[150] Savage B, Almus-Jacobs F, Ruggeri ZM. Specific synergy of multiple substrate-receptor interactions in platelet thrombus formation under flow. Cell 1998; 94(5): 657-66.
[http://dx.doi.org/10.1016/S0092-8674(00)81607-4] [PMID: 9741630]

[151] Maxwell MJ, Westein E, Nesbitt WS, Giuliano S, Dopheide SM, Jackson SP. Identification of a 2-stage platelet aggregation process mediating shear-dependent thrombus formation. Blood 2007; 109(2): 566-76.
[http://dx.doi.org/10.1182/blood-2006-07-028282] [PMID: 16990596]

[152] Ruggeri ZM, Orje JN, Habermann R, Federici AB, Reininger AJ. Activation-independent platelet adhesion and aggregation under elevated shear stress. Blood 2006; 108(6): 1903-10.
[http://dx.doi.org/10.1182/blood-2006-04-011551] [PMID: 16772609]

[153] Cattaneo M, Cerletti C, Harrison P, *et al.* Recommendations for the standardization of light transmission aggregometry: A consensus of the working party from the platelet physiology subcommittee of SSC/ISTH. J Thromb Haemost 2013; 11: 1183-9.
[http://dx.doi.org/10.1111/jth.12231] [PMID: 23574625]

[154] Hansen RR, Wufsus AR, Barton ST, Onasoga AA, Johnson-Paben RM, Neeves KB. High content evaluation of shear dependent platelet function in a microfluidic flow assay. Ann Biomed Eng 2013; 41(2): 250-62.
[http://dx.doi.org/10.1007/s10439-012-0658-5] [PMID: 23001359]

[155] Santos-Martínez MJ, Prina-Mello A, Medina C, Radomski MW. Analysis of platelet function: role of microfluidics and nanodevices. Analyst (Lond) 2011; 136(24): 5120-6.
[http://dx.doi.org/10.1039/c1an15445a] [PMID: 22029043]

[156] Sinn S, Müller L, Drechsel H, *et al.* Platelet aggregation monitoring with a newly developed quartz crystal microbalance system as an alternative to optical platelet aggregometry. Analyst (Lond) 2010; 135(11): 2930-8.
[http://dx.doi.org/10.1039/c0an00474j] [PMID: 20877907]

[157] Gresele P, Harrison P, Bury L, *et al.* Diagnosis of suspected inherited platelet function disorders: results of a worldwide survey. J Thromb Haemost 2014; 12(9): 1562-9.
[http://dx.doi.org/10.1111/jth.12650] [PMID: 24976115]

[158] Michelson AD. Methods for the measurement of platelet function. Am J Cardiol 2009; 103(3) (Suppl.): 20A-6A.
[http://dx.doi.org/10.1016/j.amjcard.2008.11.019] [PMID: 19166709]

[159] Cardinal DC, Flower RJ. The electronic aggregometer: a novel device for assessing platelet behavior in blood. J Pharmacol Methods 1980; 3(2): 135-58.

[http://dx.doi.org/10.1016/0160-5402(80)90024-8] [PMID: 7392654]

[160] Mackie IJ, Jones R, Machin SJ. Platelet impedance aggregation in whole blood and its inhibition by antiplatelet drugs. J Clin Pathol 1984; 37(8): 874-8.
[http://dx.doi.org/10.1136/jcp.37.8.874] [PMID: 6206096]

[161] Smith JW, Steinhubl SR, Lincoff AM, *et al.* Rapid platelet-function assay: an automated and quantitative cartridge-based method. Circulation 1999; 99(5): 620-5.
[http://dx.doi.org/10.1161/01.CIR.99.5.620] [PMID: 9950658]

[162] Kundu SK, Heilmann EJ, Sio R, *et al.* Characterization of an *in vitro* platelet function analyzer, PFA-100(TM). Clin Appl Thromb Hemost 1996; 2: 241-9.
[http://dx.doi.org/10.1177/107602969600200404]

[163] Podda GM, Bucciarelli P, Lussana F, Lecchi A, Cattaneo M. Usefulness of PFA-100 testing in the diagnostic screening of patients with suspected abnormalities of hemostasis: comparison with the bleeding time. J Thromb Haemost 2007; 5(12): 2393-8.
[http://dx.doi.org/10.1111/j.1538-7836.2007.02752.x] [PMID: 18034764]

[164] Bednar B, Condra C, Gould RJ, Connolly TM. Platelet aggregation monitored in a 96 well microplate reader is useful for evaluation of platelet agonists and antagonists. Thromb Res 1995; 77(5): 453-63.
[http://dx.doi.org/10.1016/0049-3848(95)93881-Y] [PMID: 7778060]

[165] De Cuyper IM, Meinders M, van de Vijver E, *et al.* A novel flow cytometry-based platelet aggregation assay. Blood 2013; 121(10): e70-80.
[http://dx.doi.org/10.1182/blood-2012-06-437723] [PMID: 23303822]

[166] Fox SC, Sasae R, Janson S, May JA, Heptinstall S. Quantitation of platelet aggregation and microaggregate formation in whole blood by flow cytometry. Platelets 2004; 15(2): 85-93.
[http://dx.doi.org/10.1080/09537100310001645979] [PMID: 15154600]

[167] Harrison P, Lordkipanidzé M. Testing platelet function. Hematol Oncol Clin North Am 2013; 27(3): 411-41.
[http://dx.doi.org/10.1016/j.hoc.2013.03.003] [PMID: 23714306]

[168] Kim D, Finkenstaedt-Quinn S, Hurley KR, Buchman JT, Haynes CL. On-chip evaluation of platelet adhesion and aggregation upon exposure to mesoporous silica nanoparticles. Analyst (Lond) 2014; 139(5): 906-13.
[http://dx.doi.org/10.1039/C3AN01679J] [PMID: 24300894]

[169] Ruslinda AR, Penmatsa V, Ishii Y, Tajima S, Kawarada H. Highly sensitive detection of platelet-derived growth factor on a functionalized diamond surface using aptamer sandwich design. Analyst (Lond) 2012; 137(7): 1692-7.
[http://dx.doi.org/10.1039/c2an15933c] [PMID: 22349046]

[170] Reimers RC, Sutera SP, Joist JH. Potentiation by red blood cells of shear-induced platelet aggregation: relative importance of chemical and physical mechanisms. Blood 1984; 64(6): 1200-6.
[http://dx.doi.org/10.1182/blood.V64.6.1200.1200] [PMID: 6498335]

[171] Miyazaki Y, Nomura S, Miyake T, *et al.* High shear stress can initiate both platelet aggregation and shedding of procoagulant containing microparticles. Blood 1996; 88(9): 3456-64.
[http://dx.doi.org/10.1182/blood.V88.9.3456.bloodjournal8893456] [PMID: 8896411]

[172] Li M, Ku DN, Forest CR. Microfluidic system for simultaneous optical measurement of platelet aggregation at multiple shear rates in whole blood. Lab Chip 2012; 12(7): 1355-62.
[http://dx.doi.org/10.1039/c2lc21145a] [PMID: 22358184]

[173] Jain A, Graveline A, Waterhouse A, Vernet A, Flaumenhaft R, Ingber DE. A shear gradient-activated microfluidic device for automated monitoring of whole blood haemostasis and platelet function. Nat Commun 2016; 7: 10176.
[http://dx.doi.org/10.1038/ncomms10176] [PMID: 26733371]

[174] Para AN, Ku DN. A low-volume, single pass in-vitro system of high shear thrombosis in a stenosis.

Thromb Res 2013; 131(5): 418-24.
[http://dx.doi.org/10.1016/j.thromres.2013.02.018] [PMID: 23535566]

[175] Westein E, van der Meer AD, Kuijpers MJ, Frimat JP, van den Berg A, Heemskerk JW. Atherosclerotic geometries exacerbate pathological thrombus formation poststenosis in a von Willebrand factor-dependent manner. Proc Natl Acad Sci USA 2013; 110(4): 1357-62.
[http://dx.doi.org/10.1073/pnas.1209905110] [PMID: 23288905]

[176] Li M, Hotaling NA, Ku DN, Forest CR. Microfluidic thrombosis under multiple shear rates and antiplatelet therapy doses. PLoS One 2014; 9(1)e82493
[http://dx.doi.org/10.1371/journal.pone.0082493] [PMID: 24404131]

[177] Jung SY, Yeom E. Microfluidic measurement for blood flow and platelet adhesion around a stenotic channel: Effects of tile size on the detection of platelet adhesion in a correlation map. Biomicrofluidics 2017; 11(2)024119
[http://dx.doi.org/10.1063/1.4982605] [PMID: 28798854]

[178] D'Silva J, Austin RH, Sturm JC. Inhibition of clot formation in deterministic lateral displacement arrays for processing large volumes of blood for rare cell capture. Lab Chip 2015; 15(10): 2240-7.
[http://dx.doi.org/10.1039/C4LC01409J] [PMID: 25855487]

[179] Yeom E, Park JH, Kang YJ, Lee SJ. Microfluidics for simultaneous quantification of platelet adhesion and blood viscosity. Sci Rep 2016; 6: 24994.
[http://dx.doi.org/10.1038/srep24994] [PMID: 27118101]

[180] Zhu J, Wen M, Wen W, *et al.* Recent progress in biosensors based on organic-inorganic hybrid nanoflowers. Biosens Bioelectron 2018; 120: 175-87.
[http://dx.doi.org/10.1016/j.bios.2018.08.058] [PMID: 30176421]

[181] Arosio P, Hu K, Aprile FA, Müller T, Knowles TP. Microfluidic diffusion viscometer for rapid analysis of complex solutions. Anal Chem 2016; 88(7): 3488-93.
[http://dx.doi.org/10.1021/acs.analchem.5b02930] [PMID: 26940224]

Point-of-Care Portable *In-vitro* Diagnostics: Smartphones, Imaging, Sensing, Connectivity, and AI

Michael G. Mauk[1,*], Jinzhao Song[1], Changchun Liu[1,2] and Xianbo Qiu[3]

[1] *Mechanical Engineering and Applied Science, School of Engineering and Applied Sciences, University of Pennsylvania, Philadelphia, PA, USA*

[2] *UCONN Health, University of Connecticut, USA*

[3] *College of Information Science and Technology, Beijing University of Chemical Technology, Beijing, China*

Abstract: Microfluidic-based ("lab-on-a-chip") bioassays and sensors enable automated or simply-operated medical diagnostic testing in near real-time at almost any location. These diagnostic devices can be connected to networks, especially using smartphones, where the smartphone camera serves as an optical detector or means of image capture. In addition, the smartphone provides connected sensors, GPS, visual displays, user-friendly interfaces, and limited electrical power. The added communications, control, and computational capabilities foster a synergism that will widen the applications of POC devices in healthcare and facilitate data acquisition for machine learning and artificial intelligence to enhance diagnostics accuracy and expand medical knowledge. Here the technological developments for microfluidic devices in combination with consumer devices, such as smartphones, for integration into the Internet of Medical Things (IoMT), are reviewed.

Keywords: Internet of Medical Things (IoMT), Lab-on-a-Chip (LOC), Microfluidics, Medical Diagnostics, Point-of-Care (POC), Smartphones.

INTRODUCTION AND OVERVIEW

New developments in point-of-care (POC) diagnostics technology offer prospects for pervasive, miniaturized, rapid or real-time medical tests that will expand the horizons of healthcare by reducing costs, improving effectiveness, and widening their access. Realistic expectations for such technology in the near future include compact palm-sized—or even postage stamp-sized—devices, at a cost of $1 to $10 per test, providing results in time frames of less than 10 minutes to 1 hour.

* **Corresponding author Michael G. Mauk:** Mechanical Engineering and Applied Science, School of Engineering and Applied Sciences, University of Pennsylvania, Philadelphia, PA, USA; E-mail: mmauk@seas.upenn.edu

Such tests will become as ubiquitous as cellphones, and will be highly advantageous—if not essential—for many users and applications. POC diagnostics will be practical in doctor's and dentist's offices, school infirmaries, nursing homes, rural clinics, at border crossings, and even for home use and sold as over-the-counter products. Moreover, POC technology finds ever increasing uses at pharmacies, walk-in 'retail' medical clinics, and other outpatient centers. Rapid diagnostics tests are also needed by first-responders, paramedics, and emergency medical technicians. Furthermore, there is a growing need for monitoring those with chronic health problems, as well as companion diagnostics tests, to assess the efficacy of various therapies, such as cancer treatments. POC tests can provide appropriate, sustainable diagnostics technology for many resource-limited areas of the world currently lacking adequate healthcare infrastructure. More generally, POC diagnostics will enable or foster new paradigms for distributed, patient-centered, customized, and precision healthcare. Other applications for such and similar technology include forensics, food safety, environmental monitoring, quality assurance in biotechnology, and detection of bioterror agents.

Biosensors can measure patients' physiological variables in real-time, and transmit the results to the user, or over networks to healthcare providers, or to remote computers for more sophisticated analysis of measurements. POC or 'lab on a chip' (LOC) *in vitro* diagnostics generally refers to device technologies that process and analyze patient specimens, such as blood or urine, using microfluidic components. POC *in vitro* tests are, thus, more invasive than passive sensors. Also, the linking and integration of distributed POC tests *via* communications technology with healthcare information networks for purposes of data archiving and analysis presents significant challenges, since most of the biosensors are inherently electronic and thus, readily couple to wireless networks, POC devices tend to be somewhat bulkier, and typically comprise hybrid combinations of diverse technologies: fluidics, chemical processing, mechanics, thermal management, optics, sensors, transducers, and electronics. As described in this Chapter, Smartphones are proving a viable, cost-effective, and versatile platform for interconnecting LOC devices for POC diagnostics and other applications. This is most often implemented through the Smartphone camera for diagnostic imaging or as an optical detector, as well as with other accessory sensors coupled to the Smartphone. This connectivity will allow POC devices, along with passive biosensors, to be wirelessly connected to computer networks for communications, computation, and various data archiving and information processing functions. POC devices will then be positioned to exploit capabilities stemming from machine learning and artificial intelligence available on networked and on-demand ('cloud') computing.

Biosensors and diagnostic devices will be components or nodes of the emerging *Internet of Medical Things* (IoMT), a network of connected medical technology, information and data resources, sensors, and portable communication devices that will transform healthcare. Connected POC diagnostics devices will be able to access more powerful computer resources, such as servers or data centers, as links to large computer networks for more intense computational analysis and access to databases. Moreover, as machine learning and artificial intelligence (AI) are applied to medical diagnostics in general, POC devices will also be able to exploit these developments to improve their accuracy and allow healthcare providers to better utilize test results. POC "testing for the masses" will also foster proactive patient-based initiatives, such as large-scale wellness pilot studies, along with direct-to-consumer testing and various self-testing services [1]. AI will enable digital health advisors or 'health coaches', using POC test data, to supplant clinicians for at least some simple or routine tasks [2].

As mentioned, it is relatively straightforward to wirelessly connect sensors that measure physiological variables, such as body temperature and heart rate, to such networks. There is less work and, as yet, no broad design consensus on the connection of *in vitro* diagnostics tests that require processing and analysis of patient specimens. For example, blood, saliva, urine, stool, vaginal swabs, or bronchial lavage.

It is instructive to consider POC LOC tests as comprising of three phases: pre-analytical, analytical, and post-analytical [3, 4]. The pre-analytical phase includes sample collection, which is specific to the type of specimen (*e.g.*, capillary whole blood vs. venous plasma) and its volume (*e.g.*, several microliters of blood finger prick vs. milliliters of urine), plus any need for immediate action to preserve sample integrity or deactivate harmful components. The analytical phase is the detection of disease biomarkers (*e.g.*, viral DNA, bacterial proteins, host antibodies), typically utilizing various immunoassays or Nucleic Acid Amplification Tests (NAATs), but also cell counting and image-based sample analysis, such as for malaria blood smears. Post-analytical steps include signal processing, data analysis, storage and transmission, and possibly clinical decision support. Tests are classified as invasive, non-invasive, or minimally invasive, and this is determined by the sample requirements and specimen collection method (*e.g.*, oral swabs, urine cup, venipuncture syringe, finger-prick blood collector) used for the test. Invasiveness is a key factor in promoting wide acceptance and use of a test, and there is much incentive to use non-invasive (*e.g.*, urine) or minimally invasive (*e.g.*, oral fluid) samples in small amounts, if feasible, rather than drawing blood. The analytical phase is addressed by an immense technology base of microfluidics [5, 6] (including 'paper based' [7, 8]) devices. However, since LOC devices are fluidic and mechanical in nature, they typically lack any built-in electronics to interface with networks. However, as reviewed here, this is being addressed by a growing trend to combine LOC devices with smartphones as optical detectors for microfluidic-based bioassays. Smartphones can offer additional integrated or accessory transducers and actuators, such as, temperature and pH sensors, microphones, LED light sources, and furthermore, can provide on-board data acquisition, computation, and control capabilities, friendly user interfaces, and small amounts of electric power. For example, Kuo *et al.* [9] demonstrated 'hijacking' power (7.4 mW) and bandwidth (8.8 kbits/s) from the mobile phone audio jack, turning an iPhone into an inexpensive oscilloscope, EKG monitor, and soil moisture sensor. More simply, to date, most Smartphone platforms, for point-of-care diagnostics, utilize merely the optical detection/imaging capabilities of the phone camera or other built-in or accessory sensors for detection, with very little or none of the control and power provision capabilities of the Smartphone. Some work in this regard includes a smartphone-controlled microscale fluidic handling system with elastomeric valves and a compact pneumatic system to implement the liquid handling functions for a bead-based immunoassay chip, with no human intervention [10]. Yafia *et al.* [11] described a smartphone system that commands a microcontroller to operate an integrated digital microfluidic (DMF) system. The low system power requirements permit the use of small lithium ion batteries. Currently, the Smartphone provides its most important contribution to the post-analytical phase of the test. By adding connectivity through the Smartphone, POC devices now have access to more powerful computation and data analysis, including machine learning and artificial intelligence.

Progress in POC diagnostics technology is enabled by advances in microfluidics, microfabrication, nanotechnology [12], polymer materials, rapid prototyping (*e.g.*, 3D printers), sensors, and biochemical assays. Wireless communication, ubiquitous cloud computing, machine learning, and artificial intelligence will substantially enhance the capabilities of POC devices and overcome technical and non-technical hurdles that have so far hindered wider applications of POC diagnostics. Because Smartphones are almost universal, their features and capabilities can help mitigate the implementation costs of POC. Also, mobile devices are already widely used in healthcare, and the Smartphone may well become the 'stethoscope of the 21st century" [13] with profound consequences in reversing the historic dependency role between patient and physician. The patient will no longer have to rely on the physician to take and interpret health-relevant data.

A typical POC *in vitro* diagnostics system will comprise a low-cost, single-use microfluidic 'chip' for sample analysis. Chips are typically credit-card sized plastic cartridges that host a miniaturized fluidic network for sample processing (*e.g.*, metering, separations, reactions) and analysis (*e.g.*, detection of target analytes). The chips have varying degrees of sophistication and may include filters, membranes, pre-loaded lyophilized reagents, integrated flow control (valves) or fluid actuation (pumps), as well as pouches and/or blister packs for fluid reservoirs. Alternatively, paper-based microfluidics, such as filter paper with flow paths defined by wax printing, offers an alternative implementation of microfluidics, especially for immunoassays and simple detection reactions. The chip is loaded with a patient sample at the point of care using a syringe, pipette, or swab. The sample-loaded chip may mate with a portable instrument or cellphone-based platform that provides heating or more sophisticated temperature regulation such as thermal cycling for PCR (polymerase chain reaction) analysis, external fluid actuation (*e.g.*, a bellows suction cup or small electric pump), optical or electrochemical detection, data acquisition, and communication. There is also a trend for non-instrumented or minimally instrumented chips that forego a companion instrument. For example, chips may utilize chemical heating methods, such as a ballasted exothermic water-activated oxidation reaction [14], to avoid the need for electrical mains or batteries, and rely on visible indicators (*e.g.*, color change) to report test results. However, such autonomous chips in themselves lack connectivity unless read with a cellphone camera.

In this review, developments of the last decade that move us closer to networked point-of-care diagnostics devices, and in particular, the leveraging of Smartphones and other portable communication and image/scanning technologies, to bring computation and connectivity to microfluidic-based bioassays, are surveyed. The focus in this review is on medical diagnostics, but much of the technology finds other uses, such as food safety [15], environmental monitoring [16], and veterinary applications [17]. Some common terminology for emerging healthcare technology and practices in this area are defined by Christodouleas *et al.* [18] and include *eHealth* (information technologies for healthcare), *telemedicine* (virtual interaction between patient and health provider, as well as remote monitoring of patients), *mobile health* or *mHealth* (technology that facilitates communication between patient and provider, and *eDiagnostics* that include low-cost medical test devices to analyze patient samples outside of laboratories, and in this context, with communication, such as provided by a mobile phone.

The Medical Diagnostics Landscape

Diagnostics, therapeutics, and discovery (research) are the triad of medicine are driven as much by technological progress such as x-rays, sensors, computers, lasers, and optics, as by expanding medical knowledge. Historically, diagnostics first used subjective interpretation of symptoms and patient medical histories. Instruments such as the sphygmomanometer, thermometer, and stethoscope made interpretation of symptoms less subjective. Microscopic examination of blood and other tissues provided reliable indicators of infections and other diseases. The wide use of blood tests began in the 1950s. *in vitro* assays included chemical analysis of blood components, serological tests based on antibody-antigen reactions (immunoassays), and later, nucleic acid-based tests based on analysis of DNA and RNA. Nucleic acid tests rely on the hybridization of labeled probes to target NAs, and often oligo primer-specific amplification of NAs, greatly increasing the signal, and thus providing the most specific and sensitive diagnostics assays. Digital (or droplet) PCR can yield absolute quantification of NA targets but involves considerably more complicated systems [19], and near-term will be probably limited in point-of-care applications. Digital LAMP (isothermal Loop-Mediated AMPlification) has also been used for antibiotic susceptibility testing in microfluidic devices, providing answers within 30 minutes [20]. Recently, there is an increasing role for nucleic acid sequencing in medical diagnostics for cancer [21] and liquid biopsies [22].

Complementary to *in vitro* tests described above, medical imaging began with x-rays and later expanded to include MRI, CAT scans, PET, and ultrasound, for which computers now enhance with image processing and analysis, machine learning, and artificial intelligence. Medical imaging was traditionally performed with expensive, bulky stationary instruments in centralized facilities, although lately, more portable instruments (mobile medical imaging) are enabling such imaging diagnostics closer to the point of care [23]. Similarly, inexpensive CCD and infrared cameras are widening the use of imaging methods, such as in dermatology and ophthalmology, allowing transmission and supplemented microscopy cellphone microscopes. Both types of diagnostics—*in vitro* and imaging—will be integrating into the IoMT, and will increasingly rely on machine learning and artificial intelligence.

POC Microfluidic *In-vitro* Diagnostic Devices

Clinical specimens, such as blood (whole, serum, or plasma), urine, oral fluid ('saliva'), stool, and less commonly used samples such as tears, sweat, bronchial lavages, or breath, can be analyzed for the presence and quantity of various disease markers, including toxins, pathogen or host nucleic acids and proteins, as well as host antibodies and metabolites. Historically, these tests were performed almost exclusively in highly-instrumented, automatized centralized facilities, often located in hospitals. Over the last three decades, such assays have been miniaturized for use outside of laboratories to bring diagnostics tests to the hospital bedside, doctor's office, or home. These labs on chip devices are realized with a variety of technology approaches using different materials (glass, plastics, silicon), fabrication methods (soft lithography, laser machining, Computer

Numerical Controlled (CNC) machining, stamping, injection molding), and methods of flow control, temperature control, fluid actuation, and detection of analytes. Sensitivity, in terms of Limits of Detection (LODs) and specificity, are the main performance metrics, but also important are: test turn-around time (time required between sample collection/introduction and test report), convenience or required skill level or needed training for operator, shelf life (especially if including pre-stored reagents), and cost of instrument and cost per test.

The simplest point-of-care devices are immunoassays, which can be realized with no instrumentation. Molecular diagnostics, such as Nucleic Acid Amplification Tests (NAATs), on the other hand, require more elaborate sample processing including lysis, NA isolation, amplification, and generally needing regulated heating, fluid actuation and flow control, such that substantially more complexity is necessary compared to immunoassays. O'Sullivan *et al.* [24] surveyed some new detection principles with potential applications to POC diagnostics including 1. Cavity-enhanced absorption spectroscopy where detection of a sample contained in an optical cavity provides a 50-fold improvement in sensitivity, 2. Plasmonic sensors based on detection of surface plasmons resulting from gold nanoparticle aggregation induced by an analyte, and 3. Digital microarrays based on particle confinement (*e.g.*, in drops or microwells) and single-molecule counting, which could provide three orders of magnitude enhancement in limits of detection.

Multiplexed tests can test for several or more pathogens, including HIV and hepatitis [25, 26]. Syndromic testing, in which groups of pathogens that produce similar symptoms are tested in a single, multiplexed test proves useful in many clinical situations where a multiplexed test can identify various agents associated with a presenting disease syndrome [27]. In addition to convenience, POC testing has other benefits over conventional diagnostics conducted in centralized laboratories or hospitals. Rapid test results feasible with POC tests are crucial in many strategies for controlling outbreaks of infectious diseases and epidemics. POC tests quickly determine infectious status allowing patients to modify their behavior to decrease spread of the infection, and also reduce patient anxiety in waiting for test results. POC testing can lead to considerable savings in healthcare costs [28]. Based on mathematical models, Ferguson *et al.* [29] surmised that anti-viral treatment of clinical cases could reduce transmission of influenza only if initiated within one day of symptoms, implying the need diagnostics tests with short (< 24 hr) turn-around times. POC real-time testing is also crucial in the monitoring and management of sepsis (severe inflammatory immune response to bacterial infection), where even an hour delay in diagnosis can significantly increase mortality [30].

The Smartphone as a Diagnostics Platform

Recently, there has been much work in combining POC devices with cellphones, and especially Smartphones (featuring an integrated microcomputer, digital camera, internet access, and GPS). Increased battery life, open source operating systems (iOS and Android) touch screens, sensors such as gyroscopes, rugged and waterproof construction, and large data storage are added and expanded features of Smartphones. The use of Smartphones is motivated in part as a means to reduce costs of implementation by leveraging ubiquitous cellphones (and their CCD camera) for detection, data acquisition and processing, control, display, and user-friendly interfaces. Smartphones have been adapted for colorimetry, microscopy, intensity-based fluorimetry, absorption or fluorescence spectroscopy, and surface-plasma based sensing, as well as electro chemoluminescence [31]. Implementations of smartphone-based instrumentation for public health safety, including water purity and food quality, are discussed by Jamalipour and Hoosain [32], who note that steady-state (rather than time-resolved) measurements are mostly the norm, and stable, uniform light sources are often technical challenges for applications based on measuring optical properties of bulk liquids or reflection from a solid surface. They also point out advantages or future prospects related to environmental monitoring, interactive maps, and 'augmented reality'.

Connectivity will add considerable diagnostics power by access to databases, cloud computing, and providing communication between healthcare networks, providers, expert systems, and patients. For instance, networked POC devices with GPS could track the spread of influenza or food poisoning. As a result, *in vitro* diagnostics tests can now become nodes of the internet of medical things (IoMT), a network of wearable sensors, home diagnostics kits, mobile healthcare (eMedicine or telemedicine) applications connected to healthcare information technology systems. Connected POC devices will likely serve a prominent role in the continued 'digital transformation' in healthcare, integrating the IoMT, advanced analytics ('big data'), machine learning, and artificial intelligence (AI) [33]. The expected benefits are improved outcomes with more timely and better targeted treatments, reduced costs, and increased accessibility. This chapter reviews the impact and potential of POC microfluidic devices with connectivity, computation, and artificial intelligence, as increasingly enabled by their integration or coupling with cellphone-based platforms.

Compared to immunoassays, such as lateral flow strips for home pregnancy (hormones in urine) tests, drugs of abuse (metabolites in saliva or urine) tests, and HIV (antibodies in saliva) tests, the pervasive use of POC tests, especially molecular tests, is still limited. POC tests are motivated by the need for more convenient diagnosis, facilitating testing and treatment at home rather than travel to hospitals, clinics, laboratories, or doctors' offices, a pressing need for an ageing population and rural areas far from healthcare services. POC testing will facilitate more frequent testing and monitoring, leading to more timely and appropriate treatments, ultimately lowering healthcare costs and helping relieve an overburdened healthcare system [34].

Although the main focus of this review is on *in vitro* diagnostics, and particularly immunoassays and NAATs, a brief survey of other diagnostics applications of Smartphones or related portable imaging/communication devices is included for perspective, and to show the versatility of smartphones in healthcare. Convenient and immediate communication and access to databases and other resources is a powerful tool for physicians in logging patient data and keeping track of therapeutic regimens. Ten years ago, physicians began using smartphones to replace personal digital assistances (PDAs), pagers, and laptops [35] for calendar and scheduling functions, accessing medical information and patient data, medical calculators, and input for patient billing data; as well as options for real-time video conferencing between patient and physician [34].

Smartphones in eMedicine/Telemedicine

Rapid infectious disease diagnostics with Smartphones are reviewed by Bates and Zumla [36], who noted that some aspects of telemedicine have a long history: such as the transmission of electrocardiograms by telephone in the 1950s. Phone cameras can capture images of patients' physical signs, such as dermatological issues, which can be transmitted for expert interpretation. Image quality is crucial in these applications. Text messages can be sent to patient smartphones to effectively improve adherence to medications and help modify patient behavior [37]. Mobile devices, including Smartphones, have transformed healthcare and are now common among healthcare professionals, and are used for information and time management, health record maintenance and access, communication and consulting, literature and drug reference data, patient management and monitoring, support for clinical decision making, and medical education and training [38]. A survey of the considerable resources for infectious disease healthcare available on iPhones, including digital media, dosage calculators, drug databases, outbreak information trackers, treatment guides, and study/review aids, has been made by Oehler *et al.* [39]. From the patient perspective, "information overload" will necessitate some types of data and information integration and co-ordination. As an indication, Friedman *et al.* [40] report that patients with chronic diseases may typically be treated by more than ten different physicians and receive over 50 drug prescriptions per year.

In allergy diagnostics, Smartphone Apps have been used to integrate traditional data (clinical history, physical examination, diagnostics tests, and patient-reported outcomes) with supplemental data from patient input regarding foods, embedded sensors in the Smartphone monitoring the environment and patient physiology, geolocation, as well as pollen and pollution data, in order to refine and personalize diagnostics [41].

Some implementations of POC devices into clinical practice have been reported. Hirst *et al.* [42] assessed the use of POC diagnostics for HbA1c (glycated hemoglobin, an indicator of blood sugar levels) in primary care settings for the management of diabetic patients. Such use of POC tests was feasible when operated by nurses who could spend 20 minutes per test, but less so by physicians when their patient face-to-face time was limited to around ten minutes. Pai *et al.* [43] described the integration of POC tests, cloud-connected Smartphone apps, laboratory testing, and healthcare data networks in providing diagnostics and engagement in screening and monitoring antenatal Indian women. The POCT and Smartphone enabled system was deemed feasible in providing screening for anemia, HIV, and other STDs and in expediting communications and linkages to clinical care for pregnant women in resource-limited settings.

A fundamental issue in distributed diagnostics relates to the location of where the sample is collected, analyzed, and archived, in proximity to the patient. Patients can provide specimens or be imaged by cellphone at almost any location. The sample specimen can be stabilized and shipped (by mail, parcel carrier, or even by drone) to a central laboratory, and the results can be communicated back *via* cellphone. For example, Whatman FTA paper (GE Healthcare) is a cellulose-based matrix on which blood samples can be blotted, dried, and stabilized for shipment to laboratories. Similarly, blood collection tubes have been developed with coated reagents that stabilize blood samples and allow transport (at room temperature) to labs within a 1-week timeframe. Alternatively, some analysis could be done at the point of care, and data can be relayed to the cloud or other networked computer resources for more intense analysis. For instance, Semret *et al.* [44] observe that despite the availability of POC devices to detect various febrile syndromes (*e.g.*, Dengue virus infection), there is a lack of such POC devices to specifically identify strains resistant to antimicrobials. Accordingly, for some healthcare, the role of such POC devices with data communication capabilities connected to centralized laboratories, or POC sample collection and transport, should be in support of leveraging laboratory capacity.

Wearable Sensors and Novel POC Sensors Strokes and cardiovascular disease are the leading cause of death worldwide, accounting for over 30% of all deaths (WHO, 2017), which has provided motivation for real-time wearable sensors to monitor vital signs.

"Lab on skin" describes a trend for wearable electronic sensors packaged in materials (*e.g.*, silicone elastomers) and with laminate shapes that can meld with the skin to provide continuous health monitoring of body temperature, blood pressure, blood oxygenation, skin modulus, and hydration, and non-invasive monitoring of blood glucose, lactate, pH, and ions, and is reviewed by Liu *et al.* [45]. They note that the provision of electric power and power management for wireless communication is the most challenging technical area. Godfrey *et al.* [46] noted that the disruptive technology aspects of wearable sensors and other devices in healthcare—often providing capabilities and features that exceed current pragmatic clinical needs,leave many unresolved issues, such as lack of knowledge regarding the effect of wearables on medical outcomes, safety, data management, and analysis, that have hindered wider adaptation and slowed their evolution. Tan *et al.* [47] and Christodouleas *et al.* [18] surveyed a variety of novel biosensors for closer integration into healthcare. These include contact lens sensors for electrochemical detection of glucose oxidase; graphene-based "tooth tattoo" sensors for saliva analysis to monitor oral health; skin-based sensors to analyze sweat and wounds, such as diabetic foot ulcers, and interstitial fluids; paper-based devices for urinalysis, such as potentiometric electrochemical sensor-based assays of creatine to assess kidney function. Smartphones, for both data storage and providing a user interface, can be interfaced with many such sensors *via* Bluetooth or other wireless technologies. These next-generation biosensors are enabled by novel materials, such as graphene, that include substrates of stretchable and flexible materials and can greatly increase sensitivity, as is crucial for the detection of many biomarkers, especially in fluids, such as saliva, sweat, and tears.

Smartphones for Medical Imaging, Microscopes, and Cytometers The potential of Smartphones for image capture in healthcare has been recognized for over a decade. The WHO estimates that three-quarters of the world does not have access to medical imaging. In the developing world, conventional medical imaging technology is expensive and difficult to maintain. Since the diagnosis of many diseases depends on some form of imaging, many compact and inexpensive imaging platforms for use outside of laboratories, both for *in vitro* and *in vivo* diagnostics, have been developed [48].

About ten years ago, improvements in phone camera image resolution, supplemented with a microscope lens, proved suitable for morphological analysis of blood films on slides, allowing a quick method of 'telehaemotology' for remote locations [49]. A practical mobile phone-based microscope with an LED light source, optical filters, lenses, and extension tubes was demonstrated for bright field imaging of blood cells for *P falciparum* (malaria parasite) and sickle cell disease, as well as fluorescence imaging of sputum for tuberculosis [50]. The potential of cellphone-enabled diagnosis, for bridging the formidable obstacles to sustainable healthcare in areas of the world, such as sub-Sahara Africa, where doctors and trained personnel are few, medical supply chains are tenuous, and conventional medical technology is difficult to maintain, was widely appreciated, including NGOs [51]. Granot *et al.* [52] developed an electrical impedance tomography (EIT) instrument with transmitted data *via* a cellphone (Fig. **1**) for patient self-testing of breast cancer tumors.

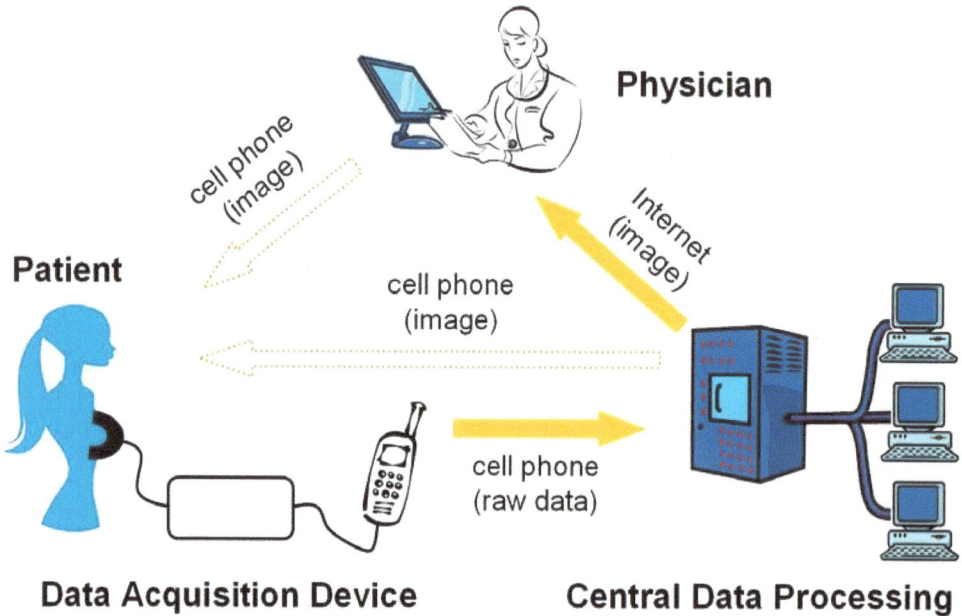

Fig. (1). System configuration for breast cancer tumors patient self-testing. (reprinted with permission from [52]; copyright 2008 PLoS ONE).

High-pixel density (5 MegaPixel) cameras on later generations of mobile phones (iPhone and Android phones such as Samsung Galaxy LG Nexus) enabled near-diffraction limited quantitative imaging of single cells, but many features were built-in to these phones, such as automatic focus, exposure, and color gain need that otherwise degrade high-resolution image quality, unless corrected [53]. In field tests in Africa, iPhone-based microscopy enabled the diagnosis of Schistosomiasis and intestinal protozoa infections in stool and urine samples [54].

Smartphone imaging, enabled by an optical attachment, is used in ophthalmic examination in primary care as an easy-to-learn alternative to the more specialized instrumentation used by opthalmologists for early detection of cataracts and diabetic retinopathy, among other eye diseases [55].

Smartphones for Chemical Analysis and Clinical Chemistry.

Grudpan *et al.* [56] surveyed the use of mobile phones, digital cameras, scanners, and webcams for colorimetric analytical chemistry for POC diagnostics and at-site detection for applications in environmental, agricultural and food processing monitoring. Meredith *et al.* [57] developed a commercial palm-sized breath carbon monoxide meter (Smokerlyzer®) that attaches to and communicates with a smartphone through its audio port to detect cigarette smoking, as part of evidence-based smoking cessation programs. Smartphone cameras can be used to 'read' pH indicator strips with pH ranges from 2 to 10, and a resolution of □0.5 pH units [58]. A recent review [59] described various Smartphone-based microfluidic devices for analytical and clinical chemistry, including paper-based schemes for water analysis of pH and nitrites, colorimetric detection of heavy metals in water samples, cholesterol [60] in blood by colorimetric changes from an enzymatic reaction on a reagent test strip.

Smartphone Immunoassays

Immunoassays offer specific detection of protein and other antigen biomarkers, requiring practically no sample preparation, as assays can function with small volumes of raw specimens, such as whole blood, saliva, or urine. A common application is to use the Smartphone camera for reading test and control lines (striped capture zones) on lateral flow strips or other paper-based devices for the purpose of improved sensitivity and quantification of a signal. More generally, colorimetric assays with paper-based microfluidic devices, such as for the detection of glucose or protein in urine, can be captured with a variety of portable imaging devices, such as cellphone cameras and scanners [61]. Cadle *et al.* [62] used a cellphone camera, as well as comparisons with webcams, scanners, digital cameras, and USB microscopes, for the imaging of test strip immunoassays for drugs of abuse analytes, such as cocaine or benzoylecgonine (BE), a metabolite of cocaine in urine. The acquired image of the test strip capture lines (with time-stamp and geo-tag information) is transmitted to a central computer *via* the internet for automated image analysis based on the ImageJ software. The analysis is based on quantitative ratiometric pixel analysis. The method proved to discriminate clinically-relevant concentrations of analyte, and was found to be robust under test conditions with variable temperature, lighting, and camera resolution and magnification, and is a viable rapid, low-cost alternative to laboratory-based methods using chromatography and/or mass spectrometry.

Preechaburana *et al.* [63] used a cellphone camera to analyze commercial lateral flow strips for detecting NT-proBNP in blood, a marker for cardiovascular disease. By controlling the light exposure and imaging parameters, and using multiple exposures sets, improvements in resolution and detection range were achieved compared to test based on a computer-screen photo-assisted technique (CSPT, *i.e.*, using a computer display screen as a light source) and web camera for a detector, thus translating the CSPT technique to a mobile phone. Meagher and Kousvelari [64] reviewed Smartphone detection of various biomarkers in saliva, for example, chemiluminescence reporter on a lateral flow strip. Salivary analytes include steroids, antibodies, and other proteins, growth factors, cytokines, and drugs, such as anticonvulsants, antibiotics, analgesics, and drugs of abuse and ethanol. Oral and systemic disease markers detectable in saliva include oral and pancreatic cancer, Crohn's disease, dental caries, and obesity.

A complete and comprehensive point-of-care diagnosis system for STDs (sexually transmitted diseases), configured as a Smartphone accessory ("dongle"), was developed by the Sia laboratory at Columbia University (Fig. 2) [65]. The Smartphone dongle comprised an autonomous microfluidic cassette for sample processing that plugs into iPod Smartphone audio jack. The sample is finger-prick whole blood and is simultaneously tested for HIV antibodies and antibodies diagnostic for syphilis infection. The immunoassay is implemented in an array of channels with immobilized antigens to capture sample antibodies, which are then bound with gold-labeled antibodies, washed, and signal amplified by silver precipitation catalyzed by the gold labels. Reagents are pre-stored on the cassette, and flow is actuated by a manually operated plunger built into the dongle. The silver precipitation is detected by LEDs and diodes, wherein the optical absorption signals are encoded and transmitted to the Smartphone through the Audio Jack, which also provides dc power to the dongle electronics. This design minimized power such that about 40 tests could be made on a single charge of the Apple iPod or Smartphone. The dongle design is in contrast to alternative approaches that use the Smartphone camera as the optical detector.

Cellphone microscopes have also been adapted for lateral electrophoretic assays for multiplexed detection of antigens and antibodies, such as antibodies against hepatitis C in serum (reprinted with permission from [65]; copyright 2015 *Science Translation Medicine.*)

Ra *et al.* [66] described a Smartphone-based multiplexed immunoassay colorimetric test for ten targets in urine with various design features to reduce the environmental effects, such as lighting as well as user-variability. In addition to imaging and colorimetry, fluorescence, and absorption intensity, Smartphones can also be adapted for spectrometers for a broad range of medical and chemical applications [67]. L-J Wang *et al.* [68] developed a multichannel smartphone spectrometer as a high-throughput optical biosensor that can quantify proteins, which are potentially useful for cancer diagnostics, for example, a LOD (limit of detection) of 10.6 mg/ml for a cancer marker (*e.g*, IL-6) in human serum. A low-cost kit for using the camera of an Android Smartphone as a spectrometer for real-time transmittance and absorbance measurements is described by Ormachea *et al.* [69].

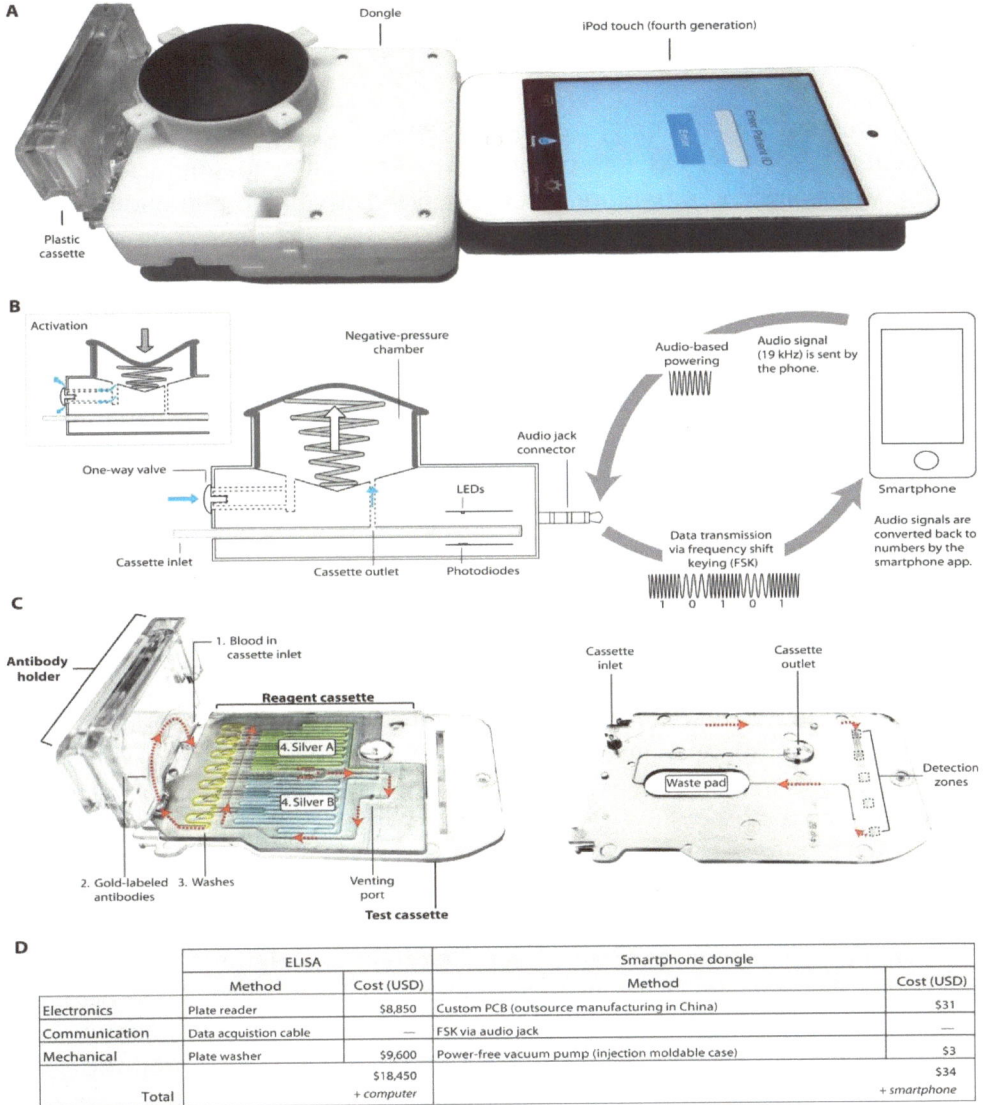

Fig. (2). Smartphone immune-assay dongle. From Laksanasopin *et al.* (2015) [65].

A mobile phone imaging and cloud computing analysis and reporting system for malaria screening was developed by Scherr *et al.* [70]. An unmodified

Smartphone (iPhone 5s) camera is used to image commercial lateral flow strips for detecting malaria antigens in the blood. The captured image is uploaded to an open-source cloud-based database management system (Redcap). Remote image analysis using MATLAB software corrects for angle and lighting effects and facilitates reproducible, objective quantitation of the test strip capture lines, and automatic reporting to the user and clinical database in less than 5 minutes.

Smartphone Molecular Diagnostics

Molecular diagnostics generally refers to the sequence-specific detection of nucleic acids (DNA or RNA), and particularly to nucleic acid amplification tests (NAATs), which are not only more specific and sensitive than immunoassays but also require more elaborate sample processing. NAATs are based on successful amplification of a pathogen-specific nucleic acid sequence extracted from the patient specimen and detection of the amplification product as a positive test result. Most approaches rely on a fluorescence or luminescence reporter to detect amplification products, which can be implemented with a CCD camera, including a smartphone camera. Varying degrees of automation for sample preparation have been reported. Protocols using manual steps (pipetting, sample transfer, centrifugation) as well as microfluidic devices that combine most of these steps in the chip are described below. The common feature is test data captured with a mobile communication device.

One of the earlier reports of smartphone molecular diagnostics was a compact device termed Gene-Z, which operated a microfluidic cartridge with an array of isothermal nucleic acid amplification chambers [71]. The real-time fluorescence was detected with LEDs and a photodiode, and the device was operated with a Smartphone *via* a wireless connection. This report also recognized the capabilities enabled by GPS and barcode reading in Smartphone platforms for POC diagnostics.

Barnes *et al.* [72] developed a Smartphone-based pathogen diagnosis system for urinary sepsis patients. Sepsis detection by culture and/or using blood samples is time consuming. The authors proposed that a more rapid diagnosis (1-hour vs 18-28 hours for culture) can be attained by isothermal amplification of pathogen nucleic acids in patient urine samples (Fig. **3**). Various Gram positive and Gram negative bacteria are assayed in parallel and stratified by concentration (Low, Medium, and High), and diagnosis based on data is provided by a freeware App. Components for the entire detection system cost about $100, making it accessible for resource-limited areas.

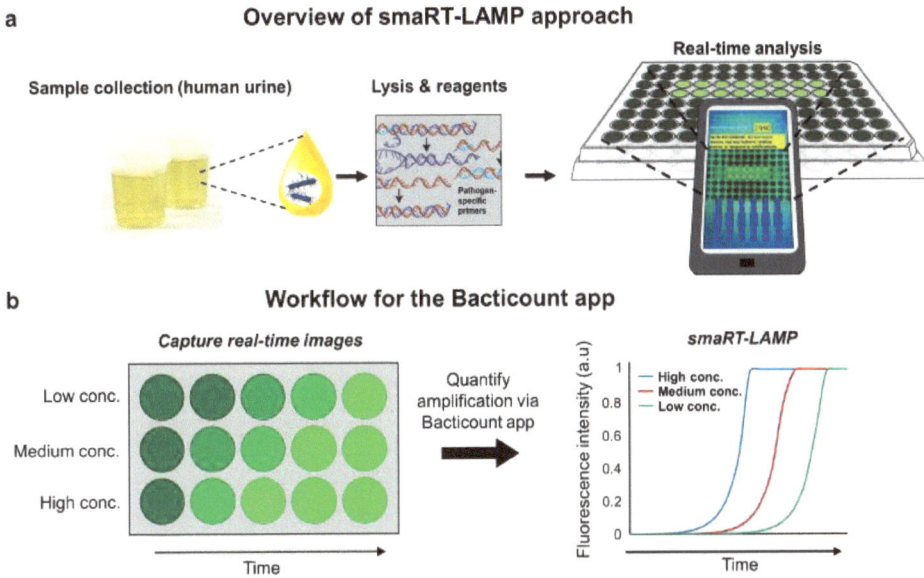

Fig. (3). Patient urine samples are lysed and amplified by isothermal LAMP in microtiter plates that are imaged with a Smartphone camera, and analyzed with a custom app. (reprinted with permission from [72]; copyright 2018 EBioMedicine).

Smartphone-based diagnostics for rapid detection of Zika, chikungunya, and dengue, for affordable diagnostics in resource-limited settings, has been demonstrated using real-time LAMP assays [73]. An apparatus for controlled heating, optical excitation, optical filtering, and Smartphone camera detection for tube-based LAMP reactions of virus-specific sequences from nucleic acids in blood, saliva, or urine samples was described. Such systems are intended to address the inadequate diagnostics capabilities that hinder Zika outbreak management strategies.

Song *et al.* [74] describe a smartphone-based mobile detection platform for molecular diagnostics and spatiotemporal disease mapping (Fig. **4**). A Smartphone is coupled with a thermos-bottle like device ("Smartcup") in which a credit-card sized microfluidic chip, loaded with the patient sample, such as saliva or urine, is inserted. The chip extracts nucleic acid from the sample and specifically amplifies pathogen sequences (*e.g.*, zika virus) using isothermal enzymatic amplification (LAMP, loop-mediated amplification) and a bioluminescence reporter (BART). The Smartcup utilizes chemical heating, such as used in ready-to-eat meals packaging, in combination with phase change materials that act as a thermal 'ballast' to incubate the LAMP reaction at 65 °C. The use of chemical heating avoids an excessive electrical load that would otherwise need to be supplied by batteries or electrical service. The fluorescence signal is detected using the smartphone camera. A custom Android App was developed for bioluminescent signal monitoring, target quantification, data sharing, and spatio-temporal disease mapping.

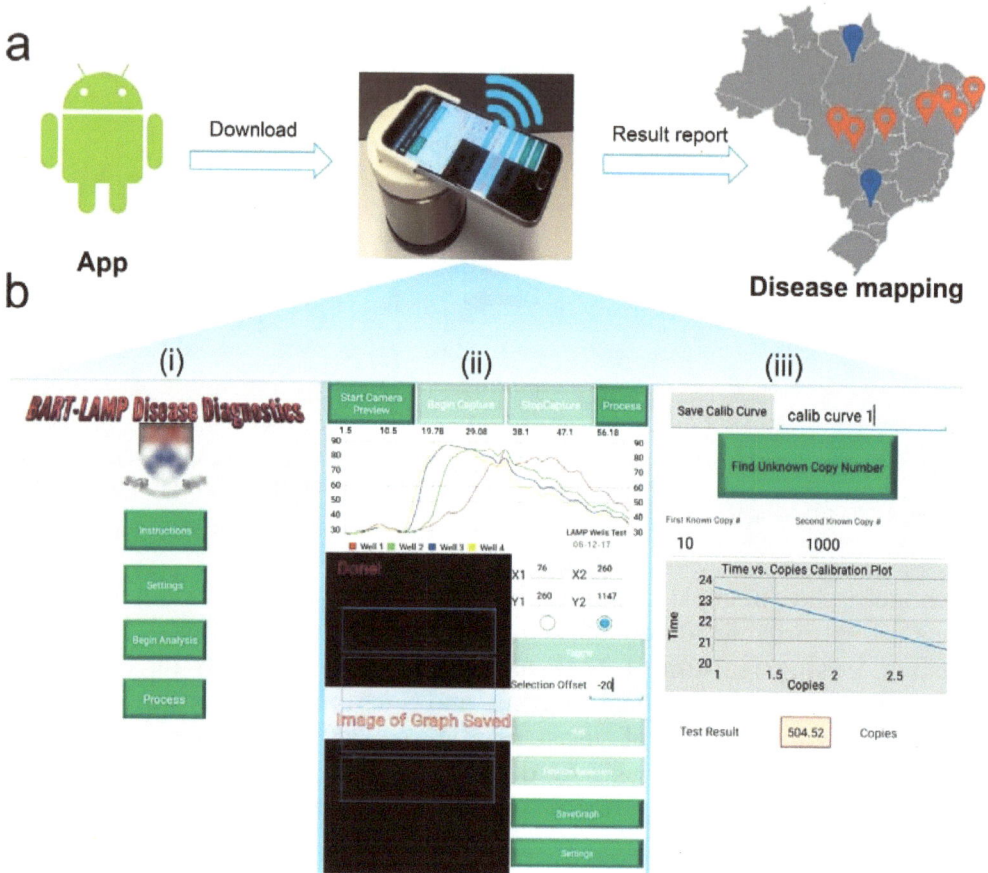

Fig. (4). Android App for smartphone-based molecular testing and disease mapping. (reprinted with permission from [74]; Copyright © 2018 American Chemical Society).

Smartphones can be used for highly multiplexed (10 parallel reactions) detection of nucleic acid sequences using the LAMP [75]. The sample is processed in a credit card-sized microfabricated fluid cartridge, preloaded with dried LAMP reagents, where it is heated in a 3D-printed cradle with optics, and a Smartphone is mounted on the cradle for detection. These workers also developed an open-source database system from the Smartphone App that wirelessly transmitted patient information (name, age, gender, location), data on heart rate, body temperature, and general health.

Smartphone-based detection for point-of-care diagnosis of H1N1 influenza by tube-based convective PCR provides results in less than 30 minutes [76].

Ming *et al.* [77] demonstrated a smartphone optical device for multiplex barcode diagnosis (Fig. **5**). Quantum dots functionalized with single-strand DNA oligos with pathogen-specific or other target sequences ('barcoded') are arrayed on a glass slide. When mixed with samples containing amplified nucleic acids derived from blood, amplicons from different viral strains were hybridized to the bead-anchored complementary oligo capture probes. These hybridized target oligos could be further hybridized with quantum dot labeled reporter oligo probes, where different reporters were conjugated with a distinct 'color'. The bead array is then scanned with a laser and images are captured with a Smartphone camera. Captured images can be transmitted to a central computer for further analysis. Such image-intensive diagnostics is attractive in its highly multiplexing capability, and furthermore, the method could be extended for protein targets by using antibody and antigen probes.

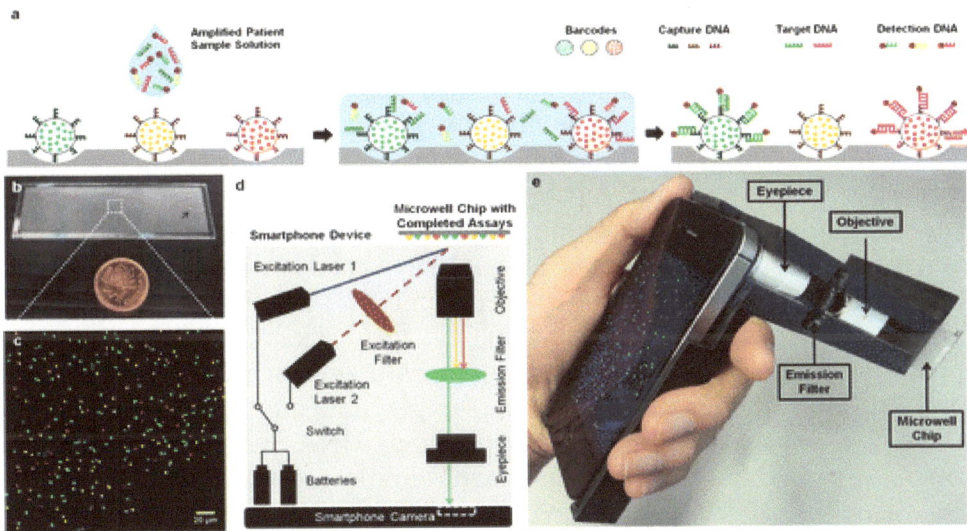

Fig. (**5**). Smartphone-based device using quantum dot barcodes. **a**) addition of patient sample to chip coated with microbeads, **b**) microwell chip, **c**) image captured by Smartphone camera, **d**) schematic of optical detection using two excitation sources and Smartphone camera as a detector, and **e**) complete device. (reprinted with permission from [77]; Copyright © 2015, American Chemical Society).

Smartphones, as well as USB digital microscopes, desktop scanners, and DVD readers, have been used to read microarray chips for DNA genotyping, as for example, used in pharmacogenomics [78]. Sequences with putative SNP (single nucleotide polymorphisms) in genomic DNA extracted from patient buccal swabs were isothermally amplified by LAMP (Loop mediated AMPlification) and hybridized to allele-specific probes immobilized on plastic slides, then imaged with the various scanning or imaging devices. All methods could support a low-cost, POC system with sufficient DNA sensitivities (100 copies) as potentially needed for patient-tailored drug therapies. Polymorphic genotyping of LAMP products, using Smartphone imaging of a colorimetric chip-based probe hybridization assay, has also been reported [79].

Nucleic Acid Sequencing with Smartphones

Smartphone-based miniature DNA sequencing devices (*e.g.*, Oxford Nanopore) have been introduced and have anticipated POC applications in physician settings for infectious disease testing, preliminary oncology testing, in vitro fertilization (IVF) clinics, wildlife species identification, and pathogen contamination testing in the food industry [80]. Kühnemund *et al.* [81] demonstrated DNA sequencing and in situ point mutation detection assays in tumor samples with mobile phone microscopy. Targeted DNA sequences in tissue samples on microscope slides were amplified by Rolling Circle Amplification (RCA) and imaged and quantified with mobile phone microscopy. RCP products were also analyzed for point mutations with NGS (next generation sequencing) reactions, such as sequencing by ligation, and imaged and quantified by Smartphone microscope. Alternatively, special oligo Padlock probes, in combination with RCP, could be used to detect rare single cell mutations in tissue sections with a Smartphone microscope. These techniques greatly expand the capabilities of Smartphones for telemedicine to include molecular marker detection, such as KRAS mutations, in clinical specimens. Challenges of real-time 'mobile' DNA analysis have been discussed by Ko *et al.* [82] in applications where time is critical (*e.g.*, response to epidemics) or where the location is critical (*e.g.*, metagenomic studies of microbes sampled directly from their native environments), and for which issues can be categorized as portable vs. benchtop, sample collection/preparation, DNA isolation, and consumables, library preparation, DNA sequencing and reads processing, power/energy requirements, and workflow management.

Non-Medical Applications of Smartphone-Platforms for Detection

In addition to the numerous medical diagnostics applications [83 - 86], smart-phones have been used for environmental sensing, food safety and testing, and veterinary applications. Smartphones combined with appropriate accessories (camera, microphone, GPS, accelerometer, temperature, light and humidity sensors), for monitoring air pollution, noise pollution, electromagnetic fields, and radiation exposure, have been used for 'opportunistic' environment sensing [87, 88].

Food testing is often done by sending samples collected in the field to centralized laboratories. There are considerable incentives in distributed food testing along the entire food chain ('farm to fork') as enabled by portable tests, particularly with regard to logistics and timeliness of responses. Rateni *et al.* [89], have reviewed a broad range of Smartphone-based diagnostics technologies for food and water testing, including fluorescence assay for bacteria (such as by immunolabeled quantum dots imaged by phone camera), colorimetric assays for various allergens, fluorides, catechols, lateral flow strips for fungal toxins, and ELISA tests for environmental contaminants often found in food. Moreover, there are various Smartphone electrochemical (amperometric, potentiometric, and impedimetric) sensors, Smartphone spectroscopy, NIR (near infrared) optical detection, and gas sensors to detect spoilage. In the area of food testing, Smartphone scanning of microtiter plates supports magnetic bead-based nanoflower (a class of highly-structured nanoparticles used as a reporter) ELISA (Enzyme-Linked Immunosorbent Assay) for detecting Salmonella in dairy products [90]. Jang *et al.* [91] developed a robust Smartphone portable diagnostic reader to measure progesterone hormone in milk. Giordano *et al* [92], described a smartphone platform for point-of-use electroanalytical (cyclic voltammetry) chemometric "fingerprinting" of honey samples according to the geographic and botanical origin. This system could internally process complex multivariate data by unsupervised principal component analysis with the aim of reducing model overfitting by novice users. Rapid detection of residual antibiotics, such as streptomycin, in foods such as chicken and milk, using digital image colorimetry with a Smartphone, has been reported [93]. A Smart 'Forensic' phone has been developed for colorimetric analysis to estimate the age of bloodstains at crime scenes [94].

For veterinary use, Smartphone *in vitro* diagnostics, using microfluidic chips, could perform the same types of tests on animals as on humans. For instance, animal parasitic diseases can be diagnosed using Smartphone-based immunoassays [95].

Zhang *et al.* [96] described a Smartphone portable biosensing system for real-time impedance-based detection of TNT (2,4,6-trinitrotoluene), an explosive monitored for threats to public safety. The system has a disposable biodetector with printed electrodes modified with TNT-specific peptides that transmits to a Smartphone *via* Bluetooth.

POC *in vitro* Diagnostics as Nodes of The Internet of Medical Things (IoMT)

As currently implemented or envisioned, the Internet of Medical Things (sometimes also called the medical Internet of Things, mIOT) is a subset of the Internet of Things (IoTs), or more specifically a network of medical devices, including, for example, smart devices such as wearable sensors and vital sign monitors, and point-of-care diagnostics devices, sited on the patient body, in the home, in clinics, hospitals, or other care facilities, as well as interfaced with healthcare workers communication devices, that can connect to healthcare information technology systems for real-time data transmission (Fig. **6**). The concept of an Internet of Things dates back to 1999, stemming from the convergence of RFID technologies, embedded systems, MEMS (micro-electromechanical systems), wireless sensors—all connected through the internet [97]. The IoT application domains can be categorized on the basis of network availability, coverage, scale, heterogeneity, availability, user involvement, and impact [98]. IoT connects millions of devices for purposes varying from agriculture, entertainment, transportation (cars), smart homes and appliances, manufacturing, business, and retail, and broadly facilitates human interaction and collaboration [99]. From a purely logistics and cost perspective, the IoMT will accelerate the adoption of EHR (Electronic Health Records) towards more efficient and error-free delivery of healthcare.

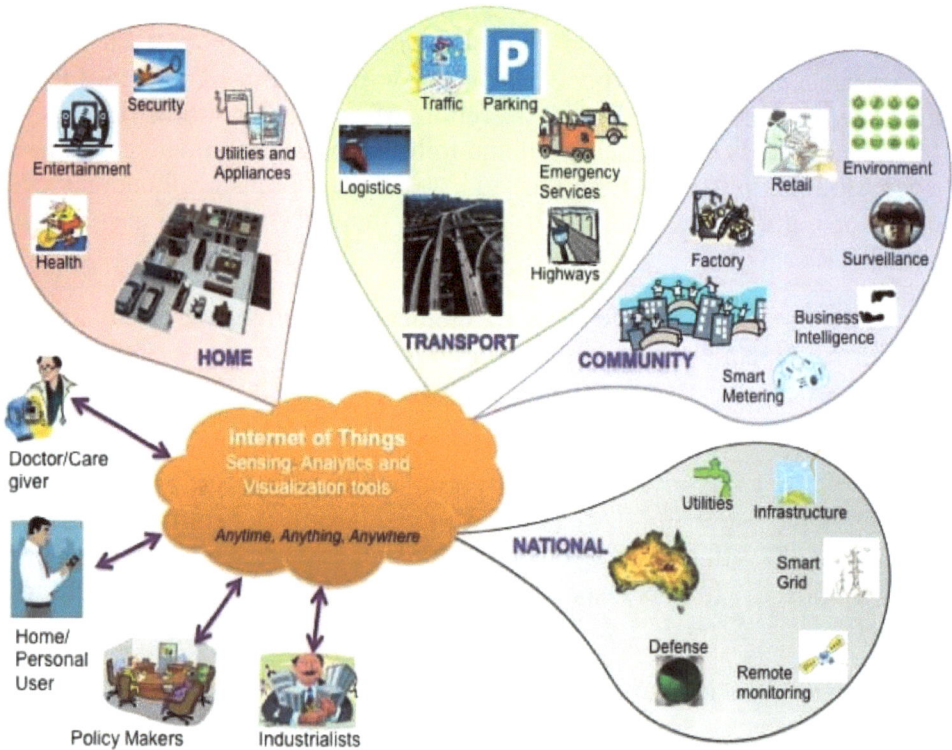

Fig. (6). Internet of Things. (reprinted with permission from [100]; Copyright © 2013 Future Generation Computer Systems).

Shelke [101] notes that the patents for pacemaker telemetry were filed as long ago as 1970, but that patent filings for such and related technologies started growing 'robustly' after 1990. Marr [102] reports that in 2018, there were 3.7 million patents connected medical devices to monitor personal health, with the number of IoMT devices projected to be between 20 to 30 billion by 2020 [103]. The wearables may be wristbands, headbands, smart garments and belts, or other flexible sensors attached to the skin. Community needs could be served by kiosks. Hospitals would have connections at the bedside (*e.g.*, intravenous pumps and monitors) and throughout the facility in clinical laboratory instruments (MRIs, CT scanners), wheelchairs, gurneys, barcode readers, as part of systems for inventory and supply chain management, environment control, and patient flow management. Singh [104] surveyed the IoMT for real-time data care systems, healthcare analytics, cost reduction, increasing patient interest and participation, error reduction, health alerts, chronic disease management, assistance to the physically challenged, and drug or therapy management, utilizing new technologies, such as digestible sensors. Home-care combining sensors, smart devices, and the internet of medical things have the potential dramatic improvements in the care of complications associated with diabetes, *e.g.*, lower extremity ulcers [105]. Martin [103] lists some of the broadly anticipated advantages of the IoMT for healthcare including improved accessibility while reducing office visits, and lower per-patient costs and fast implementation, while challenges range from high infrastructure costs, security vulnerabilities, lack of standardization, strain on existing networks, to regulatory uncertainties.

Jagadeewari *et al.* [106] discusses the recent emerging technologies for personalized healthcare systems, including cloud computing, fog computing, Big Data analytics, the IoT, and mobile devices. Some illustrative examples include sensor acquired personal health data transmitted wirelessly for cloud computing using medical knowledge bases for appropriate responses and medical alert generation. Other systems have been developed for controlling the spread of Zika and H1N1 virus. This review drew distinctions between the cloud layer (big data processing and warehousing, and access to remote users such as hospitals and doctors), the fog layer (local networks, data analysis and reduction), the edge layer (closer to the user, embedded systems, PCs, and other gateways which are connected to various wireless sensors), and of interest to this review, microfluidic devices with or without intervening smartphone platforms.

While Smartphones have excellent prospects for near-term implementation of an IoMT, other wireless network technologies, including Wi-Fi, Bluetooth, Zigbee, and LoRA, and others currently developed for smart parking, waste management, utility meters, toll roads, and vending machines, offer features complementary to Smartphone networks. For example, Catherwood *et al.* [107] reported a Low

Power Wide Area Network communications platform for connecting a microfluidic biofluid analyzer for the diagnosis of urinary tract infections (UTI). This LoRa system has subscription-free service, highly secure two-way communication with three layers of encryption, 5- to 10-year battery life, and low cost, and can operate in dense urban areas, as well as the long range ($\square$20 km) needed for rural communities. The UTI POC device is based on reading a lateral flow test strip with LED/photodiode detection. A formidable challenge for IoMT will be aggregating and normalizing data from many sources, as health data is fragmented in "institutional silos" over generations of legacy equipment [2, 108].

Machine Learning and Artificial Intelligence in POC in *vitro* Diagnostics

Artificial Intelligence,computer systems that can augment or emulate human decision making,is currently used for applications such as face, speech, and handwriting recognition, data mining, natural language processing, robotics, and virtual reality. AI can reveal important information in the massive data generated by sensors, clinician and patient input, patient traits, and diagnostics tests, to support clinical decisions, and also use feedback for self-correction and improvement of algorithms. The most basic AI, Machine Learning (ML), analyzes structured data such as images, sensor readings, gene sequences, and electrophysiological data by supervised or unsupervised learning using clustering and principal component analysis (PCA). More advanced AI encompasses NLP (natural language processing) to extract information from unstructured data. Machine Learning algorithms reported in the medical literature include support vector machines, neural networks, logistic regression, discriminant analysis, random forest, linear regression, naïve Bayes, nearest neighbor, decision trees, and hidden Markov models [109]. Applications of artificial intelligence (AI) in medicine are well established and include computer-based knowledge generation, clinical data mining, information retrieval, natural language processing, pattern recognition, image processing, data and knowledge representation, classification and filtering, clinical guidelines, machine learning, and decision support systems [110]. Diagnostic decision support systems can recommend the optimum mix of tests, automate routine aspects of clinical work with rules-based programming, and employ algorithms to provide faster and more accurate treatments [111]. Hoffmann *et al*. [112] described machine learning techniques to formulate more optimal diagnostic pathways in the form of decision trees (expert rules: "if, then, else") for differential diagnosis of Hepatitis C. POC and IoMT diagnostics tests could be nodes on such decision trees. In many areas of diagnostics and especially medical imaging, AI can provide a quantitative and objective interpretation of data, and increase 'diagnostic yield' (clinically relevant information) [113]. Machine learning, such as convolutional neural networks, is also being used for the prediction of chronic diseases based on demographics, habits (*e.g.* smoking), diagnostics tests, medical history, and geographic locale [114]. Liao *et al.* [115] developed Bayesian Belief Network (BBN), a model bases on probabilistic relationships among variables, to assess disease outbreak based on cases of virus detection.

Gopal *et al.* [116] provided some perspectives on the role of present and future information technologies, including advanced analytics and big data, IoMT, machine learning, in the digital transformation of healthcare (sources cited therein): 1) 30% of the entire world's data volume is generated by the healthcare, 2) a patient generates 80 Megabytes per year, mostly due to diagnostic imaging, but also due to omics data, 3) there are 325,000 mobile health apps, growing 25% per year, 4) global healthcare spending will reach $8.7 trillion by 2020, and 5) spending on AI and ML is expected to reach $57 billion by 2021. In addition to the immense applications of AI to medical imaging (CT, MRI, PET, SPECT, ultrasound) and scans (EEG, EMG, ECG), and mass spectrometry, Vashita *et al.* [117] list several applications of AI approaches to infectious diseases, including image processing for rotavirus, drug regimens for HIV, fog computing for Zika virus, and Artificial Neural Networks for Hepatitis B. According to one technology survey [118], AI in medical diagnosis is motivated by the large contribution of diagnostic errors to patient deaths (10%) and hospital complications (17%), as reported by the National Academies of Medicine in 2015. The survey also highlighted some impressive achievements of AI in diagnostics, such as neural networks outperforming dermatologists in diagnosing skin cancer, and recent developments such as machine learning for diagnosis of multiple sclerosis using blood tests, machine learning platforms for identifying developmental delays in children based on videos provided by parents, and machine learning algorithms to diagnose PTSD from speech patterns.

A recent review by Yu *et al.* [119] surveys applications of AI in basic biomedical research (laboratory automation, literature mining, simulation of molecular dynamics), translational research (biomarker discovery, drug discovery and repurposing, prediction of toxicity), and clinical practice (disease diagnosis, treatment selection, automated surgery, patient monitoring, and patient risk stratification for prevention). ML content has been recommended in the education of next-generation medical students and other healthcare professionals [120].

In the diagnostics arena, Machine Learning and Artificial Intelligence have mostly focused on applications of interpreting images: in radiology, for example, X-ray radiography, CAT scans, MRI, and ultrasound; in dermatology, for the diagnosis of skin lesions, including skin cancer; heart sound analysis, ophthalmology, in imaging of retina, and histopathology of biopsies. Healthcare BOTs (autonomous programs that can interact with users) in mobile messaging apps, as well as chatbots that can answer patient questions and provide, for example, guidance on taking medication, can be enhanced with AI through learning and mimicking human conversation, detecting emotions, and incorporating Natural Language Processing and Sentiment analysis [121]. Outstanding issues for healthcare AI are accuracy and safety, uncertainties when applied to novel or exceptional cases, patient acceptance, adaptation by healthcare workers, and regulatory hurdles.

Besides the large data of images, big data from patient diagnostics and outcomes offers opportunities for healthcare analytics. For example, one study implied that ovarian cancer patients who happen to be using a beta-blocker for high blood pressure lived four and a half years longer than those not taking the beta-blocker, a finding that would not likely have been discerned based on current medical science knowledge [122]. Data mining can help doctors find similar cases to help personalize treatments. Next-generation wearable biosensors and POC devices will provide measurements to train machine learning algorithms, combined with 'big data' repositories from pharmaceutical services, health surveys, medical imaging data banks, clinical registries, 'omics' databases, and electronic health record data, using methods, such as Bayesian networks, decision-learning trees, cluster analysis, graph analytics, language processing, and data visualization [117].

The direct application or incorporation of Machine Learning or AI into POC diagnostics devices or their platforms has so far been limited. The potential scope and first steps of integrating AI/ML into point-of-care diagnostics are discussed by O'Sullivan *et al.* [24] To date, most applications of AI have been applied to imaging or genome analysis, and to cancer, neurology, or cardiovascular disease types [109], rather than *in vitro* diagnostics of infectious diseases. However, it is clear that there is considerable potential for enhancing the functionality of POC technology by utilizing connectivity and computational capabilities enabled by cellphones or other wireless devices. For example, the portable XPRIZE DeepQ tricorder system [123] uses artificial intelligence to diagnose twelve common diseases, combining three modules: 1) a patient Q&A session analyzed with context-aware reinforcement learning to check patient symptoms, 2) a wireless camera to image and diagnose ear infections and melanoma, using a diagnostic algorithm that combines deep learning and transfer learning, and 3) monitoring of five vital signs (heart rate, respiration rate, blood pressure, oxygen saturation, and body temperature). Smith *et al.* [124] developed an automated interpretation of stained blood culture smears using a deep convolutional neural network (CNN) for the diagnosis of bloodstream infections. Xie *et al.* [113] review the application of deep learning, specifically CNNs, in diagnostic histopathology. CNNS have been used for image-based pattern-recognition classification for object, facial, and speech recognition. CNNs can process massive cohorts of annotated images to discover informative patterns. Specifically, image analysis with deep CNNs first analyzes images pixel by pixel to discern simple geometric patterns, *e.g.*, edges, which are then inputted to deeper levels to discern more complex features, and where features of known diagnostic importance are given more weight within the neural network. These methods have been successfully applied to radiology, histological pathology, EEG analysis, and dermatology. The FDA is currently developing standards for such computer-aided diagnostics ("Software as a medical device."). Koydemir *et al.* [125] used machine learning algorithms (bootstrap aggregating) to count and differentiate parasites imaged by mobile phone-based fluorescent microscopy.

Areas for AI applications in POC diagnostics include the human / device interface with regard to learning and mimic human conversations or other elements of natural language processing (NLP). In the arena of *in vitro* diagnostics devices, including POC tests, applications of AI and machine learning will provide useful features, such as chatbots and digital assistants for patient interaction, freeing healthcare professionals for other tasks, clinical decision support, NLP will translate complex technical language into layman's terms, automated and accurate billing for healthcare services, and in particular, enabling or fostering outcome-based (value of care) billing [116]. Vashita *et al.* [117] emphasized the need for standardizing diagnostics platforms for a meaningful comparison of disease cases by AI and ML.

Some developments in applications of AI and ML in various POC diagnostics, based on images or ultrasound with likely relevance to *in vitro* diagnostics, can be mentioned. Qiu *et al.* [126] used pattern recognition of optical signals from multiple test lines on a lateral flow strip for genotyping of the hepatitis B virus. Valderrama *et al.* [127] discuss the improvements in the use of a low-cost point-of-care Doppler ultrasound Smartphone-connected device for fetal monitoring in rural Guatemala, with regard to usability and decision support. Real-time machine learning analysis of the quality of signal and signal classification were based on extracting features by direct template matching, linear resampling, dynamic time warping, and weighted dynamic time warping, as well as sample entropy measures, wavelet features, statistical and power spectrum density features. Signal degradation could be attributed to poor cable connections, electrical interference (*e.g.*, cellphones), people talking, and other problems. Accordingly, low- and high-quality signals could be distinguished, and sources of error can be identified, suggesting corrective actions for the operator. Image analysis and machine learning to improve malaria diagnostics, based on blood smears, especially in resource-limited settings and enabled by Smartphones are surveyed by Poostchi *et al.* [128]. In particular, previous applications of machine learning have been characterized by small data sets, and lack of uniformity and consistency among different endeavors, as well a variability due to microscopes, staining, and methods of machine analysis and software. The advent of more general-purpose image analysis methods (filtering, segmentation, clustering and classification methods, and new deep learning (multilayer neural networks trained with back propagation using large training sets) will offer dramatic improvements in automated malaria microscopy, translatable to the point-of-care. While immunoassays and nucleic acid amplification tests are not as crucially dependent on image analysis, large data set deep learning will foster more standardized field use of POC devices in general. Some molecular diagnostics applications relying on image-based cell counting will no doubt benefit from deep learning image analysis. For example, S-J Kim *et al.* [129] reported a deep-*transfer* learning method to analyze hologram images of cells labeled with molecular-specific beads captured with lens-free digital in-line holography (LDIH). While LDIH hardware is technologically compatible as a low-cost, portable POC diagnostics, it conventionally requires extensive data processing, provided by on-line resources, or else circumvented by less computationally-intense algorithms. Machine learning has also been utilized for blood cell counting in lens-less (compact) microfluidic systems with a CMOS image sensor in order to improve resolution, achieving performance comparable to a conventional cytometer [130].

An inexpensive smartphone-based device has been developed for point-of-care tests for predicting ovulation [131] that incorporates artificial intelligence to interpret images of saliva smears. Current ovulation tests, as used, for example, by individuals that prefer natural family planning, utilize assays of luteinizing hormone in urine, rectal or oral basal body temperature analysis, or other ways of detecting biomarkers or signals indicating the 4-day window around ovulation. Another indicator of ovulation is saliva *ferning*, which refers to fern-like (highly-branched) crystalline structures that appear in air-dried saliva samples smeared onto a microscope slide. The ferning is due to increased salivary electrolytes that occur during the follicular phase of the menstrual cycle. Potluri developed several accessories to collect, spread and dry, and optically image (μl) saliva samples. The optical component that attaches to a smartphone has an LED light source and facilitates imaging of the dried saliva with the phone camera. A neural network analysis was used to rapidly (30 seconds) analyze ferning in saliva samples. To interpret images, MobileNet, a class of open-source models for efficient embedded vision applications in mobile devices, using depth-wise separable convolutions in deep neural networks, was utilized. The fern structures were classified with MobileNet pre-training with 1.4 million images, employing 2D convolution, average pooling, cross-entropy loss functions, and gradient calculations for classification of images. The accuracy of the test, in discriminating ovulation and non-ovulation periods, was 99.5%. The total test time is about 7 minutes. Other veterinary applications for detecting ovulation in animals are also suggested.

Regulatory Issues and Risks

The FDA gave 510(K) clearance to a mobile radiology application for viewing and diagnostic interpretation of computed tomography, magnetic resonance imaging in 2011 [132]. In the same year, 510(K) clearance was given to a Smartphone ultrasound imaging system [133]. The US FDA has approved mobile health devices that are purposed mainly to measure and transmit patient data, in which case they were regarded as accessories, but now tends to view healthcare software and applications as components or fundamental features, rather than accessories of cellphone diagnostics, and should be regulated as medical devices [134]. The FDA is currently developing regulations and standards for diagnostics software platforms under a "Software as Medical Device" model [113]. There is a consensus that the biggest hurdle for mHealth apps (and presumably related IoMT and POC technology) is a lack of standards and proper regulation to ensure accuracy and performance, as well as privacy and security concerns [135]. Young [136] lists impending issues and "key threats" to Healthcare Cybersecurity for the Internet of Medical Things which include: 1) medical records will be increasingly stolen and hacked, 2) amplified by medical devices and their potential misuse as backdoors into hospital IT networks, 3) outdated medical device technology that are easily compromised, 4) clinicians neglecting cybersecurity safeguards, 5) FDA issued security recommendations rather than mandates.

Direct Access or Direct-to-Consumer Testing, POC Devices and the IoMT

A recent trend in healthcare is the advent of laboratory tests directly available to consumers without a physician's order, referred to as Direct Access Testing (DAT) or Direct-To-Consumer (DTC) testing. The consumer-driven DAT market in the US will likely exceed $350 million in 2020 [137]. Most familiar are genetic testing services (*e.g.*, 23-and-me), based on mail-in samples to centralized labs. Diagnostics tests are also increasingly performed in pharmacies or sold over-th--counter or through the internet for home use, such as pregnancy and HIV tests. POC technology, particularly microfluidic modules for use with Smartphones, will no doubt widen the scope of such testing. Reliability will be crucial as neither consumers nor pharmacists have the means to validate test performance [138]. Connectivity will permit integration into healthcare networks, and aid users in the interpretation of test results, and assuring sample adequacy, and smartphones will likely become the repository of information gained by DAT [138]. Laboratory test results have proved difficult for consumers to understand, and only about 10% of adults have sufficient 'medical literacy' to interpret their meaning [139]. Ironically perhaps, the specifics of DAT legality in many places prohibit the test supplier from interpreting the test, as this would infringe on the physician's prerogative [140], thus leaving test results to the user to interpret. Consumers find DAT and DTC attractive due to price transparency, the low cost compared to conventional laboratory diagnostics, the ability to keep their test data confidential that might otherwise adversely affect their insurability (*e.g.*, the propensity to diseases) or prove potentially embarrassing (*e.g.*, STDs), and generally support more control of their. One aspect of such consumer testing is that it can generate commercially or scientifically valuable 'big data' for the providers of such services.

DISCUSSION AND SUMMARY

While the interconnection of wearable sensors and medical laboratory equipment into healthcare computer networks as part of an Internet of Medical Things grows apace, the inclusion of *in vitro* diagnostics devices will no doubt lag due to the mismatches of miniaturized hardware (lab on chip devices) that requires physical specimen samples, chemical processing, with purely electronic or optoelectronic systems, such as networked computers, telecommunication systems, and other instrumentation. The smartphone will provide a powerful platform and serve as a bridge between fluidic processing and analysis.

The Smartphone is the 'ultimate' IoT (and IoMT) device due to its enabling technologies for seamless interconnection built-in sensors, Bluetooth, RFID tracking, and near-field communications, high resolution screens, camera, user-friendly access, and most of all, due to its ubiquity; giving it capabilities for Big Data, cloud computing, and cross-organization integration between medical information systems, hospitals, patients, and medical care providers and personnel [141]. There are around 5 billion cellphone subscribers in the world [142], and it is estimated that in 2019, there are 3.5 billion Smartphones [143]. Smartphone/non-Smartphone cellphone penetration in some selected countries is: S Korea (94%/6%), USA (77%/17%), China (68%/30%), Nigeria (32%/48%), India (22%/51%), with a global median (59%/31%) [144].

The Smartphone-enabled POC *in vitro* diagnostic devices are poised to play a major role in the imminent paradigm shift of healthcare forecasted by Eric Topal, *The Patient Will See You Now,* and summarized by Kish [145] as: 1) decentralization of healthcare, transcending time and place, 2) democratization of medicine, where patient and care provider are equals, 3) more peer-to-peer medicine, *e.g.*, patients connected to other patients, 4) new sources of medical innovations, from unexpected areas, 5) patient-centered care and value-based payments, 6) massively open online medical education, 7) reassessment of medical risks by patients, 8) potential risk of the dominance of virtual healthcare monopolies.

Predictions concerning the future paths of healthcare in general and in medical diagnostics, in particular, are instructive even if sometimes wide of the mark. Kricka [146] lists some major developments and trends in laboratory medicine (*in vitro* diagnostics), and long term forecasts. These include past predictions such as the advent of molecular diagnostics (nucleic acid based tests), near-patient testing *via* biosensors, image analysis, robotics in clinical laboratories, information management, that have largely come to pass. Also are trends that are underway, such as widespread personal genome sequencing, smartphones as hubs of medicine, as well as long-term predictions such as medical check-ups by cellphone, and continuous monitoring of vital signs by wearable sensors. Smartphone platforms for microfluidic-based assays are moving from the laboratory to the field, and are poised to play an essential role in many of these current or predicted trends.

In summary:

- The Internet of Medical Things, a network of medical devices, databases, computational resources, and communication ports, is rapidly evolving that will transform healthcare in many ways.
- Miniaturized *in vitro* microfluidic (lab on a chip) or paper-based devices will enable automated or semi-automated, rapid or near-real-time chemical analysis, immunoassays, cell analysis, and molecular diagnostics (such as nucleic acid amplification tests) for highly specific and sensitive detection of disease markers.
- Smartphone cameras and other accessory sensors can serve as detection devices for microfluidic devices, providing the bridge between chemistry and electronic data.
- Due to the ubiquity of Smartphones, and their compatibility with many communication formats, they also serve as the most expedient means of connecting portable, field-deployed, in vitro diagnostics devices.
- Once connected to the IoMT, POC diagnostics devices will be able to exploit machine learning and artificial intelligence to improve their performance as tools for supporting medical decisions.

CONSENT FOR PUBLICATION

Not applicable.

CONFLICT OF INTEREST

The authors confirm that this chapter contents have no conflict of interest.

ACKNOWLEDGEMENTS

Declared none.

REFERENCES

[1]   Li M, Diamandis EP. Technology-driven diagnostics: From smart doctor to smartphone. Crit Rev Clin Lab Sci 2016; 53(4): 268-76.
[http://dx.doi.org/10.3109/10408363.2016.1149689] [PMID: 26857116]

[2]   Dimitrov DV. Medical internet of things and big data in healthcare. Healthc Inform Res 2016; 22(3): 156-63.
[http://dx.doi.org/10.4258/hir.2016.22.3.156] [PMID: 27525156]

[3]   Hawkins R. Managing the pre- and post-analytical phases of the total testing process. Ann Lab Med 2012; 32(1): 5-16.
[http://dx.doi.org/10.3343/alm.2012.32.1.5] [PMID: 22259773]

[4]   Xu X, Akay A, Wei H, *et al.* Advances in smart phone-based point-of-care diagnostics. Proc IEEE 2015; 103(2): 236-47.

[5]   Gale BK, Jafek AR, Lampert CJ, *et al.* A review of current methods in microfluidic device fabrication and future commercialization prospects. Inventions 2018; 3: 60.
[http://dx.doi.org/10.3390/inventions3030060]

[6]   Primiceri E, Chiriaco MS, Notarangelo FM, Crocamo A, Ardissino D, Cereda M. aP Bramanti, MA Bianchessi, G Giannelli and G Maruccio, "Key enabling technologies for point-of-care diagnostics. Sensors (Basel) 2018; 18: 3607.
[http://dx.doi.org/10.3390/s18113607]

[7]   Pandey CM, Augustine S, Kumar S, *et al.* "Microfluidics based point-of-care diagnostics" *Biotechnology Journal* (2018) 13 1700047.C Rozand, "Paper-based analytical devices for point-o--care infectious disease testing. Eur J Clin Microbiol Infect Dis 2014; 33: 147-56.
[http://dx.doi.org/10.1007/s10096-013-1945-2]

[8]   Sher M, Zhuang R, Demirci U, Asghar W. Paper-based analytical devices for clinical diagnosis: Recent advances in the fabrication techniques and sensing mechanisms. Expert Rev Molecular Diagnostics 2017; 17(4): 351-66.
[http://dx.doi.org/10.1080/14737159.2017.1285228]

[9]   Kuo Y-S, Verma S, Schmid T, Dutta P. Hijacking power and bandwidth from the mobile phone's audio interface

[10]   Li B, Li L, Guan A, *et al.* A smartphone controlled handheld microfluidic liquid handling system. Lab Chip 2014; 14(20): 4085-92.
[http://dx.doi.org/10.1039/C4LC00227J] [PMID: 25182078]

[11]   Yafia M, Ahmadi A, Hoorfar M, Najjaran H. Ultra-portable smartphone controlled integrated digital microfluidic system in a 3D-printed modular assembly. Micromachines (Basel) 2015; 6: 1289-305.
[http://dx.doi.org/10.3390/mi6091289]

[12]   Petryayeva E. RSC Advances 2015; 5: 22256-82.
[http://dx.doi.org/10.1039/C4RA15036H]

[13]   Bartmann F. Smartphone-das Stethoskop des 21 Jahrhunderts. Internist (Berl) 2018.
[http://dx.doi.org/10/1007/s00108-018-0525-z]

[14]   Liu C, Mauk MG, Hart R, Qiu X, Bau HH. A self-heating cartridge for molecular diagnostics. Lab Chip 2011; 11(16): 2686-92.
[http://dx.doi.org/10.1039/c1lc20345b] [PMID: 21734986]

[15]   Vidic J, Vizzini P, Manzano M, *et al.* Point-of-need DNA testing for detection of foodborne

pathogenic bacteria. Sensors (Basel) 2019; 19(5): 1100.
[http://dx.doi.org/10.3390/s19051100] [PMID: 30836707]

[16]   Lin Y, Gritsenko D, Feng S, Teh YC, Lu X, Xu J. Detection of heavy metal by paper-based
       microfluidics. Biosens Bioelectron 2016; 83: 256-66.
       [http://dx.doi.org/10.1016/j.bios.2016.04.061] [PMID: 27131999]

[17]   Busin V, Wells B, Kersaudy-Kerhoas M, Shu W, Burgess STG. Opportunities and challenges for the
       application of microfluidic technologies in point-of-care veterinary diagnostics. Mol Cell Probes 2016;
       30(5): 331-41.
       [http://dx.doi.org/10.1016/j.mcp.2016.07.004] [PMID: 27430150]

[18]   Christodouleas DC, Kaur B, Chorti P. From point-of-care testing to eHealth diagnostic devices
       (eDiagnostics). ACS Cent Sci 2018; 4(12): 1600-16.
       [http://dx.doi.org/10.1021/acscentsci.8b00625] [PMID: 30648144]

[19]   Sreejith KR, Ooi CH, Jin J, Dao DV, Nguyen NT. Digital polymerase chain reaction technology -
       recent advances and future perspectives. Lab Chip 2018; 18(24): 3717-32.
       [http://dx.doi.org/10.1039/C8LC00990B] [PMID: 30402632]

[20]   Schoepp NG, Schlappi TS, Curtis MS, *et al.* Rapid pathogen-specific phenotypic antibiotic
       susceptibility testing using digital LAMP quantification in clinical samples. Sci Transl Med 2017;
       9(410)eaal3693
       [http://dx.doi.org/10.1126/scitranslmed.aal3693] [PMID: 28978750]

[21]   Meldrum C, Doyle MA, Tothill RW. Next-generation sequencing for cancer diagnostics: a practical
       perspective. Clin Biochem Rev 2011; 32(4): 177-95.
       [PMID: 22147957]

[22]   Egatz-Gomez A, Wang C, Klacsmann F, *et al.* Future microfluidic and nanofluidic modular platforms
       for nucleic acid liquid biopsy in precision medicine. Biomicrofluidics 2016; 10(3)032902
       [http://dx.doi.org/10.1063/1.4948525] [PMID: 27190565]

[23]   Grzywinska   D.   Mobile   Medical   Imaging
       2013.https://healthmanagement.org/c/imaging/issuearticle/mobile-medical-imaging

[24]   O'Sullivan S, Ali Z, Jiang X, Abdolvand R. MS ünlü, H Plácido da Silva, JT Baca, B Kim, S Scott, M
       I Sajid, S Moradian, H Mansoorzare, and A Holzinger, "Developments in transduction, connectivity
       and AI/machine learning for point-of-care testing. Sensors (Basel) 2019; 19: 1917.

[25]   Pant N, Dahler J. Multiplexed testing for HIV and related bacterial and viral co-infections at the point-
       of-care: quo vadis? Expert Review of Molecular Diagnostics 2015; 15(4): 463-9.

[26]   Dincer C, Bruch R, Kling A, Dittrich PS, Urban GA. Multiplexed point-of-care testing—xPOCT
       Trends in Biotechnology 2017; 35(8): 728-42.
       [http://dx.doi.org/10.1016/j.tibtech.2017.03.013]

[27]   Relich RF, Abbott AN. Syndromic and point-of-care molecular testing. Advances in Molecular
       Pathology 2018; 1: 97-113.
       [http://dx.doi.org/10.1016/j.yamp.2018.07.007]

[28]   Loubiere S, Moatti JP. Economic evaluation of point-of-care diagnostic technologies for infectious
       diseases. Clin Microbiol Infect 2010; 16(8): 1070-6.
       [http://dx.doi.org/10.1111/j.1469-0691.2010.03280.x] [PMID: 20670289]

[29]   Ferguson NM, Cummings DAT, Fraser C, Cajka JC, Cooley PC, Burke DS. Strategies for mitigating
       an influenza epidemic Nature 2006; 442(27): 448-52.

[30]   Teggert A, Datta H, Ali Z. Biomarkers for Point-of-Care Diagnosis of Sepsis. Micromachines (Basel)
       2020; 11(3)E286
       [http://dx.doi.org/10.3390/mi11030286] [PMID: 32164268]

[31]   Doeven EH. GJ Barbante AJ Harsant, PS Donnelly, TU Connell, CF Hogan, and PS Francis, "Mobile

phone-based electrochemiluminescence sensing exploiting the 'USB On-The-Go' protocol" *Sensors and Actuators***B**. Chemical 2015; 216: 608-13.

[32]   Jamalipour A, Hossain MA. Smartphone Instrumentations for Public Health Safety. Cham, Switzerland: Springer 2019.
[http://dx.doi.org/10.1007/978-3-030-02095-8]

[33]   Davenport T, Kalakota R. The potential of artificial intelligence in healthcareFuture Healthcare J 2019; 6(2): 94-8.
[http://dx.doi.org/10.7861/futurehosp.6-2-94]

[34]   Malik NN. Integration of diagnostic and communication technologies. J Telemed Telecare 2009; 15(7): 323-6.
[http://dx.doi.org/10.1258/jtt.2009.009001] [PMID: 19815900]

[35]   Burdette SD, Herchline TE, Oehler R. Surfing the web: practicing medicine in a technological age: using smartphones in clinical practice. Clin Infect Dis 2008; 47(1): 117-22.
[http://dx.doi.org/10.1086/588788] [PMID: 18491969]

[36]   Bates M, Zumla A. Rapid infectious diseases diagnostics using Smartphones. Ann Transl Med 2015; 3(15): 215.
[PMID: 26488011]

[37]   Wei J, Hollin I, Kachnowski S. A review of the use of mobile phone text messaging in clinical and healthy behaviour interventions. J Telemed Telecare 2011; 17(1): 41-8.
[http://dx.doi.org/10.1258/jtt.2010.100322] [PMID: 21097565]

[38]   Ventola CL. Mobile devices and Apps for health care professionals: Uses and benefits P&T 2014; 39(5): 356-64.

[39]   Oehler RL, Smith K, Toney JF. Infectious diseases resources for the iPhone. Clin Infect Dis 2010; 50(9): 1268-74.
[http://dx.doi.org/10.1086/651602] [PMID: 20233061]

[40]   Friedman B, Jiang HJ, Elixhauser A, Segal A. Hospital costs for adults with multiple chronic conditions Medical Care Research Review 2006; 63(3): 327-46.
[http://dx.doi.org/10.1177/1077558706287042]

[41]   Pereira AM, Jácome C, Almeida R, Fonseca JA. How the smartphone is changing allergy diagnostics. Curr Allergy Asthma Rep 2018; 18(12): 69.
[http://dx.doi.org/10.1007/s11882-018-0824-4] [PMID: 30361774]

[42]   Hirst JA, Stevens RJ, Smith I, James T, Gudgin BC, Farmer AJ. How can point-of-care HbA1c testing be integrated into UK primary care consultations? - A feasibility study. Diabetes Res Clin Pract 2017; 130: 113-20.
[http://dx.doi.org/10.1016/j.diabres.2017.05.014] [PMID: 28602811]

[43]   Pai NP, Dhurat R, Potter M, *et al.* Will a quadruple multiplexed point-of-care screening strategy for HIV-related co-infections be feasible and impact detection of new co-infections in at-risk populations? Results from cross-sectional studies. BMJ Open 2014; 4(12)e005040
[http://dx.doi.org/10.1136/bmjopen-2014-005040] [PMID: 25510882]

[44]   Semret M, Ndao M, Jacobs J, Yansouni CP. Point-of-care and point-of-'can': leveraging reference-laboratory capacity for integrated diagnosis of fever syndromes in the tropics. Clin Microbiol Infect 2018; 24(8): 836-44.
[http://dx.doi.org/10.1016/j.cmi.2018.03.044] [PMID: 29649602]

[45]   Liu Y, Pharr M, Salvatore GA. Lab-on-skin: A review of flexible and stretchable electronics for wearable health monitoring. ACS Nano 2017; 11(10): 9614-35.
[http://dx.doi.org/10.1021/acsnano.7b04898] [PMID: 28901746]

[46]   Godfrey A, Hetherington V, Shum H, Bonato P, Lovell NH, Stuart S. From A to Z: Wearable technology explained. Maturitas 2018; 113: 40-7.

[http://dx.doi.org/10.1016/j.maturitas.2018.04.012] [PMID: 29903647]

[47]   Tan EKW, Au YZ, Moghaddam GK, Occhipinti LG, Lowe CR. Towards closed-loop integration of point-of-care technologies. Trends in Biotechnology 2019; 37(7): 775-88.
[http://dx.doi.org/10.1016/j.tibtech.2018.12.004]

[48]   Zhu H, Isikman SO, Mudanyali O, Greenbaum A, Ozcan A. Optical imaging techniques for point-o--care diagnostics. Lab Chip 2013; 13(1): 51-67.
[http://dx.doi.org/10.1039/C2LC40864C] [PMID: 23044793]

[49]   McLean R, Jury C, Bazeos A, Lewis SM. Application of camera phones in telehaematology. J Telemed Telecare 2009; 15(7): 339-43.
[http://dx.doi.org/10.1258/jtt.2009.090114] [PMID: 19815902]

[50]   Breslauer DN, Maamari RN, Switz NA, Lam WA, Fletcher DA. Mobile phone based clinical microscopy for global health applications. PLoS One 2009; 4(7):e6320.
[http://dx.doi.org/10.1371/journal.pone.0006320]

[51]   Berke A. Can you heal me now? Using cell phones to diagnose disease. Berkeley Science Review 2019; 17: 30-3.

[52]   Granot Y, Ivorra A, Rubinsky B. A new concept for medical imaging centered on cellular phone technology. PLoS ONE 2008; 3(4): e2075.
[http://dx.doi.org/10.1371/journal.pone.0002075]

[53]   Skandarajah A, Reber CD, Switz NA, Fletcher DA. Quantitative imaging with a mobile phone microscope. PLOS ONE 2014; 9(5):e96906.
[http://dx.doi.org/10.1371/journal.pone.0096906]

[54]   Coulibaly JT, Ouattara M, D'Ambrosio MV, *et al.* Accuracy of mobile phone and handheld light microscopy for the diagnosis of Schistosomiasis and intestinal protozoa infections in Côte d'Ivoire. PLOS: Neglected   Tropical   Diseases   2016.
https://journals.plos.org/plosntds/article?id=10.1371/journal.pntd.0004768
[http://dx.doi.org/DOI:10.1371/journal.pntd.0004768]

[55]   Bifolck E, Fink A, Pedersen D, Gregory T. Smartphone imaging for the ophthalmic examination in primary care. JAAPA 2018; 31(8): 34-8.
[http://dx.doi.org/10.1097/01.JAA.0000541482.54611.7c]

[56]   Grudpan K, Kolev SD, Lapanantnopakhun S, McKelvie ID, Wongwilai W. Applications of everyday IT and communications devices in modern analytical chemistry: A review. Talanta 2015; 136: 84-94.
[http://dx.doi.org/10.1016/j.talanta.2014.12.042] [PMID: 25702989]

[57]   Meredith SE, Robinson A, Erb P, *et al.* A mobile-phone-based breath carbon monoxide meter to detect cigarette smoking. Nicotine Tob Res 2014; 16(6): 766-73.
[http://dx.doi.org/10.1093/ntr/ntt275] [PMID: 24470633]

[58]   Shen L, Hagen JA, Papautsky I. Point-of-care colorimetric detection with a smartphone. Lab Chip 2012; 12(21): 4240-3.
[http://dx.doi.org/10.1039/c2lc40741h] [PMID: 22996728]

[59]   Hárendarčíková L, Petr J. Smartphones & microfluidics: Marriage for the future. Electrophoresis 2018; 39(11): 1319-28.
[http://dx.doi.org/10.1002/elps.201700389] [PMID: 29484674]

[60]   Oncescu V, Mancuso M, Erickson D. Cholesterol testing on a smartphone. Lab Chip 2014; 14(4): 759-63.
[http://dx.doi.org/10.1039/C3LC51194D] [PMID: 24336861]

[61]   Martinez AW, Phillips ST, Carrilho E, Thomas SW III, Sindi H, Whitesides GM. Simple telemedicine for developing regions: camera phones and paper-based microfluidic devices for real-time, off-site diagnosis. Anal Chem 2008; 80(10): 3699-707.
[http://dx.doi.org/10.1021/ac800112r] [PMID: 18407617]

[62]   Cadle BA, Rasmus KC, Varela JA, *et al.* Cellular phone-based image acquisition and quantitative ratiometric method for detecting cocaine and benzoylecgonine for biological and forensic applications. Subst Abuse 2010; 4: 21-33.
[http://dx.doi.org/10.4137/SART.S5025] [PMID: 22879741]

[63]   Preechaburana P, Macken S, Suska A, Filippini D. Mobile phone analysis of NT-proBNP using high dynamic range (HDR) imaging. Procedia Eng 2010; 5: 584-7.
[http://dx.doi.org/10.1016/j.proeng.2010.09.177]

[64]   Meagher RJ, Kousvelari E. Mobile oral heath technologies based on saliva. Oral Dis 2018; 24(1-2): 194-7.
[http://dx.doi.org/10.1111/odi.12775] [PMID: 29480598]

[65]   Laksanasopin TW, S Nayak Guo , *et al.* A smartphone dongle for diagnosis of infectious diseases at the point of care" Science Translation Medicine 2015; 7(273):273re1.
[http://dx.doi.org/10.1126/scitranslmed.aaa0056] [PMID: 25653222]

[66]   Ra M, Muhammad MS, Lim C, Han S, Jung C, Kim W-Y. Smartphone-based point-of-care urinalysis under variable illumination. IEEE J Transl Eng Health Med 2017; 62800111
[PMID: 29333352]

[67]   McGonigle AJS, Wilkes TC, Pering TD, *et al.* Smartphone Spectrometers. Sensors (Basel) 2018; 18(1): 223.
[http://dx.doi.org/10.3390/s18010223] [PMID: 29342899]

[68]   Wang LJ, Chang Y-C, Sun R, Li L. A multichannel smartphone optical biosensor for high-throughput point-of-care diagnostics. Biosens Bioelectron 2017; 87: 686-92.
[http://dx.doi.org/10.1016/j.bios.2016.09.021] [PMID: 27631683]

[69]   Ormachea A, Escalera R , *et al.* A spectrometer based on smartphones and a low-cost kit for transmittance and absorbance measurements in real time Óptica Pura Y Applicada 2017; 50(3): 239-49.

[70]   Scherr TF, Gupta S, Wright DW, Haselton FR. Mobile phone imaging and cloud-based analysis for standardized malaria detection and reporting. Sci Rep 2016; 6: 28645.
[http://dx.doi.org/10.1038/srep28645] [PMID: 27345590]

[71]   Stedtfeld RD, Tourlousse DM, Seyrig G, *et al.* Gene-Z: a device for point of care genetic testing using a smartphone. Lab Chip 2012; 12(8): 1454-62.
[http://dx.doi.org/10.1039/c2lc21226a] [PMID: 22374412]

[72]   Barnes L, Heithoff DM, Mahan SP, *et al.* Smartphone-based pathogen diagnosis in urinary sepsis patients. EBioMedicine 2018; 36: 73-82.
[http://dx.doi.org/10.1016/j.ebiom.2018.09.001] [PMID: 30245056]

[73]   Priye A, Bird SW, Light YK, Ball CS, Negrete OA, Meagher RJ. A smartphone-based diagnostic platform for rapid detection of Zika, chikungunya, and dengue viruses. Sci Rep 2017; 7: 44778.
[http://dx.doi.org/10.1038/srep44778] [PMID: 28317856]

[74]   Song J, Pandian V, Mauk MG, *et al.* Smartphone-based mobile detection platform for molecular diagnostics and spatiotemporal disease mapping. Anal Chem 2018; 90(7): 4823-31.
[http://dx.doi.org/10.1021/acs.analchem.8b00283] [PMID: 29542319]

[75]   Chen W, Yu H, Sun F, *et al.* Mobile Platform for Multiplexed Detection and Differentiation of Disease-Specific Nucleic Acid Sequences, Using Microfluidic Loop-Mediated Isothermal Amplification and Smartphone Detection. Anal Chem 2017; 89(21): 11219-26.
[http://dx.doi.org/10.1021/acs.analchem.7b02478] [PMID: 28819973]

[76]   Qiu X, Ge S, Gao P, *et al.* A smartphone-based point-of-care diagnosis of H1N1 with microfluidic convection PCR. Microsyst Technol 2017; 23: 2951-6.
[http://dx.doi.org/10.1007/s00542-016-2979-z]

[77]   Ming K, Kim J, Biondi MJ, Syed A, Chen K, Lam A. "Integrated quantum dot barcode smartphone optical device for wireless multiplexed diagnosis of infected patients" ACS Nano 2015; 9(3): 3060-74.

[78]   Tortajada-Genaro LA, Yamanaka ES, Maquieira Á. Consumer electronics devices for DNA genotyping based on loop-mediated isothermal amplification and array hybridisation. Talanta 2019; 198: 424-31.
[http://dx.doi.org/10.1016/j.talanta.2019.01.124] [PMID: 30876582]

[79]   Yamanaka ES, Tortajada-Genaro LA, Pastor N, Maquieira Á. Polymorphism genotyping based on loop-mediated isothermal amplification and smartphone detection. Biosens Bioelectron 2018; 109: 177-83.
[http://dx.doi.org/10.1016/j.bios.2018.03.008] [PMID: 29558731]

[80]   Karow J. Oxford Nanopore developing Smartphone-powered device, launches New Pore 2016.https://www.genomeweb.com/sequencing/oxford-nanopore-developing-smartph-ne-powered-device-launches-new-pore#.XKq3DJhKiUk

[81]   Kühnemund M, Wei Q, Daria E, Wang Y, Hernándex-Nueta I. Z yang, D Tseng, A Ahlford, L Mathot, T Sjöblom, A Ozcan, and M Nilsson, "Target DNA sequencing and in situ mutation analysis using mobile phone microscopy. Nat Commun 2017; 8: 13913.
[http://dx.doi.org/10.1038/ncomms13913] [PMID: 28094784]

[82]   Ko SY, Sassoubre L, Zola J. Applications and challenges of real-time mobile DNA analysis Proceedings of the 19th International Workshop on Mobile Computing Systems & Applications. 1-6.
[http://dx.doi.org/10.1145/3177102.3177114]

[83]   Huang X, Xu D, Chen J, *et al.* Smartphone-based analytical biosensors. Analyst (Lond) 2018; 143(22): 5339-51.
[http://dx.doi.org/10.1039/C8AN01269E] [PMID: 30327808]

[84]   Xu D, Huang X, Guo J, Ma X. Automatic smartphone-based microfluidic biosensor system at the point of care. Biosens Bioelectron 2018; 110: 78-88.
[http://dx.doi.org/10.1016/j.bios.2018.03.018] [PMID: 29602034]

[85]   Kanchi S, Sabela MI, Mdluli PS, Inamuddin , Bisetty K. Smartphone based bioanalytical and diagnosis applications: A review. Biosens Bioelectron 2018; 102: 136-49.
[http://dx.doi.org/10.1016/j.bios.2017.11.021] [PMID: 29128716]

[86]   Yang K, Peretz-Soroka H, Liu Y, Lin F. Novel developments in mobile sensing based on the integration of microfluidic devices and smartphones. Lab Chip 2016; 16(6): 943-58.
[http://dx.doi.org/10.1039/C5LC01524C] [PMID: 26899264]

[87]   Nemati E, Batteate C, Jerrett M. Opportunistic environmental sensing with Smartphones: A critical review of current literature and applications. Curr Environ Health Rep 2017; 4(3): 306-18.
[http://dx.doi.org/10.1007/s40572-017-0158-8] [PMID: 28879432]

[88]   Chaix B. Mobile sensing in environmental health and neighborhood research. Annu Rev Public Health 2018; 39: 367-84.
[http://dx.doi.org/10.1146/annurev-publhealth-040617-013731] [PMID: 29608869]

[89]   Rateni G, Dario P, Cavallo F. Smartphone-based food diagnostic technologies: A Review. Sensors (Basel) 2017; 17(6): 1453.
[http://dx.doi.org/10.3390/s17061453] [PMID: 28632188]

[90]   Zeinhom MMA, Wang Y, Sheng L, *et al.* "Smart phone based immunosensor coupled with nanoflower signal amplification for rapid detection of Salmonella Enteritidis in milk, cheese and water" *Sensors and ActuatorsB.* Chemical 2018; 261: 75-82.
[http://dx.doi.org/10.1016/j.snb.2017.11.093]

[91]   Jang H, Ahmed SR, Neethirajan S. GryphSens: A smartphone-based portable diagnostic reader for rapid detection of progesterone in milk. Sensors (Basel) 2017; 17(5): 1079.
[http://dx.doi.org/10.3390/s17051079] [PMID: 28489036]

[92]   Giordano GF, Vincentini MBR, Murer RC, *et al.* Point-of-use electroanalytical platform on home made potentiostat and smartphone for multivariate data processing. Electrochim Acta 2016; 219: 170-7.
[http://dx.doi.org/10.1016/j.electacta.2016.09.157]

[93]   Lin B, Yu Y, Cao Y. M guo, D Zhu, J Dai, and M Zheng, "Point-of-care testing for streptomycin based on aptamer recognized and digital image colorimetry by smartphone. Biosens Bioelectron 2018; 100: 482-9.
[http://dx.doi.org/10.1016/j.bios.2017.09.028] [PMID: 28965053]

[94]   Shin J, Choi S, Ynag J-S, Song J, Choi J-S, Jung H-I. "Smart forensic phone: Colorimetric analysis of a bloodstain for age and estimation using a smartphone" *Sensors and Actuators B*. Chemical 2017; 243: 221-5.

[95]   Saaed MA, Jabbar A. 'Smart diagnosis' of parasitic diseases by use of smartphones J Clinical Microbiology 2018; 56(1)e01469.

[96]   Zhang D, Jiang J, Chen J, *et al.* Smartphone-based portable biosensing system using impedance measurement with printed electrodes for 2,4,6-trinitrotoluene (TNT) detection. Biosens Bioelectron 2015; 70: 81-8.
[http://dx.doi.org/10.1016/j.bios.2015.03.004] [PMID: 25796040]

[97]   Kulkarni A, Sathe S. Healthcare applications of the Internet of Things: A review Int J Computer Science and Information Technologies 2014; 5(5): 6229-32.

[98]   Gluhak A, Krco S, Nati M, Pfisterer D, Mitton N, Razafindralambo T. A survey of facilities for experimental internet of things research. IEEE Communications 2011; 49: 58-67.
[http://dx.doi.org/10.1109/MCOM.2011.6069710]

[99]   Sethi P, Sarangi SR. Internet of Things: Architectures, Protocols, and Applications. J Electr Comput Eng 2017.: 9324035.
[http://dx.doi.org/10.1155/2017/9324035]

[100]   Gubbi J, Buyya R, Marusic S. Internet of Things (IoT): A vision, architectural elements, and future directions. Future Generation Computer Systems 2013; 29(7): 1645-1660.
[http://dx.doi.org/10.1016/j.future.2013.01.010]

[101]   Shelke Y. The internet of medical things in healthcare 2017. https://www.healthcaretechnologies.com

[102]   Marr B. Why the internet of medical things (IoMT) will start to transform healthcare in 2018. 2018.

[103]   Martin R. The internet of medical things (IoMT)- The future of healthcare 2018. https://igniteoutsourcing.com

[104]   Singh H. Internet of medical things (IoMT): The future of the medical world 2018.http://customerthink.com/internet

[105]   Basatneh R, Najafi B, Armstrong DG. Health sensors, smart home devices, and the internet of medical things: An opportunity for dramatic improvement in care for the lower extremity complictions of diabetes. J Diabetes Sci Technol 2018; 12(3): 577-86.
[http://dx.doi.org/10.1177/1932296818768618] [PMID: 29635931]

[106]   Jagadeeswari V, Subramaniyaswamy V, Logesh R, Vijayakumar V. A study on medical Internet of Things and Big Data in personalized healthcare system. Health Inf Sci Syst 2018; 6(1): 14.
[http://dx.doi.org/10.1007/s13755-018-0049-x] [PMID: 30279984]

[107]   Catherwood PA, Steele D, Little M, Mccomb S, Mclaughlin J. A community-based IoT personalized wireless healthcare solution trial. IEEE J Transl Eng Health Med 2018; 6: 2800313.
[http://dx.doi.org/10.1109/JTEHM.2018.2822302] [PMID: 29888145]

[108]   Chang H, Choi M. Big data and healthcare: Building an augmented world. Healthc Inform Res 2016; 22(3): 153-5.
[http://dx.doi.org/10.4258/hir.2016.22.3.153] [PMID: 27525155]

[109] Jiang F, Jiang Y, Zhi H, *et al.* Artificial intelligence in healthcare: past, present and future. Stroke Vasc Neurol 2017; 2(4): 230-43.
[http://dx.doi.org/10.1136/svn-2017-000101] [PMID: 29507784]

[110] Patel VL, Shortliffe EH, Stefanelli M, *et al.* The coming of age of artificial intelligence in medicine. Artif Intell Med 2009; 46(1): 5-17.
[http://dx.doi.org/10.1016/j.artmed.2008.07.017] [PMID: 18790621]

[111] Siemens Healthcare Diagnostics. From automating muscle to augmenting the brain: How artificial intelligence will change the clinical laboratory. Siemens Healthcare Diagnostics, Inc. 2018.

[112] Hoffmann G, Bietenbeck A, Lichtinghagen R, Klawonn F. Using machine learning techniques to generate laboratory diagnostic pathways- a case study. J Lab Precis Med 2018; 3: 58.
[http://dx.doi.org/10.21037/jlpm.2018.06.01]

[113] Xie Q, Faust K, Van Ommeren R, Sheikh A, Djuric U, Diamandis P. Deep learning for image analysis: Personalizing medicine closer to the point of care. 2019.
[http://dx.doi.org/10.1080/10408363.2018.1536111]

[114] Saiful Islam M, Hasan MM, Wang X, Germack HD, Noor-E MD. -Alam, "A systematic review on healthcare analytics: Application and theoretical perspective of data mining. Health Care (Don Mills) 2018; 6: 54.

[115] Liao Y, Xu B, Wang J, Liu X. A new method for assessing the risk of infectious disease outbreak. Sci Rep 2017; 7: 40084.
[http://dx.doi.org/10.1038/srep40084] [PMID: 28067258]

[116] Gopal G, Suter-Crazzolara C, Toldo L, Eberhardt W. Digital transformation in healthcare - architectures of present and future information technologies. Clin Chem Lab Med 2019; 57(3): 328-35.
[http://dx.doi.org/10.1515/cclm-2018-0658] [PMID: 30530878]

[117] Vashistha R, Dangi AK, Kumar A, Chhabra D, Shukla P. Futuristic biosensors for cardiac health care: An artificial intelligence approach 2018.
[http://dx.doi.org/10.1007/s13205-018-1368-y]

[118] 13D Research, "Artificial intelligence is on the precipice of revolutionizing medical diagnosis" [2017] http://latest.13d.com/artificial

[119] Yu K-H, Beam AL, Kohane IS. Artificial intelligence in healthcare. Nat Biomed Eng 2018; 2(10): 719-31.
[http://dx.doi.org/10.1038/s41551-018-0305-z] [PMID: 31015651]

[120] Kolachalama VB, Garg PS. Machine learning and medical education. NPJ Digit Med 2018; 1: 54.
[http://dx.doi.org/10.1038/s41746-018-0061-1] [PMID: 31304333]

[121] Raval S. Natural Language Processing and Sentiment Analysis 2017.https://medium.com/udacity/natural-language-processing-and-sentiment-analysis-43111c33c27e

[122] Kennedy LP. Health care's hard drive 2019.

[123] Chang EY, Wu M-H, Tang K-F, Kao H-C, Chou C-N. Artificial intelligence in XPRIZE DeepQ Tricorder MMHealth'17: Proceedings of the 2nd International Workshop on Multimedia for Personal Health and Health Care. 11-8.
[http://dx.doi.org/10.1145/3132635.3132637]

[124] Smith KP, Kang AD, Kirby JE. "Automated interpretation of blood culture Gram stains by use of a deep convolutional neural network" J Clinical Chemistry (2018) 56, 3 e1521-17

[125] Koydemir HC, Gorocs Z, Tseng D, *et al.* Rapid imaging, detection and quantification of Giardia lamblia cysts using mobile-phone based fluorescent microscopy and machine learning. Lab Chip 2015; 15(5): 1284-93.
[http://dx.doi.org/10.1039/C4LC01358A] [PMID: 25537426]

[126] Qiu X, Song L, Yang S, *et al.* A fast and low-cost genotyping method for hepatitis B virus based on pattern recognition in point-of-care settings. Sci Rep 2016; 6: 28274.
[http://dx.doi.org/10.1038/srep28274] [PMID: 27306485]

[127] Valderrama CE, Marzbanrad F, Stroux L, *et al.* Improvement in quality of point-of-care diagnostics with real-time machine learning in low literacy LMIC settings https://doi.org/https://doi.org/https://doi.org/10.1145/3209811.3209811.3209815

[128] Poostchi M, Silamut K, Maude RJ, Jaeger S, Thoma G. Image analysis and machine learning for detecting malaria. Transl Res 2018; 194: 36-55.
[http://dx.doi.org/10.1016/j.trsl.2017.12.004] [PMID: 29360430]

[129] Kim S-J, Wang C, Zhao B, *et al.* Deep transfer learning based hologram classification for molecular diagnostics. 2018.
[http://dx.doi.org/10.1038/s41598-018-35274-x]

[130] Huang X, Jiang Y, Liu X, *et al.* Machine learning based single-frame super-resolution processing for lensless blood cell counting. Sensors (Basel) 2016; 16(11): 1836.
[http://dx.doi.org/10.3390/s16111836] [PMID: 27827837]

[131] Potluri V, Kathiresan PS, Kandula H, *et al.* "An inexpensive smartphone-based device for point-o--care ovulation testing" Lab Chip (2018) 19,1 59-67

[132] Dolan BF. FDA clears first diagnosticradiology app, Mobile MIM https://mobilehealthnews.com/10173/2011.

[133] Dolan BF. FDA approves Mobisante;s smartphone ultrasound https://mobilehealthnews.com/10165/2011.

[134] Kumar R. The FDA's regulation of mobile technology as medical devices 2010.https://www.law.uh.edu/healthlaw/perspectives/2010/kumar-fdamobile.pdf

[135] Kao C-K, Liebovitz DM. Consumer mobile health apps: Current state, barriers, and future directions. PM R 2017; 9(5S): S106-15.
[http://dx.doi.org/10.1016/j.pmrj.2017.02.018] [PMID: 28527495]

[136] Young A. What internet of medical things (IoMT) devices means for healthcare cybersecurity https://healthtechmagazine.net/article/2018/04/The-Internet-of-Medical-Things-Opens--ealth-Organizations-Up-to-More-Threats2018.

[137] Gronowski AM, Haymond S, Master SR. Improving Direct-to-Consumer Medical Testing. 2017.
[http://dx.doi.org/10.1001/jama.2017.13733]

[138] Li M, Diamandis EP, Grenache D, Joyner MJ, Holmes DT, Seccombe R. Direct-to-Consumer Testing 2017.
[http://dx.doi.org/10.1373/clinchem.2016.260349]

[139] Tolan NV. Direct-to-Consumer testing: A new paradigm for point-of-care testing. Point Care 2017; 16: 108-1111.
[http://dx.doi.org/10.1097/POC.0000000000000137]

[140] Lovett Rockwell K. Direct-to-consumer medical testing in the era of value-based care 2017.

[141] El Khaddar MA, Boulmalf M. 2017.

[142] Ozcan A. Mobile phones democratize and cultivate next-generation imaging, diagnostics and measurement tools. Lab Chip 2014; 14(17): 3187-94.
[http://dx.doi.org/10.1039/C4LC00010B] [PMID: 24647550]

[143] https://www.statista.com/statistics/330695/number-of-smartphone-users-worldwide/

[144] https://www.statista.com/topics/840/smartphones/

[145] Kish L. 8 takeaways from Topal's 1 atest: 'The Patient Will See You Now'

2015.http://healthstandards.com/nlog/2015/01/28/future-of-medicine-is-in-your-hands/

[146] Kricka LJ. History of disruptions in laboratory medicine: What have we learned from predictions? Clin Chem Lab Med 2018.
[http://dx.doi.org/10.1515/ccim-2018-0518] [PMID: 29927745]

Frontiers in Nanobiotechnology, 2020, Vol. 1, 347-386

CHAPTER 9

Biomarkers and Applications in Alzheimer's Disease

Ru-Yi Youh[1], Po-Yen Chen[1], Yen-Cheng Chao[4], Di-Hua Luo[2], Hao-Hsiang Chang[3], Yu-Ling Chang[2], Wei-Min Liu[4] and Dean Chou[1,†]

[1] *Department of Mechanical Engineering, National Central University, Taoyuan, Taiwan*

[2] *Department of Psychology, College of Science, National Taiwan University, Taipei, Taiwan*

[3] *Department of Family Medicine, National Taiwan University Hospital, Taipei, Taiwan*

[4] *Department of Chemistry, Fu Jen Catholic University, New Taipei City, Taiwan*

Abstract: In this chapter, we will review some methods and platforms related to the diagnosis of Alzheimer's disease (AD). The global prevalence of dementia and AD shows the urgent requirement of effective treatment, where an accurate and early diagnosis plays an important role. Apart from cognitive diagnosis that clarifies the cognitive deterioration of AD, abundant clinical studies have consistently recognised the core neuropathological features and related fluid biomarkers as utile indicators for the diagnosis and prognosis of AD and its preclinical stages. In order to enhance the accuracy of detecting these biomarkers, convinced methods and platforms are essential. Here, we summarised associated platforms, including imaging platforms (*e.g.*, positron emission tomography (PET) and structural imaging), enzyme-linked immunosorbent assays (ELISA), and matrix-assisted laser desorption/ionisation – time of flight – mass spectrometry (MALDI-TOF-MS).

Keywords: Amyloid-β (Aβ), Alzheimer's Disease, Biomedical Modelling, Biomarker, Cerebroporomehcaincs, Dementia, Enzyme-linked Immunosorbent Assays (ELISA), Matrix-Assisted Laser Desorption/Ionisation – Time of Flight – Mass Spectrometry (MALDI-TOF-MS), MultipleNetwork Poroelastic Theory (MPET), Tau, Neuroimaging, Virtual Physiological Human (VPH).

INTRODUCTION

Though medical advances have enhanced both health and life expectancy, it also brought about new challenges. According to the World Population Ageing 2017 Report, life expectancy at birth has been increasing worldwide for both males and females [1]. Whereas the 2018 revision of world population prospects shows,

* **Corresponding author Dean Chou:** National Central University, Department of Mechanical Engineering Taiwan; E-mail:dean@ncu.edu.tw

Han-Sheng Chuang & Yi-Ping Ho (Eds.)

the number of older persons in the world is projected to be billion in 2050, and could rise to 3.1 billion in 2100 [2]. However, while the world's population is ageing, ageing has been demonstrated as a significant risk factor of neurodegenerative diseases. These neurodegenerative diseases affect millions of people worldwide, and the prevalence is still rising [3 - 6]. It is a challenging task to accurately distinguish different diseases due to the similarity of their clinical and pathological features [7 - 10]. Consequently, the scientist has spent much effort to discriminate these diseases through bio-molecular diagnosis [11, 12] and genetic variabilities [13, 14] in the past few decades.

Dementia is one of the influential outcomes in an ageing society. The cause of long term decreases in the cogitable ability, and retentivity affects a person's daily functioning and therefore becomes a financial burden of both family and country. The prevalence of dementia increases through age, and the number of people estimated suffering from dementia is expected to double every 20 years [15 - 17]. Based on the World Dementia Report 2018, there is an estimation of 50 million people worldwide living with dementia and the population is projected to rise to about 152 million people by 2050 which may be presented as a trillion-dollar question [18].

Dementia can be divided into several subtypes according to the related disease such as AD, vascular dementia, dementia with Lewy bodies and frontotemporal dementia. In comparison with other subtypes of dementia, AD is the most common subtype that is approximately two-thirds of cases of dementia [19]. Patients with AD may experience difficulty in daily activity, language problems, memory loss, depression, hallucination and other behavioural disturbances [20]. Vascular dementia is the second most common subtype of dementia, which is caused by cerebrovascular diseases, standard forms of vascular dementia, *e.g.*, multi-infarct dementia, and subcortical ischemic vascular dementia. Large vessel diseases generally cause multi-infarct dementia. Major strokes or a series of minor strokes may occur and lead to widespread infarcts around the brain. Subcortical ischemic vascular dementia is caused by small vessel disease and accompanies changes in white matter and lacunar infarction [21 - 24]. Among all subtypes of dementia, a single type of dementia rarely occurs alone. Patients may have one or more pathologies coexisting and symptoms may be similar. The coexistence of pathology is called mixed dementia and raises the difficulty in diagnosis of various types of dementia [25 - 27]. Here, we will focus on the most common subtype dementia – AD in further discussion.

Alzheimer's Disease

As mentioned previously, around 50 million people live with dementia worldwide and that AD, one of the most common neurodegenerative diseases, comprises 70 per centum of all dementia [19, 28]. Reports show that new patients appear every three seconds on average, owing to the rising population of older adults [19, 28]. Despite the urgency, AD is temporary incurable, and that the aetiology is incompletely known. Studies have given attempts to understand the pathogenesis of AD and to develop diagnosis methodology with higher precision. Research advances have enabled extensive comprehension of the pathophysiology of this disorder. A summary of the pathogenesis of AD will be shown in the next section "biomarkers of AD".

Risk Factors

Risk factors of AD have been widely studied where ageing and genetic are mostly discussed. The prevalence of AD increases exponentially, which doubles every five years after the age of 60 and the incidence rate is estimated to double approximately every 4.4 years [29, 30]. Besides ageing, other risk factors have also been proposed. Some of the risk factors are behaviour-related, including smoking [31 - 39]. Others may be related to vascular systems, including diabetes, hypertension, and metabolic syndromes [40 - 43]. Factors related to cerebro-vascular diseases, namely vascular factors, not only affect vascular dementia but also affect AD. Studies show that dementia in 50% of demented-patients may be influenced by vascular pathologies [44]. These vascular risk factors include raised systolic blood pressure, high serum cholesterol concentration, and high total cholesterol level in midlife [45, 46]. Moreover, the presence of specific diseases also exhibits a higher risk of AD, including obesity, hypertension diabetes, and heart diseases [46 - 48]. Though some factors are presented, the mechanism between vascular risk factors and AD is uncertain. Some metal ions are also considered as important AD risk factors. These metal ions not only accelerate protein aggregation and stabilize amyloid fibrils, but also enhance the interaction between aggregated protein with cell's membranes causing neuronal cell dysfunction. In addition, metal protein complex, Fe^{2+} and Cu^{2+} in particular, lead to H_2O_2 production resulting in oxidative stress-damaging [49].

Four genetic factors associated with AD include amyloid precursor protein (APP), presenilin 1 presenilin 2, and apolipoprotein E. The genes encoding APP, presenilin 1, presenilin 2, and apolipoprotein E are respectively mapped on chromosome 21, chromosome 14, chromosome 1, and chromosome 19. Among these genetic factors, APP, presenilin one, and presenilin two are identified as autosomal-dominant and deterministic genes involving in early-onset AD [50 - 54], whereas apolipoprotein E is determined as an influential factor for both early-onset and late-onset AD [55 - 59]. Early-onset AD generally affects patients in the age of 40s to 60s and exhibits similar pathological features to late-onset

AD. Although early-onset AD is a rare form of AD, the understanding of early-onset AD brought about useful clinical information for the pathophysiology of AD [60]. Late-onset AD generally affects patients aged over 65, and that is associated with Apolipoprotein E [58, 61]. Apolipoprotein E has three alleles, including type 2, type 3, and type 4 alleles. Studies show that apolipoprotein E type 4 allele is a strong risk factor for AD, while apolipoprotein E type 2 allele is protective against AD [59].

In comparison with genetic variabilities, abnormal protein aggregation processes, including amyloidopathies and tauopathies are standard molecular features of AD. As a result, AD has also been classified as amyloidosis. Amyloidosis is a group of diseases caused by systemic or localised misfolded insoluble protein aggregates [62 - 64]. Amyloidopathies and tauopathies in AD result in amyloid plaques and neurofibrillary tangles deposits, respectively. Amyloid plaques are formed from amyloid-β (Aβ) and neurofibrillary tangles are made of tau protein within the brain. Tauopathies accompany the phosphorylation of tau protein. These abnormal microtubule-associated tau proteins are hyperphosphorylated and cause tau protein to dissociate from microtubules forming neurofibrillary tangles in the human brain. Moreover, studies showed that tau fibrils, transferring between neurons, link with the tau propagation, whereas tau oligomers correlate with the neurodegeneration [65 - 69]. Therefore, Aβ and tau protein are considered as the main biomarkers for AD diagnosis.

BIOMARKERS OF ALZHEIMER'S DISEASE

To our limited knowledge, no disease-modifying drugs for AD are fully validated temporarily in commercialisation or phase III clinical trials. The reason may partially lie in the fact that some clinically diagnosed patients exhibit no evidence of amyloid pathology [70]. The high accuracy rate of 80–90% applying clinical criteria are reported based on diagnosis in later stages of the disease. However, diagnostic accuracy is lower at the earlier clinical stages of the disease, especially preclinical stages [71]. Literature reports have suggested that diagnostic criteria for the preclinical stages of AD based on biomarkers, which is objectively measured and evaluated as an indicator of normal biological processes, pathogenic processes, or pharmacologic responses to therapeutic intervention, enhances the sensitivity and the specificity compared with conventionally clinical diagnosis [72 - 74]. Therefore, biomarkers may create a possible solution aiding early diagnosis with high accuracy of AD. The following features keep an ideal diagnosis biomarker: high sensitivity detecting AD, high specificity for distinguishing other dementias, reliable, reproducible, and non-invasive [71, 75].

Aβ and Tau

The neuropathological feature of AD is commonly characterized by: (1) extracellular plaque deposits of amyloid beta (Aβ) peptides and (2) intraneuronal hyperphosphorylated tau-containing neurofibrillary tangles (NFTs), which collectively induce neuronal loss in specific brain regions – primarily the medial temporal lobe structures and the temporal-parietal association cortices — of affected individuals [76, 77]. A longitudinal study showed that Aβ might link with the detection of the earliest pathologic change, while tau protein is more closely related to the clinical progression of AD [78]. Other abundant clinical studies have consistently recognised these core neuropathological features and their related fluid biomarkers as utile indicators for the diagnosis and prognosis of AD and its preclinical stages. The following section will give a summary update on the research of the core biomarkers of AD, highlighting the evidence derived from recent studies of fluid biomarkers, such as toxic protein in cerebrospinal fluid (CSF) and plasma. In the CSF, 42 amino acid form of amyloid-β (Aβ42), phosphorylated tau (p-tau), and total tau (t-tau) are the most convinced biomarkers for AD [79]. In plasma, plasma Aβ, plasma t-tau, and plasma p-tau are the potential biomarkers for AD.

CSF Aβ and Tau

One of the core biomarkers of AD is associated with Aβ peptides. Aβ peptides arise from the metabolic degradation of the APP, an 87-kDa transmembrane protein with a large extracellular domain. APP undergoes two different metabolic digestion pathways: the non-amyloidogenic pathway and the amyloidogenic pathway (Fig. 1) [80]. For the non-amyloidogenic pathway, APP is firstly cleaved by α-secretases resulting in two fragments. One of these two fragments called sAPPα is released into the extracellular space, and the other smaller fragment is further digested by γ-secretases to yield a soluble N-terminal fragment (p3) and a membrane-bound C-terminal fragment (AICD, or APP intracellular domain). In this non-amyloidogenic pathway, no Aβ peptides are produced. In the amyloidogenic pathway, APP is initially processed by the β-secretases to form sAPPβ that is also released into the extracellular space. The rest of the APP is subsequently cleaved by γ-secretases to give several peptide fragments varying in length. Generally, these peptides contain 39-43 amino-acids. Within these peptides, Aβ40 and Aβ42 are two major Aβ peptides, and that has only two amino acid differences at C-terminal. Both the Aβ40 and Aβ42 alloforms are significant components of the extracellular plaques found in Alzheimer's disease brain tissue. The concentrations of these peptides in CSF of AD patients is correlated with the presence of amyloid plaques, and that is also an essential indicator for AD diagnosis.

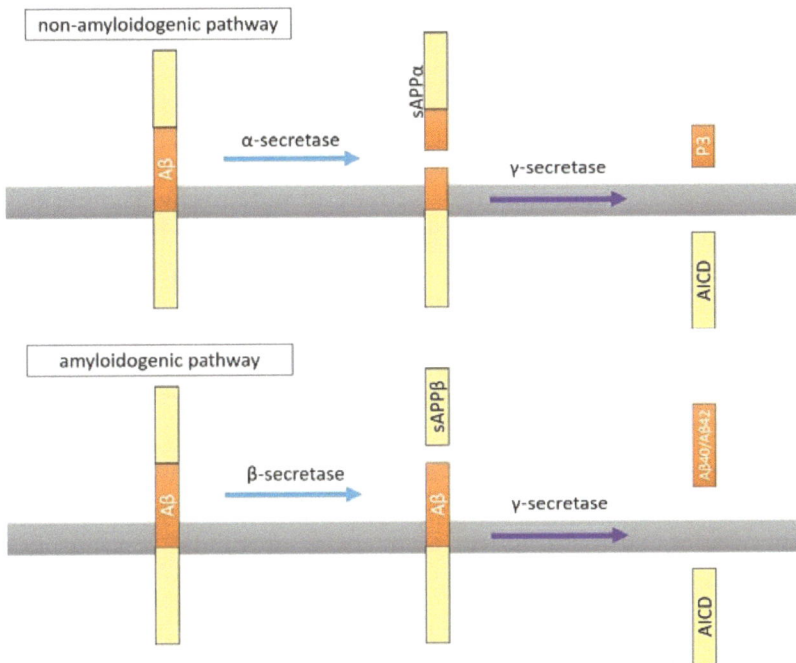

Fig. (1). Two different metabolic digestion pathways of amyloid precursor protein (APP) [80, 81].

In early studies, the total concentration of Aβ polypeptides including its isoforms was considered as a candidate biomarker for diagnosis of AD. However, slight or no differences are shown between patients and controls utilising total Aβ as an indicator

for AD [82 - 84]. Lately, two specific Aβ polypeptides, Aβ40 and Aβ42, were studied as a candidate biomarker in the CSF. The Aβ42 is the major component of the senile plaques in AD brains [85], but a minor component of Aβ peptides in the CSF [86] and plasma [87]. Decreases in CSF Aβ42 levels in AD patients have been well verified and replicated [88 - 92], which reflect sequestration of Aβ42 in senile plaques in the brain, as evidenced by autopsy and *In vivo* amyloid PET imaging studies [93]. Attenuation of CSF Aβ42 levels has also been observed in mild cognitive impairment (MCI) patients and individuals in the pre-clinical stages of AD [88, 94]. Studies showed the mean sensitivity and specificity of discriminating patients with AD and healthy ageing utilising CSF Aβ42 is between 86% and 90% [73, 95]. Furthermore, evidence suggests that CSF Aβ42 may be prognostic of further cognitive decline in both cognitively normal individuals and MCI patients [96].

CSF Aβ42 has been shown to remain relatively stable over time in patients with

AD dementia and may have limited utility for monitoring disease progression once AD is established [96]. Also, studies have suggested that the ratio of Aβ42/Aβ40, which corrects for inter-individual differences in CSF dynamics, may be a superior predictor of Aβ deposition in the brain measured than CSF Aβ42 alone and may help reduce misdiagnosis [96].

Low concentrations of CSF Aβ42 are also found in patients with other dementia disorders, and consequently render limitations for distinguishing AD from other subtypes of dementia [95, 97]. In order to achieve a more accurate differential diagnosis, the discovery of other biomarkers is essential. Studies show that a combined analysis of two or more biomarkers enhances the accuracy of AD diagnosis compared to a single biomarker alone [97 - 101].

Another hallmark of AD is the formation of neurofibrillary tangles, which is a sign of neurological injury [77]. Neurofibrillary tangles are caused by abnormally hyperphosphorylated tau protein. The role of a healthy axonal tau protein is to stabilise microtubules assembling through its microtubule-binding domains. When tau protein abnormally hyperphosphorylated, which has been hypothesised to be driven by Aβ pathology [102], the phosphorylated protein becomes prone to aggregation to form fibrils in tangles further damaging neuronal function (Fig. 2). As a consequence, the well-organised microtubules disassemble and thus impair axonal transport, compromising neuronal and synaptic function.

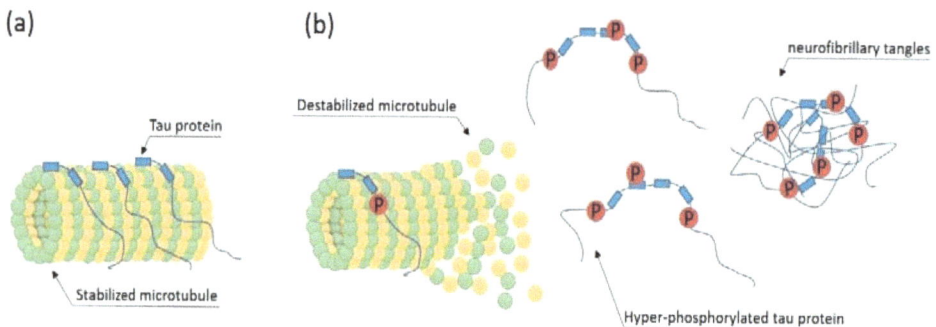

Fig. (2). Tauopathies pathway. **(a)** Normal tau protein stabilises microtubule. **(b)** Hyper-phosphorylated tau might diminish the stability of microtubule structure, entailing axonal transport failure and neurodegeneration, and further form neurofibrillary tangles [103].

The two fluid tau biomarkers in the most widespread use are t-tau and p-tau with the presence of the 4-repeat (4R) or the 3-repeat (3R) tau isoforms. Measurement of t-tau in CSF is based on recognising all six tau isoforms irrespective of phosphorylation state, while that of p-tau is based on recognising phosphorylated residues that may reflect tau pathology. Some research suggests that both CSF t-tau and CSF p-tau are biomarkers linked to neuronal damage in patients with AD, where CSF p-tau may further reflect the formation of neurofibrillary tangles [95]. Marked increases in both CSF t-tau and p-tau in AD patients have been replicated in abundant studies [88]. In the AD spectrum, both higher concentration of t-tau and p-tau have also been shown to predict a more rapid disease progression, such as faster progression of cognitive deficits and higher mortality [104, 105] — also, both CSF t-tau and p-tau show utility in the differentiation of AD from healthy controls. Studies showed the sensitivity and specificity discriminating patients with AD, and healthy ageing is between 80% and 90% for CSF t-tau and CSF p-tau [73, 95, 106]. Although the sensitivity and specificity above show t-tau as a reliable core biomarker, the increasing concentration of CSF t-tau is also presented in patients with other dementia disorders [97, 101]. In contrast to CSF Aβ42 or CSF t-tau, CSF p-tau levels remain standard in most other types of dementia, and thus, CSF p-tau may be particularly crucial for differential diagnosis [106 - 108].

Despite being well established as AD biomarkers, the utility of CSF t-tau and p-tau for diagnosis of AD and prediction of disease progression may be further improved when combined with CSF Aβ42 [96 - 98, 106, 109 - 111]. For example, both CSF t-tau/Aβ42 and p-tau/Aβ42 ratios have been shown to surpass any of the individual biomarkers in discerning Aβ pathology [32] and predicting progression from MCI to AD [112]. Indeed, CSF t-tau and p-tau, in combination with CSF Aβ42, are currently recognised as the three core CSF biomarkers for supporting the diagnosis of AD [109]. Explicitly, the 'Alzheimer's CSF profile' is often represented by a biomarker pattern with increased levels of t-tau and p-tau together with decreased Aβ42.

Plasma Aβ and Tau

Though core CSF biomarkers of AD including CSF Aβ42, CSF t-tau, and CSF p-tau provide methods to the diagnosis of AD, CSF collection requiring lumbar puncture is relatively high invasive and expensive [113, 114]. Therefore, CSF collection is unsuitable for routine clinical practice, and attempts are made to develop blood-based biomarkers or plasma biomarkers [115]. Blood testing, in contrast, is less invasive and only requires a simple procedure. It has been globally established as a clinical routine that is no further training for health-care professionals are required [116, 117]. However, in the detection of plasma biomarker, challenges are faced. The blood-brain barrier limits molecules to pass between the central nervous system and peripheral circulation; as a consequence, plasma biomarkers present relatively low concentrations in blood compartments [118, 119]. Moreover, the presence of heterophilic antibodies in the blood may lead to false results in immunochemical tests measuring biomarkers [120].

Despite the current difficulties, plasma biomarkers still may provide possibilities to develop precise and accurate early diagnosis of AD.

In contrast to the promising diagnostic utility of CSF Aβ42 for AD, studies on plasma Aβ42 as a biomarker have shown inconsistent results [88, 94, 121]. Most studies have failed to show an association between plasma Aβ42 and risk of AD or cerebral PET Aβ. No or minor changes and significant overlaps in both Aβ42 and Aβ40 levels between AD patients and controls have been revealed [88, 107]. Meanwhile, other studies show a decrease in plasma Aβ42 and Aβ42/Aβ40 ratio [79, 122, 123]. Nevertheless, recent studies using ultrasensitive immunoassay technique suggest that plasma Aβ still could be a useful screening biomarker [96, 124, 125]. Apart from plasma Aβ42, plasma tau proteins, including plasma t-tau and p-tau, has also been evaluated as potential biomarkers for clinical utility. A systematic review shows that the increase of plasma t-tau in AD may provide the possibility to discriminate patients with AD [88]. Elevated plasma t-tau is demonstrated to be both cross-sectionally and longitudinally associated with higher brain atrophy, cognitive decline, and risk of MCI in several large-scale studies, such as the Alzheimer's Disease Neuroimaging Initiative (ADNI) and the Mayo Clinic Study of Aging (MCSA) studies [126 - 128]. Besides, studies show that the plasma t-tau is correlated with rapid progression in later stages of AD [127, 129, 130]. Compared with plasma t-tau, plasma p-tau is closer correlated to the severity of AD and presents a higher sensitivity and specificity [131 - 133]. Moreover, plasma p-tau has also been found to be elevated in AD patients as well as MCI patients in several recent studies [131, 134]. Even though the decrease of plasma Aβ42 and Aβ42/Aβ40 ratio and the increase of plasma t-tau and plasma p-tau showed similar trends respectively to CSF Aβ42, CSF t-tau, and CSF p-tau in patients with AD, further validation of the diagnosis in early stages of AD is still required [114, 123].

Other Candidate Biomarkers

Candidate biomarkers other than Aβ and tau is also studied, including neurofilament light protein (NFL), soluble Aβ oligomers (AβOs) and β-secretase 1 (BACE 1), also known as β-site APP-cleaving enzyme 1 (BACE 1). As mentioned above, BACE 1 participates in the process of Aβ formation. Consequently, BACE 1 is a potential biomarker for AD diagnosis. In a comparison with healthy controls, CSF BACE1 levels have been demonstrated to be higher in AD patients [135]. Another study also points out that the plasma BACE 1 activity may be an indicator for predicting the progression from MCI to AD [136].

NFL is one of the subunits of neurofilaments in the mature nervous system and that neurofilaments are crucial components of neural cytoskeleton appearing in axons [137 - 139]. Due to the damage of axons and death of neurons, the NFL is released into CSF and provides indications of neurodegeneration [140 - 142]. Therefore, CSF NFL has been supported as a general marker of neurodegeneration correlating to the severity of cognitive impairment [141 - 144]. Studies show high CSF NFL concentrations in both patients with MCI and AD [141, 143, 145]. Besides high concentrations of NFL in CSF, the NFL is also found to elevate in plasma, which provides possibilities to utilise simple blood tests instead of invasive CSF collections [142, 145, 146]. However, the increase of NFL is also found in other neurodegenerative diseases and thus raised the difficulty for the NFL as a single biomarker for differential diagnosis [140, 147]. Despite the overlap of NFL existence among neurodegenerative diseases, the NFL is still a candidate progression marker with the advantage of diagnosing early clinical stages [141, 144].

Despite that Aβ have long been supposed as one of the hallmarks of AD and presents as the causation of synapse loss and memory loss, a hypothesis regards that AβOs account for dementia in AD [148 - 150]. In order to explain the controversy, a study estimates that more than one species may play a role in synapse loss [151], while another shows that senile plaques may be a potential reservoir of AβOs [150]. Due to the hypothesis, AβOs have been instigated to trigger the dysfunction of neural signalling and the inhibition of long-term potentiation (LTP) of synapses, which are both related to memory loss and dementia [107, 148, 151 - 154]. However, the level of AβOs in CSF is lower compared with Aβ monomers and thus increased the difficulty in detection [107, 155]. As a result, the comparison of AβOs level in CSF varies in different studies and that the exact relation between AβOs and AD is unclear [148, 151, 155]. Despite the unknown, since memory loss and the pathologic AβOs both appear in the early stage of AD, studies still postulate AβOs as a candidate biomarker for AD which requires further validations [107, 148, 149, 151].

Some synaptic proteins are also reported as candidate biomarkers, such as synaptosomal-associated protein 25 (SNAP-25), synaptotagmin-1 (SYT1) and neurogranin (Ng) [121, 156]. SNAP-25 is a presynaptic plasma membrane protein, whereas neurogranin is a dendritic protein. SYT1 is a presynaptic vesicle protein. Ng is a calmodulin-binding postsynaptic protein and that is highly expressed in brain region involved in synaptic plasticity and long-term potentiation. These synaptic proteins showed an increase in CSF levels differentiating MCI patients and AD patients [157 - 159]. Moreover, a systematic study showed that some other synaptic proteins, which are Thy-1, Syntaxin-1B, Neurexin-2A, Neurexin-3A, GluR4 and Calsynten in-1 peptides, exhibit changes before neurodegeneration actualising in the preclinical stage of AD [156]. As a consequence, synaptic biomarkers may respond to the progression of AD in the early stages, since synaptic dysfunction is related to cognitive deterioration [160]. These synaptic proteins show potential to aid the diagnosis in the preclinical stage AD. Nevertheless, further studies are required to uncover more discriminative features of various synaptic biomarkers for AD diagnosis.

Aβ plague deposition in the AD brain triggers the activation of microglia, resulting in a broad range of inflammatory responses [161]. As a result, inflammation markers have been considered as candidate biomarkers for AD. Recently, Chitinase-3-like protein 1 (CHI3L1), known as YKL-40, is an indicator of microglia activity and that as a potential biomarker for AD has been investigated. The amount of CSF YKL-40 of AD patients is higher than healthy controls and the level of CSF YKL-40 could also be used to predict the progression of MCI to AD [49, 162]. Besides YKL-40, other chemokines concentration in AD has also been assessed in a comparison with healthy control group or MCI group. For example, both the concentration of CCL2 and CXCL8 are increased in the serum and CSF of patients with AD [163, 164].

DIAGNOSE PLATFORM OF ALZHEIMER'S DISEASE

Platforms associated with the diagnosis of AD are summarised in three sections, including imaging platforms (*e.g.*, positron emission tomography (PET) and structural imaging), enzyme-linked immunosorbent assays (ELISA), and matrix-assisted laser desorption/ionisation – time of flight – mass spectrometry (MALDI-TOF-MS).

Imaging Platforms

The following section will give a summary update highlighting the evidence derived from recent studies of *In vivo* neuroimaging, such as PET and structural imaging.

Cerebral Amyloid Imaging

Amyloid imaging agents typically bind to insoluble Aβ42 and Aβ40 deposits. 11C-Pittsburgh Compound B (PiB) was the first amyloid imaging PET agent used in human subjects (Fig. **3**). 11C-PiB compound was later replaced with 18F-labeled Aβ tracers, such as 18F-Florbetapir, 18F-Florbetaben, and 18F-Flutemetamol (Fig. **3**), to overcome the limitation of short half-life. Aβ tracer retention is usually higher in AD patients than in healthy controls [165]. Amyloid scans from different stages of disease progression also demonstrate a pattern of tracer retention that coincides with amyloid deposition found in postmortem AD patients [166]. Besides, approximately 50% of MCI patients have been shown to have a high Aβ load on 18F-Florbetapir PET [167].

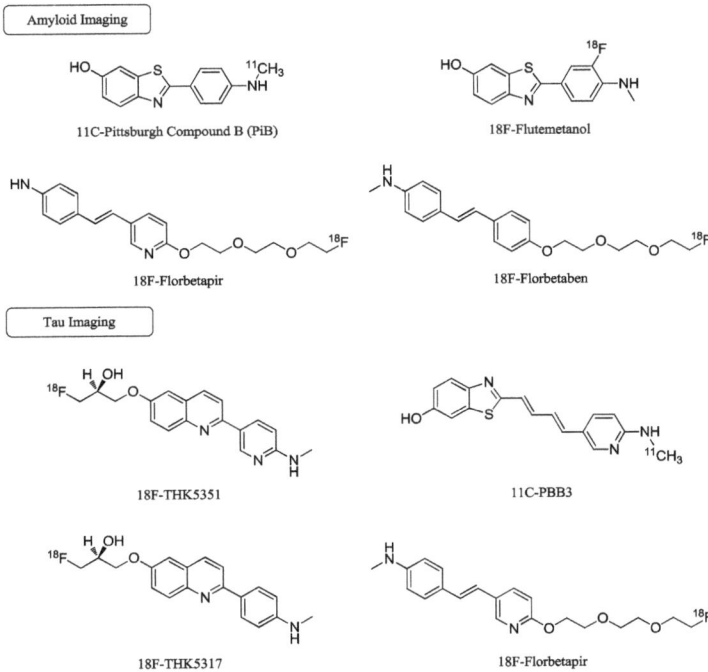

Fig. (3). The structures of PET reagents.

Autopsy studies confirm a significant correlation between antemortem cognitive impairment and neocortical Aβ plaques [168]. Furthermore, multicenter studies have demonstrated that a high Aβ load on 18F-Florbetapir PET was associated with poor memory performance in healthy older adults [169]. Nonetheless, it has been demonstrated that amyloid PET imaging does not correlate with cognitive decline and is weak in monitoring disease progression once early AD is established [170].

Specifically, amyloid deposition may have already peaked in the stage of MCI and reached a plateau by early clinical stages of AD. As such, the amyloid imaging might play a role more in facilitating the early diagnosis of AD, while being insufficient for the disease progression monitoring.

Cerebral Tau Imaging

In the very recent past few years, several tau-selective PET tracers, such as 18F-flortaucipir, 18F-THK5351, 18F-THK5317, and 11C-PBB3 (Fig. **3**), have just been developed and extensively used in research studies while have yet to be applied to clinical practice. The regional topography of tau accumulation observed from *In vivo* tau PET imaging is conspicuously consistent with the well-established spreading patterns of NFTs and neurodegeneration derived from post-mortem studies [171, 172]. It has been revealed that AD patients showed higher tau tracer retention in the hippocampus, temporal, parietal, and orbitofrontal cortices, compared with healthy controls [173]. Elevated tau accumulation in predominantly temporal-parietal cortices in AD patients has been consistently revealed, demonstrating extraordinary discrimination from healthy controls [174].

It is suggested that tau PET imaging could be a valid tool for monitoring disease progression and cognitive decline in AD [175], which is also in line with earlier clinicopathological studies showing that the number and density of neocortical NFTs are both strongly related to the severity of dementia and cognitive impairment [168, 176, 177]. In this regard, numerous PET studies have demonstrated moderate to strong correlations between tau and cognition in both patients with MCI and AD, involving episodic memory, verbal and visual memory, language, visuospatial performance, as well as global cognition [178, 179]. Furthermore, several groups have indicated that despite Aβ plaques may play a key role in AD pathogenesis, the burden of neocortical neurofibrillary tangles correlates more closely with the severity of cognitive impairment [168], and tau imaging may serve better for disease staging and disease progression prediction of AD than amyloid imaging [180, 181].

Structural Changes in AD

MRI-derived markers allow accurate tracking of the grey matter and white matter degeneration in AD, providing practical information for supporting the clinical diagnosis and monitoring disease progression in clinical trials.

Gray Matter Atrophy

Numerous MRI studies have demonstrated a degeneration pattern of neocortices concurring with the classical neuropathological staging of NFT pathology [171]. Specifically, cortical atrophy occurs initially in the medial temporal lobe (MTL) (*i.e.*, the entorhinal cortex (EC) and hippocampus), subsequently extending to the association areas following a temporal-parietal-frontal trajectory, with motor areas relatively preserved until late disease stages [182, 183]. This topographical neurodegeneration progression relates closely with the disease severity and course of clinical symptoms, in which memory impairments usually precede other forms of cognitive deficits in AD when the degeneration is initially confined to MTL [182].

Among the regional grey matter atrophy measured by MRI, hippocampal atrophy is the best established and validated marker of AD pathology [184]. Recent studies progress towards an investigation into subfields atrophy of the hippocampus and have revealed an apparent involvement of the head of the hippocampus, especially in the sector 1 of the cornu ammonis (CA1), in AD patients [185]. Similarly, when comparing MCI patients to healthy controls, CA1 consistently demonstrated shape alteration or volume reduction among different studies [186, 187]. It is suggested that the differential pattern of hippocampal subfields atrophy may have more sensitivity and accuracy in predicting pathological alterations [188]. Other cortical regions, such as entorhinal cortex, frontal, parietal, lateral temporal regions, and subcortical regions, including the amygdala, thalamus, and basal ganglia, and basal forebrain, have also been demonstrated to be potential biomarkers in AD [189 - 191]. Interested readers are referred to recent reviews for further information [185, 192].

White Matter Abnormality

White matter lesions are commonly found on the T2-weighted or fluid-attenuated inversion recovery (FLAIR) MRI in elderly individuals and AD patients. The causative mechanism of white matter pathology in AD remains a contentious research issue. Wallerian degeneration [193], retrogenesis progression [194], prion-like propagation [195], neuroinflammation [196], and local microvascular changes [197] are considered as possible underlying mechanisms.

Owing to the advances in structural neuroimaging, new imaging techniques, such as diffusion tensor imaging (DTI) and diffusion spectrum imaging (DSI), enable further insights and resolution to the white matter pathology of AD. In concordance with patterns of grey matter atrophy, Diffusion imaging studies have revealed that white matter pathology in AD usually locates within white matter tracts connecting the temporal lobe with other brain regions [192]. Both regions of interest and voxel-based studies have exhibited a prominent involvement of temporoparietal regions and, to a lesser extent, the frontal lobes in AD [198]. Tractography studies in AD patients revealed that diffusion abnormalities commonly appear in the significant limbic tracts, such as fornix and cingulum, the corpus callosum, and the association tracts, such as uncinate fasciculus, inferior fronto-occipital fasciculus, superior longitudinal fasciculus, and inferior longitudinal fasciculus [198]. Involvement of white matter tract abnormalities seemed to appear in a similar pattern in MCI patients [199 - 201]. Longitudinal studies in MCI and AD patients indicated that cingulum, fornix, and corpus callosum might be the best indicators of disease progression [200, 202].

Enzyme-Linked Immunosorbent Assays (ELISA)

ELISA, also named enzyme immunoassay (EIA), is a standard method to detect target proteins, peptides, antibodies and hormones. Because of its sensitivity and specificity, this technology is a prevalent choice for the evaluation of various research and diagnostic targets [203]. When executing ELISA, the antigen must be immobilised on a solid surface and then complexed with an antibody that is linked to an enzyme. Detection is accomplished by assessing the conjugated enzyme activity *via* incubation with a substrate to produce a measurable product. The most crucial element of the detection strategy is a highly specific antibody-antigen interaction [204].

Detection of Amyloid-beta by ELISA

ELISA based methods provided more results and application in research and clinical practice, *e.g.*, the AD diagnosis targeting Aβ peptide and AβOs. For the detection of Aβ monomers such as Aβ42, ELISA is commonly used. The detection limit usually reaches 1–10 pM in about 100 μL of the sample [205]. Apart from Aβ monomer detection, AβOs detection is also available utilising solid-phase sandwich ELISA. Usually, two different types of antibodies for sequence-specific recognition and conformation-specific, respectively, are employed [206]. These target-specific antibodies have been pre-coated in the wells of the supplied microplate. However, the application of the only usage of conformation-specific approach was unsuccessful to quantify the amount of AβOs in biofluids because other amyloid oligomers with similar conformation, such as α-synuclein, prion, and heat shock proteins, are also captured by antibodies [206] (Fig. **4a**). By contrast, the double usage of the same sequence-specific antibody twice in the system (Fig. **4b**), for capturing as well as for detection is a more reliable method for quantifying the concentration of AβOs independently instead of all Aβ isoforms [207]. A variety of ELISA-based tools were published. Those include N-terminal binding BAN50, or MOAB-2, HJ3.4 for capture and detection oligomers [208 - 210]. For example, the limit of quantification for AbOs detection is two pg/mL by using N-terminal monoclonal antibody 82E1 [211].

Amyloid Beta Detection on Luminex Platform with the Bead in CSF

Though solid-phase sandwich ELISA is a reliable method quantifying AβOs, the multistep process causes solid-phase sandwich ELISA to be labour-intensive [206]. The assay may last between a few hours and a day, and usually requires an overnight incubation [207]. However, the bead-based method dramatically reduced the analysis time and simplified the complicated preparation procedure compared with solid-phase sandwich ELISA [106, 206, 212]. This method is a fluid-phase assay approach, and that combines ELISA and Luminex xMAP technology. The Luminex xMAP technology is a flow cytometric method where different antibodies couple to spectrally specific fluorescent microspheres [213,

214]. The antibodies of the target are coated on bead rather than on the solid supported utilising in a solid-phase sandwich ELISA. This method allows for the simultaneous detection of several target peptides or chemicals at the same time (Fig. **5**). The operation of the test is similar to ELISA. Commercial Kit,

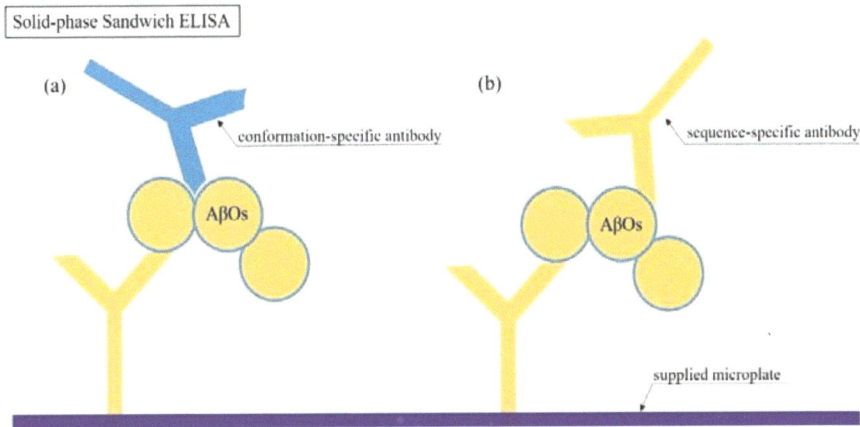

Fig. (4). Strategies used for solid-phase sandwich ELISA. **(a)** The only usage of conformation-specific antibody was unsuccessful to quantify the amount of AβOs. **(b)** The double usage of the same sequence-specific antibody is a more reliable method to detect AβOs.

MILLIPLEX MAP Human Amyloid Beta Tau Magnetic Bead Panel utilises Luminex xMAP technology and is used for the simultaneous quantification of Aβ40, Aβ42, t-tau, and p-tau [214]. As mentioned previously, a combined analysis of two or more biomarkers enhances the accuracy of AD diagnosis compared to a single biomarker alone [97 - 101]. The bead-based method may be beneficial for the AD diagnosis with the allowance of simultaneously quantifying different biomarkers. Moreover, it is convenient to detect multiple biomarkers in a test with the volume of sample reduced, mainly when the sample is hard to access, *e.g.*, CSF [214]. The detection of molecules, including high-molecular-weight amyloid, oligomer, and monomer in a varied body fluid such as CSF, plasma or nasal discharge, is fundamental for application to screening, diagnosis and treatment of AD. Apart from solid-phase sandwich ELISA, the bead-based method combining ELISA and Luminex system is becoming more feasible for clinical use. Some novel methods, like biosensors, have the potential to provide rapid, real-time, and accurate results. The application of these methods lacks mandates the evidence in longitudinal or extensive cohort studies.

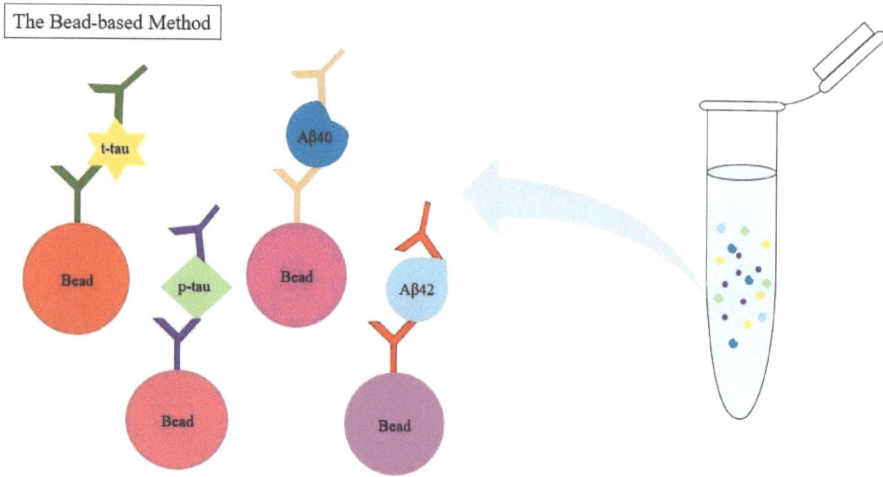

Fig. (5). The bead-based method is a fluid-phase assay approach allowing simultaneous quantification of Aβ40, Aβ42, t-tau, and p-tau, which is compared to the solid-phase sandwich ELISA running one assay at a time.

ELISA methods provide adequate sensitivity for detection of AβOs and quantification by using standard AβOs preparations. However, only one signal for all oligomers in the sample is provided, and the oligomers cannot be characterised in details such as aggregate size distribution. Recently, some methods were described which claim single molecule sensitivity. These methods are based on fluorescence correlation spectroscopy (FCS), flow cytometry, or confocal laser scanning microscopy (LSM) [215]. These methods offer a more precise, rapid and convenient measurement of AβOs. More studies recruited longitudinal larger population cohort are necessary before they could be commonly applied in clinical practice.

MALDI-TOF Mass Spectrometry

MALDI-TOF-MASS

Matrix-assisted laser desorption/ionisation (MALDI) and electrospray ionisation (ESI) is the commonly used soft ionisation methods for mass spectrometry-based biomolecules analyses [216]. In contrast to MALDI, ESI analysis usually combined with liquid chromatography-mass spectrometry (LC-MS), as a consequence, the analysis process is time-consuming. Nevertheless, the advantages of MALDI are widely practised for quality control during sample preparation and qualitative analysis due to its speed, sensitivity, and low sample consumption [217]. For MALDI analysis process, sample preparation plays a pivotal role. The sample preparation starts with matrix selection, and this critical step may have a decisive influence on the analysis results [218, 219]. The selected matrix will be mixed or coated with the analyte, and then the matrix and analyte complex will be stimulated by laser triggering desorption and ionisation of the analyte with the matrix. As a result, the analyte is transformed into a gaseous phase and is protonated or deprotonated. During this step, any existence of contaminants can seriously interfere with the co-crystallization of the analyte molecules and the matrix. Besides that, it is equally important to decrease the risk of segregation during analyte and matrix co-crystallisation [220, 221].

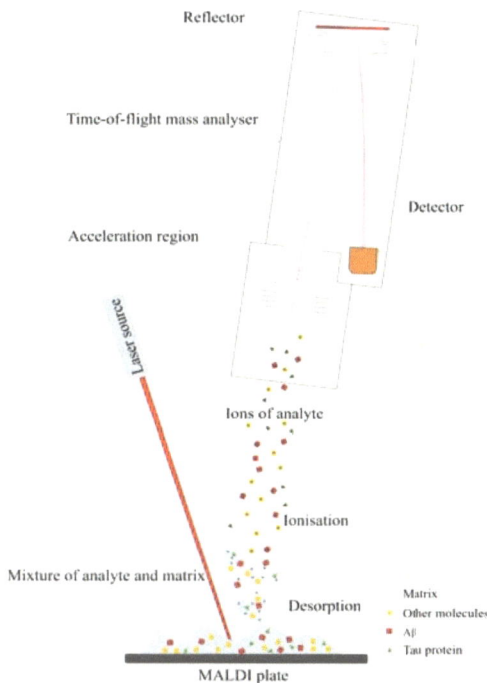

Fig. (6). General schematic for MALDI-TOF.

These ionised analytes will be measured and analysed using distinct types of mass detectors. Among all kinds of mass detectors, Time-of-flight (TOF) [222 - 224] is the most widely used one. The fundamental principle of TOF is that ionised analytes with different mass-to-charge ratios are dispersed over a field-free drifting path of known length in time during their flight. To be more precisely, after the sample is stimulated, ionised analytes are expelled from the source. These ionised analytes are then accelerated by applying a potential difference between the electrode and the extraction grid to move towards the flight tube [225]. After leaving the acceleration zone, ionised analytes enter into the magnetic field-free region and are separated according to their speeds. In the end, the ionised analytes will reach the detector and produce a mass spectrum (Fig. **6**) [226 - 229].

Aβ and Tau Protein

As mentioned previously, Aβ and tau protein are the main biomarkers for the diagnosis of Alzheimer's disease and that can be found in CSF and plasma. Due to the low abundance of these biomarkers in body fluids, efficient sample preparation is essential. Herein, immunoprecipitation (IP) was employed for isolating the desired biomarkers with sufficient sensitivity from body fluids. In general, the biomarkers are captured by antibodies functionalized magnetic beads and the most frequently used antibodies are 6E10 and 4G8, targeting Aβ epitopes 4-9 and 18-22, respectively [86, 219]. Besides analysing the captured biomarkers by MALDI-TOF-MS, the amount of the analytes can also be quantified by adding isotopically-labelled peptides as an internal reference standard (IRS). Herein, Aβ 1-15 $Arg^{13}C^{15}N$ and Aβ 1-34 $Arg^{13}C^{15}N$ are two commonly used IRS for Aβ quantification [218, 219].

Fania *et al.* provided some tests by MALDI profiling. In their study, the level of biomarkers in CSF and plasma from 36 ADs, 32 iNPHs (idiopathic normal pressure hydrocephalus), and 12 controls were compared. In addition to detecting Aβ and tau protein, they introduced another diagnostic marker, apolipoprotein A-1 (Apo A-1), which enables more effective diagnosis of AD. At the beginning of the examination, they mixed the samples from three different targets with DHAP (2,5-dihydroxyacetophenone) matrix and repeated the analysis four times. Comparing to iNPH samples, the CSF and plasma samples from AD patients give a particular protein profile. They observed an aberrant change in Apo A-1 levels in AD and a specific disorder in the Apo A-1 proteoform. The results indicate that a characteristic Apo A-1 may be a potential marker and which can help the diagnosis of AD [230].

CURRENT LIMITATIONS AND FUTURE PERSPECTIVES

So far, early-onset AD diagnosis with high accuracy, sensitivity, and specificity remains a challenge due to several reasons. First, AD and other neurodegenerative diseases share a common pathological hallmark which is toxic proteins accumulation and synaptic dysfunction, resulting in non-specificity of biomarkers to distinguish AD from others. For example, NFL is a candidate biomarker for AD diagnosis. However, a high level of NFL can also be found in Parkinson's diseases, Huntington's disease, and Creutzfeldt-Jakob disease [231]. Second, most of the AD-related biomarkers are inside the brain. Although CSF biomarkers can be obtained by lumbar puncture, the use of lumbar puncture is not applicable in all cases and has some side effects, such as headaches, nausea, and low blood pressure *et al.*, in the following few days. Furthermore, this technique is invasiveness and lack of accessibility [232]. Blood, urine, or other biofluids are more accessible compared to CSF. However, the concentration of biomarkers outside CSF is extremely low due to the blood-brain barrier. For instance, the concentration of biomarkers in CSF is 10- to 10^2- fold higher than in plasma [233]. Besides the issue of low concentration, blood or urine sample usually contains high levels of various interfering agents, leading to difficulties for blood- or urine-based biomarkers seeking. Consequently, it is urgent need to seek new biomarkers in other biofluids for AD diagnosis and to develop new methodologies for accurate and reliable early AD diagnosis.

Since no single biomarker is likely be an accurate and reliable biomarker for early AD diagnosis, simultaneous consideration of multi-biomarker models is necessary. Recently, Nakamura *et al.* have demonstrated a first example that can analyze the ratios of blood-based Aβ related biomarkers *via* immunoprecipitation-mass spectrometry (IP-MS) assays. This technology can investigate the concentration of desired biomarkers from plasma. The sensitivity and specificity of Aβ detection are exceeded 90% by checking with PIB-PET imaging. In this study, the ratio of APP $_{669-711}$ to Aβ $_{1-42}$ was measured. They discovered that the proportion of Aβ $_{1-40}$/Aβ $_{1-42}$ also achieved at the same rate in comparison with the ratio of APP $_{699-711}$/Aβ $_{1-42}$, and the incorporated biomarker scores of these two can further enhance the accuracy. Besides, they have also investigated the interrelationship between the plasma Aβ and Aβ-PET burden as well as the correlation between plasma Aβ and CSF Aβ, showing the potential utility of the plasma biomarker for early AD diagnosis [122].

Kim *et al.* designed a multiplexed electrical sensing platform for detecting multiple AD biomarkers (t-tau, p-tau $_{181}$, Aβ $_{1-42}$ and Aβ $_{1-40}$) in blood plasma. A densely aligned single-walled carbon nanotube thin film as a transducer was applied in the sensor array. This sensor array enables to accurately detect the AD biomarkers in ultra-low concentration (femtomolar). By comparing the ratios of biomarkers (t-tau/Aβ $_{1-42}$, p-tau $_{181}$/Aβ $_{1-42}$, Aβ $_{1-42}$/Aβ $_{1-40}$), this sensing platform can improve the accuracy to differentiate the clinically diagnosed AD patients from healthy controls [234].

SOME ALZHEIMER'S DISEASE MODELS IN SILICO

With the rapid development of manufacturing process technology and semiconductor technology, the capability of computing has a tremendous improvement, *e.g.*, CPU clock speed and storage capacity. Such advances will lead us into a world of precision medical care in the future and enable us to explore unknown medical fields or to gain an in-depth understanding of existing physiology and pathology. Among them, utilising the computational frameworks [235 - 237], *e.g.*, mathematical modelling or big data technique, to seek other potential biomarkers has been developed to explore AD.

The pathology of AD is somehow to occur in the human brain where the abnormal aggregation of specific protein and the dysfunction or death of neurons happen. Blood pressure has been read as an index of AD as well. It has been announced the relationship between age and AD development. However, the direct correlation between blood pressure and AD is still an open question [238, 239]. So far, the human brain has been identified as one of the most complex organs, and thus enhances the complexity to understand AD fully. At the same time, medical experts and policy makers are increasingly aware that the efficacy and economy of therapy are strongly connected with the personalisation of treatment.

On the one hand, the white house in the USA announced the Brain Research through Advancing Innovative Neurotechnologies (BRAIN) Initiative. It was launched to revolutionise the understanding of the human brain. While some of the current imaging techniques provide a static picture of the human brain, BRAIN Initiative aimed to produce a dynamic picture of the human brain, showing both space and time, through innovative techniques [240]. BRAIN Initiative may deliver a clearer insight into AD, which is associated with a better diagnosis. On the other hand, a European initiative was proposed to investigate the human body *in silico,* which is called Virtual Physiological Human (VPH). It was initially proposed to translate the computational physiology into clinical practice [241]. One of the long term expectation of VPH is to utilise patient models and test drugs or medical devices [241]. The VPH projects that tackle the neuroscience topic may potentially enable effective medicines for AD in the future with high impact.

Constructing associated mathematical models may provide a possible method to describe the complex progression of AD and further aid the process of discoveries. For example, the dementia prevalence model was proposed to explore the disease processes, foresee effects of future demographics, and evaluate combination of interventions *via* virtual experimentation [242]. Moreover, the PredictAD, which is one of the VPH projects, aims explicitly at the early diagnosis of AD. Instead of finding a single biomarker of AD, this project developed a methodology for biomarker discovery [243]. This project reprocessed collected data and visualised the individual contributions of different biomarkers. Moreover, the construction of analysis software from the PredictAD project proved that tools, *e.g.* models, may improve the diagnosis of AD in an earlier stage with high accuracy [244, 245].

Furthermore, one of the goal of the Virtual Physiological Human: DementiA Research Enabled by IT (VPH-DARE@IT) project, similar to that of the PredictAD project, is to enable a better diagnosis for dementia in an earlier stage. While doctors rely on cognitive tests and scanning results from imaging platforms, the early stage of AD could hardly be recognised. Therefore, VPH-DARE@IT provides a research platform to monitor the progression of dementia and develops a clinical decision-support tool based on the PredictAD project for disease modelling. Apart from the improvement for clinical diagnosis, VPH-DARE@IT additionally designs tools for personal use that help evaluate the risk of dementia.

These research projects mentioned above brings possibilities to improve the current understanding and diagnosis of AD. To combine the computational framework with the experimental process may be the next generation of precision medicine shown in Fig. (7). Meanwhile, the utilisation of computational models may potentially reduce not only the number of animal testing but also the implementation of expensive or risky tests and collections such as MRI and lumbar puncture. Hence, we should positively face the computational technologies and bring them as the assistant schemes to bridge the gap between current and future.

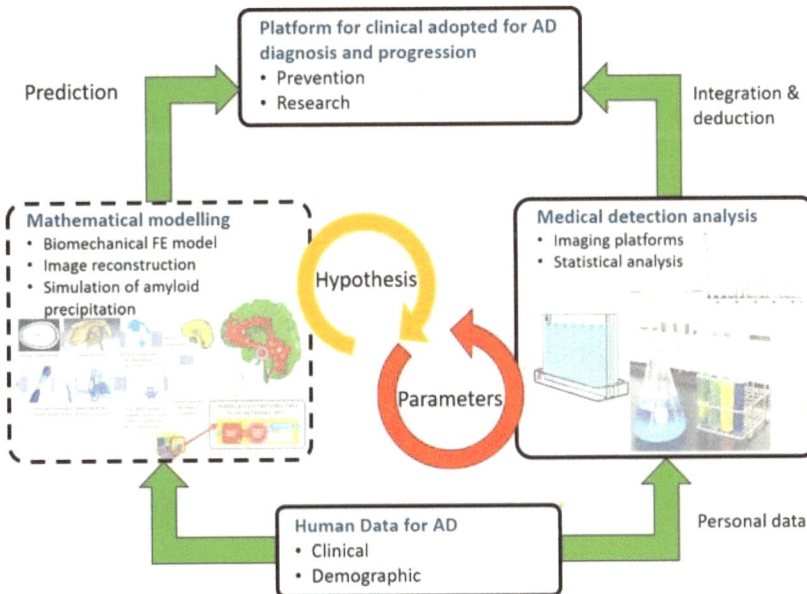

Fig. (7). A prospective AD diagnosis process for the next generation.

CONCLUDING REMARKS

Abundant clinical studies have consistently recognised the core neuropathological features and related fluid biomarkers as utile indicators for the diagnosis and prognosis of AD and its preclinical stages. The neuropathological feature of AD is commonly characterised by (1) extracellular plaque deposits of amyloid beta (Aβ) peptides and (2) intraneuronal hyperphosphorylated tau-containing neurofibrillary tangles (NFTs). The related fluid biomarkers summarised in this chapter include convinced biomarkers (Aβ42, t-tau, and p-tau in both CSF and plasma) and other candidate biomarkers. Moreover, methods and platforms utilised to detect these biomarkers including imaging platforms (positron emission tomography (PET) and structural imaging), enzyme-linked immunosorbent assays (ELISA), and matrix-assisted laser desorption/ionisation – time of flight – mass spectrometry (MALDI-TOF-MS) are also summarised.

CONFLICT OF INTEREST

We wish to confirm that there are no known conflicts of interest associated with this publication, and there has been no significant financial support for this work that could have influenced its outcome.

ACKNOWLEDGEMENTS

We gratefully thank Miss Hsiu-Han Chang, who is one of our co-author Dr. Hao-Hsiang Chang's assistant at NTUH to collect the information regarding ELISA in this chapter. Meanwhile, we also would like to thank the funding, MOST 106-2218-E-008-012-MY3 and 108-2113-M-030-001, from Ministry of Science and Technology (MOST) in Taiwan. Finally, this review was done by co-author Di-Hua Luo and Yu-Ling Chang who worked on imaging issue and was done by co-author Hao-Hsiang Chang who worked on ELISA issue and was done by co-author Po-Yen Chen who worked on MALDI-TOF-MS issue and was done by co-author Yen-Cheng Chao who worked on biomarkers issue. The first author, Ru-Yi Youh, integrated and wrote this review. The correspondence authors, Wei-Min Liu and Dean Chou, gave the idea, revised the article and handle the whole review work.

REFERENCES

[1]   World Population Prospects 2008: Department of Economic and Social Affairs, Population Division, United Nations 2008.

[2]   Hindle JV. Ageing, neurodegeneration and Parkinson's disease. Age Ageing 2010; 39(2): 156-61.
       [http://dx.doi.org/10.1093/ageing/afp223] [PMID: 20051606]

[3]   Heemels MT. Neurodegenerative diseases. Nature 2016; 539(7628): 179.
       [http://dx.doi.org/10.1038/539179a] [PMID: 27830810]

[4]   Reeve A, Simcox E, Turnbull D. Ageing and Parkinson's disease: why is advancing age the biggest risk factor? Ageing Res Rev 2014; 14: 19-30.
[http://dx.doi.org/10.1016/j.arr.2014.01.004] [PMID: 24503004]

[5]   Niccoli T, Partridge L. Ageing as a risk factor for disease. Curr Biol 2012; 22(17): R741-52.
[http://dx.doi.org/10.1016/j.cub.2012.07.024] [PMID: 22975005]

[6]   Hung CW, Chen YC, Hsieh WL, Chiou SH, Kao CL. Ageing and neurodegenerative diseases. Ageing Res Rev 2010; 9 (Suppl. 1): S36-46.
[http://dx.doi.org/10.1016/j.arr.2010.08.006] [PMID: 20732460]

[7]   Armstrong RA, Lantos PL, Cairns NJ. Overlap between neurodegenerative disorders. Neuropathology 2005; 25(2): 111-24.
[http://dx.doi.org/10.1111/j.1440-1789.2005.00605.x] [PMID: 15875904]

[8]   Uitti RJ, Berry K, Yasuhara O, *et al.* Neurodegenerative 'overlap' syndrome: Clinical and pathological features of Parkinson's disease, motor neuron disease, and Alzheimer's disease. Parkinsonism Relat Disord 1995; 1(1): 21-34.
[http://dx.doi.org/10.1016/1353-8020(95)00004-P] [PMID: 18590998]

[9]   McKee AC, Robinson ME. Military-related traumatic brain injury and neurodegeneration. Alzheimers Dement 2014; 10(3) (Suppl.): S242-53.
[http://dx.doi.org/10.1016/j.jalz.2014.04.003] [PMID: 24924675]

[10]   Ahmed RM, Devenney EM, Irish M, *et al.* Neuronal network disintegration: common pathways linking neurodegenerative diseases. J Neurol Neurosurg Psychiatry 2016; 87(11): 1234-41.
[http://dx.doi.org/10.1136/jnnp-2014-308350] [PMID: 27172939]

[11]   Dugger BN, Dickson DW. Pathology of Neurodegenerative Diseases. Cold Spring Harb Perspect Biol 2017; 9(7)a028035
[http://dx.doi.org/10.1101/cshperspect.a028035] [PMID: 28062563]

[12]   Koo EH, Lansbury PT Jr, Kelly JW. Amyloid diseases: abnormal protein aggregation in neurodegeneration. Proc Natl Acad Sci USA 1999; 96(18): 9989-90.
[http://dx.doi.org/10.1073/pnas.96.18.9989] [PMID: 10468546]

[13]   Hardy J, Gwinn-Hardy K. Genetic classification of primary neurodegenerative disease. Science 1998; 282(5391): 1075-9.
[http://dx.doi.org/10.1126/science.282.5391.1075] [PMID: 9804538]

[14]   Price DL, Sisodia SS, Borchelt DR. Genetic neurodegenerative diseases: the human illness and transgenic models. Science 1998; 282(5391): 1079-83.
[http://dx.doi.org/10.1126/science.282.5391.1079] [PMID: 9804539]

[15]   Prince M, *et al.* The global prevalence of dementia: a systematic review and metaanalysis 2013.
[http://dx.doi.org/10.1016/j.jalz.2012.11.007]

[16]   Forette F, Boller F. Hypertension and the risk of dementia in the elderly. Am J Med 1991; 90(3A): 14S-9S.
[http://dx.doi.org/10.1016/0002-9343(91)90430-6] [PMID: 2006654]

[17]   Rizzi L, Rosset I, Roriz-Cruz M. Global epidemiology of dementia: Alzheimer's and vascular types. BioMed Res Int 2014; 2014908915
[http://dx.doi.org/10.1155/2014/908915] [PMID: 25089278]

[18]   Nepal B, Brown LJ, Anstey KJ. Rising midlife obesity will worsen future prevalence of dementia. PLoS One 2014; 9(9)e99305
[http://dx.doi.org/10.1371/journal.pone.0099305] [PMID: 25184830]

[19]   Fratiglioni L, De Ronchi D, Agüero-Torres H. Worldwide prevalence and incidence of dementia. Drugs Aging 1999; 15(5): 365-75.
[http://dx.doi.org/10.2165/00002512-199915050-00004] [PMID: 10600044]

[20]   Burns A, Iliffe S. Alzheimer's disease. BMJ 2009; 338: b158.
        [http://dx.doi.org/10.1136/bmj.b158] [PMID: 19196745]

[21]   Román GC, Erkinjuntti T, Wallin A, Pantoni L, Chui HC. Subcortical ischaemic vascular dementia.
        Lancet Neurol 2002; 1(7): 426-36.
        [http://dx.doi.org/10.1016/S1474-4422(02)00190-4] [PMID: 12849365]

[22]   Chui HC. Subcortical ischemic vascular dementia. Neurol Clin 2007; 25(3): 717-740, vi. [vi.].
        [http://dx.doi.org/10.1016/j.ncl.2007.04.003] [PMID: 17659187]

[23]   Jellinger KA. The pathology of "vascular dementia": a critical update. J Alzheimers Dis 2008; 14(1):
        107-23.
        [http://dx.doi.org/10.3233/JAD-2008-14110] [PMID: 18525132]

[24]   Thal DR, Grinberg LT, Attems J. Vascular dementia: different forms of vessel disorders contribute to
        the development of dementia in the elderly brain. Exp Gerontol 2012; 47(11): 816-24.
        [http://dx.doi.org/10.1016/j.exger.2012.05.023] [PMID: 22705146]

[25]   Jellinger KA, Attems J. Neuropathological evaluation of mixed dementia. J Neurol Sci 2007; 257(1-2):
        80-7.
        [http://dx.doi.org/10.1016/j.jns.2007.01.045] [PMID: 17324442]

[26]   Langa KM, Foster NL, Larson EB. Mixed dementia: emerging concepts and therapeutic implications.
        JAMA 2004; 292(23): 2901-8.
        [http://dx.doi.org/10.1001/jama.292.23.2901] [PMID: 15598922]

[27]   Zekry D, Hauw JJ, Gold G. Mixed dementia: epidemiology, diagnosis, and treatment. J Am Geriatr
        Soc 2002; 50(8): 1431-8.
        [http://dx.doi.org/10.1046/j.1532-5415.2002.50367.x] [PMID: 12165002]

[28]   Colton CA, Mott RT, Sharpe H, Xu Q, Van Nostrand WE, Vitek MP. Expression profiles for
        macrophage alternative activation genes in AD and in mouse models of AD. J Neuroinflammation
        2006; 3: 27.
        [http://dx.doi.org/10.1186/1742-2094-3-27] [PMID: 17005052]

[29]   Kawas C, Gray S, Brookmeyer R, Fozard J, Zonderman A. Age-specific incidence rates of
        Alzheimer's disease: the Baltimore Longitudinal Study of Aging. Neurology 2000; 54(11): 2072-7.
        [http://dx.doi.org/10.1212/WNL.54.11.2072] [PMID: 10851365]

[30]   Cornutiu G. The Epidemiological Scale of Alzheimer's Disease. J Clin Med Res 2015; 7(9): 657-66.
        [http://dx.doi.org/10.14740/jocmr2106w] [PMID: 26251678]

[31]   López-Arrieta JM, Rodríguez JL, Sanz F. Efficacy and safety of nicotine on Alzheimer's disease
        patients. Cochrane Database Syst Rev 2001; (2): CD001749
        [PMID: 11406005]

[32]   Fagan AM, Shaw LM, Xiong C, *et al.* Comparison of analytical platforms for cerebrospinal fluid
        measures of β-amyloid 1-42, total tau, and p-tau181 for identifying Alzheimer disease amyloid plaque
        pathology. Arch Neurol 2011; 68(9): 1137-44.
        [http://dx.doi.org/10.1001/archneurol.2011.105] [PMID: 21555603]

[33]   Almeida OP, Hulse GK, Lawrence D, Flicker L. Smoking as a risk factor for Alzheimer's disease:
        contrasting evidence from a systematic review of case-control and cohort studies. Addiction 2002;
        97(1): 15-28.
        [http://dx.doi.org/10.1046/j.1360-0443.2002.00016.x] [PMID: 11895267]

[34]   Durazzo TC, Mattsson N, Weiner MW. Smoking and increased Alzheimer's disease risk: a review of
        potential mechanisms. Alzheimers Dement 2014; 10(3) (Suppl.): S122-45.
        [http://dx.doi.org/10.1016/j.jalz.2014.04.009] [PMID: 24924665]

[35]   Ott A, Slooter AJ, Hofman A, *et al.* Smoking and risk of dementia and Alzheimer's disease in a
        population-based cohort study: the Rotterdam Study. Lancet 1998; 351(9119): 1840-3.

[http://dx.doi.org/10.1016/S0140-6736(97)07541-7] [PMID: 9652667]

[36] Reitz C, den Heijer T, van Duijn C, Hofman A, Breteler MM. Relation between smoking and risk of dementia and Alzheimer disease: the Rotterdam Study. Neurology 2007; 69(10): 998-1005.
      [http://dx.doi.org/10.1212/01.wnl.0000271395.29695.9a] [PMID: 17785668]

[37] Anstey KJ, von Sanden C, Salim A, O'Kearney R. Smoking as a risk factor for dementia and cognitive decline: a meta-analysis of prospective studies. Am J Epidemiol 2007; 166(4): 367-78.
      [http://dx.doi.org/10.1093/aje/kwm116] [PMID: 17573335]

[38] Cataldo JK, Prochaska JJ, Glantz SA. Cigarette smoking is a risk factor for Alzheimer's Disease: an analysis controlling for tobacco industry affiliation. J Alzheimers Dis 2010; 19(2): 465-80.
      [http://dx.doi.org/10.3233/JAD-2010-1240] [PMID: 20110594]

[39] Rolland Y, Abellan van Kan G, Vellas B. Physical activity and Alzheimer's disease: from prevention to therapeutic perspectives. J Am Med Dir Assoc 2008; 9(6): 390-405.
      [http://dx.doi.org/10.1016/j.jamda.2008.02.007] [PMID: 18585641]

[40] Barnes DE, Yaffe K. The projected effect of risk factor reduction on Alzheimer's disease prevalence. Lancet Neurol 2011; 10(9): 819-28.
      [http://dx.doi.org/10.1016/S1474-4422(11)70072-2] [PMID: 21775213]

[41] Luchsinger JA, Reitz C, Honig LS, Tang MX, Shea S, Mayeux R. Aggregation of vascular risk factors and risk of incident Alzheimer disease. Neurology 2005; 65(4): 545-51.
      [http://dx.doi.org/10.1212/01.wnl.0000172914.08967.dc] [PMID: 16116114]

[42] Gorelick PB. Risk factors for vascular dementia and Alzheimer disease. Stroke 2004; 35(11) (Suppl. 1): 2620-2.
      [http://dx.doi.org/10.1161/01.STR.0000143318.70292.47] [PMID: 15375299]

[43] Van Cauwenberghe C, Van Broeckhoven C, Sleegers K. The genetic landscape of Alzheimer disease: clinical implications and perspectives. Genet Med 2016; 18(5): 421-30.
      [http://dx.doi.org/10.1038/gim.2015.117] [PMID: 26312828]

[44] Breteler MM. Vascular risk factors for Alzheimer's disease: an epidemiologic perspective. Neurobiol Aging 2000; 21(2): 153-60.
      [http://dx.doi.org/10.1016/S0197-4580(99)00110-4] [PMID: 10867200]

[45] Kivipelto M, Helkala EL, Laakso MP, et al. Midlife vascular risk factors and Alzheimer's disease in later life: longitudinal, population based study. BMJ 2001; 322(7300): 1447-51.
      [http://dx.doi.org/10.1136/bmj.322.7300.1447] [PMID: 11408299]

[46] Kivipelto M, Ngandu T, Fratiglioni L, et al. Obesity and vascular risk factors at midlife and the risk of dementia and Alzheimer disease. Arch Neurol 2005; 62(10): 1556-60.
      [http://dx.doi.org/10.1001/archneur.62.10.1556] [PMID: 16216938]

[47] Kalaria RN, Maestre GE, Arizaga R, et al. Alzheimer's disease and vascular dementia in developing countries: prevalence, management, and risk factors. Lancet Neurol 2008; 7(9): 812-26.
      [http://dx.doi.org/10.1016/S1474-4422(08)70169-8] [PMID: 18667359]

[48] Sparks DL, Scheff SW, Liu H, Landers TM, Coyne CM, Hunsaker JC III. Increased incidence of neurofibrillary tangles (NFT) in non-demented individuals with hypertension. J Neurol Sci 1995; 131(2): 162-9.
      [http://dx.doi.org/10.1016/0022-510X(95)00105-B] [PMID: 7595642]

[49] Muszyński P, Groblewska M, Kulczyńska-Przybik A, Kułakowska A, Mroczko B. YKL-40 as a Potential Biomarker and a Possible Target in Therapeutic Strategies of Alzheimer's Disease. Curr Neuropharmacol 2017; 15(6): 906-17.
      [http://dx.doi.org/10.2174/1570159X15666170208124324] [PMID: 28183245]

[50] Jonsson T, Atwal JK, Steinberg S, et al. A mutation in APP protects against Alzheimer's disease and age-related cognitive decline. Nature 2012; 488(7409): 96-9.
      [http://dx.doi.org/10.1038/nature11283] [PMID: 22801501]

[51] Chartier-Harlin MC, Crawford F, Houlden H, *et al.* Early-onset Alzheimer's disease caused by mutations at codon 717 of the beta-amyloid precursor protein gene. Nature 1991; 353(6347): 844-6.
[http://dx.doi.org/10.1038/353844a0] [PMID: 1944558]

[52] Goate A, Chartier-Harlin MC, Mullan M, *et al.* Segregation of a missense mutation in the amyloid precursor protein gene with familial Alzheimer's disease. Nature 1991; 349(6311): 704-6.
[http://dx.doi.org/10.1038/349704a0] [PMID: 1671712]

[53] Rogaev EI, Sherrington R, Rogaeva EA, *et al.* Familial Alzheimer's disease in kindreds with missense mutations in a gene on chromosome 1 related to the Alzheimer's disease type 3 gene. Nature 1995; 376(6543): 775-8.
[http://dx.doi.org/10.1038/376775a0] [PMID: 7651536]

[54] Campion D, Dumanchin C, Hannequin D, *et al.* Early-onset autosomal dominant Alzheimer disease: prevalence, genetic heterogeneity, and mutation spectrum. Am J Hum Genet 1999; 65(3): 664-70.
[http://dx.doi.org/10.1086/302553] [PMID: 10441572]

[55] Strittmatter WJ, Saunders AM, Schmechel D, *et al.* Apolipoprotein E: high-avidity binding to beta-amyloid and increased frequency of type 4 allele in late-onset familial Alzheimer disease. Proc Natl Acad Sci USA 1993; 90(5): 1977-81.
[http://dx.doi.org/10.1073/pnas.90.5.1977] [PMID: 8446617]

[56] Saunders AM, Strittmatter WJ, Schmechel D, *et al.* Association of apolipoprotein E allele epsilon 4 with late-onset familial and sporadic Alzheimer's disease. Neurology 1993; 43(8): 1467-72.
[http://dx.doi.org/10.1212/WNL.43.8.1467] [PMID: 8350998]

[57] Corder EH, Saunders AM, Strittmatter WJ, *et al.* Gene dose of apolipoprotein E type 4 allele and the risk of Alzheimer's disease in late onset families. Science 1993; 261(5123): 921-3.
[http://dx.doi.org/10.1126/science.8346443] [PMID: 8346443]

[58] Liu CC, Liu CC, Kanekiyo T, Xu H, Bu G. Apolipoprotein E and Alzheimer disease: risk, mechanisms and therapy. Nat Rev Neurol 2013; 9(2): 106-18.
[http://dx.doi.org/10.1038/nrneurol.2012.263] [PMID: 23296339]

[59] Kim J, Basak JM, Holtzman DM. The role of apolipoprotein E in Alzheimer's disease. Neuron 2009; 63(3): 287-303.
[http://dx.doi.org/10.1016/j.neuron.2009.06.026] [PMID: 19679070]

[60] Bateman RJ, Aisen PS, De Strooper B, *et al.* Autosomal-dominant Alzheimer's disease: a review and proposal for the prevention of Alzheimer's disease. Alzheimers Res Ther 2011; 3(1): 1.
[http://dx.doi.org/10.1186/alzrt59] [PMID: 21211070]

[61] Gatz M, Reynolds CA, Fratiglioni L, *et al.* Role of genes and environments for explaining Alzheimer disease. Arch Gen Psychiatry 2006; 63(2): 168-74.
[http://dx.doi.org/10.1001/archpsyc.63.2.168] [PMID: 16461860]

[62] Hazenberg BP. Amyloidosis: a clinical overview. Rheum Dis Clin North Am 2013; 39(2): 323-45.
[http://dx.doi.org/10.1016/j.rdc.2013.02.012] [PMID: 23597967]

[63] Sipe JD, Benson MD, Buxbaum JN, *et al.* Nomenclature 2014: Amyloid fibril proteins and clinical classification of the amyloidosis. Amyloid 2014; 21(4): 221-4.
[http://dx.doi.org/10.3109/13506129.2014.964858] [PMID: 25263598]

[64] Knowles TP, Vendruscolo M, Dobson CM. The amyloid state and its association with protein misfolding diseases. Nat Rev Mol Cell Biol 2014; 15(6): 384-96.
[http://dx.doi.org/10.1038/nrm3810] [PMID: 24854788]

[65] Goedert M, Spillantini MG, Jakes R, Rutherford D, Crowther RA. Multiple isoforms of human microtubule-associated protein tau: sequences and localization in neurofibrillary tangles of Alzheimer's disease. Neuron 1989; 3(4): 519-26.
[http://dx.doi.org/10.1016/0896-6273(89)90210-9] [PMID: 2484340]

[66] Goedert M, Eisenberg DS, Crowther RA. Propagation of Tau Aggregates and Neurodegeneration. Annu Rev Neurosci 2017; 40: 189-210.
[http://dx.doi.org/10.1146/annurev-neuro-072116-031153] [PMID: 28772101]

[67] Goedert M, Spillantini MG. Propagation of Tau aggregates. Mol Brain 2017; 10(1): 18.
[http://dx.doi.org/10.1186/s13041-017-0298-7] [PMID: 28558799]

[68] Andorfer C, Kress Y, Espinoza M, *et al.* Hyperphosphorylation and aggregation of tau in mice expressing normal human tau isoforms. J Neurochem 2003; 86(3): 582-90.
[http://dx.doi.org/10.1046/j.1471-4159.2003.01879.x] [PMID: 12859672]

[69] Williams DR. Tauopathies: classification and clinical update on neurodegenerative diseases associated with microtubule-associated protein tau. Intern Med J 2006; 36(10): 652-60.
[http://dx.doi.org/10.1111/j.1445-5994.2006.01153.x] [PMID: 16958643]

[70] Salloway S, Sperling R, Fox NC, *et al.* Two phase 3 trials of bapineuzumab in mild-to-moderate Alzheimer's disease. N Engl J Med 2014; 370(4): 322-33.
[http://dx.doi.org/10.1056/NEJMoa1304839] [PMID: 24450891]

[71] Frank RA, Galasko D, Hampel H, *et al.* Biological markers for therapeutic trials in Alzheimer's disease. Proceedings of the biological markers working group; NIA initiative on neuroimaging in Alzheimer's disease. Neurobiol Aging 2003; 24(4): 521-36.
[http://dx.doi.org/10.1016/S0197-4580(03)00002-2] [PMID: 12714109]

[72] McKhann GM, Knopman DS, Chertkow H, *et al.* The diagnosis of dementia due to Alzheimer's disease: recommendations from the National Institute on Aging-Alzheimer's Association workgroups on diagnostic guidelines for Alzheimer's disease. Alzheimers Dement 2011; 7(3): 263-9.
[http://dx.doi.org/10.1016/j.jalz.2011.03.005] [PMID: 21514250]

[73] Dubois B, Feldman HH, Jacova C, *et al.* Research criteria for the diagnosis of Alzheimer's disease: revising the NINCDS-ADRDA criteria. Lancet Neurol 2007; 6(8): 734-46.
[http://dx.doi.org/10.1016/S1474-4422(07)70178-3] [PMID: 17616482]

[74] Sperling RA, Aisen PS, Beckett LA, *et al.* Toward defining the preclinical stages of Alzheimer's disease: recommendations from the National Institute on Aging-Alzheimer's Association workgroups on diagnostic guidelines for Alzheimer's disease. Alzheimers Dement 2011; 7(3): 280-92.
[http://dx.doi.org/10.1016/j.jalz.2011.03.003] [PMID: 21514248]

[75] Consensus report of the Working Group on: "Molecular and Biochemical Markers of Alzheimer's Disease". Neurobiol Aging 1998; 19(2): 109-16.
[PMID: 9558143]

[76] Scheltens P, Blennow K, Breteler MM, *et al.* Alzheimer's disease. Lancet 2016; 388(10043): 505-17.
[http://dx.doi.org/10.1016/S0140-6736(15)01124-1] [PMID: 26921134]

[77] Blennow K, de Leon MJ, Zetterberg H. Alzheimer's disease. Lancet 2006; 368(9533): 387-403.
[http://dx.doi.org/10.1016/S0140-6736(06)69113-7] [PMID: 16876668]

[78] Hanseeuw BJ, Betensky RA, Jacobs HIL, *et al.* Association of Amyloid and Tau With Cognition in Preclinical Alzheimer Disease: A Longitudinal Study. JAMA Neurol 2019.
[http://dx.doi.org/10.1001/jamaneurol.2019.1424] [PMID: 31157827]

[79] Hampel H, Bürger K, Teipel SJ, Bokde AL, Zetterberg H, Blennow K. Core candidate neurochemical and imaging biomarkers of Alzheimer's disease. Alzheimers Dement 2008; 4(1): 38-48.
[http://dx.doi.org/10.1016/j.jalz.2007.08.006] [PMID: 18631949]

[80] Cavallucci V, D'Amelio M, Cecconi F. Aβ toxicity in Alzheimer's disease. Mol Neurobiol 2012; 45(2): 366-78.
[http://dx.doi.org/10.1007/s12035-012-8251-3] [PMID: 22415442]

[81] Wang H, Megill A, He K, Kirkwood A, Lee HK. Consequences of inhibiting amyloid precursor protein processing enzymes on synaptic function and plasticity. Neural Plast 2012; 2012272374

[http://dx.doi.org/10.1155/2012/272374] [PMID: 22792491]

[82]   Tabaton M, Nunzi MG, Xue R, Usiak M, Autilio-Gambetti L, Gambetti P. Soluble amyloid beta-protein is a marker of Alzheimer amyloid in brain but not in cerebrospinal fluid. Biochem Biophys Res Commun 1994; 200(3): 1598-603.
[http://dx.doi.org/10.1006/bbrc.1994.1634] [PMID: 8185615]

[83]   Van Nostrand WE, Wagner SL, Shankle WR, *et al.* Decreased levels of soluble amyloid beta-protein precursor in cerebrospinal fluid of live Alzheimer disease patients. Proc Natl Acad Sci USA 1992; 89(7): 2551-5.
[http://dx.doi.org/10.1073/pnas.89.7.2551] [PMID: 1557359]

[84]   Motter R, Vigo-Pelfrey C, Kholodenko D, *et al.* Reduction of beta-amyloid peptide42 in the cerebrospinal fluid of patients with Alzheimer's disease. Ann Neurol 1995; 38(4): 643-8.
[http://dx.doi.org/10.1002/ana.410380413] [PMID: 7574461]

[85]   Masters CL, Simms G, Weinman NA, Multhaup G, McDonald BL, Beyreuther K. Amyloid plaque core protein in Alzheimer disease and Down syndrome. Proc Natl Acad Sci USA 1985; 82(12): 4245-9.
[http://dx.doi.org/10.1073/pnas.82.12.4245] [PMID: 3159021]

[86]   Portelius E, Westman-Brinkmalm A, Zetterberg H, Blennow K. Determination of β-amyloid peptide signatures in cerebrospinal fluid using immunoprecipitation-mass spectrometry. J Proteome Res 2006; 5(4): 1010-6.
[http://dx.doi.org/10.1021/pr050475v] [PMID: 16602710]

[87]   Pannee J, Törnqvist U, Westerlund A, *et al.* The amyloid-β degradation pattern in plasma--a possible tool for clinical trials in Alzheimer's disease. Neurosci Lett 2014; 573: 7-12.
[http://dx.doi.org/10.1016/j.neulet.2014.04.041] [PMID: 24796810]

[88]   Olsson B, Lautner R, Andreasson U, *et al.* CSF and blood biomarkers for the diagnosis of Alzheimer's disease: a systematic review and meta-analysis. Lancet Neurol 2016; 15(7): 673-84.
[http://dx.doi.org/10.1016/S1474-4422(16)00070-3] [PMID: 27068280]

[89]   Kanai M, Matsubara E, Isoe K, *et al.* Longitudinal study of cerebrospinal fluid levels of tau, A beta1-40, and A beta1-42(43) in Alzheimer's disease: a study in Japan. Ann Neurol 1998; 44(1): 17-26.
[http://dx.doi.org/10.1002/ana.410440108] [PMID: 9667589]

[90]   Mehta PD, Pirttilä T, Mehta SP, Sersen EA, Aisen PS, Wisniewski HM. Plasma and cerebrospinal fluid levels of amyloid beta proteins 1-40 and 1-42 in Alzheimer disease. Arch Neurol 2000; 57(1): 100-5.
[http://dx.doi.org/10.1001/archneur.57.1.100] [PMID: 10634455]

[91]   Strozyk D, Blennow K, White LR, Launer LJ. CSF Abeta 42 levels correlate with amyloid-neuropathology in a population-based autopsy study. Neurology 2003; 60(4): 652-6.
[http://dx.doi.org/10.1212/01.WNL.0000046581.81650.D0] [PMID: 12601108]

[92]   Tapiola T, Alafuzoff I, Herukka SK, *et al.* Cerebrospinal fluid beta-amyloid 42 and tau proteins as biomarkers of Alzheimer-type pathologic changes in the brain. Arch Neurol 2009; 66(3): 382-9.
[http://dx.doi.org/10.1001/archneurol.2008.596] [PMID: 19273758]

[93]   Blennow K, Mattsson N, Schöll M, Hansson O, Zetterberg H. Amyloid biomarkers in Alzheimer's disease. Trends Pharmacol Sci 2015; 36(5): 297-309.
[http://dx.doi.org/10.1016/j.tips.2015.03.002] [PMID: 25840462]

[94]   Bateman RJ, Xiong C, Benzinger TL, *et al.* Dominantly Inherited Alzheimer Network. Clinical and biomarker changes in dominantly inherited Alzheimer's disease. N Engl J Med 2012; 367(9): 795-804.
[http://dx.doi.org/10.1056/NEJMoa1202753] [PMID: 22784036]

[95]   Blennow K, Hampel H. CSF markers for incipient Alzheimer's disease. Lancet Neurol 2003; 2(10): 605-13.
[http://dx.doi.org/10.1016/S1474-4422(03)00530-1] [PMID: 14505582]

[96]   Molinuevo JL, Ayton S, Batrla R, *et al.* Current state of Alzheimer's fluid biomarkers. Acta Neuropathol 2018; 136(6): 821-53.
[http://dx.doi.org/10.1007/s00401-018-1932-x] [PMID: 30488277]

[97]   Mattsson N, Zetterberg H, Hansson O, *et al.* CSF biomarkers and incipient Alzheimer disease in patients with mild cognitive impairment. JAMA 2009; 302(4): 385-93.
[http://dx.doi.org/10.1001/jama.2009.1064] [PMID: 19622817]

[98]   Hansson O, Zetterberg H, Buchhave P, Londos E, Blennow K, Minthon L. Association between CSF biomarkers and incipient Alzheimer's disease in patients with mild cognitive impairment: a follow-up study. Lancet Neurol 2006; 5(3): 228-34.
[http://dx.doi.org/10.1016/S1474-4422(06)70355-6] [PMID: 16488378]

[99]   Maddalena A, Papassotiropoulos A, Müller-Tillmanns B, *et al.* Biochemical diagnosis of Alzheimer disease by measuring the cerebrospinal fluid ratio of phosphorylated tau protein to beta-amyloid peptide42. Arch Neurol 2003; 60(9): 1202-6.
[http://dx.doi.org/10.1001/archneur.60.9.1202] [PMID: 12975284]

[100]   Sunderland T, Linker G, Mirza N, *et al.* Decreased beta-amyloid1-42 and increased tau levels in cerebrospinal fluid of patients with Alzheimer disease. JAMA 2003; 289(16): 2094-103.
[http://dx.doi.org/10.1001/jama.289.16.2094] [PMID: 12709467]

[101]   Shaw LM, Korecka M, Clark CM, Lee VM, Trojanowski JQ. Biomarkers of neurodegeneration for diagnosis and monitoring therapeutics. Nat Rev Drug Discov 2007; 6(4): 295-303.
[http://dx.doi.org/10.1038/nrd2176] [PMID: 17347655]

[102]   Bakota L, Brandt R. Tau Biology and Tau-Directed Therapies for Alzheimer's Disease. Drugs 2016; 76(3): 301-13.
[http://dx.doi.org/10.1007/s40265-015-0529-0] [PMID: 26729186]

[103]   Sanabria-Castro A, Alvarado-Echeverría I, Monge-Bonilla C. Molecular Pathogenesis of Alzheimer's Disease: An Update. Ann Neurosci 2017; 24(1): 46-54.
[http://dx.doi.org/10.1159/000464422] [PMID: 28588356]

[104]   Wallin ÅK, Blennow K, Zetterberg H, Londos E, Minthon L, Hansson O. CSF biomarkers predict a more malignant outcome in Alzheimer disease. Neurology 2010; 74(19): 1531-7.
[http://dx.doi.org/10.1212/WNL.0b013e3181dd4dd8] [PMID: 20458070]

[105]   Hertze J, Minthon L, Zetterberg H, Vanmechelen E, Blennow K, Hansson O. Evaluation of CSF biomarkers as predictors of Alzheimer's disease: a clinical follow-up study of 4.7 years. J Alzheimers Dis 2010; 21(4): 1119-28.
[http://dx.doi.org/10.3233/JAD-2010-100207] [PMID: 21504133]

[106]   Kang JH, Korecka M, Toledo JB, Trojanowski JQ, Shaw LM. Clinical utility and analytical challenges in measurement of cerebrospinal fluid amyloid-β(1-42) and τ proteins as Alzheimer disease biomarkers. Clin Chem 2013; 59(6): 903-16.
[http://dx.doi.org/10.1373/clinchem.2013.202937] [PMID: 23519967]

[107]   Blennow K, Hampel H, Weiner M, Zetterberg H. Cerebrospinal fluid and plasma biomarkers in Alzheimer disease. Nat Rev Neurol 2010; 6(3): 131-44.
[http://dx.doi.org/10.1038/nrneurol.2010.4] [PMID: 20157306]

[108]   Hampel H, Buerger K, Zinkowski R, *et al.* Measurement of phosphorylated tau epitopes in the differential diagnosis of Alzheimer disease: a comparative cerebrospinal fluid study. Arch Gen Psychiatry 2004; 61(1): 95-102.
[http://dx.doi.org/10.1001/archpsyc.61.1.95] [PMID: 14706948]

[109]   Dubois B, Feldman HH, Jacova C, *et al.* Advancing research diagnostic criteria for Alzheimer's disease: the IWG-2 criteria. Lancet Neurol 2014; 13(6): 614-29.
[http://dx.doi.org/10.1016/S1474-4422(14)70090-0] [PMID: 24849862]

[110]   Zetterberg H, Wahlund LO, Blennow K. Cerebrospinal fluid markers for prediction of Alzheimer's

disease. Neurosci Lett 2003; 352(1): 67-9.
[http://dx.doi.org/10.1016/j.neulet.2003.08.011] [PMID: 14615052]

[111] De Meyer G, Shapiro F, Vanderstichele H, *et al.* Alzheimer's Disease Neuroimaging Initiative. Diagnosis-independent Alzheimer disease biomarker signature in cognitively normal elderly people. Arch Neurol 2010; 67(8): 949-56.
[http://dx.doi.org/10.1001/archneurol.2010.179] [PMID: 20697045]

[112] Ferreira D, Rivero-Santana A, Perestelo-Pérez L, *et al.* Improving CSF Biomarkers' Performance for Predicting Progression from Mild Cognitive Impairment to Alzheimer's Disease by Considering Different Confounding Factors: A Meta-Analysis. Front Aging Neurosci 2014; 6(287): 287.
[PMID: 25360114]

[113] Schneider P, Hampel H, Buerger K. Biological marker candidates of Alzheimer's disease in blood, plasma, and serum. CNS Neurosci Ther 2009; 15(4): 358-74.
[http://dx.doi.org/10.1111/j.1755-5949.2009.00104.x] [PMID: 19840034]

[114] Goudey B, Fung BJ, Schieber C, Faux NG. Alzheimer's Disease Metabolomics Consortium; Alzheimer's Disease Neuroimaging Initiative. A blood-based signature of cerebrospinal fluid $A\beta_{1-42}$ status. Sci Rep 2019; 9(1): 4163.
[http://dx.doi.org/10.1038/s41598-018-37149-7] [PMID: 30853713]

[115] de Almeida SM, Shumaker SD, LeBlanc SK, *et al.* Incidence of post-dural puncture headache in research volunteers. Headache 2011; 51(10): 1503-10.
[http://dx.doi.org/10.1111/j.1526-4610.2011.01959.x] [PMID: 21797856]

[116] Hampel H, O'Bryant SE, Molinuevo JL, *et al.* Blood-based biomarkers for Alzheimer disease: mapping the road to the clinic. Nat Rev Neurol 2018; 14(11): 639-52.
[http://dx.doi.org/10.1038/s41582-018-0079-7] [PMID: 30297701]

[117] Thambisetty M, Lovestone S. Blood-based biomarkers of Alzheimer's disease: challenging but feasible. Biomarkers Med 2010; 4(1): 65-79.
[http://dx.doi.org/10.2217/bmm.09.84] [PMID: 20387303]

[118] Snyder HM, Carrillo MC, Grodstein F, *et al.* Developing novel blood-based biomarkers for Alzheimer's disease. Alzheimers Dement 2014; 10(1): 109-14.
[http://dx.doi.org/10.1016/j.jalz.2013.10.007] [PMID: 24365657]

[119] Henriksen K, O'Bryant SE, Hampel H, *et al.* Blood-Based Biomarker Interest Group. The future of blood-based biomarkers for Alzheimer's disease. Alzheimers Dement 2014; 10(1): 115-31.
[http://dx.doi.org/10.1016/j.jalz.2013.01.013] [PMID: 23850333]

[120] Zetterberg H, Burnham SC. Blood-based molecular biomarkers for Alzheimer's disease. Mol Brain 2019; 12(1): 26.
[http://dx.doi.org/10.1186/s13041-019-0448-1] [PMID: 30922367]

[121] Blennow K, Zetterberg H. Biomarkers for Alzheimer's disease: current status and prospects for the future. J Intern Med 2018; 284(6): 643-63.
[http://dx.doi.org/10.1111/joim.12816] [PMID: 30051512]

[122] Nakamura A, Kaneko N, Villemagne VL, *et al.* High performance plasma amyloid-β biomarkers for Alzheimer's disease. Nature 2018; 554(7691): 249-54.
[http://dx.doi.org/10.1038/nature25456] [PMID: 29420472]

[123] Janelidze S, Stomrud E, Palmqvist S, *et al.* Plasma β-amyloid in Alzheimer's disease and vascular disease. Sci Rep 2016; 6: 26801.
[http://dx.doi.org/10.1038/srep26801] [PMID: 27241045]

[124] Verberk IMW, Slot RE, Verfaillie SCJ, *et al.* Plasma Amyloid as Prescreener for the Earliest Alzheimer Pathological Changes. Ann Neurol 2018; 84(5): 648-58.
[http://dx.doi.org/10.1002/ana.25334] [PMID: 30196548]

[125] Lashley T, Schott JM, Weston P, *et al.* Molecular biomarkers of Alzheimer's disease: progress and

prospects. Dis Model Mech 2018; 11(5)dmm031781
[http://dx.doi.org/10.1242/dmm.031781] [PMID: 29739861]

[126] Deters KD, Risacher SL, Kim S, *et al*. Alzheimer Disease Neuroimaging Initiative. Plasma Tau Association with Brain Atrophy in Mild Cognitive Impairment and Alzheimer's Disease. J Alzheimers Dis 2017; 58(4): 1245-54.
[http://dx.doi.org/10.3233/JAD-161114] [PMID: 28550246]

[127] Mattsson N, Zetterberg H, Janelidze S, *et al*. ADNI Investigators. Plasma tau in Alzheimer disease. Neurology 2016; 87(17): 1827-35.
[http://dx.doi.org/10.1212/WNL.0000000000003246] [PMID: 27694257]

[128] Mielke MM, Hagen CE, Wennberg AMV, *et al*. Association of Plasma Total Tau Level With Cognitive Decline and Risk of Mild Cognitive Impairment or Dementia in the Mayo Clinic Study on Aging. JAMA Neurol 2017; 74(9): 1073-80.
[http://dx.doi.org/10.1001/jamaneurol.2017.1359] [PMID: 28692710]

[129] Zetterberg H, Wilson D, Andreasson U, *et al*. Plasma tau levels in Alzheimer's disease. Alzheimers Res Ther 2013; 5(2): 9.
[http://dx.doi.org/10.1186/alzrt163] [PMID: 23551972]

[130] Mielke MM, Hagen CE, Wennberg AMV, *et al*. Association of Plasma Total Tau Level With Cognitive Decline and Risk of Mild Cognitive Impairment or Dementia in the Mayo Clinic Study on Aging. JAMA Neurol 2017; 74(9): 1073-80.
[http://dx.doi.org/10.1001/jamaneurol.2017.1359] [PMID: 28692710]

[131] Yang CC, Chiu MJ, Chen TF, Chang HL, Liu BH, Yang SY. Assay of Plasma Phosphorylated Tau Protein (Threonine 181) and Total Tau Protein in Early-Stage Alzheimer's Disease. J Alzheimers Dis 2018; 61(4): 1323-32.
[http://dx.doi.org/10.3233/JAD-170810] [PMID: 29376870]

[132] Tatebe H, Kasai T, Ohmichi T, *et al*. Quantification of plasma phosphorylated tau to use as a biomarker for brain Alzheimer pathology: pilot case-control studies including patients with Alzheimer's disease and down syndrome. Mol Neurodegener 2017; 12(1): 63.
[http://dx.doi.org/10.1186/s13024-017-0206-8] [PMID: 28866979]

[133] Mielke MM, Hagen CE, Xu J, *et al*. Plasma phospho-tau181 increases with Alzheimer's disease clinical severity and is associated with tau- and amyloid-positron emission tomography. Alzheimers Dement 2018; 14(8): 989-97.
[http://dx.doi.org/10.1016/j.jalz.2018.02.013] [PMID: 29626426]

[134] Shekhar S, Kumar R, Rai N, *et al*. Estimation of Tau and Phosphorylated Tau181 in Serum of Alzheimer's Disease and Mild Cognitive Impairment Patients. PLoS One 2016; 11(7)e0159099
[http://dx.doi.org/10.1371/journal.pone.0159099] [PMID: 27459603]

[135] Zetterberg H, Andreasson U, Hansson O, *et al*. Elevated cerebrospinal fluid BACE1 activity in incipient Alzheimer disease. Arch Neurol 2008; 65(8): 1102-7.
[http://dx.doi.org/10.1001/archneur.65.8.1102] [PMID: 18695061]

[136] Shen Y, Wang H, Sun Q, *et al*. Increased Plasma Beta-Secretase 1 May Predict Conversion to Alzheimer's Disease Dementia in Individuals With Mild Cognitive Impairment. Biol Psychiatry 2018; 83(5): 447-55.
[http://dx.doi.org/10.1016/j.biopsych.2017.02.007] [PMID: 28359566]

[137] Khalil M, Teunissen CE, Otto M, *et al*. Neurofilaments as biomarkers in neurological disorders. Nat Rev Neurol 2018; 14(10): 577-89.
[http://dx.doi.org/10.1038/s41582-018-0058-z] [PMID: 30171200]

[138] Lee MK, Cleveland DW. Neuronal intermediate filaments. Annu Rev Neurosci 1996; 19: 187-217.
[http://dx.doi.org/10.1146/annurev.ne.19.030196.001155] [PMID: 8833441]

[139] Yilmaz A, Blennow K, Hagberg L, *et al*. Neurofilament light chain protein as a marker of neuronal

injury: review of its use in HIV-1 infection and reference values for HIV-negative controls. Expert Rev Mol Diagn 2017; 17(8): 761-70.
[http://dx.doi.org/10.1080/14737159.2017.1341313] [PMID: 28598205]

[140] Varhaug KN, Torkildsen Ø, Myhr KM, Vedeler CA. Neurofilament Light Chain as a Biomarker in Multiple Sclerosis. Front Neurol 2019; 10: 338.
[http://dx.doi.org/10.3389/fneur.2019.00338] [PMID: 31024432]

[141] Zetterberg H, Skillbäck T, Mattsson N, *et al.* Alzheimer's Disease Neuroimaging Initiative. Association of Cerebrospinal Fluid Neurofilament Light Concentration With Alzheimer Disease Progression. JAMA Neurol 2016; 73(1): 60-7.
[http://dx.doi.org/10.1001/jamaneurol.2015.3037] [PMID: 26524180]

[142] Chatterjee P, Goozee K, Sohrabi HR, *et al.* Association of Plasma Neurofilament Light Chain with Neocortical Amyloid-β Load and Cognitive Performance in Cognitively Normal Elderly Participants. J Alzheimers Dis 2018; 63(2): 479-87.
[http://dx.doi.org/10.3233/JAD-180025] [PMID: 29630554]

[143] Skillbäck T, Farahmand B, Bartlett JW, *et al.* CSF neurofilament light differs in neurodegenerative diseases and predicts severity and survival. Neurology 2014; 83(21): 1945-53.
[http://dx.doi.org/10.1212/WNL.0000000000001015] [PMID: 25339208]

[144] Zetterberg H. Neurofilament Light: A Dynamic Cross-Disease Fluid Biomarker for Neurodegeneration. Neuron 2016; 91(1): 1-3.
[http://dx.doi.org/10.1016/j.neuron.2016.06.030] [PMID: 27387643]

[145] Ashton NJ, Leuzy A, Lim YM, *et al.* Increased plasma neurofilament light chain concentration correlates with severity of post-mortem neurofibrillary tangle pathology and neurodegeneration. Acta Neuropathol Commun 2019; 7(1): 5.
[http://dx.doi.org/10.1186/s40478-018-0649-3] [PMID: 30626432]

[146] Lewczuk P, Ermann N, Andreasson U, *et al.* Plasma neurofilament light as a potential biomarker of neurodegeneration in Alzheimer's disease. Alzheimers Res Ther 2018; 10(1): 71.
[http://dx.doi.org/10.1186/s13195-018-0404-9] [PMID: 30055655]

[147] Teunissen CE, Khalil M. Neurofilaments as biomarkers in multiple sclerosis. Mult Scler 2012; 18(5): 552-6.
[http://dx.doi.org/10.1177/1352458512443092] [PMID: 22492131]

[148] Mroczko B, Groblewska M, Litman-Zawadzka A, Kornhuber J, Lewczuk P. Amyloid β oligomers (AβOs) in Alzheimer's disease. J Neural Transm (Vienna) 2018; 125(2): 177-91.
[http://dx.doi.org/10.1007/s00702-017-1820-x] [PMID: 29196815]

[149] Lacor PN, Buniel MC, Chang L, *et al.* Synaptic targeting by Alzheimer's-related amyloid beta oligomers. J Neurosci 2004; 24(45): 10191-200.
[http://dx.doi.org/10.1523/JNEUROSCI.3432-04.2004] [PMID: 15537891]

[150] Koffie RM, Meyer-Luehmann M, Hashimoto T, *et al.* Oligomeric amyloid beta associates with postsynaptic densities and correlates with excitatory synapse loss near senile plaques. Proc Natl Acad Sci USA 2009; 106(10): 4012-7.
[http://dx.doi.org/10.1073/pnas.0811698106] [PMID: 19228947]

[151] Viola KL, Klein WL. Amyloid β oligomers in Alzheimer's disease pathogenesis, treatment, and diagnosis. Acta Neuropathol 2015; 129(2): 183-206.
[http://dx.doi.org/10.1007/s00401-015-1386-3] [PMID: 25604547]

[152] Lesné S, Kotilinek L, Ashe KH. Plaque-bearing mice with reduced levels of oligomeric amyloid-beta assemblies have intact memory function. Neuroscience 2008; 151(3): 745-9.
[http://dx.doi.org/10.1016/j.neuroscience.2007.10.054] [PMID: 18155846]

[153] Gandy S, Simon AJ, Steele JW, *et al.* Days to criterion as an indicator of toxicity associated with human Alzheimer amyloid-beta oligomers. Ann Neurol 2010; 68(2): 220-30.

[PMID: 20641005]

[154] Townsend M, Shankar GM, Mehta T, Walsh DM, Selkoe DJ. Effects of secreted oligomers of amyloid beta-protein on hippocampal synaptic plasticity: a potent role for trimers. J Physiol 2006; 572(Pt 2): 477-92.
[http://dx.doi.org/10.1113/jphysiol.2005.103754] [PMID: 16469784]

[155] Santos AN, Ewers M, Minthon L, *et al.* Amyloid-β oligomers in cerebrospinal fluid are associated with cognitive decline in patients with Alzheimer's disease. J Alzheimers Dis 2012; 29(1): 171-6.
[http://dx.doi.org/10.3233/JAD-2012-111361] [PMID: 22214781]

[156] Lleó A, Núñez-Llaves R, Alcolea D, *et al.* Changes in Synaptic Proteins Precede Neurodegeneration Markers in Preclinical Alzheimer's Disease Cerebrospinal Fluid. Mol Cell Proteomics 2019; 18(3): 546-60.
[http://dx.doi.org/10.1074/mcp.RA118.001290] [PMID: 30606734]

[157] Öhrfelt A, Brinkmalm A, Dumurgier J, *et al.* The pre-synaptic vesicle protein synaptotagmin is a novel biomarker for Alzheimer's disease. Alzheimers Res Ther 2016; 8(1): 41.
[http://dx.doi.org/10.1186/s13195-016-0208-8] [PMID: 27716408]

[158] Brinkmalm A, Brinkmalm G, Honer WG, *et al.* SNAP-25 is a promising novel cerebrospinal fluid biomarker for synapse degeneration in Alzheimer's disease. Mol Neurodegener 2014; 9: 53.
[http://dx.doi.org/10.1186/1750-1326-9-53] [PMID: 25418885]

[159] Thorsell A, Bjerke M, Gobom J, *et al.* Neurogranin in cerebrospinal fluid as a marker of synaptic degeneration in Alzheimer's disease. Brain Res 2010; 1362: 13-22.
[http://dx.doi.org/10.1016/j.brainres.2010.09.073] [PMID: 20875798]

[160] Duits FH, Brinkmalm G, Teunissen CE, *et al.* Synaptic proteins in CSF as potential novel biomarkers for prognosis in prodromal Alzheimer's disease. Alzheimers Res Ther 2018; 10(1): 5.
[http://dx.doi.org/10.1186/s13195-017-0335-x] [PMID: 29370833]

[161] Reitz C, Mayeux R. Alzheimer disease: epidemiology, diagnostic criteria, risk factors and biomarkers. Biochem Pharmacol 2014; 88(4): 640-51.
[http://dx.doi.org/10.1016/j.bcp.2013.12.024] [PMID: 24398425]

[162] Baldacci F, Lista S, Cavedo E, Bonuccelli U, Hampel H. Diagnostic function of the neuroinflammatory biomarker YKL-40 in Alzheimer's disease and other neurodegenerative diseases. Expert Rev Proteomics 2017; 14(4): 285-99.
[http://dx.doi.org/10.1080/14789450.2017.1304217] [PMID: 28281838]

[163] Zhang R, Miller RG, Madison C, *et al.* Systemic immune system alterations in early stages of Alzheimer's disease. J Neuroimmunol 2013; 256(1-2): 38-42.
[http://dx.doi.org/10.1016/j.jneuroim.2013.01.002] [PMID: 23380586]

[164] Alsadany MA, Shehata HH, Mohamad MI, Mahfouz RG. Histone deacetylases enzyme, copper, and IL-8 levels in patients with Alzheimer's disease. Am J Alzheimers Dis Other Demen 2013; 28(1): 54-61.
[http://dx.doi.org/10.1177/1533317512467680] [PMID: 23242124]

[165] Femminella GD, Thayanandan T, Calsolaro V, *et al.* Imaging and Molecular Mechanisms of Alzheimer's Disease: A Review. Int J Mol Sci 2018; 19(12): 3702.
[http://dx.doi.org/10.3390/ijms19123702] [PMID: 30469491]

[166] Braak H, Braak E. Frequency of stages of Alzheimer-related lesions in different age categories. Neurobiol Aging 1997; 18(4): 351-7.
[http://dx.doi.org/10.1016/S0197-4580(97)00056-0] [PMID: 9330961]

[167] Fleisher AS, Chen K, Liu X, *et al.* Using positron emission tomography and florbetapir F18 to image cortical amyloid in patients with mild cognitive impairment or dementia due to Alzheimer disease. Arch Neurol 2011; 68(11): 1404-11.
[http://dx.doi.org/10.1001/archneurol.2011.150] [PMID: 21747008]

[168] Nelson PT, Alafuzoff I, Bigio EH, *et al.* Correlation of Alzheimer disease neuropathologic changes with cognitive status: a review of the literature. J Neuropathol Exp Neurol 2012; 71(5): 362-81.
[http://dx.doi.org/10.1097/NEN.0b013e31825018f7] [PMID: 22487856]

[169] Sperling RA, Johnson KA, Doraiswamy PM, *et al.* AV45-A05 Study Group. Amyloid deposition detected with florbetapir F 18 ((18)F-AV-45) is related to lower episodic memory performance in clinically normal older individuals. Neurobiol Aging 2013; 34(3): 822-31.
[http://dx.doi.org/10.1016/j.neurobiolaging.2012.06.014] [PMID: 22878163]

[170] Engler H, Forsberg A, Almkvist O, *et al.* Two-year follow-up of amyloid deposition in patients with Alzheimer's disease. Brain 2006; 129(Pt 11): 2856-66.
[http://dx.doi.org/10.1093/brain/awl178] [PMID: 16854944]

[171] Braak H, Braak E. Neuropathological stageing of Alzheimer-related changes. Acta Neuropathol 1991; 82(4): 239-59.
[http://dx.doi.org/10.1007/BF00308809] [PMID: 1759558]

[172] Schwarz AJ, Yu P, Miller BB, *et al.* Regional profiles of the candidate tau PET ligand 18F-AV-1451 recapitulate key features of Braak histopathological stages. Brain 2016; 139(Pt 5): 1539-50.
[http://dx.doi.org/10.1093/brain/aww023] [PMID: 26936940]

[173] Villemagne VL, Furumoto S, Fodero-Tavoletti MT, *et al. In vivo* evaluation of a novel tau imaging tracer for Alzheimer's disease. Eur J Nucl Med Mol Imaging 2014; 41(5): 816-26.
[http://dx.doi.org/10.1007/s00259-013-2681-7] [PMID: 24514874]

[174] Hall B, Mak E, Cervenka S, Aigbirhio FI, Rowe JB, O'Brien JT. *In vivo* tau PET imaging in dementia: Pathophysiology, radiotracer quantification, and a systematic review of clinical findings. Ageing Res Rev 2017; 36: 50-63.
[http://dx.doi.org/10.1016/j.arr.2017.03.002] [PMID: 28315409]

[175] Wilson H, Pagano G, Politis M. Dementia spectrum disorders: lessons learnt from decades with PET research. J Neural Transm (Vienna) 2019; 126(3): 233-51.
[http://dx.doi.org/10.1007/s00702-019-01975-4] [PMID: 30762136]

[176] Arriagada PV, Growdon JH, Hedley-Whyte ET, Hyman BT. Neurofibrillary tangles but not senile plaques parallel duration and severity of Alzheimer's disease. Neurology 1992; 42(3 Pt 1): 631-9.
[http://dx.doi.org/10.1212/WNL.42.3.631] [PMID: 1549228]

[177] Giannakopoulos P, Gold G, Kövari E, *et al.* Assessing the cognitive impact of Alzheimer disease pathology and vascular burden in the aging brain: the Geneva experience. Acta Neuropathol 2007; 113(1): 1-12.
[http://dx.doi.org/10.1007/s00401-006-0144-y] [PMID: 17036244]

[178] Ossenkoppele R, Schonhaut DR, Schöll M, *et al.* Tau PET patterns mirror clinical and neuroanatomical variability in Alzheimer's disease. Brain 2016; 139(Pt 5): 1551-67.
[http://dx.doi.org/10.1093/brain/aww027] [PMID: 26962052]

[179] Cho H, Choi JY, Hwang MS, *et al.* Tau PET in Alzheimer disease and mild cognitive impairment. Neurology 2016; 87(4): 375-83.
[http://dx.doi.org/10.1212/WNL.0000000000002892] [PMID: 27358341]

[180] Johnson KA, Schultz A, Betensky RA, *et al.* Tau positron emission tomographic imaging in aging and early Alzheimer disease. Ann Neurol 2016; 79(1): 110-9.
[http://dx.doi.org/10.1002/ana.24546] [PMID: 26505746]

[181] Lockhart SN, Baker SL, Okamura N, *et al.* Dynamic PET Measures of Tau Accumulation in Cognitively Normal Older Adults and Alzheimer's Disease Patients Measured Using [18F] THK-5351. PLoS One 2016; 11(6)e0158460
[http://dx.doi.org/10.1371/journal.pone.0158460] [PMID: 27355840]

[182] Apostolova LG, Steiner CA, Akopyan GG, *et al.* Three-dimensional gray matter atrophy mapping in mild cognitive impairment and mild Alzheimer disease. Arch Neurol 2007; 64(10): 1489-95.

[http://dx.doi.org/10.1001/archneur.64.10.1489] [PMID: 17923632]

[183] Prestia A, Drago V, Rasser PE, Bonetti M, Thompson PM, Frisoni GB. Cortical changes in incipient Alzheimer's disease. J Alzheimers Dis 2010; 22(4): 1339-49.
[http://dx.doi.org/10.3233/JAD-2010-101191] [PMID: 20930288]

[184] Jack CR Jr, *et al.* Steps to standardization and validation of hippocampal volumetry as a biomarker in clinical trials and diagnostic criterion for Alzheimer's disease 2011.
[http://dx.doi.org/10.1016/j.jalz.2011.04.007]

[185] Pini L, Pievani M, Bocchetta M, *et al.* Brain atrophy in Alzheimer's Disease and aging. Ageing Res Rev 2016; 30: 25-48.
[http://dx.doi.org/10.1016/j.arr.2016.01.002] [PMID: 26827786]

[186] Apostolova LG, Green AE, Babakchanian S, *et al.* Hippocampal atrophy and ventricular enlargement in normal aging, mild cognitive impairment (MCI), and Alzheimer Disease. Alzheimer Dis Assoc Disord 2012; 26(1): 17-27.
[http://dx.doi.org/10.1097/WAD.0b013e3182163b62] [PMID: 22343374]

[187] Pluta J, Yushkevich P, Das S, Wolk D. *In vivo* analysis of hippocampal subfield atrophy in mild cognitive impairment *via* semi-automatic segmentation of T2-weighted MRI. J Alzheimers Dis 2012; 31(1): 85-99.
[http://dx.doi.org/10.3233/JAD-2012-111931] [PMID: 22504319]

[188] Apostolova LG, Thompson PM, Green AE, *et al.* 3D comparison of low, intermediate, and advanced hippocampal atrophy in MCI. Hum Brain Mapp 2010; 31(5): 786-97.
[http://dx.doi.org/10.1002/hbm.20905] [PMID: 20143386]

[189] Chang YL, Fennema-Notestine C, Holland D, *et al.* Alzheimer's Disease Neuroimaging Initiative. APOE interacts with age to modify rate of decline in cognitive and brain changes in Alzheimer's disease. Alzheimers Dement 2014; 10(3): 336-48.
[http://dx.doi.org/10.1016/j.jalz.2013.05.1763] [PMID: 23896613]

[190] Chang YL, Jacobson MW, Fennema-Notestine C, *et al.* Alzheimer's Disease Neuroimaging Initiative. Level of executive function influences verbal memory in amnestic mild cognitive impairment and predicts prefrontal and posterior cingulate thickness. Cereb Cortex 2010; 20(6): 1305-13.
[http://dx.doi.org/10.1093/cercor/bhp192] [PMID: 19776343]

[191] Chang YL, Bondi MW, McEvoy LK, *et al.* Alzheimer's Disease Neuroimaging Initiative. Global clinical dementia rating of 0.5 in MCI masks variability related to level of function. Neurology 2011; 76(7): 652-9.
[http://dx.doi.org/10.1212/WNL.0b013e31820ce6a5] [PMID: 21321338]

[192] Bozzali M, Serra L, Cercignani M. Quantitative MRI to understand Alzheimer's disease pathophysiology. Curr Opin Neurol 2016; 29(4): 437-44.
[http://dx.doi.org/10.1097/WCO.0000000000000345] [PMID: 27228309]

[193] Coleman M. Axon degeneration mechanisms: commonality amid diversity. Nat Rev Neurosci 2005; 6(11): 889-98.
[http://dx.doi.org/10.1038/nrn1788] [PMID: 16224497]

[194] Reisberg B, Franssen EH, Souren LE, Auer SR, Akram I, Kenowsky S. Evidence and mechanisms of retrogenesis in Alzheimer's and other dementias: management and treatment import. Am J Alzheimers Dis Other Demen 2002; 17(4): 202-12.
[http://dx.doi.org/10.1177/153331750201700411] [PMID: 12184509]

[195] Frost B, Diamond MI. Prion-like mechanisms in neurodegenerative diseases. Nat Rev Neurosci 2010; 11(3): 155-9.
[http://dx.doi.org/10.1038/nrn2786] [PMID: 20029438]

[196] Krstic D, Knuesel I. Deciphering the mechanism underlying late-onset Alzheimer disease. Nat Rev Neurol 2013; 9(1): 25-34.

[http://dx.doi.org/10.1038/nrneurol.2012.236] [PMID: 23183882]

[197] Sjöbeck M, Haglund M, Englund E. White matter mapping in Alzheimer's disease: A neuropathological study. Neurobiol Aging 2006; 27(5): 673-80.
[http://dx.doi.org/10.1016/j.neurobiolaging.2005.03.007] [PMID: 15894407]

[198] Caso F, Agosta F, Filippi M. Insights into White Matter Damage in Alzheimer's Disease: From Postmortem to *In vivo* Diffusion Tensor MRI Studies. Neurodegener Dis 2016; 16(1-2): 26-33.
[http://dx.doi.org/10.1159/000441422] [PMID: 26618812]

[199] Sexton CE, *et al.* A meta-analysis of diffusion tensor imaging in mild cognitive impairment and Alzheimer's disease 2011.
[http://dx.doi.org/10.1016/j.neurobiolaging.2010.05.019]

[200] Chang YL, Yen YS, Chen TF, Yan SH, Tseng WY. Clinical Dementia Rating Scale Detects White Matter Changes in Older Adults at Risk for Alzheimer's Disease. J Alzheimers Dis 2016; 50(2): 411-23.
[http://dx.doi.org/10.3233/JAD-150599] [PMID: 26639963]

[201] Chang YL, Chen TF, Shih YC, Chiu MJ, Yan SH, Tseng WY. Regional cingulum disruption, not gray matter atrophy, detects cognitive changes in amnestic mild cognitive impairment subtypes. J Alzheimers Dis 2015; 44(1): 125-38.
[http://dx.doi.org/10.3233/JAD-141839] [PMID: 25190630]

[202] Nowrangi MA, Lyketsos CG, Leoutsakos JM, *et al.* Longitudinal, region-specific course of diffusion tensor imaging measures in mild cognitive impairment and Alzheimer's disease. Alzheimers Dement 2013; 9(5): 519-28.
[http://dx.doi.org/10.1016/j.jalz.2012.05.2186] [PMID: 23245561]

[203] Lequin RM. Enzyme immunoassay (EIA)/enzyme-linked immunosorbent assay (ELISA). Clin Chem 2005; 51(12): 2415-8.
[http://dx.doi.org/10.1373/clinchem.2005.051532] [PMID: 16179424]

[204] Crowther JR. ELISA. Theory and practice. Methods Mol Biol 1995; 42: 1-218.
[PMID: 7655571]

[205] Giljohann DA, Mirkin CA. Drivers of biodiagnostic development. Nature 2009; 462(7272): 461-4.
[http://dx.doi.org/10.1038/nature08605] [PMID: 19940916]

[206] Zhou Y, Liu L, Hao Y, Xu M. Detection of Aβ Monomers and Oligomers: Early Diagnosis of Alzheimer's Disease. Chem Asian J 2016; 11(6): 805-17.
[http://dx.doi.org/10.1002/asia.201501355] [PMID: 26994700]

[207] Bruggink KA, Müller M, Kuiperij HB, Verbeek MM. Methods for analysis of amyloid-β aggregates. J Alzheimers Dis 2012; 28(4): 735-58.
[http://dx.doi.org/10.3233/JAD-2011-111421] [PMID: 22156047]

[208] Tai LM, Bilousova T, Jungbauer L, *et al.* Levels of soluble apolipoprotein E/amyloid-β (Aβ) complex are reduced and oligomeric Aβ increased with APOE4 and Alzheimer disease in a transgenic mouse model and human samples. J Biol Chem 2013; 288(8): 5914-26.
[http://dx.doi.org/10.1074/jbc.M112.442103] [PMID: 23293020]

[209] Fukumoto H, Tokuda T, Kasai T, *et al.* High-molecular-weight beta-amyloid oligomers are elevated in cerebrospinal fluid of Alzheimer patients. FASEB J 2010; 24(8): 2716-26.
[http://dx.doi.org/10.1096/fj.09-150359] [PMID: 20339023]

[210] Esparza TJ, Zhao H, Cirrito JR, *et al.* Amyloid-β oligomerization in Alzheimer dementia *versus* high-pathology controls. Ann Neurol 2013; 73(1): 104-19.
[http://dx.doi.org/10.1002/ana.23748] [PMID: 23225543]

[211] Hölttä M, Hansson O, Andreasson U, *et al.* Evaluating amyloid-β oligomers in cerebrospinal fluid as a biomarker for Alzheimer's disease. PLoS One 2013; 8(6)e66381
[http://dx.doi.org/10.1371/journal.pone.0066381] [PMID: 23799095]

[212] Kim JA, Kim M, Kang SM, Lim KT, Kim TS, Kang JY. Magnetic bead droplet immunoassay of oligomer amyloid β for the diagnosis of Alzheimer's disease using micro-pillars to enhance the stability of the oil-water interface. Biosens Bioelectron 2015; 67: 724-32.
[http://dx.doi.org/10.1016/j.bios.2014.10.042] [PMID: 25459055]

[213] Olsson A, Vanderstichele H, Andreasen N, *et al.* Simultaneous measurement of beta-amyloid(1-42), total tau, and phosphorylated tau (Thr181) in cerebrospinal fluid by the xMAP technology. Clin Chem 2005; 51(2): 336-45.
[http://dx.doi.org/10.1373/clinchem.2004.039347] [PMID: 15563479]

[214] Le Bastard N, Coart E, Vanderstichele H, Vanmechelen E, Martin JJ, Engelborghs S. Comparison of two analytical platforms for the clinical qualification of Alzheimer's disease biomarkers in pathologically-confirmed dementia. J Alzheimers Dis 2013; 33(1): 117-31.
[http://dx.doi.org/10.3233/JAD-2012-121246] [PMID: 22936010]

[215] Funke SA. Detection of Soluble Amyloid-β Oligomers and Insoluble High-Molecular-Weight Particles in CSF: Development of Methods with Potential for Diagnosis and Therapy Monitoring of Alzheimer's Disease. Int J Alzheimers Dis 2011; 2011151645
[http://dx.doi.org/10.4061/2011/151645] [PMID: 22114742]

[216] Diehn S, Zimmermann B, Bağcıoğlu M, *et al.* Matrix-assisted laser desorption/ionization time-o--flight mass spectrometry (MALDI-TOF MS) shows adaptation of grass pollen composition. Sci Rep 2018; 8(1): 16591.
[http://dx.doi.org/10.1038/s41598-018-34800-1] [PMID: 30409982]

[217] Pekov S, Indeykina M, Popov I, *et al.* Application of MALDI-TOF/TOF-MS for relative quantitation of α- and β-Asp7 isoforms of amyloid-β peptide. Eur J Mass Spectrom (Chichester) 2018; 24(1): 141-4.
[http://dx.doi.org/10.1177/1469066717730544] [PMID: 29232976]

[218] Trenchevska O, Nelson RW, Nedelkov D. Mass spectrometric immunoassays for discovery, screening and quantification of clinically relevant proteoforms. Bioanalysis 2016; 8(15): 1623-33.
[http://dx.doi.org/10.4155/bio-2016-0060] [PMID: 27396364]

[219] Bros P, *et al.* Quantitative detection of amyloid-β peptides by mass spectrometry: state of the art and clinical applications.Clinical Chemistry and Laboratory Medicine. CCLM 2015; p. 1483.
[http://dx.doi.org/10.1515/cclm-2014-1048]

[220] Hosseini S, Martinez-Chapa SO. Principles and Mechanism of MALDI-ToF-MS Analysis.Fundamentals of MALDI-ToF-MS Analysis: Applications in Bio-diagnosis, Tissue Engineering and Drug Delivery. Singapore: Springer Singapore 2017; pp. 1-19.
[http://dx.doi.org/10.1007/978-981-10-2356-9_1]

[221] Jackson SN, Woods AS. The Development of Matrix-Assisted Laser Desorption Ionization (MALDI) Mass Spectrometry.The Encyclopedia of Mass Spectrometry. Boston: Elsevier 2016; pp. 124-31.
[http://dx.doi.org/10.1016/B978-0-08-043848-1.00015-8]

[222] Anonymous . Proceedings of the American Physical Society. Phys Rev 1946; 69(11-12): 674-702.
[http://dx.doi.org/10.1103/PhysRev.69.674]

[223] Wolff MM, Stephens WE. A Pulsed Mass Spectrometer with Time Dispersion. Rev Sci Instrum 1953; 24(8): 616-7.
[http://dx.doi.org/10.1063/1.1770801]

[224] Wiley WC, McLaren IH. Time☐of☐Flight Mass Spectrometer with Improved Resolution. Rev Sci Instrum 1955; 26(12): 1150-7.
[http://dx.doi.org/10.1063/1.1715212]

[225] O'Connor B. P and F Hillenkamp, MALDI Mass Spectrometry Instrumentation. Weinheim: Wiley-VCH 2007; pp. 29-82.

[226] Satoh T, Tsuno H, Iwanaga M, Kammei Y. The design and characteristic features of a new time-o-

-flight mass spectrometer with a spiral ion trajectory. J Am Soc Mass Spectrom 2005; 16(12): 1969-75.
[http://dx.doi.org/10.1016/j.jasms.2005.08.005] [PMID: 16246577]

[227] Liu R, Li Q, Smith LM. Detection of large ions in time-of-flight mass spectrometry: effects of ion mass and acceleration voltage on microchannel plate detector response. J Am Soc Mass Spectrom 2014; 25(8): 1374-83.
[http://dx.doi.org/10.1007/s13361-014-0903-2] [PMID: 24789774]

[228] Price D. Time-of-Flight Mass Spectrometry 1993.
[http://dx.doi.org/10.1021/bk-1994-0549.ch001]

[229] Boesl U. Time-of-flight mass spectrometry: Introduction to the basics. Mass Spectrom Rev 2017; 36(1): 86-109.
[http://dx.doi.org/10.1002/mas.21520] [PMID: 27859457]

[230] Fania C, Arosio B, Capitanio D, *et al.* Protein signature in cerebrospinal fluid and serum of Alzheimer's disease patients: The case of apolipoprotein A-1 proteoforms. PLoS One 2017; 12(6)e0179280
[http://dx.doi.org/10.1371/journal.pone.0179280] [PMID: 28628634]

[231] Obrocki P, Khatun A, Ness D, *et al.* Perspectives in fluid biomarkers in neurodegeneration from the 2019 biomarkers in neurodegenerative diseases course-a joint PhD student course at University College London and University of Gothenburg. Alzheimers Res Ther 2020; 12(1): 20.
[http://dx.doi.org/10.1186/s13195-020-00586-6] [PMID: 32111242]

[232] Duits FH, Martinez-Lage P, Paquet C, *et al.* Performance and complications of lumbar puncture in memory clinics: Results of the multicenter lumbar puncture feasibility study. Alzheimers Dement 2016; 12(2): 154-63.
[http://dx.doi.org/10.1016/j.jalz.2015.08.003] [PMID: 26368321]

[233] Song F, Poljak A, Valenzuela M, Mayeux R, Smythe GA, Sachdev PS. Meta-analysis of plasma amyloid-β levels in Alzheimer's disease. J Alzheimers Dis 2011; 26(2): 365-75.
[http://dx.doi.org/10.3233/JAD-2011-101977] [PMID: 21709378]

[234] Kim K, Kim MJ, Kim DW, Kim SY, Park S, Park CB. Clinically accurate diagnosis of Alzheimer's disease*via* multiplexed sensing of core biomarkers in human plasma. Nat Commun 2020; 11(1): 119.
[http://dx.doi.org/10.1038/s41467-019-13901-z] [PMID: 31913282]

[235] Greco I, Day N, Riddoch-Contreras J, *et al.* Alzheimer's disease biomarker discovery using in silico literature mining and clinical validation. J Transl Med 2012; 10: 217.
[http://dx.doi.org/10.1186/1479-5876-10-217] [PMID: 23113945]

[236] Yao F, Zhang K, Zhang Y, *et al.* Identification of Blood Biomarkers for Alzheimer's Disease Through Computational Prediction and Experimental Validation. Front Neurol 2019; 9: 1158.
[http://dx.doi.org/10.3389/fneur.2018.01158] [PMID: 30671019]

[237] Yao F, Hong X, Li S, *et al.* Urine-Based Biomarkers for Alzheimer's Disease Identified Through Coupling Computational and Experimental Methods. J Alzheimers Dis 2018; 65(2): 421-31.
[http://dx.doi.org/10.3233/JAD-180261] [PMID: 30040720]

[238] Kennelly S, Collins O. Walking the cognitive "minefield" between high and low blood pressure. J Alzheimers Dis 2012; 32(3): 609-21.
[http://dx.doi.org/10.3233/JAD-2012-120748] [PMID: 22810098]

[239] Ostergaard SD, *et al.* Associations between Potentially Modifiable Risk Factors and Alzheimer Disease: A Mendelian Randomization Study. Eur Neuropsychopharmacol 2017; 27: S166-7.

[240] Insel TR, Landis SC, Collins FS. The NIH BRAIN Initiative. Research priorities. Science 2013; 340(6133): 687-8.
[http://dx.doi.org/10.1126/science.1239276] [PMID: 23661744]

[241] Viceconti M, Hunter P. The Virtual Physiological Human: Ten Years After. Annu Rev Biomed Eng

2016; 18: 103-23.
[http://dx.doi.org/10.1146/annurev-bioeng-110915-114742] [PMID: 27420570]

[242] Vickland V, McDonnell G, Werner J, Draper B, Low LF, Brodaty H. In silico modeling systems: learning about the prevalence and dynamics of dementia through virtual experimentation. Alzheimers Dement 2011; 7(4): e77-83.
[http://dx.doi.org/10.1016/j.jalz.2010.11.011] [PMID: 21784345]

[243] Antila K, Lötjönen J, Thurfjell L, *et al.* The PredictAD project: development of novel biomarkers and analysis software for early diagnosis of the Alzheimer's disease. Interface Focus 2013; 3(2)20120072
[http://dx.doi.org/10.1098/rsfs.2012.0072] [PMID: 24427524]

[244] Mattila J, Soininen H, Koikkalainen J, *et al.* Optimizing the diagnosis of early Alzheimer's disease in mild cognitive impairment subjects. J Alzheimers Dis 2012; 32(4): 969-79.
[http://dx.doi.org/10.3233/JAD-2012-120934] [PMID: 22890102]

[245] Mattila J, Koikkalainen J, Virkki A, *et al.* Alzheimer's Disease Neuroimaging Initiative. A disease state fingerprint for evaluation of Alzheimer's disease. J Alzheimers Dis 2011; 27(1): 163-76.
[http://dx.doi.org/10.3233/JAD-2011-110365] [PMID: 21799247]

Frontiers in Nanobiotechnology, 2020, *Vol. 1*, 387-435 **387**

CHAPTER 10

Diagnostics for Neurodegenerative Disorders

Wen-Wei Tseng[1], Ching-Hua Lu[2,3], Zih-Hua Chen[1], Yu-De Lin[1], Ko-Hong Lin[1], Yi-Chia Wei[4] and An-Chi Wei[1,*]

[1] Graduate Institute of Biomedical Electronics and Bioinformatics, National Taiwan University, Taipei, Taiwan

[2] Department of Neurology, China Medical University Hospital, Taiwan

[3] School of Medicine, China Medical University, Taiwan

[4] Department of Neurology, Keelung Chang Gung Memorial Hospital, and Chang Gung University College of Medicine, Keelung, Taiwan

Abstract: Neurodegenerative diseases (NDDs) stem from the loss of neurons and related progressive disruption of psychological, cognitive, and motor functions. The development of NDDs results from either disruption or dysfunction of normal nervous tissues or the accumulation of pathologically altered proteins in the brain. Traditionally, the diagnoses are based on clinical presentations, with limited sensitivity for early diagnosis and specificity for differential diagnosis. However, advancements in the research of biomarkers and biosensing techniques have led to additional promising strategies for the molecular diagnosis of NDDs.

In this chapter, we have reviewed the clinical features, diagnostic criteria and known genetic and protein biomarkers of common NDDs. We have also discussed the importance of bioenergetics in the development of NDDs. Finally, we have placed emphasis on current developments in the detection and diagnosis of NDDs, including neuroimaging, metabolome profiling, and biosensors for NDD biomarkers. Biosensing provides a noninvasive way to diagnose NDDs at an early stage to detect alterations and abnormal products in the blood and brain tissues with high sensitivity and selectivity. This chapter is expected to provide an overview of the recent advances in diagnosing NDDs, as well as pointing out the current progress and challenges in the evaluation and treatment of NDDs and beyond.

Keywords: Biomarkers, Biosensing, Neurodegenerative diseases.

INTRODUCTION TO NEURODEGENERATIVE DISEASES

Neurodegenerative diseases (NDDs) stem from the loss of neurons and related progressive disruption of psychological, cognitive, and motor functions [1, 2].

* **Corresponding author An-Chi Wei:** Graduate Institute of Biomedical Electronics and Bioinformatics, National Taiwan University, Taipei, Taiwan; E-mail: acwei86@ntu.edu.tw

Han-Sheng Chuang & Yi-Ping Ho (Eds.)
All rights reserved-© 2020 Bentham Science Publishers

These disorders are traditionally detected and diagnosed by their clinical features (Fig. 1). Based on detailed medical and family histories, neurological examinations and cognitive tests, medical professionals can identify and differentiate various types of NDDs and their mimics. However, the pathophysiology of NDDs involves an interplay among genetic mutations, abnormal processing of misfolded proteins, neuroinflammation, increased oxidative stress, mitochondrial dysfunction, and other mechanisms [3 - 5]. Understanding these underlying mechanisms could lead to the development of novel methods for the diagnosis of NDDs, even before the onset of symptoms, which may be beneficial to research related to the prevention, intervention, and treatment of NDDs.

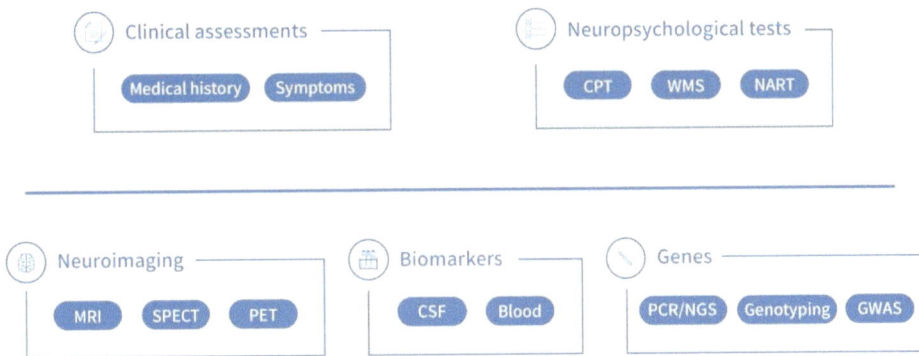

Fig. (1). Diagnosis of neurodegenerative diseases. Multiple aspects from the clinical assessments, neurophysiological tests, neuroimaging, biomarker detection, and gene mutation tests are combined to diagnose neurodegenerative diseases. CPT, continuous performance task; CSF, cerebrospinal fluid; GWAS, genome-wide association studies; IMR, immunomagnetic reduction; MRI, magnetic resonance imaging; NART, National Adult Reading Test; PET, positron emission tomography; NGS, next-generation sequencing; SPECT, single photon emission computerized tomography; WMS, Wechsler Memory Scale.

In this chapter, we focus on the following four most common NDDs: Alzheimer's disease (AD), Parkinson's disease (PD), Huntington's disease (HD), and amyotrophic lateral sclerosis (ALS). The clinical aspects, the proteinopathy and metabolism and the known and potential biomarkers for the diagnosis of these four NDDs are reviewed. Finally, we introduce the technologies utilized in biosensors to detect these biomarkers.

CLINICAL ASPECTS OF NEURODEGENERATIVE DISEASES

Alzheimer's Disease

AD is a chronic progressive neurodegenerative disorder characterized by the following three primary groups of symptoms: cognitive dysfunction, psychobehavioral disturbances, and difficulties in daily activities [6, 7]. Cognitive dysfunction includes memory loss, language difficulties, such as difficulties in finding words, and executive dysfunction, such as difficulties in planning. Psychobehavioral disturbances include depression, hallucinations, delusions, and agitation. Finally, patients with AD experience difficulties in performing daily activities ranging from complex activities, such as driving and shopping, to simple activities, such as dressing and eating unaided [6].

AD is also characterized by its insidious onset and gradual progression, representing a continuum from normal aging to symptomatic AD rather than a well-defined illness [8]. Thus, distinguishing between normal aging and the early preclinical stage of AD based solely on symptoms and cognitive tests is challenging. The accuracy of the clinical diagnosis of AD is approximately 70-90% during the middle and late stages of AD [9]. AD slowly progresses from the preclinical stage, which is characterized by proteinopathy signs without clinical symptoms, to mild cognitive impairment (MCI) within approximately a decade. The conversion from MCI to bedbound, very severe AD occurs within approximately 8-9 years (Fig. **2**) [10].

The most accepted criteria for the diagnosis of AD are the National Institutes of Aging and Alzheimer's Association (NIA-AA) criteria proposed by the Alzheimer's Disease and Related Disorders Association (ADRDA) workgroup in 2011 [11, 12]. The NIA-AA criteria define asymptomatic status, MCI, and dementia based on clinical symptoms of cognitive and neuropsychiatric disorders; furthermore, these criteria describe probable, possible, and other differential diagnoses by tracing disease progression (insidious onset or not) and excluding secondary causes (*e.g.*, delirium) and mimics (*e.g.*, dementia with Lewy bodies). At the time these criteria were developed, biomarkers were used in a complementary manner to increase confidence in the clinical diagnosis. Recently, however, the trend has shifted to the use of biomarkers for an independent molecular diagnosis of AD using the so-called **ATN** system [13, 14]. It was suggested by the NIA-AA that the AD continuum classification system should be based on biomarkers rather than clinical symptoms. This biomarker classification, the ATN system, binarizes three biomarker outcomes as positive or negative: the presence of amyloid-beta (Aβ) biomarkers (designated **A**), tau biomarkers (designated **T**), and neurodegeneration or neuronal injury (designated **N**). Aβ biomarkers can typically be detected using amyloid positron emission tomography (PET) and cerebrospinal fluid (CSF) Aβ42; tau biomarkers can typically be detected using CSF p-tau or tau PET; and neurodegenerative biomarkers can typically be detected using CSF total tau (t-tau), structural magnetic resonance imaging (MRI) or [18F]-fluorodeoxyglucose (FDG) PET in the clinical setting [8, 14].

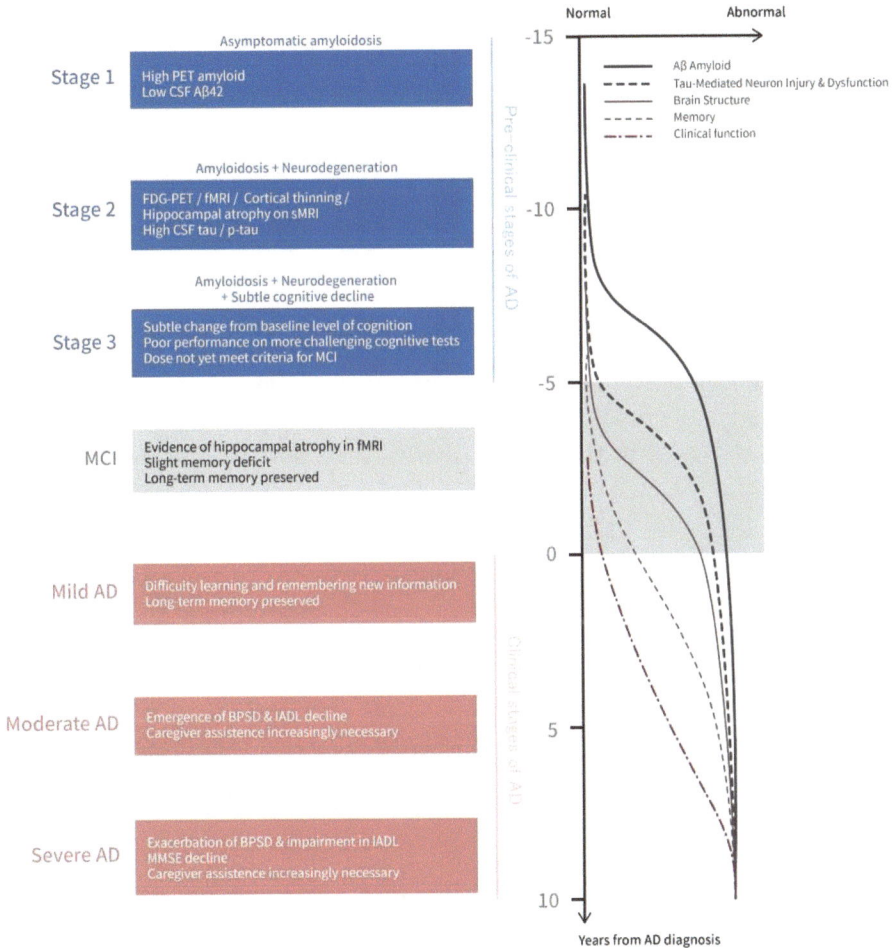

Fig. (2). Progression of Alzheimer's disease (AD) from NC (normal cognition) to MCI (mild cognitive impairment) and AD. Temporal changes in AD core biomarkers are correlated with the progression of AD along the cognitive continuum from healthy to dementia. BPSD, behavioral and psychological symptoms of dementia; IADL, instrumental activities of daily living; ADL, activities of daily living; MMSE, Mini-Mental Status Examination. This figure was adapted from Trojanowski *et al.* and other related papers [15 - 18].

Pathologically, amyloidosis induces or facilitates the spread of pathological tau, and tauopathy is a proximate cause of neurodegeneration. Therefore, the logical biomarker sequence of AD could be A+T-N-, followed by A+T+N- and A+T+N+. For example, a person who is Aβ positive (A+) might be diagnosed with AD continuum. A person who is A+ but T- might be diagnosed with Alzheimer's pathological change. A person who is A+ and T+ might be diagnosed with AD. However, some arguments state that the ATN system may be an oversimplified system and may need to extend its consideration of other pathological factors, such as neuroinflammation, vascular small vessel disease, and Lewy body pathology [19]. Sabbagh and coworkers [20] proposed a stepwise approach, including informant-based questionnaires, risk factor analysis, bedside cognitive screening, physical and neurologic examinations, and laboratory screening tests, as well as the immunomagnetic reduction (IMR) assay to analyze the levels of plasma tau and beta-amyloid 42 (Aβ42), to distinguish AD from clinically similar conditions such as Lewy body disease (LBD) and frontotemporal degeneration (FTD).

Parkinson's Disease

PD is characterized by both motor and nonmotor symptoms. The motor symptoms are best described as TRAP, essentially as follows: 4-6 Hz Tremor at rest, Rigidity of muscles, Akinesia (or bradykinesia), and Postural instability. In addition, a unilateral onset, flexed posture, freezing (motor blocks), and response to levodopa are significant signs and symptoms of PD [5].

The stages of Parkinson's disease arise from pathology in particular structures within the nervous system; Braak *et al.* [21] proposed that the clinical manifestations range from nonmotor symptoms in the early stages to motor symptoms in the middle stages and cognitive symptoms in the final Braak stages. Nonmotor dysfunctions in PD are recognized less than motor dysfunctions but can also significantly affect patients' lives. These nonmotor symptoms include autonomic, cognitive, behavioral, sleep, and sensory dysfunctions. Autonomic dysfunctions include constipation, orthostatic hypotension, abnormal sweating, sphincter dysfunction, and erectile dysfunction. The cognitive and behavioral dysfunctions include depression, apathy, anxiety, hallucinations, and obsessive-compulsive and impulsive behavior (*e.g.*, craving for sweets). Rapid eye movement sleep behavioral disorder (REM SBD) involves violent dream content accompanied by talking, yelling, swearing, grabbing, punching, kicking, and/or jumping. The sensory abnormalities include olfactory dysfunction (hyposmia), pain, paresthesia, akathisia, oral pain, and genital pain [5, 22].

PD is currently diagnosed entirely by clinical criteria, such as the most popular criteria by the UK Parkinson's Disease Society Brain Bank (UKPDSBB) in 1988 [5, 22]. The UKPDSBB criteria emphasize bradykinesia as a core feature of PD with the inclusion of supporting features and exclusion of differential diagnoses and mimics, such as dementia with Lewy bodies (DLB). To assess disability and impairment among people with PD, the Unified Parkinson's Disease Rating Scale (UPDRS) is the most well-established scale [23 - 25].

Huntington's Disease

HD is characterized by progressive motor, behavioral, and cognitive disorders [26]. Motor disorders include chorea, abnormal saccadic eye movement, dystonia, and Parkinsonism-like bradykinesia and progress to life-threatening injuries ranging from falls to aspiration and dysphagia [27].

Dementia is a less noted component of HD, but the impairment inflicted is no less than the motor dysfunctions. Dementia in patients with HD is largely subcortical and characterized by slow thought processes, executive dysfunction, inattention and difficulties in sequencing, but the memory impairment is less severe than the dementia associated with AD. The psychological problems experienced by HD patients include anxiety, apathy, delusion, hallucinations, depression, obsessive-compulsive behaviors, irritability, and outbursts.

HD is diagnosed both clinically and genetically [27]. The motor symptoms are stratified according to the "Diagnostic Confidence Level" (DCL) of the Unified Huntington's Disease Rating Scale (UHDRS) and range from asymptomatic (score of 0) to unequivocal signs of HD (score of 4). Genetically, HD is an autosomal dominant inherited disease associated with excessive CAG trinucleotide repeats in the huntingtin gene (*HTT*) on chromosome 4 [26]. The longer the repeat, the earlier the age at onset. Because the diagnosis of HD is relatively straightforward and DNA sequencing methods to detect CAG repeats are relatively mature, we refrain from a discussion of the biosensors used for the diagnosis of HD.

Amyotrophic Lateral Sclerosis

ALS is characterized by the progressive loss of upper and lower motor neurons and is associated with muscle weakness and atrophy [28]. The symptoms eventually progress to paralysis and lethal respiratory failure with a median survival of 2-3 years. There are several subtypes of ALS with different clinical presentations and prognoses. Among these subtypes, primary bulbar palsy is associated with the worst survival due to swallowing difficulty. In contrast, symmetrical weakness of the limbs (flail arm or flail leg) has the best prognosis.

The diagnosis of ALS is based on clinical symptoms, electrophysiological studies, and exclusion of differential diagnosis. The El Escorial criteria for ALS [27] define the signs of lower and upper motor neuron degeneration and disease spread. The Awaji criteria are useful for the early diagnosis of ALS patients with bulbar onset disease and are important for arranging palliative measures, such as gastrostomy for swallowing difficulty.

Nonmotor symptoms are also present in ALS. Frontotemporal cognitive impairment can be observed in 30~50% of patients. Advanced tools, such as the Edinburgh Cognitive and Behavioural ALS Screen (ECAS) [28, 29], are useful for detecting these symptoms.

Mutations in more than 25 genes are associated with ALS [28]. Among the familial cases of ALS (fALS), approximately 70% are from the mutated genes of superoxide dismutase 1 (*SOD1*), TAR DNA-binding protein 43 (*TARDBP*; TDP-43), FUS RNA binding protein (*FUS*), and chromosome 9 open reading frame 72 (*C9orf72*) [28]. A mutation in the *C9orf72* gene is the most frequent cause of ALS, accounting for approximately 40% of familial and approximately 7% of sporadic ALS cases [30], and consists of an expansion of a GGGGCC (G4C2) hexanucleotide repeat between the noncoding exons 1a and 1b [31, 32]. In addition to diagnosis, the hexanucleotide GGGGCC(G4C2) repeat expansion in the *C9orf72* gene has prompted the development of a treatment based on antisense oligonucleotides, small molecules and genetic modifiers that target *C9orf72* repeat RNA [33]. The RNA product transcribed by a mutant *C9orf72* gene is translated to dipeptides, called dipeptide repeat proteins (DPRs), by repeat-associated non-ATG translation. Five polypeptides, poly(GA), poly(GR), poly(GP), poly(PR), and poly(PA), are produced by using the open reading frame from both directions. Poly(GP) has been shown to be a potential pharmacodynamic biomarker for C9FTD/ALS [34].

In addition to genetic mutations, other genetic variations represent a substantial proportion of ALS genetic research. With the advent of high-throughput DNA sequencing, global projects, such as Project MinE, have been launched to unveil the genetic differences between ALS patients and controls [35, 36].

With the increasing understanding of the functions of genes related to ALS, it has become clear that these genes can be stratified into three major groups: RNA metabolism, cytoskeletal dynamics, and protein homeostasis. Dysregulation in one subgroup of genes may lead to serious consequences in other domains. For example, perturbations in RNA metabolism may increase cellular stress with respect to proteostasis (mechanisms include autophagy, increased ER stress, lysosomal dysfunction, and the formation of protein aggregates), which may result in the formation of toxic cytoplasmic aggregates and further interrupt cytoskeletal dynamics in the delivery of important signals and nutrients to distal cellular compartments [37].

The key pathological hallmark of ALS is the deposition of proteins into ubiquitinated cytoplasmic inclusions, which are immunoreactive for either SOD1 [38], TDP-43 [39] or FUS [40]. As the majority (97% of cases), TDP-43 aggregates can be formed from both sporadic ALS and TDP-43 mutated fALS or as a downstream consequence of other mutations (*e.g.*, C9orf72), while SOD1 (2%) and FUS (1%) aggregation is contributed to by mutations in cognate genes [37]. Furthermore, these pathological features spread between cells to the conjunct body parts, consistent with the clinical propagation of symptoms; hence, as in PD and AD, it has been suggested that prion-like spread of protein misfolding and aggregates is a key mechanism in neurodegenerative disease pathobiology [41].

BIOENERGETIC ASPECTS OF NEURODEGENERATIVE DISEASES

Neurons constantly consume energy to pump ions and maintain their membrane potentials for electrophysiological excitability, as well as to release and recycle neurotransmitters at the synapse [42]. Cellular energy credit is primarily provided in the form of adenosine triphosphate (ATP), which is mostly synthesized in the mitochondria, *i.e.*, the powerhouse of cells, through oxidative phosphorylation (OXPHOS) [43]. Mitochondria are double-membrane bound organelles that are hypothesized to have originated from endosymbiosis, a process in which a eukaryotic cell incorporates a free-living aerobic prokaryote. The outer mitochondrial membrane (OMM) separates the cytosol and the intermembrane space (IMS) compartments. Small molecules such as ions, ATP, creatine, and various metabolites are allowed to freely pass through the porins on the OMM, whereas the trafficking of larger molecules such as proteins and long-chain fatty acids is restricted. The inner mitochondrial membrane (IMM) separates the mitochondrial matrix and the IMS into two compartments. The IMM comprises inward-folded structures called cristae that increase the surface-to-volume ratio for the membrane-bound respiratory complexes, which consist of the electron transport chain (ETC) and ATP synthase. The ETC is a redox pipeline that consumes hydrogen equivalents in the form of NADH or $FADH_2$ from catabolic processes such as glycolysis, lipid oxidation, and the citric acid cycle and transfers the electron in a step-by-step manner to oxygen molecules to form water. The free energy released by this redox process is utilized to pump hydrogen ions (protons) out of the matrix and into the intermembrane space, generating both electrical and concentration gradients called the proton motive force (PMF). In this process, ATP synthase acts as a turbo generator, converting the energy from the inward proton flux driven by the PMF to synthesize ATP from ADP and inorganic phosphate (Pi). The process of converting metabolites and oxygen to generate ATP is called OXPHOS, which is much more efficient than other means used to produce ATP. For instance, the catabolism of one glucose molecule can generate 2 ATP molecules through oxygen-independent glycolysis, whereas approximately 30 ATP molecules can be generated via OXPHOS. In addition to ATP production and metabolism, mitochondria participate in several key cellular physiological functions, such as calcium homeostasis, cell survival, apoptosis, and cellular signaling [44]. For instance, mitochondria play a crucial role in cellular calcium hemostasis due to their close proximity to the endoplasmic reticulum (ER), the reservoir for calcium, at specific sites named mitochondria-associated membranes (MAMs) [45]. Calcium ions enter the mitochondria via ion channels in the IMM, primarily through the mitochondrial calcium uniporter (MCU), which is driven by the mitochondrial membrane potential across the IMM. Calcium ions physiologically facilitate the citric acid cycle and OXPHOS, increasing ATP output from the mitochondria. Calcium ions can be transported back to the cytosol via a sodium-calcium-lithium exchanger (NCLX, also called mitochondrial sodium-calcium exchanger), involving the influx of three sodium ions in exchange for the efflux of one calcium ion. However, pathological calcium dynamics may lead to calcium overload in the mitochondria, encouraging the prolonged opening of mitochondrial permeability transition pore (mPTP), a non-selective channel in the IMM, causing the loss of mitochondrial membrane potential and the production of ATP, ultimately leading to cell death [45]. Mitochondria are also dynamic organelles that constantly undergo fission, fusion, biogenesis, mitophagy, and trafficking across the cell. These processes are vital to maintaining their shape, distribution, and quality [43]. Mitochondrial dysfunction plays an important role in the pathogenesis of NDDs [44]. Genetic mutations in mitochondria-related proteins, such as Parkin, PINK1, DJ-1, α-synuclein, LRRK2, and SOD1 have been linked to mitochondrial biogenesis, mitochondrial transport, mitochondrial turnover, dynamics, and respiration (Fig. 3), and these mutations may disrupt normal mitochondrial function and could eventually lead to energy failure and neuronal death [46, 47]. Impaired mitochondrial function not only reduces the production of ATP and results in energy deficiency but also increases the production of mitochondria-derived reactive oxygen species (mtROS), causing excessive oxidative stress and detrimental effects on biomolecules, such as lipids, protein, and DNA, as well as on mitochondrial signaling and calcium homeostasis [46]. The destruction of mitochondrial DNA (mtDNA) further exacerbates the overproduction of mtROS, the deficiency of ATP, and the altered calcium homeostasis, causing a vicious cycle and ultimately leading to neuron dysfunction and death [48]. In major NDDs, such as AD, PD, HD, and ALS, excessive levels of ROS and genetic defects related to mitochondrial functions and dynamics have been observed in some hereditary forms of NDDs [49].

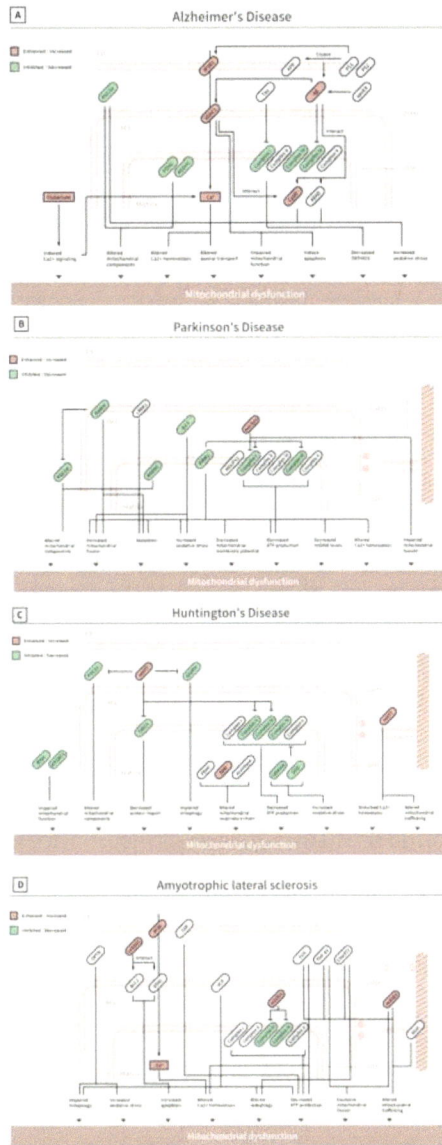

Fig. (3). The molecular mechanism through which mitochondrial dysfunction mediates the pathophysiology of neurodegenerative disorders. Proteinopathies are related to mitochondrial dysfunction. Proteins observed to be altered or aggregated are present in the mitochondrial membrane and matrix in neurons. Abnormal mitochondrial transport machinery, mitochondrial bioenergetics, ROS production, and calcium regulation are also related to NDDs. NDDs have been linked to impairment in mitochondrial respiratory chain complex activity by increasing the expression of hyperphosphorylated tau and Aβ plaques, mα-synuclein, mHTT, and mSOD. The combined mitochondrial complex deficiencies caused by the increases in the expression levels of the related proteins result in a feedforward accumulation of aggregated/misfolded proteins through inhibited proteasome activity observed in NDD patients. **(A)** In AD, APP or Aβ is present in mitochondrial membranes and the matrix of neurons. Amyloid proteins enter mitochondria and interact with other proteins to induce free radicals, decrease cytochrome oxidase activity, and inhibit ATP production. The N-terminus of ApoE4 causes mitochondrial oxidative damage. Presenilin (PS) mutants exhibit altered intracellular Ca^{2+} homeostasis through inositol trisphosphate receptors (IP3R) that may lead to mitochondrial dysfunction and neuronal death. Mutations in presenilin 1 (PS1) affect mitochondrial axonal transport by affecting the ability of GSK3β to phosphorylate the kinesin light chain. Peroxisome proliferator-activated receptor gamma coactivator 1-alpha (PGC-1α; a master regulator of mitochondrial biogenesis) is downregulated in AD patients, as are the enzyme activities of pyruvate dehydrogenase complex (PDHC) and α-ketoglutarate dehydrogenase complex (KGDHC) in the tricarboxylic acid cycle (TCA). **(B)** In PD, α-synuclein in mitochondrial membranes can cause mitochondrial dysfunction. PINK 1 and Parkin participate in mitochondrial dynamics regulation. PINK1 is a nuclear-encoded, mitochondrial kinase protein, and the overexpression of PINK1 causes reduced mitochondrial membrane potential. Parkin, which is a mitochondrial outer membrane protein and a gene product of ubiquitin E3 ligase, induces free radical production. Protein deglycase DJ-1 is located in the mitochondrial intermembrane space, and the matrix is a sensor of oxidative stress. LRRK2, which is associated with the outer mitochondrial membrane, regulates mitochondrial trafficking, and is involved in inducing free radical production. **(C)** In HD, mutant huntingtin binds to the outer mitochondrial membrane that induces free radical production, affects calcium uptake, alters PGC1α activity, inhibits mitochondrial protein import through TIM23, and impedes GAPDH-mediated mitophagy. Mitochondrial trafficking in axons is also interrupted. Defects in the enzymes pyruvate dehydrogenase complex (PDHC), aconitase and succinate dehydrogenase (SDH) as well as impaired Rhes/mTORC1 metabolic signaling pathway activity have been reported in HD patients. **(D)** In ALS, mutant superoxide dismutase 1 (SOD1) aggregates are present in the outer mitochondrial membrane, the inner mitochondrial membrane space, and the matrix. SOD1 is a cytosolic ROS scavenging enzyme, and mutant SOD1 induces free radicals and mitochondrial dysfunction in ALS patients. Mutant SOD1, TDP-43, SigR1, VAPB and FUS are associated with disruptions in ER-mitochondrial interactions, calcium homeostasis, mitochondrial respiration and quality control in ALS [75]. This figure was adapted from Schon *et al.* [76] and Jha *et al.* [58].

Furthermore, in NDD pathogenesis, dysfunctional proteins and mitochondria could reinforce each other, creating a vicious cycle of neurodegeneration [50]. For example, in AD, toxic Aβ oligomers and phosphorylated tau protein (p-tau) contribute to the disruption of mitochondrial fission and fusion, and increased mtROS production by impaired mitochondria triggers more APP proteolysis and more Aβ oligomers as a result.

Oxidative stress has been implicated in the progression of several NDDs [51]. Several NDD-related proteins located in the mitochondrial inner or outer membrane have been reported to participate in ROS production. Trans-4-hydro-y-2-nonenal (4-HNE) and malondialdehyde (MDA), which are products of lipid peroxidation, are the most investigated biomarkers related to oxidative stress; however, the ability to reliably measure their plasma levels and their validity and accuracy still needs more research [52, 53].

Mitochondrial bioenergetics and metabolism are components of the metabolic network. Neurometabolic alterations and metabolic reprogramming are expected phenotypes in NDDs [54]. Glucose is the predominant source of energy in the brain. However, glucose hypometabolism has been observed in presymptomatic AD patients, indicating that energy-deprived neurons and metabolic dysfunction contribute to AD development, as detected by fluorodeoxyglucose PET and metabolomics approaches such as mass spectrometry and nuclear magnetic resonance platforms [55]. In addition, emerging evidence suggests that lipid and glucose metabolism modulates β-amyloid, tau, and neurodegeneration during the pathogenesis of AD. For example, diabetes is associated with reduced volumes of the hippocampus, gray matter, and white matter. In addition, ApoE, the strongest genetic risk factor for AD, as well as other risk genes revealed by GWAS (BIN1, CLU, ABCA7, TREM2, and PICALM), modulates lipid metabolism. Moreover, high levels of low-density cholesterol (LDL) and/or low levels of high-density cholesterol (HDL) are associated with higher amyloid content, which can be reduced by statins (LDL-lowering medication) in an experimental setting. Furthermore, impaired glucose or cholesterol metabolism is related to the hyperphosphorylation of tau protein, which is associated with the formation of neurofibrillary tangles (NFTs) [56]. Metabolic syndrome is also interlinked with the pathophysiology of neurodegenerative disorders [57 - 59]. For example, reduced glucose and pyruvate metabolism have been reported in AD and PD, and both have been linked to type 2 diabetes mellitus (T2DM) [60].

Metabolites are small molecules formed from the intermediate end products of metabolism. The sum of all metabolites comprises the metabolome, and the human metabolome consists of more than 100,000 metabolites [61]. Metabolomic methodologies have been developed to study potential perturbations in biochemical pathways linked to neurodegeneration and are widely used to investigate NDDs [62, 63]. Recent research has shown that uric acid, choline, creatine, L-glutamine, alanine, creatinine, and N-acetyl-L-aspartate are shared metabolite signatures among AD, PD and ALS and that alanine, aspartate, glutamate, and purine metabolism might provide alternative metabolic pathways to compensate for the altered glucose metabolism in neurodegeneration [64]. Several metabolomic studies have attempted to identify metabolic biomarkers for NDDs [55, 65, 66]. However, although promising and powerful metabolic biomarkers have been identified, they have not been validated for clinical use.

Nuclear magnetic resonance (NMR) spectroscopy and mass spectrometry (MS) are two primary platforms typically used for metabolic profiling. NMR spectroscopy is a technique used by scientists to investigate compound structures and dynamics. This technique can also be used to quantify all compounds in biological samples. This nondestructive technique has the advantages of high reproducibility and low processing time over MS-based approaches [67]. Several studies using (1)H NMR reveal abnormal serum or CSF metabolite patterns in NDD patients and model animals [68 - 71].

MS-based approaches rely on highly sensitive and broad spectrum equipment capable of analyzing a large number of compounds in biological samples and, therefore, have become widely used techniques in metabolomics studies [72]. MS uses the mass to charge (m/z) ratio to identify small molecules. A mass spectrometer, which comprises an ion source, analyzer, and detector system, ionizes the samples, separates the ionized molecules by their mass to charge ratio and determines the relative abundance of these molecules. In addition to direct injection, a mass spectrum of a sample is typically generated in tandem with sample separation techniques, such as liquid or gas chromatography (LC or GC, respectively) or capillary electrophoresis/electrospray ionization. LC-MS consists of high-performance liquid chromatography (HPLC) and MS. This approach is typically applied to samples that cannot endure high temperatures. Several metabolomic studies investigating NDDs were successfully conducted using LC-MS [73]. In GC–MS, the combination of gas chromatography and MS is primarily used to detect and quantify amino acids, lipids, organic acids, sugars, and amines. Although this method is characterized by its high reproducibility, sensitivity, and resolution, sample processing is more difficult than other methods.

Capillary electrophoresis (CE) is another MS-based method and a powerful tool used to separate charged metabolites. The advantages of using CE-MS include the following: (1) fewer required samples, (2) higher resolution and (3) reduced matrix effect. Due to its high performance in detecting organic acids, amino acids, nucleotides, and saccharides, CE-MS is a good metabolomic technique. For example. An untargeted metabolomics approach based on CE-MS has been used to study metabolic differences in CSF samples from AD subjects with different cognitive statuses [74].

NEUROIMAGING OF NEURODEGENERATIVE DISEASES

In addition to biotransducers, neuroimaging is another common method used to detect biomarkers for NDDs [77, 78]. Various neuroimaging techniques play an important role in the early and relative noninvasive diagnosis of NDDs. For example, structural changes, such as atrophy in certain brain regions, are diagnostic of different types of NDDs. Furthermore, glucose metabolism, which is an indicator of energy expenditure, could be measured via fluorodeoxyglucose (FDG)-labeled PET. Moreover, the advent of selective radioligands has enabled the *in vivo* detection of biochemical biomarkers, such as protein aggregates and dopamine transporters, aiding in the early detection and diagnosis of NDDs [9].

Alzheimer's Disease

Regarding AD, Pittsburgh compound B (PiB) is the first selective PET ligand for detecting Aβ deposits, differentiating AD patients from cognitively unimpaired subjects predicting MCI-to-AD conversion and even identifying cognitively normal people with a high risk of AD. However, due to the short half-life of PiB (20 minutes), it is available only at medical centers with cyclotrons. An alternative to PiB with similar biochemical properties is [18F]-flutemetamol, which has a longer half-life (110 minutes). Other compounds targeting Aβ deposits, such as [18F]-florbetapir, [18F]-AV-45, and Amyvid ([18F]-florbetapir injection), are under active investigation. However, the topographical distribution of amyloid deposition is not relevant to clinical symptoms. The topographical-clinical mismatch of amyloid PET is especially observed in atypical AD, such as the frontal variant, posterior cortical atrophy (PCA), corticobasal syndrome (CBS) and logopenic variant of primary progressive aphasia (lvPPA) subtypes. Therefore, tracers that bind to hyperphosphorylated paired helical filament (PHF) tau were developed to increase the clinical value of PET in diagnosing AD. The tracers currently under development are classified as quinolone derivatives, benzothiazole derivatives, and benzimidazole pyrimidines. The clinical utility of these tracers remains under investigation [79, 80].

Glucose metabolism is reduced in the parietotemporal cortex in AD patients, as detected by [18F]-FDG-PET [77, 78]. Structural MRI shows atrophy in the hippocampal and entorhinal cortex in AD patients. Dementia mimicking AD can be differentiated by neuroimaging. In frontotemporal dementia (FTD), structural MRI and FDG-PET show atrophy and hypometabolism in the frontal lobe and temporal lobe, respectively. Given the pathological tauopathy of FTD, PET imaging of abnormal tau also helps to identify FTD. Abnormal dopamine transporter imaging can differentiate AD from DLB and PDD. In DLB, DaTscan, which is a technique used to detect dopamine transporters, shows a reduced quantity of these transporters, similar to what can be observed in PD. Assessments of functional connectivity and white matter integrity by functional MR imaging and diffusion tensor imaging, respectively, can also be used to evaluate the functional and structural perturbations caused by pathological processes in AD.

Parkinson's Disease

Regarding PD, dopamine transporter (DAT) single-photon emission computerized tomography (SPECT) is approved by the Food and Drug Administration (FDA) to evaluate suspected PD. Transcranial sonography (TCS) shows increased signal intensity (hyperechogenicity) in the substantia nigra of PD patients. Other technologies, such as PET ligands for PD and diffusion imaging in MRI, are under investigation [77]. For example, [18F]9-fluoropropyl-(+)-dihydrotet-rabenazine (18F-(+)DTBZ), also known as 18F-AV-133, is a novel tracer for vesicular monoamine transporter type 2 (VMAT2) imaging to evaluate the integrity of the dopaminergic system; this tracer has the advantages of high sensitivity and a long half-life [81, 82].

Huntington's Disease

Structural MRI and PET studies have been robustly explored in HD. Two large prospective multisite studies, TRACK-HD and PREDICT-HD, reported strong associations between striatal atrophy/volume and measures of both motor and cognitive impairment as well as estimated time to symptomatic onset and disease burden [83]. A number of molecular targets have been explored in HD. For instance, targeting PDE10A (phosphodiesterase 10A), which plays an important role in modulating the activity of the direct and indirect striatal pathways, using [^{11}C]IMA107 PET can show the earliest changes in PreHD, prior to striatal atrophy detected from structural MRI, suggesting its potential role in prognostic onset of symptoms and monitoring disease progression [84].

NEUROPHYSIOLOGY OF NEURODEGENERATIVE DISORDERS

Emerging evidence indicates that the pathogenesis of neurodegeneration is related to widespread and progressive changes in brain networking, which could be in structural (focal and tract neural degeneration) and functional (brain connectivity, neural and neuromotor transmission) terms. While brain MRI and PET scans have improved our understanding of the pathogenesis and spreading during progression in these neurodegenerative disorders, applying advanced quantitative electroencephalography and magnetoencephalography (qEEG/MEG) and transcranial magnetic stimulation (TMS) can help capture abnormal neural transmissions and networking associated with clinical symptoms [85].

EEG can capture activity in cortical sources oriented both tangentially and radially to the scalp surface as a result of electric field propagation and electrical conduction in the volume. MEG signals are captured exclusively by cortical sources oriented tangentially to the scalp surface, which are not affected by the propagation of electric currents through head tissues with different resistance [86]. EEG/MEG signals reflect the spatial summation of relatively long-lasting (ten to hundreds of milliseconds) excitatory/inhibitory postsynaptic potentials and dendritic influences of neurons (*e.g.*, cortical pyramidal neurons), summed together in adjacent regions [87], and in longer-range pathways. (*e.g.*, thalamo-cortical connections and loops) [88, 89]. Moreover, it has also been shown that the fast spiking activity of cortical neurons may also appear at higher EEG/MEG frequencies in the high gamma band (>40 Hz) [90]. The recording could be divided into resting-state and event-related. With the advanced techniques of careful application of blind source separation, independent component analysis, nonparametric statistics [91] and cortical source localization methods [92], the level of noise and artifacts in the EEG/MEG signals have been dramatically reduced and hence may increase the sensitivity of the changes due to disease progression.

TMS, by delivering magnetic stimuli to the motor cortex, invokes muscle responses (motor evoked potentials; MEP), is a non-invasive method of brain stimulation. Primarily originating from the activation of the upper motor neurons and related cortical interneurons, the descending pathways activate spinal cord networks, including lower motor neurons' connections to associated muscles. Therefore, MEPs can provide information about the integrity of the corticospinal tract, quantified by motor threshold (the minimum stimulation intensity required to achieve a target MEP amplitude). This technology has already been commercialized for use in diagnostics and clinical outcome measures for neuromuscular disorders [93].

TMS can provide single-pulse measures, paired-pulse measures, dual-coil paired pulse measures, afferent inhibition measures and threshold tracking. The use of precisely timed 'conditioning' magnetic or electrical pulses can activate network components such as interneurons [94 - 97], while conditioning sub- and supra-threshold stimuli over non-primary motor areas, such as the supplementary motor areas, premotor cortices, dorsolateral prefrontal or posterior parietal regions, can reveal the connectivity of these regions to the primary motor cortices and the other brain areas [98].

Alzheimer's Disease

Candidate biomarkers of AD (at clinical (dementia) or prodromal (mild cognitive impairment: MCI) stages) have been generated using frequency domain spectral analysis from eyes-closed resting state (rs) EEG/MEG [99]. RS cortical delta and alpha rhythms in particular reveal compromised network synchronization and connectivity in AD at both group and individual levels [100, 101], by reduced posterior cortical alpha (8–12 Hz) and beta (13–30 Hz) rsEEG rhythm intensity and diffuse increases in the intensity of cortical delta (<4 Hz) and theta (4–7 Hz) oscillations [102]. These rsEEG findings have been cross-validated by rsMEG [103 - 105].

Parkinson's Disease

Spectral EEG revealed an increase in basal ganglia-cortical beta power, as these oscillations represent the probability of a voluntary movement [106]. Beta oscillations increase longitudinally [107]. Levodopa and deep brain stimulation (DBS) of the subthalamic nucleus reduced beta power, correlating with therapeutic effects on bradykinesia and rigidity [106, 108].

In a recent systematic review, Geraedts *et al* examined the relevance of qEEG measurements as outcomes of disease severity in PD. After a systematic search of the primary databases, 36 out of 605 identified studies were included. Clinical outcome could be categorized into cognition (23 studies), motor function (13 studies), responsiveness to interventions (7 studies) and other (10 studies). In cross-sectional and longitudinal studies, qEEG slowing (decreased dominant frequency and increased θ power) correlated with cognitive impairment and deterioration over time, suggesting its potential in the early recognition of nonmotor symptoms and monitoring the progression of PD. However, there were no conclusive findings in motor dysfunction and treatment response [109].

TMS can detect a reduction in resting motor threshold (RMT) that correlates with poorer Unified Parkinson's Disease Rating Scale motor score, which is indicative of pathological corticospinal hyperexcitability [110]. Furthermore, reduced SICI (short intracortical inhibition) and increased ICF (intracortical-facilitation) in the off state of PD point to additional abnormalities in intracortical inhibitory and facilitatory cortical network activity [111]. as drivers of motor hyperexcitability.

Amyotrophic Lateral Sclerosis

Resting-state EEG/MEG in ALS can reliably identify increases in intra- and inter-motor cortical functional connectivity [112, 113], which is consistent with evidence of motor hyperexcitability as defined by threshold tracking TMS in ALS. Using TMS, hyperexcitability in ALS is quantified by reduced motor threshold, a measure of corticospinal excitability. SICI, a measure of GABAergic interneuron function, is also consistently reduced in ALS, implying loss of inhibition as a source of network hyperexcitability [114]. This decrease in SICI can distinguish ALS from mimicking neuromuscular syndromes with 73% sensitivity and 80% specificity. Decreased SICI may also be presymptomatically present [115], providing a prodromal biomarker.

As cognitive impairment in ALS correlates with poorer prognosis [116], subgrouping based on domains of network impairment has the potential to improve early prognostic accuracy and facilitate recruitment to cognition-targeted therapeutic trials. Application of quantitative EEG analysis of event-related potentials (ERP) in ALS patients has shown increased average delay in the mismatch negativity ERP, a measure of involuntary attention switching, which echoes the findings in Stroop task performance, a psychological test of inhibitory control and attention shifting [29]. Regarding the source localization of this EEG signal, ALS patients exhibited excessive left frontoparietal activity, which correlates with poorer inhibitory control and decreased bilateral inferior frontal activity [85]. Cognitive impairment is not biased by learning effects or physical disability.

Huntington's Disease

According to Painold *et al* [117, 118], reduced alpha power seems to be a trait marker of HD, whereas increased prefrontal delta power seems to reflect worsening of the disease; moreover, in these studies, motor and cognitive functions deteriorated together with a decrease in alpha and theta power. Modification in the alpha-theta border suggests that EEG alterations in pre-HD individuals may be related to the course of the pathological process [119]. Decreased alpha power and increased slow frequencies (delta and theta) were generally accepted EEG findings in HD and in presymptomatic subjects. EEG modifications have been related to clinical state, cognitive impairment, cortical atrophy, CAG repeats, and revolution with age [120].

In a recent study, Odish *et al.* constructed an automatic classifier for distinguishing healthy controls from HD gene carriers using qEEG and derived qEEG features that correlate with clinical markers known to change with disease progression in HD, including UHDRS-TMS, TFC, Symbol Digit Modalities Test (SDMT), Stroop Word Reading (SWR) and Beck Depression Inventory-II (BDI-II) scores [121]. EEG was recorded for three minutes with subjects at rest. An EEG index was created by applying statistical pattern recognition to a large set of EEG features, which was subsequently tested using 10-fold cross-validation. Analysis of subsets of electrophysiological features resulted in highly significant correlations with SDMT and UHDRS-TMS scores. These results show potential for qEEG to serve as a biomarker in HD progression, which may be further utilized in monitoring therapeutic effects.

BIOCHEMICAL BIOMARKERS OF NEURODEGENERATIVE DISEASES

Biomarkers have become an essential component of diagnosing NDDs and clinical research (Table **1**) [76 - 78, 122 - 125]. Because biomarkers reflect the progress of the pathogenesis of NDDs, they aid in a more rapid, accurate disease diagnosis; stratify the patient population to identify good responders to treatments; and help studies targeting new drug development. In addition to the image-based biomarkers mentioned above, other types exist, such as nucleic acid and biochemical biomarkers (Fig. **4**).

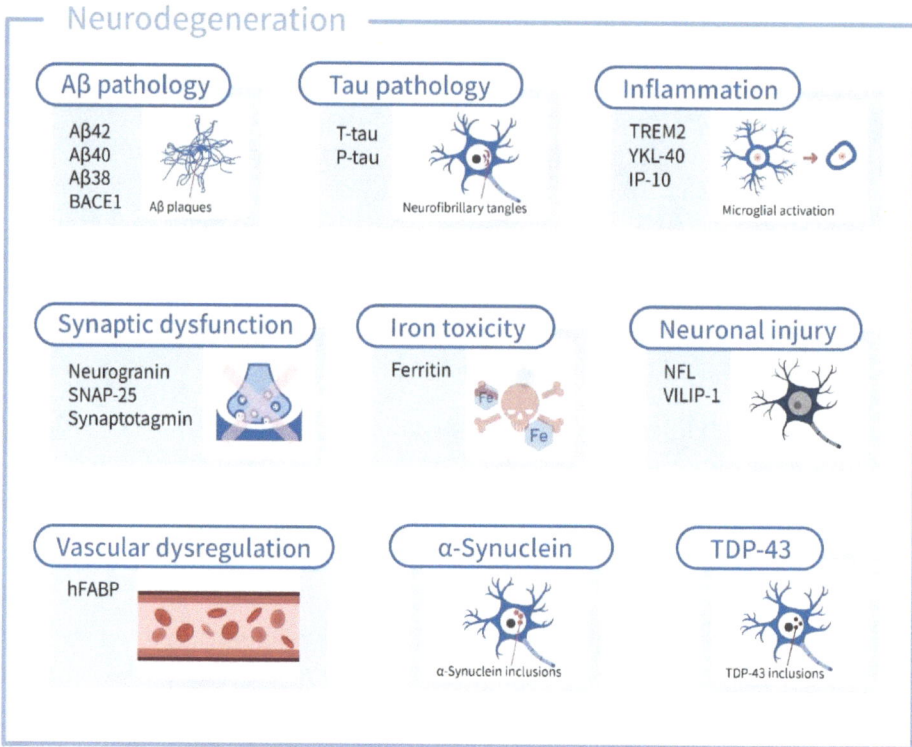

Fig. (4). Fluidic biomarkers of neural degenerative diseases. Multiple pathological mechanisms, including proteinopathies, synapse dysfunction, inflammation, vascular dysregulation, and neuronal injury, are related to NDDs. The corresponding proteins or biomolecules are potential biomarkers that can be detected in body fluids. This figure is adapted from Molinuevo *et al.* [192].

HD, familial AD, familial PD, and some forms of ALS are related to DNA mutations, and genetic biomarkers currently have the greatest clinical utility for diagnosis. Other types of nucleic acid biomarkers, such as RNAs and epigenetic changes, are also related to certain NDDs and are vigorously investigated.

Regarding biochemical biomarkers, obtaining tissue-based biopsies for diagnosis and research can be difficult in living humans; thus, biofluids, such as blood and cerebrospinal fluid (CSF), are of interest. CSF is the closest biofluid to the diseased site, *i.e.*, the central nervous system (CNS); however, obtaining CSF requires an invasive lumbar puncture, limiting its acceptance. In contrast, blood samples are easier to collect, but their compositions are far more complex, containing proteins and nucleic acids from all tissues.

Among the biochemical biomarkers, protein-based biomarkers are the most investigated; nonetheless, RNA-based and exosome-based biomarkers of NDDs have also been identified [77].

MicroRNAs (miRNAs) are noncoding small RNAs ranging from 21-25 nucleotides long that act as post-transcriptional regulators of genes by binding complementary target mRNAs to inhibit their translation or degradation [126]. MicroRNAs often play central roles in cell differentiation and proliferation, and in the neuronal system, miRNAs regulate synaptic plasticity, neurogenesis, and neural stem cell renewal and proliferation. The altered expression of miRNAs has been associated with neurodegenerative diseases, possibly via the involvement of the increased accumulation of toxic proteins, neural survival and the immune response [127, 128]. MicroRNAs are stable and easily detectable in biofluids as either circulating in serum or plasma in free form or encapsulated in vesicles (exosomes, microparticles, or apoptotic bodies). Several studies have investigated deregulated miRNAs in experimental models and/or human samples of NDDs, and two miRNAs, *i.e.*, miR-132 and miR-22, have been shown to be commonly deregulated in NDDs [129]. Several different miRNA families have been reported to be upregulated or downregulated in AD, PD, ALD, and HD [130 - 132].

Exosomes are extracellular vesicles 40-150 nm in diameter. These vesicles are secreted by cells as a way of communication among cells. Exosomes are carriers of biomolecules, such as proteins, lipids, and nucleic acids (including microRNA) and are able to carry both neurotrophic factors and misfolded proteins. Exosomes participate in neuroprotection and the spread of misfolded proteins. Thus, exosomes are a double-edged sword in NDDs [133]. Exosomes are attractive candidates as biomarkers and treatment for NDDs due to their ability to cross the blood-brain barrier and the high specificity of surface markers. Therefore, we can detect misfolded proteins and deliver therapeutic agents using exosomes traveling from and to the CNS.

Alzheimer's Disease

Regarding AD, the major biomarkers under investigation are Aβ42, tau, including t-tau and p-tau (phosphorylated at threonine 181), and neurofilament light chain (NFL) [77, 134 - 136]. The ratio of the CSF levels of T-181 to Aβ42 has a sensitivity of 86% and specificity of 97% in differentiating AD patients from healthy controls and other NDD patients [77]. Neurofilament light chain (NFL) levels are an indicator of axonal injury, and higher levels of NFL are associated with faster cognitive decline and brain and hippocampal atrophy [77]. In addition to t-tau, p-tau, Aβ42, and NFL in CSF, which are regularly used in clinical practice and clinical research, several other AD markers, such as the CSF biomarkers NSE, VLP-1, HFABP, and YKL-40, are potential biomarkers since they are moderately associated with AD [136]. Neurogranin is another potential CSF biomarker of AD because AD and prodromal AD are marked by an increase in CSF neurogranin. This molecule is abundant in the cortex, hippocampus, and amygdala and concentrated in dendritic spines. Since neurogranin is an indicator of synaptic dysfunction and degeneration, CSF neurogranin might be a progression marker [137, 138].

Additionally, low baseline Aβ42 and high baseline t-tau and p-tau levels are associated with cognitive decline during follow-up and predict the conversion from no cognitive impairment (NCI) to MCI, followed by AD. However, the plasma Aβ42 and tau levels do not accurately match their levels in CSF for the diagnosis of AD. The use of other brain-derived biomarkers along with ultrasensitive detection techniques is under active research. Exosomes from the CNS in the blood represent another potential biomarker. Compared with controls, higher levels of Aβ42, t-tau, and two types of p-tau (T-181 and S-396) have been detected in blood exosomes from AD patients [77].

The current diagnosis of AD is based solely on clinical symptoms and cognitive testing, and the use of biomarkers is complementary [11]. However, with refinement of the sensitivity and specificity of both imaging and biochemical biomarkers, the paradigm is shifting toward biomarker-based staging and diagnosis independent of the clinical manifestations of dementia [14]. Combining neuroimaging and biofluid biomarkers enables diagnostic predictions in the clinical and prodromal stages of AD and assessments of disease progression [9].

Parkinson's Disease

In PD, α-synuclein is the major biomarker under rigorous research. Decreased total α-synuclein levels but increased oligomeric and phosphorylated α-synuclein levels have been observed in CSF from PD patients compared with healthy controls [143]. The ratio of α-synuclein oligomers to total α-synuclein is a PD diagnosis indicator with optimal sensitivity and specificity (89.3 and 90.6%, respectively) [144]. However, α-synuclein is highly abundant in blood cells; therefore, blood samples are prone to contamination from red blood cell hemolysis. Thus, deducing the CSF levels of α-synuclein from blood samples is challenging. Another type of biomarker is related to oxidative stress. For example, higher plasma levels of uric acid are related to slower disease progression and better prognosis in PD patients. Some growth factors could also be utilized for disease diagnosis and evaluation of prognosis. Lower levels of neuroprotective factors, such as brain-derived neurotrophic factor (BDNF) and insulin-like growth factor-1 (IGF-1), are associated with worse motor dysfunction and a poorer prognosis [77].

Table 1. Summary of biomarkers currently used for diagnosing NDDs.

Neurodegenerative Diseases				
	Alzheimer's Disease (AD)	**Parkinson's Disease (PD)**	**Amyotrophic Lateral Sclerosis (ALS)**	**Huntington's Disease (HD)**
Major symptoms	*Cognitive:* memory loss and executive dysfunction *Psychiatric:* Delusions and depression	*Motor:* bradykinesia and resting tremor *Nonmotor:* autonomous, cognitive, psychiatric, and sensory dysfunctions	*Motor:* muscle weakness and atrophy	*Motor:* chorea *Nonmotor:* Cognitive impairment
Vulnerable neuron region	Pyramidal neurons in layer II of the entorhinal cortex (EC-II) and the hippocampal CA1 (HP-CA1); cholinergic neurons in the basal forebrain (FB), and noradrenergic neurons in the locus coeruleus (LC)	Dopaminergic neurons in the substantia nigra	Upper and lower motor neurons Fast-fatigable motor neurons	Caudate nucleus and putamen Medium spiny GABA neurons (MSNs)
Genetics	APP, PSEN-1, PSEN-2, and ApoE4	LRRK2 (PARK8), Parkin (PARK2), SNCA (PARK1), PINK1 (PARK6), and DJ1 (PARK7)	SOD1, ALS2, DCTN1, VAPB, SETX, ANG, CMP2B, FIG4, FUS, OPTN, PFN1, SQSTM1, TARDBP, VCP, SIGMAR1, UBQLN2, C9ORF72.	Excessive (>34) CAG repeats in HTT

(Table 1) cont.....

Neurodegenerative Diseases				
	Alzheimer's Disease (AD)	**Parkinson's Disease (PD)**	**Amyotrophic Lateral Sclerosis (ALS)**	**Huntington's Disease (HD)**
Neuroimaging and electrophysiology	***Aβ:*** [11C]-PiB and [18F]-Flutemetamol ***Molecular Imaging:*** [18F]-FDG-PET ***Structural Imaging:*** Volumetric MRI	***Dopamine:*** DaTscan ***Structure Imaging:*** Volumetric MRI and Transcranial sonography (TCS)	***Structure Imaging:*** Brain MRI (SBM), multimodal MRI, DTI; Muscle and peripheral nerve MRI; ***Molecular Imaging:*** [11C]-PBR28, and [18F]-FDG-PET; ***Electrophysiology:*** Muscle ultrasound; Electrical impedance myography (EIM); Transcranial magnetic stimulation (TMS); Neurophysiological index; Motor uni number estimation (MUNE and MUNIX)	***Molecular Imaging:*** PET, including striatal [18F]FDG binding, postsynaptic dopaminergic function ([11C]SCH22390, [11C]raclopride) and PDE10A levels ([11C]IMA107) ***Structural Imaging:*** Volumetric MRI; DTI; MTR(Magnetization transfer imaging)
Biofluids				
CSF	Aβ42, p-tau, t-tau, and NFL	α-synuclein (oligomeric/total)	pNFH, NFL, dipeptide repeat proteins, IL-8, and MCP-1	Tau, pTau, NFL Mutant HTT, MBP, Clusterin
Blood		Plasma uric acid (UA), serum BDNF, and IGF-1, NFL	Serum creatinine/cystatin C, UA, and MCP-1, NFL	NFL, HTT protein, Mutant HTT protein, S100B, Clusterin, 24-hydroxycholesterol
Exosome	Aβ42	α-syn, LRRK2, and VPS35	SOD1, TDP-43, FUS	Mutant Huntingtin
miRNA	miRNA137 [139]	miRNA195 [140]	miRNA143-3p, miRNA206 [141]	CSF miR-520f-3p, miR-135b-3p, miR-4317, miR-3928-5p, miR-8082, miR-140-5p [142]

Amyotrophic Lateral Sclerosis

Abnormal accumulation of neurofilaments (NFs) in neurons has been shown in postmortem spinal cords of ALS patients and mouse models, and mutations of neurofilament heavy chain are also associated with ALS [145]. NFs are intermediate filaments in neurons that are composed of heteropolymers of four subunits: neurofilament heavy chain, neurofilament medium chain, neurofilament light chain and alpha-internexin [146]. They are involved in radial growth and stability of axons, axonal transport and interaction with microtubules and mitochondria. NFs have been extensively studied in ALS, with assays ranging from in-house and commercial traditional ELISA assays to newer generation immunoassays employing novel technologies such as electrochemiluminescence (ECL) and single molecule array (Simoa). NFs have demonstrated diagnostic value, prognostic value and potential in tracking treatment response in patient stratification [124, 147, 148] and in monitoring disease onset in mutant carriers of ALS [149].

Huntington's Disease

It is currently lacking disease-modifying treatment for HD, even though there has been a great advance in potential treatment and clinical trials targeting processes close to its genetic cause in the last decade. Easily accessible biomarkers for HD, early detection of symptoms for premanifest patients and monitoring of therapeutic effects would be of great value for HD. Byrne *et al.* [150] observed elevated plasma NFL levels in premanifest HD (PreHD) patients compared with controls and observed that the NFL level was associated with the onset time in the 3-year follow-up, while that observed in manifest HD patients correlated with their clinical decline and MRI findings. Utilizing the Simoa system, plasma NFL levels showed its potential to be a prognostic blood biomarker of disease onset and progression in Huntington's disease [151].

Despite the long hunt, successful quantification of soluble CSF mutant huntingtin (mHTT) at femtomolar sensitivity was only achieved in early 2015 [152], utilizing a single molecule counting (SMC) immunoassay (Singulex). There is a roughly threefold difference in mHTT levels in PreHD and manifest HD patients. These levels also correlate with motor and cognitive scores as well as the levels of NFL and Tau, suggesting its neuronal origin. The CSF mHTT level shows potential as a prognostic indicator of disease onset and reflects a therapeutic effect.

BIOSENSORS FOR NEURODEGENERATIVE DISEASES

NDDs, such as AD, PD and HD, are the most common causes of dementia in elderly people worldwide. Thus far, effective therapeutic treatments for NDDs are lacking, and disease development is irreversible. In 2010, the total estimated social care cost of dementia was US$604 billion. Wimo [153] suggests that there is considerable potential for cost increases in the coming years as the gap between diagnosis and treatment is narrowed.

In addition to clinical trials, various analytical approaches have been proposed for the identification of potential biomarkers of NDDs, including MS, MRI, Western blotting, and enzyme-linked immunosorbent assay (ELISA). Compared to biosensors, many of these technologies are relatively expensive and time consuming [154]. Several advantages of biosensors, such as their simplicity, low cost, high sensitivity and selectivity, low detection limits, and excellent reproducibility, suggest that biosensors are favorable tools for the early detection of NDDs [155].

In general, a biosensor comprises the following two parts: bioreceptor and biotransducer. Bioreceptors are compounds, such as antibodies, enzymes, or nucleic acids, that bind specific biomarkers (Fig. **5**). For example, as mentioned in the previous section, tau protein, amyloid β (Aβ), and apolipoprotein E4 (APOE4) are the top three recognized biomarkers used for the clinical diagnosis of AD in human CSF and blood [154]. Corresponding bioreceptors utilized in recent studies include anti-tau antibodies and ssDNA. Qualified bioreceptors require high selectivity and stability. These molecular recognition elements are based on bioaffinity (dissociation constant, Kd). After selective recognition events, the intrinsic properties of the biosensor that could be considered an input signal are changed. Biotransducers convert these input signals to measurable output signals. Biotransducers can be classified according to the types of input signals, such as electrochemical, optical, piezoelectric, mass-based, acoustic waves, or thermal signals.

Several electrochemical, optical, and electromagnetic biotransducers have been proposed for the detection of NDDs. In the next section, we introduce recent advances in biosensors for the detection of NDD biomarkers.

Electrochemical Biosensors for NDDs

Owing to advances in material science, new types of conductive materials, such as graphene, graphene oxide (GO), gold nanowires (AuNWs), or gold nanoparticles (AuNPs), have been employed to develop electrochemical biosensors. In an electrochemical biosensor, the most common setup is a three-electrode system that includes a working electrode, a reference electrode, and a counter electrode. Counter electrodes serve as polarized electrodes and enable dynamic or time-transient measurements [156]. Working electrodes are functionalized through surface immobilization. The capture of biomarkers changes certain intrinsic characteristics of the working electrodes. To detect NDDs, impedimetric, potentiometric, and amperometric methods are common electrochemical modes used in biosensors. Typically, the characteristic change is linearly correlated with the total amount of the target in its detection range. The common electrochemical analysis techniques applied to NDD biosensors include cyclic voltammetry (CV), differential pulse voltammetry (DPV), and electrochemical impedance spectrometry (EIS). These powerful electroanalytical tools provide real-time, highly sensitive and highly specific measurements of target biomarkers. Many electrochemical biosensors have been reported for the detection of AD or PD [157].

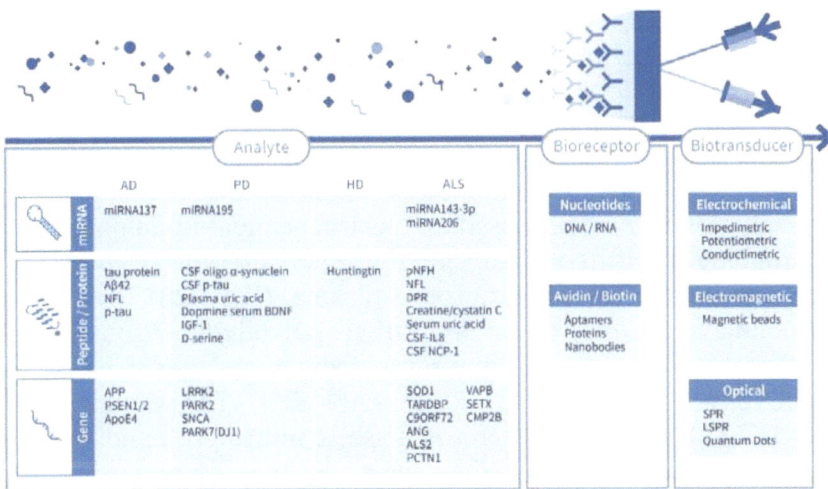

Fig (5). The workflow of biosensing in neurodegenerative diseases. Biosensing involves the following three major components: analyte (or biomarker), bioreceptor and biotransducer. Regarding NDDs, potential biomarkers can be classified as miRNAs, peptides/proteins, and genes. Bioreceptors and biotransducers constitute the core components of biosensors. Bioreceptors are chosen or designed according to their target analytes. For example, complementary sequences and antibodies are often used due to their high specificity. The detection area of biotransducers is functionalized by immobilizing bioreceptors. Electrochemical, electromagnetic, and optical biotransducers have been proposed as biosensors for the detection of NDD biomarkers.

Electrochemical Biosensors for the Detection of Alzheimer's Disease

The tau protein is a significant early detection biomarker of AD. Wang *et al.* developed a sensitive biosensor with four gold microband electrodes for the detection of the full-length 2N4R tau protein [155]. The compound 3,3'-dithiobis (sulfosuccinimidyl propionate) (DTSSP) was first applied as a cross linker, forming a self-assembled monolayer (SAM) on electrodes. Then, protein G (a bacterial immunoglobulin-binding protein often used as the basis for preparing probes or affinity media for antibodies) and anti-tau antibody were coated separately. The limit of detection (LOD) reached 0.03 pM, which is much lower than the critical cut-off value (4.3 pM) of CSF tau protein. Western blotting and commercially available ELISA were carried out to prove the selectivity, specificity, and LOD of tau protein. The performance of this electrochemical biosensor in human serum samples was similar to that of tau in phosphate buffered saline (PBS).

In addition to detection methods requiring sample labeling, Rushworth and her group developed a label-free electrical impedimetric biosensor to detect the concentration of Aβ oligomers (AβO) in the conditional medium. (Rushworth 2014) The AβO recognition elements were biotin-LC-PrPC [95 - 110] indirectly immobilized on gold electrodes with copolymer, NHS-biotin, and NeutrAvidin. EIS measurements verified that the attachment of AβO decreased the impedance of the biosensor surface. The linear range of the response to AβO detection could be as low as ~0.5 pM.

In a recent study, Diba *et al.* proposed an electrochemical immunosensor with a gold nanoparticle (Au NP)-modified screen-printed carbon electrode (SPCE) to detect Aβ1-42 in diluted human serum and plasma. (Diba 2017) A mixed self-assembled monolayer (SAM) of thiol-modified polyethylene glycol (PEG-SH) and mercaptopropionic acid (MPA) was coated on AuNP-SPCEs to increase selectivity and form a covalent bond with anti-Aβ(12F4). The secondary antibody, *i.e.*, anti-Aβ(1E11)-ALP (alkaline phosphatase) conjugate, bound target Aβ on another binding site, forming the anti-Aβ(12F4)/Aβ/anti-Aβ(1E11)-ALP sandwich complex. CV and DPV were conducted to measure the site-specific redox reaction between ALP and the substrate. Impressively, the LOD could reach the femtomolar level in diluted serum and plasma samples.

Additionally, Azimzadeh *et al.* [140] developed a biosensor based on electrochemical-reduced graphene oxidation (ERGO) and gold nanowires (AuNWs) to detect miRNA-137 for the early diagnosis of ADAn SPCE was used, and GO solution and gold nanowires were applied for surface modification before immobilizing the ssDNA thiolated probe. This three-electrode system further applied doxorubicin as an intercalated label. The electrochemical signals were measured by cyclic voltammetry (CV) and EIS, and the linear range was 5.0 to 750.0 fM. The LOD was 1.7 fM. The biosensor showed a high relative recovery percentage and acceptable relative standard deviation values when evaluating actual human serum samples. This finding reveals the potential of miRNA-137 in the clinical detection of early AD.

Electrochemical Biosensors for the Detection of Parkinson's Disease

For PD detection, Yue *et al.* [158] reported a ZnO nanowire array (ZnO NWA) grown on graphene foam by chemical vapor deposition. The ZnO NWA/GF electrode was used to selectively detect uric acid (UA), dopamine, and ascorbic acid by a DPV method for the early detection of PD; specifically, the UA level in human serum from PD patients is 25% lower than that in healthy individuals. Moreover, An *et al.* employed Au-doped TiO_2 nanotubes to develop a photoelectrochemical immunosensor for the quantitative detection of α-synuclein (α-SYN) using an anodic oxidation technique with a highly ordered TiO_2 nanotube array grown on Ti foil [159]. The Au nanoparticles were deposited in TiO_2 nanotubes, and then, primary antibody immobilization was applied on one side of the Ti foil. EIS was used to analyze the performance of the electrode surface modification.

In addition, Sierks and his group [160] developed a label-free impedimetric biosensor composed of a printed circuit board (PCB), a nanoporous alumina membrane and a silicon microfluidic chamber to detect the level of α-synuclein in CSF A nanoporous alumina membrane was soldered onto the PCB, creating numerous nanowells. The alumina membrane also served as a filter to prevent cell debris or impurities from blocking the working surface while maintaining good biocompatibility. As a recognition element, a nanobody was immobilized onto the electrode surface through chemical linkers. The presence of different α-synuclein morphologies in CSF might be measured using morphology-specific nanobodies, with a lower limit of detection in the femtomolar range.

Optical Biosensors for NDDs

Optical biosensors transfer photonic information into an electrical signal. In contrast to electrochemical biosensors, no reference electrode is needed in optical biosensors. Optical biosensors take advantage of multiwavelength measurements and, therefore, have potential in real-time high content sensing. However, although the size of biosensing chips is generally small, the peripheral instruments required for spectral analysis are large and difficult to miniaturize. Three common optical sensing techniques used for NDDs are surface plasmon resonance (SPR), localized surface plasmon resonance (LSPR), and quantum dots (QDs).

SPR

The working principle of SPR is based on the change in the surface resonance signal, which is related to the binding of the analyte. The mass change on the metal sensing surface can be detected and quantified by analyzing the SPR angle shift.

Ryu *et al*. combined *in situ* SPR optical biosensors with *ex situ* atomic force microscopy (AFM) to analyze Aβ1-42 aggregation from monomers to fibrils [161]. A surface consisting of an SAM of 11-mercaptoundecanoic acid (MUA) was chosen to decrease nonspecific binding. Compared to the bare MUA surface, a significant and steady increase in the SPR angle shift was observed on the Aβ-bound MUA surface during the 10 h time-lapse monitoring.

Yi *et al*. [162] developed a real-time SPR biosensor for the analysis of Aβ aggregation. The SPR chips were coated with A11 and OC antibodies in channels 1 and 2, respectively, through amide bond formation. Aβ oligomers can be captured by A11 antibodies, while Aβ fibrils can be recognized by OC antibodies. The other types of Aβ, including monomers, dimers, trimers, and tetramers, that are less toxic in disease development are not sensed by this device. The time-lapse SPR was investigated in this article to study the influence of curcumin, Cu^{2+} and methylene blue on Aβ aggregation, and the results show that curcumin is a potential inhibitor of Aβ(1–42) oligomer formation; on the other hand, Cu^{2+} is an accelerator of the aggregation process of Aβ. Methylene blue shows mixed effects of decreasing the aggregation rate from monomers to oligomers and increasing the aggregation rate of oligomers to fibrils, which leads to the reduction of toxic Aβ(1–42) oligomers. In addition, a recent study conducted by Palladino and his group [163] proposed another SPR optical biosensor for the detection of Aβ aggregation from monomers to oligomers. IgG1 monoclonal antibodies 82E1 and 12F4 were used to recognize the N-terminus and C-terminus of Aβ1-42, respectively.

LSPR

The LSPR chip is fabricated with a dielectric material, typically glass, instead of a metal material. The capture of biomarkers is reflected by a characteristic change in the wavelength of the maximum absorbance or absorbance value [164].

Vestergaard *et al*. developed the first immunochip based on LSPR for the detection of tau protein [165]. The gold-capped nanoparticle LSPR chips were functionalized by SAM, linker, and tau-mAb. The capture of tau protein resulted in the augmentation of the maximum absorbance value. The LSPR spectral analysis showed high selectivity and high sensitivity as low as 10 pg/ml.

Kang *et al*. used ApoE4 to induce Aβ aggregation and AuNPs to fabricate an LSPR biosensor [166]. Rayleigh scattering spectra of single AuNPs were recorded, and the characteristics of the absorbance distribution changed following an aggregation event. The authors. also provided evidence that ApoE4 is more specific in promoting the aggregation of Aβ42 than Aβ40.

Recently, Kim *et al.* presented a multidetection LSPR chip based on gold nanoparticles [167]. Three different and specific antibodies were linked to AuNPs for the detection of Aβ 1-40, Aβ 1-42, and tau protein. The nanoplasmonic biosensor enabled the lower LOD to reach the fM level without a cross-talk effect.

Quantum Dots

QDs are nanometer-scale semiconductor crystals with a size and shape that can be controlled by temperature, duration and chemical reagents during the fabrication process [168]. The principle behind the fluorescence of QDs is utilizing photons to excite QDs and create electron-hole pairs. Fluorescence is emitted during the recombination process of electrons and holes. QDs feature high fluorescence intensity, high sensitivity to changes in the surface charge, and high stability against photobleaching [169]. Due to these optical properties, QDs have high potential as materials for optical biosensors.

Ma *et al.* reported an optical biosensor for detecting the activity of mitochondrial complex I utilizing semiconductor QDs [170]. CdSe/ZnS QDs were immobilized and functionalized by ubiquinone-terminated ligands. Xia *et al.* developed quantum dot biosensors to detect the concentration of the Aβ oligomer [171]. The principle was based on the inner filter effect of AuNPs and the quenching effect of CdTe QDs.

To study the influence of ascorbic acid (AA) in detecting dopamine (DA), Ankireddy and Kim proposed an optical biosensor based on L-cysteine (L-Cys)-capped InP/ZnS QDs [169]. The surface of the InP/ZnS QDs was modified with L-Cys to increase the selectivity of DA. The fluorescence-quenching effect of QDs reflected the levels of DA and AA. Fourier transform infrared spectroscopy (FTIR) spectra and photoluminescence (PL) spectra were employed for both AA and DA, indicating the difference in their electron transformance. PL spectra of different concentrations of DA in the presence of AA were assessed.

Electromagnetic Biosensors for NDDs

Electromagnetic beads represent another widely used material for biosensors. Here, we introduce two commercial products used for detecting biomarkers of NDDs.

A single-molecule array (Simoa) has been launched by the US-based company Quanterix [172], and the Simoa digital immunoassay platform has been applied to detect serum NFL, plasma total tau, and plasma Aβ42 [173]. This instrument provides a detection limit as low as a femtomolar concentration with conventional ELISA reagents. Paramagnetic beads with capture agents can be used to detect the corresponding target in various biofluids. These beads were subsequently loaded into femtoliter-sized well arrays for fluorescent imaging. Although the principle is similar to that of conventional ELISA, the femtoliter-size well arrays enable the detection of a single-molecule signal. As a result, the sensitivity is much higher than that of conventional ELISA [174]).

MagQu, an immunomagnetic reduction (IMR) system, was developed by a Taiwanese research team and used for early detection of AD through assays of plasma amyloid and total Tau protein. The principle behind IMR is the analysis of the change in the magnetic oscillation properties. Magnetic beads with surface bioreceptors oscillate according to multiple external ac magnetic fields named mixed-frequency ac magnetic susceptibility. When binding events occurred, magnetic beads unite with each other and become larger. Larger beads show different magnetic properties and, thus, could be used as a norm for the concentration of the analyte (Fig. **6**) [175]. A high-Tc superconducting-quantu--interference-device (SQUID) ac magnetosusceptometer can be applied to achieve ultra-high sensitivity with over 80% accuracy, providing the possibility of screening for prodromal AD [176, 177].

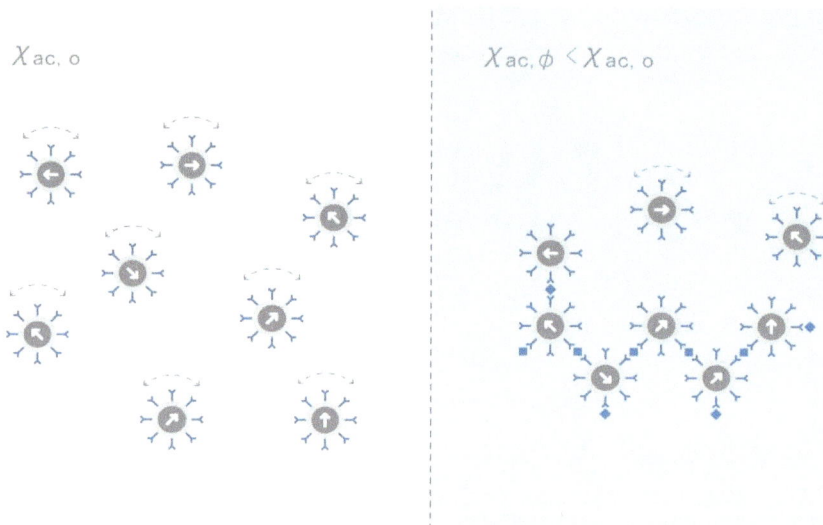

Fig. (6). Illustration of the immunomagnetic reduction (IMR) technique. IMR is an electromagnetic-based approach that uses antibody-functionalized magnetic nanoparticles as an acceptor and measures their magnetic oscillation properties by applying external magnetic fields. The nanoparticles aggregate as they capture analytes. The capture events lead to an increase in the diameter of these magnetic beads and a change in their magnetic oscillation properties, which can be analyzed to infer the quantity of the analyte. This figure is adapted from Yang *et al.* [177].

Biosensors for Exosome Detection

As mentioned in the previous section, exosomes have been recently discovered to play important roles in NDDs as prominent mediators of NDDs. Biomarkers, such as Aβ-42, huntingtin protein, and α-syn, spread and transport to other tissues from their cells of origin to other cells through exosome secretion [178]. Exosomes are nanometer-scale lipid bilayer vesicles containing message molecules. Distant cells can recognize specific protein markers on the surface of exosomes and then absorb these exosomes.

Currently, the standard exosome isolation protocol is differential ultracentrifugation [179]. With multiple steps of centrifugation, whole-mount exosomes with diameters ranging from 50-90 nm can be collected for further investigation, such as MS, Western blotting or electron microscopic analyses. However, the entire ultracentrifugation process requires approximately 5 h to complete, which is considered to be time-consuming and inefficient [180, 181].

Because the details of the influence of exosomes on NDD development remain unclear, few biosensors have been developed for detecting NDD-related exosomes. However, many microfluidic devices have been proposed for exosome isolation, detection, and analysis [180, 182]. Here, we review microfluidic-based biosensors used to detect exosomes, which might inspire the development of biosensors for the detection of NDD-related exosomes.

Exosomes in biofluids can be captured according to their immunoaffinity, physical size, surface charge, density or a combination of several physical properties [180]. For example, Fraikin *et al.* developed a high-throughput exosome analyzer composed of electrodes, nanoconstriction, fluidic resistance and a fluid channel. Constant external voltages are applied to bias the electrodes, forming an ionic electrical current along the fluid channel. When analytes pass through the nanoconstriction, the sensing electrode detects the potential change due to the voltage division between nanoconstriction and fluidic resistance (Fig. 7) [183].

In addition to physical properties, the recognition elements are typically designed for immunoaffinity capture to increase specificity. Zhou *et al.* reported an electrochemical biosensor with aptamers immobilized onto a gold electrode array. These aptamers are specific for CD63 proteins, which are commonly present on the surface of exosomes. When exosomes interact with single-stranded DNA probes through CD63 proteins, the complementary sequences are replaced, and the electrochemical signals are reduced [184].

The SPR platform can also be applied for the detection of exosomes with specific surface immobilization. Sina *et al.* developed a nanoplasmonic sensor based on transmission SPR through periodic nanohole arrays for the detection of exosomes derived from ovarian cancer cells [185]. Im *et al.* utilized a sandwich approach to implement an SPR chip for the detection of cancer-related exosomes [186].

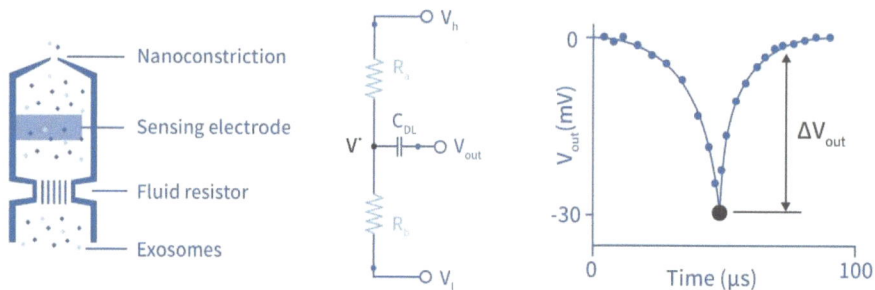

Fig. (7). Illustration of a voltage-based nanoparticle analyzer for potential exosome detection. The microfluidic device comprises two voltage-bias electrodes and a single lithographed sensing electrode between the fluidic resistor and the nanoconstriction. The nanoconstriction is for particle detection, while the fluidic restriction is for providing balancing electrical resistance. When a nanoparticle enters the constriction, the ionic electrical current is altered, reflecting the electrical potential of the fluid adjacent to the nanoconstriction. The voltage change is capacitively coupled and detected by the sensing electrode. This figure is adapted from Fraikin *et al.* [183].

Beadbased techniques are often used in biosensors detecting exosomes. The rapid inertial solution exchange (RInSE) method utilizes biotin-coated polystyrene beads to capture exosomes in biofluids and then collects target beads with the three-end microchannel, and the collected solution can be used for subsequent analysis [187]. Ko *et al.* proposed a microfluidic-based mobile exosome detector (μMED). The disposable optofluidic chip contains the following three inlets: sample, enrichment microbeads, and ELISA reagents. First, the target exosomes bind to the positively enriched microbeads, whereas the background exosomes bind to the negatively enriched microbeads. Then, the negatively enriched microbeads are blocked by porous membranes due to their larger size. Finally, ELISA reagents are applied to the target exosomes and microbeads, and fluorescence is measured using a smartphone camera [188].

Many microfluidic platforms have been developed for exosome detection based on immunocapture. Electrochemical, optical and bead-based technologies are feasible for analyzing exosomes. Thus, the first step may be identifying the appropriate recognition elements and surface markers to develop biosensors for the detection of NDD-related exosomes.

CONCLUDING REMARKS

NDDs are multifactorial conditions with different etiologies that present various pathologies, including gene mutations, protein misfolding and aggregation, mitochondrial dysfunction, oxidative stress, neuroinflammation and neuronal death. In this review, we have focused on AD, PD, ALS, and HD and discussed the current trends and methods used for the early detection and diagnosis of NDDs. The current biomolecular diagnostic markers and potential protein biomarkers in CSF and blood in the forms of miRNA and exosomes are also discussed. Since the pathologies of NDDs can begin years before the onset of clinical symptoms, the long preclinical period provides an opportunity for protective and preventive interventions regarding disease progression. Nonetheless, applications of molecular diagnostic techniques for early detection with minimally invasive and cost- and time-effective techniques are still needed. The current challenges include the determination of biomarkers at the early stage and the establishment of diagnostic criteria for disease recognition during this prodromal phase. Nanotechnology has been employed for both the diagnosis and therapeutics of NDDs. Various biosensing techniques have been applied to achieve the goal of early detection in blood biosamples, especially electromagnetic applications in reduction assays, single-molecule assays and exosome/miRNA detection.

CSF is a logical site to search for biomarkers of NDDs; the content of CSF potentially reflects pathophysiological alterations due to its direct interaction with the extracellular space in the brain. However, a major limitation is the relative invasiveness of CSF collection by lumbar puncture, prompting researchers to develop and validate diagnostic or prognostic biomarkers in blood. The challenge to develop protein blood biomarkers of brain pathophysiology includes very low levels (~35 pg/ml) of brain-derived protein compared to CSF protein levels (~350 pg/ml) and the need for a very sensitive and specific method to detect protein blood biomarkers (Hampel 2018), which might be difficult to detect using conventional immunochemical technologies, such as ELISA. The current methods used to detect NDD biomarkers in blood can be primarily classified into the following four categories: MS, metabolomics, ultrasensitive immunoassay techniques, and lab-on-a-chip technologies (Fig. **8**). Factors, such as blood-brain barrier (BBB) permeability and differences in concentrations in different compartments, are among the considerations necessary while searching for a biomarker, especially a blood-based biomarker, for a CNS disease [189 - 191].

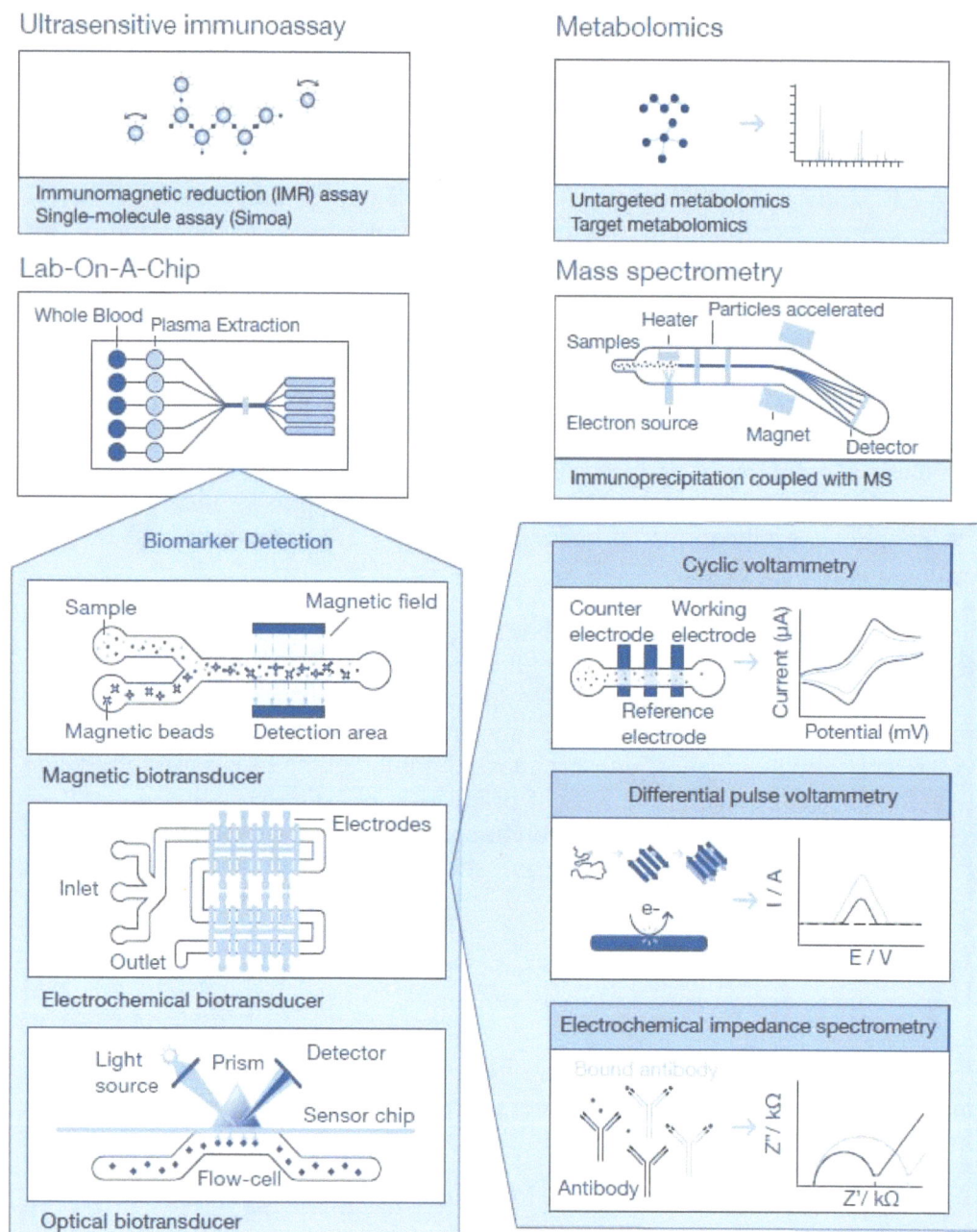

Fig. (8). Methods used for NDD-related blood biomarker discovery and molecular diagnosis. Recent advances in developing ultrasensitive immunoassays, metabolomic techniques, mass spectrometry methods and microfluidic technologies show promise for screening blood biomarkers of NDDs. Cyclic voltammetry (CV), differential pulse voltammetry (DPV), and electrochemical impedance spectrometry (EIS) are common electrochemical analysis techniques applied to NDD molecular diagnosis.

Overall, blood biomarkers can be used in first stage screening to select patients for second-grade diagnostic evaluations, such as CSF biomarkers, PET scans, and MRI scans. Developing molecular diagnostics based on circulating miRNAs or exosomes is also a highly promising approach due to their neuronal site specificity and BBB permeability. Ultimately, individualized and preventive strategies combining neuropsychological evaluations, clinical history examinations, analyses of multiple biomolecular diagnostic biomarkers, and specialized medical imaging techniques will improve the prognosis and quality of life of NDD patients.

CONSENT FOR PUBLICATION

Not applicable.

CONFLICT OF INTEREST

The authors confirm that this chapter contents have no conflict of interest.

ACKNOWLEDGEMENTS

The work was supported by MOST grants (MOST-107-2636-B-002-001, and MOST-108-2636-B-002-001).

REFERENCES

[1]   Kovacs GG. Concepts and classification of neurodegenerative diseases. Handb Clin Neurol 2017; 145: 301-7.
[http://dx.doi.org/10.1016/B978-0-12-802395-2.00021-3] [PMID: 28987178]

[2]   Kovacs GG, Lee VM, Trojanowski JQ. Protein astrogliopathies in human neurodegenerative diseases and aging. Brain Pathol 2017; 27(5): 675-90.
[http://dx.doi.org/10.1111/bpa.12536] [PMID: 28805003]

[3]   Gan L, Cookson MR, Petrucelli L, La Spada AR. Converging pathways in neurodegeneration, from genetics to mechanisms. Nat Neurosci 2018; 21(10): 1300-9.
[http://dx.doi.org/10.1038/s41593-018-0237-7] [PMID: 30258237]

[4]   García J-C, Bustos R-H. The genetic diagnosis of neurodegenerative diseases and therapeutic perspectives. Brain Sci 2018; 8(12)E222
[http://dx.doi.org/10.3390/brainsci8120222] [PMID: 30551598]

[5]   Jankovic J. Parkinson's disease: clinical features and diagnosis. J Neurol Neurosurg Psychiatry 2008; 79(4): 368-76.
[http://dx.doi.org/10.1136/jnnp.2007.131045] [PMID: 18344392]

[6]   Burns A, Iliffe S. Alzheimer's disease. BMJ 2009; 338: b158.
[http://dx.doi.org/10.1136/bmj.b158] [PMID: 19196745]

[7]   Scheltens P, Blennow K, Breteler MMB, *et al*. Alzheimer's disease. Lancet 2016; 388(10043): 505-17.
[http://dx.doi.org/10.1016/S0140-6736(15)01124-1] [PMID: 26921134]

[8]   Aisen PS, Cummings J, Jack CR Jr, *et al*. On the path to 2025: understanding the Alzheimer's disease continuum. Alzheimers Res Ther 2017; 9(1): 60.
[http://dx.doi.org/10.1186/s13195-017-0283-5] [PMID: 28793924]

[9]   Villemagne VL, Doré V, Burnham SC, Masters CL, Rowe CC. Imaging tau and amyloid-β proteinopathies in Alzheimer disease and other conditions. Nat Rev Neurol 2018; 14(4): 225-36.
[http://dx.doi.org/10.1038/nrneurol.2018.9] [PMID: 29449700]

[10] Long JM, Holtzman DM. Alzheimer disease: an update on pathobiology and treatment strategies. Cell 2019; 179(2): 312-39.
[http://dx.doi.org/10.1016/j.cell.2019.09.001] [PMID: 31564456]

[11] Jack CR Jr, Albert MS, Knopman DS, *et al.* Introduction to the recommendations from the National Institute on Aging-Alzheimer's Association workgroups on diagnostic guidelines for Alzheimer's disease. Alzheimers Dement 2011; 7(3): 257-62.
[http://dx.doi.org/10.1016/j.jalz.2011.03.004] [PMID: 21514247]

[12] McKhann GM, Knopman DS, Chertkow H, *et al.* The diagnosis of dementia due to Alzheimer's disease: recommendations from the National Institute on Aging-Alzheimer's Association workgroups on diagnostic guidelines for Alzheimer's disease. Alzheimers Dement 2011; 7(3): 263-9.
[http://dx.doi.org/10.1016/j.jalz.2011.03.005] [PMID: 21514250]

[13] Jack CR Jr, Bennett DA, Blennow K, *et al.* A/T/N: An unbiased descriptive classification scheme for Alzheimer disease biomarkers. Neurology 2016; 87(5): 539-47.
[http://dx.doi.org/10.1212/WNL.0000000000002923] [PMID: 27371494]

[14] Jack CR Jr, Bennett DA, Blennow K, *et al.* NIA-AA Research Framework: Toward a biological definition of Alzheimer's disease. Alzheimers Dement 2018; 14(4): 535-62.
[http://dx.doi.org/10.1016/j.jalz.2018.02.018] [PMID: 29653606]

[15] Jack CR Jr, Wiste HJ, Vemuri P, *et al.* Brain beta-amyloid measures and magnetic resonance imaging atrophy both predict time-to-progression from mild cognitive impairment to Alzheimer's disease. Brain 2010; 133(11): 3336-48.
[http://dx.doi.org/10.1093/brain/awq277] [PMID: 20935035]

[16] Trojanowski JQ, Vandeerstichele H, Korecka M, *et al.* Update on the biomarker core of the Alzheimer's Disease Neuroimaging Initiative subjects. Alzheimers Dement 2010; 6(3): 230-8.
[http://dx.doi.org/10.1016/j.jalz.2010.03.008] [PMID: 20451871]

[17] Weiner MW, Veitch DP, Aisen PS, *et al.* 2014 Update of the Alzheimer's Disease Neuroimaging Initiative: A review of papers published since its inception. Alzheimers Dement 2015; 11(6): e1-e120.
[http://dx.doi.org/10.1016/j.jalz.2014.11.001] [PMID: 26073027]

[18] Jack CR Jr, Knopman DS, Jagust WJ, *et al.* Hypothetical model of dynamic biomarkers of the Alzheimer's pathological cascade. Lancet Neurol 2010; 9(1): 119-28.
[http://dx.doi.org/10.1016/S1474-4422(09)70299-6] [PMID: 20083042]

[19] Gauthier S, Zhang H, Ng KP, Pascoal TA, Rosa-Neto P. Impact of the biological definition of Alzheimer's disease using amyloid, tau and neurodegeneration (ATN): what about the role of vascular changes, inflammation, Lewy body pathology? Transl Neurodegener 2018; 7: 12.
[http://dx.doi.org/10.1186/s40035-018-0117-9] [PMID: 29876101]

[20] Sabbagh MN, Lue L-F, Fayard D, Shi J. Increasing precision of clinical diagnosis of alzheimer's disease using a combined algorithm incorporating clinical and novel biomarker data. Neurol Ther 2017; 6 (Suppl. 1): 83-95.
[http://dx.doi.org/10.1007/s40120-017-0069-5] [PMID: 28733959]

[21] Braak H, Del Tredici K, Rüb U, de Vos RA, Jansen Steur EN, Braak E. Staging of brain pathology related to sporadic Parkinson's disease. Neurobiol Aging 2003; 24(2): 197-211.
[http://dx.doi.org/10.1016/S0197-4580(02)00065-9] [PMID: 12498954]

[22] Marsili L, Rizzo G, Colosimo C. Diagnostic criteria for parkinson's disease: from james parkinson to the concept of prodromal disease. Front Neurol 2018; 9: 156.
[http://dx.doi.org/10.3389/fneur.2018.00156] [PMID: 29628907]

[23] Goetz CG, Tilley BC, Shaftman SR, *et al.* Movement Disorder Society-sponsored revision of the

Unified Parkinson's Disease Rating Scale (MDS-UPDRS): scale presentation and clinimetric testing results. Mov Disord 2008; 23(15): 2129-70.
[http://dx.doi.org/10.1002/mds.22340] [PMID: 19025984]

[24] The Unified Parkinson's Disease Rating Scale (UPDRS): status and recommendations. Mov Disord 2003; 18(7): 738-50.
[http://dx.doi.org/10.1002/mds.10473] [PMID: 12815652]

[25] Goetz CG, Fahn S, Martinez-Martin P, *et al.* Movement Disorder Society-sponsored revision of the Unified Parkinson's Disease Rating Scale (MDS-UPDRS): Process, format, and clinimetric testing plan. Mov Disord 2007; 22(1): 41-7.
[http://dx.doi.org/10.1002/mds.21198] [PMID: 17115387]

[26] Dayalu P, Albin RL. Huntington disease: pathogenesis and treatment. Neurol Clin 2015; 33(1): 101-14.
[http://dx.doi.org/10.1016/j.ncl.2014.09.003] [PMID: 25432725]

[27] Reilmann R, Leavitt BR, Ross CA. Diagnostic criteria for Huntington's disease based on natural history. Mov Disord 2014; 29(11): 1335-41.
[http://dx.doi.org/10.1002/mds.26011] [PMID: 25164527]

[28] Martin S, Al Khleifat A, Al-Chalabi A. What causes amyotrophic lateral sclerosis? F1000 Res 2017; 6: 371. [version 1; peer review: 3 approved].
[http://dx.doi.org/10.12688/f1000research.10476.1] [PMID: 28408982]

[29] Iyer PM, Mohr K, Broderick M, *et al.* Mismatch Negativity as an Indicator of Cognitive Sub-Domain Dysfunction in Amyotrophic Lateral Sclerosis. Front Neurol 2017; 8: 395.
[http://dx.doi.org/10.3389/fneur.2017.00395] [PMID: 28861032]

[30] Majounie E, Renton AE, Mok K, *et al.* Frequency of the C9orf72 hexanucleotide repeat expansion in patients with amyotrophic lateral sclerosis and frontotemporal dementia: a cross-sectional study. Lancet Neurol 2012; 11(4): 323-30.
[http://dx.doi.org/10.1016/S1474-4422(12)70043-1] [PMID: 22406228]

[31] DeJesus-Hernandez M, Mackenzie IR, Boeve BF, *et al.* Expanded GGGGCC hexanucleotide repeat in noncoding region of C9ORF72 causes chromosome 9p-linked FTD and ALS. Neuron 2011; 72(2): 245-56.
[http://dx.doi.org/10.1016/j.neuron.2011.09.011] [PMID: 21944778]

[32] Renton AE, Majounie E, Waite A, *et al.* A hexanucleotide repeat expansion in C9ORF72 is the cause of chromosome 9p21-linked ALS-FTD. Neuron 2011; 72(2): 257-68.
[http://dx.doi.org/10.1016/j.neuron.2011.09.010] [PMID: 21944779]

[33] Floeter MK, Gendron TF. Biomarkers for amyotrophic lateral sclerosis and frontotemporal dementia associated with hexanucleotide expansion mutations in c9orf72. Front Neurol 2018; 9: 1063.
[http://dx.doi.org/10.3389/fneur.2018.01063] [PMID: 30568632]

[34] Gendron TF, Chew J, Stankowski JN, *et al.* Poly(GP) proteins are a useful pharmacodynamic marker for *C9ORF72*-associated amyotrophic lateral sclerosis. Sci Transl Med 2017; 9(383)eaai7866
[http://dx.doi.org/10.1126/scitranslmed.aai7866] [PMID: 28356511]

[35] Project MinE: study design and pilot analyses of a large-scale whole-genome sequencing study in amyotrophic lateral sclerosis. Eur J Hum Genet 2018; 26(10): 1537-46.
[http://dx.doi.org/10.1038/s41431-018-0177-4] [PMID: 29955173]

[36] van Rheenen W, Shatunov A, Dekker AM, *et al.* Genome-wide association analyses identify new risk variants and the genetic architecture of amyotrophic lateral sclerosis. Nat Genet 2016; 48(9): 1043-8.
[http://dx.doi.org/10.1038/ng.3622] [PMID: 27455348]

[37] McAlary L, Plotkin SS, Yerbury JJ, Cashman NR. Prion-Like Propagation of Protein Misfolding and Aggregation in Amyotrophic Lateral Sclerosis. Front Mol Neurosci 2019; 12: 262.
[http://dx.doi.org/10.3389/fnmol.2019.00262] [PMID: 31736708]

[38]   Rosen DR, Siddique T, Patterson D, *et al*. Mutations in Cu/Zn superoxide dismutase gene are associated with familial amyotrophic lateral sclerosis. Nature 1993; 362(6415): 59-62.
[http://dx.doi.org/10.1038/362059a0] [PMID: 8446170]

[39]   Neumann M, Sampathu DM, Kwong LK, *et al*. Ubiquitinated TDP-43 in frontotemporal lobar degeneration and amyotrophic lateral sclerosis. Science 2006; 314(5796): 130-3.
[http://dx.doi.org/10.1126/science.1134108] [PMID: 17023659]

[40]   Kwiatkowski TJ Jr, Bosco DA, Leclerc AL, *et al*. Mutations in the FUS/TLS gene on chromosome 16 cause familial amyotrophic lateral sclerosis. Science 2009; 323(5918): 1205-8.
[http://dx.doi.org/10.1126/science.1166066] [PMID: 19251627]

[41]   Farrawell NE, Lambert-Smith IA, Warraich ST, *et al*. Distinct partitioning of ALS associated TDP-43, FUS and SOD1 mutants into cellular inclusions. Sci Rep 2015; 5: 13416.
[http://dx.doi.org/10.1038/srep13416] [PMID: 26293199]

[42]   Camandola S, Mattson MP. Brain metabolism in health, aging, and neurodegeneration. EMBO J 2017; 36(11): 1474-92.
[http://dx.doi.org/10.15252/embj.201695810] [PMID: 28438892]

[43]   Tilokani L, Nagashima S, Paupe V, Prudent J. Mitochondrial dynamics: overview of molecular mechanisms. Essays Biochem 2018; 62(3): 341-60.
[http://dx.doi.org/10.1042/EBC20170104] [PMID: 30030364]

[44]   Panchal K, Tiwari AK. Mitochondrial dynamics, a key executioner in neurodegenerative diseases. Mitochondrion 2018.
[PMID: 30408594]

[45]   Müller M, Ahumada-Castro U, Sanhueza M, Gonzalez-Billault C, Court FA, Cárdenas C. Mitochondria and calcium regulation as basis of neurodegeneration associated with aging. Front Neurosci 2018; 12: 470.
[http://dx.doi.org/10.3389/fnins.2018.00470] [PMID: 30057523]

[46]   Lin MT, Beal MF. Mitochondrial dysfunction and oxidative stress in neurodegenerative diseases. Nature 2006; 443(7113): 787-95.
[http://dx.doi.org/10.1038/nature05292] [PMID: 17051205]

[47]   Pathak D, Berthet A, Nakamura K. Energy failure: does it contribute to neurodegeneration? Ann Neurol 2013; 74(4): 506-16.
[http://dx.doi.org/10.1002/ana.24014] [PMID: 24038413]

[48]   Cha M-Y, Kim DK, Mook-Jung I. The role of mitochondrial DNA mutation on neurodegenerative diseases. Exp Mol Med 2015; 47e150
[http://dx.doi.org/10.1038/emm.2014.122] [PMID: 25766619]

[49]   Jafri MS, Kumar R. Modeling mitochondrial function and its role in disease. Prog Mol Biol Transl Sci 2014; 123: 103-25.
[http://dx.doi.org/10.1016/B978-0-12-397897-4.00001-2] [PMID: 24560142]

[50]   Grimm A, Friedland K, Eckert A. Mitochondrial dysfunction: the missing link between aging and sporadic Alzheimer's disease. Biogerontology 2016; 17(2): 281-96.
[http://dx.doi.org/10.1007/s10522-015-9618-4] [PMID: 26468143]

[51]   Barnham KJ, Masters CL, Bush AI. Neurodegenerative diseases and oxidative stress. Nat Rev Drug Discov 2004; 3(3): 205-14.
[http://dx.doi.org/10.1038/nrd1330] [PMID: 15031734]

[52]   Frijhoff J, Winyard PG, Zarkovic N, *et al*. Clinical relevance of biomarkers of oxidative stress. Antioxid Redox Signal 2015; 23(14): 1144-70.
[http://dx.doi.org/10.1089/ars.2015.6317] [PMID: 26415143]

[53]   Niedzielska E, Smaga I, Gawlik M, *et al*. Oxidative stress in neurodegenerative diseases. Mol

Neurobiol 2016; 53(6): 4094-125.
[http://dx.doi.org/10.1007/s12035-015-9337-5] [PMID: 26198567]

[54]   Ibáñez C, Cifuentes A, Simó C. Recent advances and applications of metabolomics to investigate neurodegenerative diseases. Int Rev Neurobiol 2015; 122: 95-132.
[http://dx.doi.org/10.1016/bs.irn.2015.05.015] [PMID: 26358892]

[55]   Wilkins JM, Trushina E. Application of metabolomics in alzheimer's disease. Front Neurol 2018; 8: 719.
[http://dx.doi.org/10.3389/fneur.2017.00719] [PMID: 29375465]

[56]   Sato N, Morishita R. The roles of lipid and glucose metabolism in modulation of β-amyloid, tau, and neurodegeneration in the pathogenesis of Alzheimer disease. Front Aging Neurosci 2015; 7: 199.
[http://dx.doi.org/10.3389/fnagi.2015.00199] [PMID: 26557086]

[57]   Gizem Y, Abdullah Y. Metabolic syndrome and neurodegenerative diseases. J Geriatr Med Gerontol 2018; 4(2)
[http://dx.doi.org/10.23937/2469-5858/1510042]

[58]   Jha SK, Jha NK, Kumar D, Ambasta RK, Kumar P. Linking mitochondrial dysfunction, metabolic syndrome and stress signaling in Neurodegeneration. Biochim Biophys Acta Mol Basis Dis 2017; 1863(5): 1132-46.
[http://dx.doi.org/10.1016/j.bbadis.2016.06.015] [PMID: 27345267]

[59]   Procaccini C, Santopaolo M, Faicchia D, *et al.* Role of metabolism in neurodegenerative disorders. Metabolism 2016; 65(9): 1376-90.
[http://dx.doi.org/10.1016/j.metabol.2016.05.018] [PMID: 27506744]

[60]   Area-Gomez E, Guardia-Laguarta C, Schon EA, Przedborski S. Mitochondria, OxPhos, and neurodegeneration: cells are not just running out of gas. J Clin Invest 2019; 129(1): 34-45.
[http://dx.doi.org/10.1172/JCI120848] [PMID: 30601141]

[61]   Wishart DS, Feunang YD, Marcu A, *et al.* HMDB 4.0: the human metabolome database for 2018. Nucleic Acids Res 2018; 46(D1): D608-17.
[http://dx.doi.org/10.1093/nar/gkx1089] [PMID: 29140435]

[62]   Botas A, Campbell HM, Han X, Maletic-Savatic M. Metabolomics of neurodegenerative diseases. Int Rev Neurobiol 2015; 122: 53-80.
[http://dx.doi.org/10.1016/bs.irn.2015.05.006] [PMID: 26358890]

[63]   Zhang AH, Sun H, Wang XJ. Recent advances in metabolomics in neurological disease, and future perspectives. Anal Bioanal Chem 2013; 405(25): 8143-50.
[http://dx.doi.org/10.1007/s00216-013-7061-4] [PMID: 23715678]

[64]   Kori M, Aydın B, Unal S, Arga KY, Kazan D. Metabolic biomarkers and neurodegeneration: A pathway enrichment analysis of alzheimer's disease, parkinson's disease, and amyotrophic lateral sclerosis. OMICS 2016; 20(11): 645-61.
[http://dx.doi.org/10.1089/omi.2016.0106] [PMID: 27828769]

[65]   Havelund JF, Heegaard NHH, Færgeman NJK, Gramsbergen JB. Biomarker research in parkinson's disease using metabolite profiling. Metabolites 2017; 7(3)E42
[http://dx.doi.org/10.3390/metabo7030042] [PMID: 28800113]

[66]   Lanznaster D, de Assis DR, Corcia P, Pradat P-F, Blasco H. Metabolomics biomarkers: A strategy toward therapeutics improvement in ALS. Front Neurol 2018; 9: 1126.
[http://dx.doi.org/10.3389/fneur.2018.01126] [PMID: 30619076]

[67]   Markley JL, Brüschweiler R, Edison AS, *et al.* The future of NMR-based metabolomics. Curr Opin Biotechnol 2017; 43: 34-40.
[http://dx.doi.org/10.1016/j.copbio.2016.08.001] [PMID: 27580257]

[68]   Blasco H, Corcia P, Moreau C, *et al.* 1H-NMR-based metabolomic profiling of CSF in early amyotrophic lateral sclerosis. PLoS One 2010; 5(10)e13223

[http://dx.doi.org/10.1371/journal.pone.0013223] [PMID: 20949041]

[69] Kumar A, Bala L, Kalita J, *et al.* Metabolomic analysis of serum by (1) H NMR spectroscopy in amyotrophic lateral sclerosis. Clin Chim Acta 2010; 411(7-8): 563-7.
[http://dx.doi.org/10.1016/j.cca.2010.01.016] [PMID: 20096678]

[70] Tsang TM, Woodman B, McLoughlin GA, *et al.* Metabolic characterization of the R6/2 transgenic mouse model of Huntington's disease by high-resolution MAS 1H NMR spectroscopy. J Proteome Res 2006; 5(3): 483-92.
[http://dx.doi.org/10.1021/pr050244o] [PMID: 16512662]

[71] Verwaest KA, Vu TN, Laukens K, *et al.* (1)H NMR based metabolomics of CSF and blood serum: a metabolic profile for a transgenic rat model of Huntington disease. Biochim Biophys Acta 2011; 1812(11): 1371-9.
[http://dx.doi.org/10.1016/j.bbadis.2011.08.001] [PMID: 21867751]

[72] Han J, Datla R, Chan S, Borchers CH. Mass spectrometry-based technologies for high-throughput metabolomics. Bioanalysis 2009; 1(9): 1665-84.
[http://dx.doi.org/10.4155/bio.09.158] [PMID: 21083110]

[73] Shao Y, Le W. Recent advances and perspectives of metabolomics-based investigations in Parkinson's disease. Mol Neurodegener 2019; 14(1): 3.
[http://dx.doi.org/10.1186/s13024-018-0304-2] [PMID: 30634989]

[74] Ibáñez C, Simó C, Martín-Álvarez PJ, *et al.* Toward a predictive model of Alzheimer's disease progression using capillary electrophoresis-mass spectrometry metabolomics. Anal Chem 2012; 84(20): 8532-40.
[http://dx.doi.org/10.1021/ac301243k] [PMID: 22967182]

[75] Smith EF, Shaw PJ, De Vos KJ. The role of mitochondria in amyotrophic lateral sclerosis. Neurosci Lett 2019; 710132933
[http://dx.doi.org/10.1016/j.neulet.2017.06.052] [PMID: 28669745]

[76] Schon EA, Przedborski S. Mitochondria: the next (neurode)generation. Neuron 2011; 70(6): 1033-53.
[http://dx.doi.org/10.1016/j.neuron.2011.06.003] [PMID: 21689593]

[77] Jeromin A, Bowser R. Biomarkers in neurodegenerative diseases. Adv Neurobiol 2017; 15: 491-528.
[http://dx.doi.org/10.1007/978-3-319-57193-5_20] [PMID: 28674995]

[78] Stoessl AJ. Neuroimaging in the early diagnosis of neurodegenerative disease. Transl Neurodegener 2012; 1(1): 5.
[http://dx.doi.org/10.1186/2047-9158-1-5] [PMID: 23211024]

[79] Leuzy A, Chiotis K, Lemoine L, *et al.* Tau PET imaging in neurodegenerative tauopathies-still a challenge. Mol Psychiatry 2019; 24(8): 1112-34.
[http://dx.doi.org/10.1038/s41380-018-0342-8] [PMID: 30635637]

[80] Villemagne VL, Fodero-Tavoletti MT, Masters CL, Rowe CC. Tau imaging: early progress and future directions. Lancet Neurol 2015; 14(1): 114-24.
[http://dx.doi.org/10.1016/S1474-4422(14)70252-2] [PMID: 25496902]

[81] Lin K-J, Weng Y-H, Hsieh C-J, *et al.* Brain imaging of vesicular monoamine transporter type 2 in healthy aging subjects by 18F-FP-(+)-DTBZ PET. PLoS One 2013; 8(9)e75952
[http://dx.doi.org/10.1371/journal.pone.0075952] [PMID: 24098749]

[82] Pagano G, Niccolini F, Politis M. Current status of PET imaging in Huntington's disease. Eur J Nucl Med Mol Imaging 2016; 43(6): 1171-82.
[http://dx.doi.org/10.1007/s00259-016-3324-6] [PMID: 26899245]

[83] Wilson H, Dervenoulas G, Politis M. Structural magnetic resonance imaging in huntington's disease. Int Rev Neurobiol 2018; 142: 335-80.
[http://dx.doi.org/10.1016/j.bs.irn.2018.09.006] [PMID: 30409258]

[84] Wilson H, Politis M. Molecular imaging in huntington's disease. Int Rev Neurobiol 2018; 142: 289-333.
[http://dx.doi.org/10.1016/bs.irn.2018.08.007] [PMID: 30409256]

[85] McMackin R, Dukic S, Broderick M, *et al*. Dysfunction of attention switching networks in amyotrophic lateral sclerosis. Neuroimage Clin 2019; 22101707
[http://dx.doi.org/10.1016/j.nicl.2019.101707] [PMID: 30735860]

[86] Muthuraman M, Hellriegel H, Hoogenboom N, *et al*. Beamformer source analysis and connectivity on concurrent EEG and MEG data during voluntary movements. PLoS One 2014; 9(3)e91441
[http://dx.doi.org/10.1371/journal.pone.0091441] [PMID: 24618596]

[87] Murakami S, Okada Y. Contributions of principal neocortical neurons to magnetoencephalography and electroencephalography signals. J Physiol 2006; 575(Pt 3): 925-36.
[http://dx.doi.org/10.1113/jphysiol.2006.105379] [PMID: 16613883]

[88] Vuckovic A, Hasan MA, Osuagwu B, *et al*. The influence of central neuropathic pain in paraplegic patients on performance of a motor imagery based Brain Computer Interface. Clin Neurophysiol 2015; 126(11): 2170-80.
[http://dx.doi.org/10.1016/j.clinph.2014.12.033] [PMID: 25698307]

[89] Neuper C, Klimesch W. Event-Related Dynamics of Brain Oscillations. 1st ed. 2006; Vol. 159.

[90] Teleńczuk B, Baker SN, Kempter R, Curio G. Correlates of a single cortical action potential in the epidural EEG. Neuroimage 2015; 109: 357-67.
[http://dx.doi.org/10.1016/j.neuroimage.2014.12.057] [PMID: 25554430]

[91] Dukic S, Iyer PM, Mohr K, Hardiman O, Lalor EC, Nasseroleslami B. Estimation of coherence using the median is robust against EEG artefacts. Conf Proc IEEE Eng Med Biol Soc 2017; 2017: 3949-52.
[http://dx.doi.org/10.1109/EMBC.2017.8037720] [PMID: 29060761]

[92] Darvas F, Pantazis D, Kucukaltun-Yildirim E, Leahy RM. Mapping human brain function with MEG and EEG: methods and validation. Neuroimage 2004; 23 (Suppl. 1): S289-99.
[http://dx.doi.org/10.1016/j.neuroimage.2004.07.014] [PMID: 15501098]

[93] Groppa S, Oliviero A, Eisen A, *et al*. A practical guide to diagnostic transcranial magnetic stimulation: report of an IFCN committee. Clin Neurophysiol 2012; 123(5): 858-82.
[http://dx.doi.org/10.1016/j.clinph.2012.01.010] [PMID: 22349304]

[94] Menon P, Geevasinga N, Yiannikas C, Howells J, Kiernan MC, Vucic S. Sensitivity and specificity of threshold tracking transcranial magnetic stimulation for diagnosis of amyotrophic lateral sclerosis: a prospective study. Lancet Neurol 2015; 14(5): 478-84.
[http://dx.doi.org/10.1016/S1474-4422(15)00014-9] [PMID: 25843898]

[95] Ibey RJ, Bolton DAE, Buick AR, Staines WR, Carson RG. Interhemispheric inhibition of corticospinal projections to forearm muscles. Clin Neurophysiol 2015; 126(10): 1934-40.
[http://dx.doi.org/10.1016/j.clinph.2014.12.006] [PMID: 25561164]

[96] Di Lazzaro V, Oliviero A, Pilato F, *et al*. Neurophysiological predictors of long term response to AChE inhibitors in AD patients. J Neurol Neurosurg Psychiatry 2005; 76(8): 1064-9.
[http://dx.doi.org/10.1136/jnnp.2004.051334] [PMID: 16024879]

[97] Agarwal S, Koch G, Hillis AE, *et al*. Interrogating cortical function with transcranial magnetic stimulation: insights from neurodegenerative disease and stroke. J Neurol Neurosurg Psychiatry 2019; 90(1): 47-57.
[http://dx.doi.org/10.1136/jnnp-2017-317371] [PMID: 29866706]

[98] Ruddy KL, Leemans A, Woolley DG, Wenderoth N, Carson RG. Structural and functional cortical connectivity mediating cross education of motor function. J Neurosci 2017; 37(10): 2555-64.
[http://dx.doi.org/10.1523/JNEUROSCI.2536-16.2017] [PMID: 28154150]

[99] Babiloni C, Lizio R, Marzano N, *et al*. Brain neural synchronization and functional coupling in

Alzheimer's disease as revealed by resting state EEG rhythms. Int J Psychophysiol 2016; 103: 88-102.
[http://dx.doi.org/10.1016/j.ijpsycho.2015.02.008] [PMID: 25660305]

[100] Babiloni C, De Pandis MF, Vecchio F, *et al.* Cortical sources of resting state electroencephalographic rhythms in Parkinson's disease related dementia and Alzheimer's disease. Clin Neurophysiol 2011; 122(12): 2355-64.
[http://dx.doi.org/10.1016/j.clinph.2011.03.029] [PMID: 21924950]

[101] Andersson M, Hansson O, Minthon L, Rosén I, Londos E. Electroencephalogram variability in dementia with lewy bodies, Alzheimer's disease and controls. Dement Geriatr Cogn Disord 2008; 26(3): 284-90.
[http://dx.doi.org/10.1159/000160962] [PMID: 18841014]

[102] Vecchio F, Babiloni C, Lizio R, De Vico Fallani F, Blinowska K, Verrienti G, *et al.* Resting state cortical EEG rhythms in Alzheimer's disease.
[http://dx.doi.org/10.1016/B978-0-7020-5307-8.00015-6]

[103] Franciotti R, Iacono D, Della Penna S, *et al.* Cortical rhythms reactivity in AD, LBD and normal subjects: a quantitative MEG study. Neurobiol Aging 2006; 27(8): 1100-9.
[http://dx.doi.org/10.1016/j.neurobiolaging.2005.05.027] [PMID: 16076512]

[104] Mandal PK, Banerjee A, Tripathi M, Sharma A. A comprehensive review of magnetoencephalography (MEG) studies for brain functionality in healthy aging and alzheimer's disease (AD). Front Comput Neurosci 2018; 12: 60.
[http://dx.doi.org/10.3389/fncom.2018.00060] [PMID: 30190674]

[105] Olde Dubbelink KTE, Stoffers D, Deijen JB, *et al.* Resting-state functional connectivity as a marker of disease progression in Parkinson's disease: A longitudinal MEG study. Neuroimage Clin 2013; 2: 612-9.
[http://dx.doi.org/10.1016/j.nicl.2013.04.003] [PMID: 24179812]

[106] Jenkinson N, Brown P. New insights into the relationship between dopamine, beta oscillations and motor function. Trends Neurosci 2011; 34(12): 611-8.
[http://dx.doi.org/10.1016/j.tins.2011.09.003] [PMID: 22018805]

[107] Caviness JN, Hentz JG, Belden CM, *et al.* Longitudinal EEG changes correlate with cognitive measure deterioration in Parkinson's disease. J Parkinsons Dis 2015; 5(1): 117-24.
[http://dx.doi.org/10.3233/JPD-140480] [PMID: 25420672]

[108] Muthuraman M, Koirala N, Ciolac D, *et al.* Deep Brain Stimulation and L-DOPA Therapy: Concepts of Action and Clinical Applications in Parkinson's Disease. Front Neurol 2018; 9: 711.
[http://dx.doi.org/10.3389/fneur.2018.00711] [PMID: 30210436]

[109] Geraedts VJ, Boon LI, Marinus J, *et al.* Clinical correlates of quantitative EEG in Parkinson disease: A systematic review. Neurology 2018; 91(19): 871-83.
[http://dx.doi.org/10.1212/WNL.0000000000006473] [PMID: 30291182]

[110] Park J, Chang WH, Cho JW, *et al.* Usefulness of transcranial magnetic stimulation to assess motor function in patients with parkinsonism. Ann Rehabil Med 2016; 40(1): 81-7.
[http://dx.doi.org/10.5535/arm.2016.40.1.81] [PMID: 26949673]

[111] Ni Z, Bahl N, Gunraj CA, Mazzella F, Chen R. Increased motor cortical facilitation and decreased inhibition in Parkinson disease. Neurology 2013; 80(19): 1746-53.
[http://dx.doi.org/10.1212/WNL.0b013e3182919029] [PMID: 23576626]

[112] Nasseroleslami B, Dukic S, Broderick M, *et al.* Characteristic increases in EEG connectivity correlate with changes of structural MRI in amyotrophic lateral sclerosis. Cereb Cortex 2019; 29(1): 27-41.
[http://dx.doi.org/10.1093/cercor/bhx301] [PMID: 29136131]

[113] Proudfoot M, Colclough GL, Quinn A, *et al.* Increased cerebral functional connectivity in ALS: A resting-state magnetoencephalography study. Neurology 2018; 90(16): e1418-24.
[http://dx.doi.org/10.1212/WNL.0000000000005333] [PMID: 29661904]

[114] Grieve SM, Menon P, Korgaonkar MS, *et al.* Potential structural and functional biomarkers of upper motor neuron dysfunction in ALS. Amyotroph Lateral Scler Frontotemporal Degener 2015; 17(1-2): 85-92.
[http://dx.doi.org/10.3109/21678421.2015.1074707] [PMID: 26458122]

[115] Vucic S, Nicholson GA, Kiernan MC. Cortical hyperexcitability may precede the onset of familial amyotrophic lateral sclerosis. Brain 2008; 131(Pt 6): 1540-50.
[http://dx.doi.org/10.1093/brain/awn071] [PMID: 18469020]

[116] Elamin M, Phukan J, Bede P, *et al.* Executive dysfunction is a negative prognostic indicator in patients with ALS without dementia. Neurology 2011; 76(14): 1263-9.
[http://dx.doi.org/10.1212/WNL.0b013e318214359f] [PMID: 21464431]

[117] Painold A, Anderer P, Holl AK, *et al.* Comparative EEG mapping studies in Huntington's disease patients and controls. J Neural Transm (Vienna) 2010; 117(11): 1307-18.
[http://dx.doi.org/10.1007/s00702-010-0491-7] [PMID: 20931245]

[118] Painold A, Anderer P, Holl AK, *et al.* EEG low-resolution brain electromagnetic tomography (LORETA) in Huntington's disease. J Neurol 2011; 258(5): 840-54.
[http://dx.doi.org/10.1007/s00415-010-5852-5] [PMID: 21161261]

[119] Ponomareva N, Klyushnikov S, Abramycheva N, *et al.* Alpha-theta border EEG abnormalities in preclinical Huntington's disease. J Neurol Sci 2014; 344(1-2): 114-20.
[http://dx.doi.org/10.1016/j.jns.2014.06.035] [PMID: 25015843]

[120] Piano C, Mazzucchi E, Bentivoglio AR, *et al.* Wake and Sleep EEG in Patients With Huntington Disease: An eLORETA Study and Review of the Literature. Clin EEG Neurosci 2017; 48(1): 60-71.
[http://dx.doi.org/10.1177/1550059416632413] [PMID: 27094758]

[121] Odish OFF, Johnsen K, van Someren P, Roos RAC, van Dijk JG. EEG may serve as a biomarker in Huntington's disease using machine learning automatic classification. Sci Rep 2018; 8(1): 16090.
[http://dx.doi.org/10.1038/s41598-018-34269-y] [PMID: 30382138]

[122] Agrawal M, Biswas A. Molecular diagnostics of neurodegenerative disorders. Front Mol Biosci 2015; 2: 54.
[http://dx.doi.org/10.3389/fmolb.2015.00054] [PMID: 26442283]

[123] Fu H, Hardy J, Duff KE. Selective vulnerability in neurodegenerative diseases. Nat Neurosci 2018; 21(10): 1350-8.
[http://dx.doi.org/10.1038/s41593-018-0221-2] [PMID: 30250262]

[124] Verber NS, Shepheard SR, Sassani M, *et al.* Biomarkers in motor neuron disease: A state of the art review. Front Neurol 2019; 10: 291.
[http://dx.doi.org/10.3389/fneur.2019.00291] [PMID: 31001186]

[125] Sproviero D, La Salvia S, Giannini M, *et al.* Pathological proteins are transported by extracellular vesicles of sporadic amyotrophic lateral sclerosis patients. Front Neurosci 2018; 12: 487.
[http://dx.doi.org/10.3389/fnins.2018.00487] [PMID: 30072868]

[126] He L, Hannon GJ. MicroRNAs: small RNAs with a big role in gene regulation. Nat Rev Genet 2004; 5(7): 522-31.
[http://dx.doi.org/10.1038/nrg1379] [PMID: 15211354]

[127] Eacker SM, Dawson TM, Dawson VL. Understanding microRNAs in neurodegeneration. Nat Rev Neurosci 2009; 10(12): 837-41.
[http://dx.doi.org/10.1038/nrn2726] [PMID: 19904280]

[128] Maciotta S, Meregalli M, Torrente Y. The involvement of microRNAs in neurodegenerative diseases. Front Cell Neurosci 2013; 7: 265.
[http://dx.doi.org/10.3389/fncel.2013.00265] [PMID: 24391543]

[129] Quinlan S, Kenny A, Medina M, Engel T, Jimenez-Mateos EM. Micrornas in neurodegenerative

diseases. Int Rev Cell Mol Biol 2017; 334: 309-43.
[http://dx.doi.org/10.1016/bs.ircmb.2017.04.002] [PMID: 28838542]

[130] Sheinerman KS, Umansky SR. Circulating cell-free microRNA as biomarkers for screening, diagnosis
and monitoring of neurodegenerative diseases and other neurologic pathologies. Front Cell Neurosci
2013; 7: 150.
[http://dx.doi.org/10.3389/fncel.2013.00150] [PMID: 24058335]

[131] Sheinerman KS, Umansky SR. Early detection of neurodegenerative diseases: circulating brain-
enriched microRNA. Cell Cycle 2013; 12(1): 1-2.
[http://dx.doi.org/10.4161/cc.23067] [PMID: 23255116]

[132] Sheinerman KS, Toledo JB, Tsivinsky VG, *et al.* Circulating brain-enriched microRNAs as novel
biomarkers for detection and differentiation of neurodegenerative diseases. Alzheimers Res Ther 2017;
9(1): 89.
[http://dx.doi.org/10.1186/s13195-017-0316-0] [PMID: 29121998]

[133] Lee JY, Kim H-S. Extracellular Vesicles in Neurodegenerative Diseases: A Double-Edged Sword.
Tissue Eng Regen Med 2017; 14(6): 667-78.
[http://dx.doi.org/10.1007/s13770-017-0090-x] [PMID: 30603519]

[134] Blennow K. A Review of Fluid Biomarkers for Alzheimer's Disease: Moving from CSF to Blood.
Neurol Ther 2017; 6 (Suppl. 1): 15-24.
[http://dx.doi.org/10.1007/s40120-017-0073-9] [PMID: 28733960]

[135] Blennow K, Zetterberg H. Biomarkers for Alzheimer's disease: current status and prospects for the
future. J Intern Med 2018; 284(6): 643-63.
[http://dx.doi.org/10.1111/joim.12816] [PMID: 30051512]

[136] Olsson B, Lautner R, Andreasson U, *et al.* CSF and blood biomarkers for the diagnosis of Alzheimer's
disease: a systematic review and meta-analysis. Lancet Neurol 2016; 15(7): 673-84.
[http://dx.doi.org/10.1016/S1474-4422(16)00070-3] [PMID: 27068280]

[137] Casaletto KB, Elahi FM, Bettcher BM, *et al.* Neurogranin, a synaptic protein, is associated with
memory independent of Alzheimer biomarkers. Neurology 2017; 89(17): 1782-8.
[http://dx.doi.org/10.1212/WNL.0000000000004569] [PMID: 28939668]

[138] Wellington H, Paterson RW, Portelius E, *et al.* Increased CSF neurogranin concentration is specific to
Alzheimer disease. Neurology 2016; 86(9): 829-35.
[http://dx.doi.org/10.1212/WNL.0000000000002423] [PMID: 26826204]

[139] Aghili Z, Nasirizadeh N, Divsalar A, Shoeibi S, Yaghmaei P. A highly sensitive miR-195
nanobiosensor for early detection of Parkinson's disease. Artif Cells Nanomed Biotechnol 2017; •••:
1-9.
[PMID: 29214873]

[140] Azimzadeh M, Nasirizadeh N, Rahaie M, Naderi-Manesh H. Early detection of Alzheimer's disease
using a biosensor based on electrochemically-reduced graphene oxide and gold nanowires for the
quantification of serum microRNA-137. RSC Advances 2017; 7(88): 55709-19.
[http://dx.doi.org/10.1039/C7RA09767K]

[141] Joilin G, Leigh PN, Newbury SF, Hafezparast M. An overview of micrornas as biomarkers of ALS.
Front Neurol 2019; 10: 186.
[http://dx.doi.org/10.3389/fneur.2019.00186] [PMID: 30899244]

[142] Reed ER, Latourelle JC, Bockholt JH, *et al.* MicroRNAs in CSF as prodromal biomarkers for
Huntington disease in the PREDICT-HD study. Neurology 2018; 90(4): e264-72.
[http://dx.doi.org/10.1212/WNL.0000000000004844] [PMID: 29282329]

[143] Atik A, Stewart T, Zhang J. Alpha-Synuclein as a Biomarker for Parkinson's Disease. Brain Pathol
2016; 26(3): 410-8.
[http://dx.doi.org/10.1111/bpa.12370] [PMID: 26940058]

[144] Tokuda T, Qureshi MM, Ardah MT, *et al.* Detection of elevated levels of α-synuclein oligomers in CSF from patients with Parkinson disease. Neurology 2010; 75(20): 1766-72.
[http://dx.doi.org/10.1212/WNL.0b013e3181fd613b] [PMID: 20962290]

[145] Hardiman O, Al-Chalabi A, Chio A, *et al.* Amyotrophic lateral sclerosis. Nat Rev Dis Primers 2017; 3: 17071.
[http://dx.doi.org/10.1038/nrdp.2017.71] [PMID: 28980624]

[146] Khalil M, Teunissen CE, Otto M, *et al.* Neurofilaments as biomarkers in neurological disorders. Nat Rev Neurol 2018; 14(10): 577-89.
[http://dx.doi.org/10.1038/s41582-018-0058-z] [PMID: 30171200]

[147] Lu C-H, Macdonald-Wallis C, Gray E, *et al.* Neurofilament light chain: A prognostic biomarker in amyotrophic lateral sclerosis. Neurology 2015; 84(22): 2247-57.
[http://dx.doi.org/10.1212/WNL.0000000000001642] [PMID: 25934855]

[148] Steinacker P, Feneberg E, Weishaupt J, *et al.* Neurofilaments in the diagnosis of motoneuron diseases: a prospective study on 455 patients. J Neurol Neurosurg Psychiatry 2016; 87(1): 12-20.
[PMID: 26296871]

[149] Benatar M, Wuu J, Andersen PM, Lombardi V, Malaspina A. Neurofilament light: A candidate biomarker of presymptomatic amyotrophic lateral sclerosis and phenoconversion. Ann Neurol 2018; 84(1): 130-9.
[http://dx.doi.org/10.1002/ana.25276] [PMID: 30014505]

[150] Byrne LM, Rodrigues FB, Blennow K, *et al.* Neurofilament light protein in blood as a potential biomarker of neurodegeneration in Huntington's disease: a retrospective cohort analysis. Lancet Neurol 2017; 16(8): 601-9.
[http://dx.doi.org/10.1016/S1474-4422(17)30124-2] [PMID: 28601473]

[151] Soylu-Kucharz R, Sandelius Å, Sjögren M, *et al.* Neurofilament light protein in CSF and blood is associated with neurodegeneration and disease severity in Huntington's disease R6/2 mice. Sci Rep 2017; 7(1): 14114.
[http://dx.doi.org/10.1038/s41598-017-14179-1] [PMID: 29074982]

[152] Wild EJ, Boggio R, Langbehn D, *et al.* Quantification of mutant huntingtin protein in cerebrospinal fluid from Huntington's disease patients. J Clin Invest 2015; 125(5): 1979-86.
[http://dx.doi.org/10.1172/JCI80743] [PMID: 25844897]

[153] Wimo A, Jönsson L, Bond J, Prince M, Winblad B. The worldwide economic impact of dementia 2010. Alzheimers Dement 2013; 9(1): 1-11.e3.
[http://dx.doi.org/10.1016/j.jalz.2012.11.006] [PMID: 23305821]

[154] Shui B, Tao D, Florea A, *et al.* Biosensors for Alzheimer's disease biomarker detection: A review. Biochimie 2018; 147: 13-24.
[http://dx.doi.org/10.1016/j.biochi.2017.12.015] [PMID: 29307704]

[155] Wang SX, Acha D, Shah AJ, *et al.* Detection of the tau protein in human serum by a sensitive four-electrode electrochemical biosensor. Biosens Bioelectron 2017; 92: 482-8.
[http://dx.doi.org/10.1016/j.bios.2016.10.077] [PMID: 27829556]

[156] Hammond JL, Rosamond MC, Sivaraya S, Marken F, Estrela P. Fabrication of a horizontal and a vertical large surface area nanogap electrochemical sensor. Sensors (Basel) 2016; 16(12)E2128
[http://dx.doi.org/10.3390/s16122128] [PMID: 27983655]

[157] Veloso A, Kerman K. Advances in electrochemical detection for study of neurodegenerative disorders. Anal Bioanal Chem 2013; 405(17): 5725-41.
[http://dx.doi.org/10.1007/s00216-013-6904-3] [PMID: 23529415]

[158] Yue HY, Huang S, Chang J, *et al.* ZnO nanowire arrays on 3D hierachical graphene foam: biomarker detection of Parkinson's disease. ACS Nano 2014; 8(2): 1639-46.
[http://dx.doi.org/10.1021/nn405961p] [PMID: 24405012]

[159] An Y, Tang L, Jiang X, *et al.* A photoelectrochemical immunosensor based on Au-doped TiO2 nanotube arrays for the detection of α-synuclein. Chemistry 2010; 16(48): 14439-46.
[http://dx.doi.org/10.1002/chem.201001654] [PMID: 21038326]

[160] Sierks MR, Chatterjee G, McGraw C, Kasturirangan S, Schulz P, Prasad S. CSF levels of oligomeric alpha-synuclein and beta-amyloid as biomarkers for neurodegenerative disease. Integr Biol 2011; 3(12): 1188-96.
[http://dx.doi.org/10.1039/c1ib00018g] [PMID: 22076255]

[161] Ryu J, Joung H-A, Kim M-G, Park CB. Surface plasmon resonance analysis of Alzheimer's beta-amyloid aggregation on a solid surface: from monomers to fully-grown fibrils. Anal Chem 2008; 80(7): 2400-7.
[http://dx.doi.org/10.1021/ac7019514] [PMID: 18303863]

[162] Yi X, Feng C, Hu S, Li H, Wang J. Surface plasmon resonance biosensors for simultaneous monitoring of amyloid-beta oligomers and fibrils and screening of select modulators. Analyst (Lond) 2016; 141(1): 331-6.
[http://dx.doi.org/10.1039/C5AN01864A] [PMID: 26613550]

[163] Palladino P, Aura AM, Spoto G. Surface plasmon resonance for the label-free detection of Alzheimer's β-amyloid peptide aggregation. Anal Bioanal Chem 2016; 408(3): 849-54.
[http://dx.doi.org/10.1007/s00216-015-9172-6] [PMID: 26558762]

[164] Haes AJ, Van Duyne RP. A unified view of propagating and localized surface plasmon resonance biosensors. Anal Bioanal Chem 2004; 379(7-8): 920-30.
[http://dx.doi.org/10.1007/s00216-004-2708-9] [PMID: 15338088]

[165] Vestergaard M, Kerman K, Kim D-K, Ha MH, Tamiya E. Detection of Alzheimer's tau protein using localised surface plasmon resonance-based immunochip. Talanta 2008; 74(4): 1038-42.
[http://dx.doi.org/10.1016/j.talanta.2007.06.009] [PMID: 18371746]

[166] Kang MK, Lee J, Nguyen AH, Sim SJ. Label-free detection of ApoE4-mediated β-amyloid aggregation on single nanoparticle uncovering Alzheimer's disease. Biosens Bioelectron 2015; 72: 197-204.
[http://dx.doi.org/10.1016/j.bios.2015.05.017] [PMID: 25982728]

[167] Kim H, Lee JU, Song S, Kim S, Sim SJ. A shape-code nanoplasmonic biosensor for multiplex detection of Alzheimer's disease biomarkers. Biosens Bioelectron 2018; 101: 96-102.
[http://dx.doi.org/10.1016/j.bios.2017.10.018] [PMID: 29054022]

[168] Michalet X, Pinaud FF, Bentolila LA, *et al.* Quantum dots for live cells, *in vivo* imaging, and diagnostics. Science 2005; 307(5709): 538-44.
[http://dx.doi.org/10.1126/science.1104274] [PMID: 15681376]

[169] Ankireddy SR, Kim J. Selective detection of dopamine in the presence of ascorbic acid via fluorescence quenching of InP/ZnS quantum dots. Int J Nanomedicine 2015; 10(Spec Iss): 113-9.
[PMID: 26347250]

[170] Ma W, Qin L-X, Liu F-T, *et al.* Ubiquinone-quantum dot bioconjugates for *in vitro* and intracellular complex I sensing. Sci Rep 2013; 3: 1537.
[http://dx.doi.org/10.1038/srep01537] [PMID: 23524384]

[171] Xia N, Zhou B, Huang N, Jiang M, Zhang J, Liu L. Visual and fluorescent assays for selective detection of beta-amyloid oligomers based on the inner filter effect of gold nanoparticles on the fluorescence of CdTe quantum dots. Biosens Bioelectron 2016; 85: 625-32.
[http://dx.doi.org/10.1016/j.bios.2016.05.066] [PMID: 27240009]

[172] Wilson DH, Rissin DM, Kan CW, *et al.* The Simoa HD-1 Analyzer: A Novel Fully Automated Digital Immunoassay Analyzer with Single-Molecule Sensitivity and Multiplexing. J Lab Autom 2016; 21(4): 533-47.
[http://dx.doi.org/10.1177/2211068215589580] [PMID: 26077162]

[173] Strydom A, Heslegrave A, Startin CM, *et al.* Neurofilament light as a blood biomarker for neurodegeneration in Down syndrome. Alzheimers Res Ther 2018; 10(1): 39.
[http://dx.doi.org/10.1186/s13195-018-0367-x] [PMID: 29631614]

[174] Rissin DM, Kan CW, Campbell TG, *et al.* Single-molecule enzyme-linked immunosorbent assay detects serum proteins at subfemtomolar concentrations. Nat Biotechnol 2010; 28(6): 595-9.
[http://dx.doi.org/10.1038/nbt.1641] [PMID: 20495550]

[175] Hong C-Y, Wu CC, Chiu YC, Yang SY, Horng HE, Yang HC. Magnetic susceptibility reduction method for magnetically labeled immunoassay. Appl Phys Lett 2006; 88(21)212512
[http://dx.doi.org/10.1063/1.2206557]

[176] Yang S-Y, Chiu M-J, Chen T-F, Horng H-E. Detection of plasma biomarkers using immunomagnetic reduction: A promising method for the early diagnosis of alzheimer's disease. Neurol Ther 2017; 6 (Suppl. 1): 37-56.
[http://dx.doi.org/10.1007/s40120-017-0075-7] [PMID: 28733955]

[177] Yang S-Y, Chiu M-J, Chen T-F, *et al.* Analytical performance of reagent for assaying tau protein in human plasma and feasibility study screening neurodegenerative diseases. Sci Rep 2017; 7(1): 9304.
[http://dx.doi.org/10.1038/s41598-017-09009-3] [PMID: 28839167]

[178] Kalani A, Tyagi A, Tyagi N. Exosomes: mediators of neurodegeneration, neuroprotection and therapeutics. Mol Neurobiol 2014; 49(1): 590-600.
[http://dx.doi.org/10.1007/s12035-013-8544-1] [PMID: 23999871]

[179] Théry C, Amigorena S, Raposo G, Clayton A. Isolation and characterization of exosomes from cell culture supernatants and biological fluids. 2006.
[http://dx.doi.org/10.1002/0471143030.cb0322s30]

[180] Contreras-Naranjo JC, Wu H-J, Ugaz VM. Microfluidics for exosome isolation and analysis: enabling liquid biopsy for personalized medicine. Lab Chip 2017; 17(21): 3558-77.
[http://dx.doi.org/10.1039/C7LC00592J] [PMID: 28832692]

[181] Liga A, Vliegenthart ADB, Oosthuyzen W, Dear JW, Kersaudy-Kerhoas M. Exosome isolation: a microfluidic road-map. Lab Chip 2015; 15(11): 2388-94.
[http://dx.doi.org/10.1039/C5LC00240K] [PMID: 25940789]

[182] Yoo YK, Lee J, Kim H, Hwang KS, Yoon DS, Lee JH. Toward Exosome-Based Neuronal Diagnostic Devices. Micromachines (Basel) 2018; 9(12)E634
[http://dx.doi.org/10.3390/mi9120634] [PMID: 30501125]

[183] Fraikin J-L, Teesalu T, McKenney CM, Ruoslahti E, Cleland AN. A high-throughput label-free nanoparticle analyser. Nat Nanotechnol 2011; 6(5): 308-13.
[http://dx.doi.org/10.1038/nnano.2011.24] [PMID: 21378975]

[184] Zhou Q, Rahimian A, Son K, Shin D-S, Patel T, Revzin A. Development of an aptasensor for electrochemical detection of exosomes. Methods 2016; 97: 88-93.
[http://dx.doi.org/10.1016/j.ymeth.2015.10.012] [PMID: 26500145]

[185] Sina AAI, Vaidyanathan R, Dey S, Carrascosa LG, Shiddiky MJA, Trau M. Real time and label free profiling of clinically relevant exosomes. Sci Rep 2016; 6: 30460.
[http://dx.doi.org/10.1038/srep30460] [PMID: 27464736]

[186] Im H, Shao H, Park YI, *et al.* Label-free detection and molecular profiling of exosomes with a nano-plasmonic sensor. Nat Biotechnol 2014; 32(5): 490-5.
[http://dx.doi.org/10.1038/nbt.2886] [PMID: 24752081]

[187] Dudani JS, Gossett DR, Tse HTK, Lamm RJ, Kulkarni RP, Carlo DD. Rapid inertial solution exchange for enrichment and flow cytometric detection of microvesicles. Biomicrofluidics 2015; 9(1)014112
[http://dx.doi.org/10.1063/1.4907807] [PMID: 25713694]

[188] Ko J, Hemphill MA, Gabrieli D, *et al.* Smartphone-enabled optofluidic exosome diagnostic for concussion recovery. Sci Rep 2016; 6: 31215.
[http://dx.doi.org/10.1038/srep31215] [PMID: 27498963]

[189] Hampel H, O'Bryant SE, Molinuevo JL, *et al.* Blood-based biomarkers for Alzheimer disease: mapping the road to the clinic. Nat Rev Neurol 2018; 14(11): 639-52.
[http://dx.doi.org/10.1038/s41582-018-0079-7] [PMID: 30297701]

[190] Kawata K, Liu CY, Merkel SF, Ramirez SH, Tierney RT, Langford D. Blood biomarkers for brain injury: What are we measuring? Neurosci Biobehav Rev 2016; 68: 460-73.
[http://dx.doi.org/10.1016/j.neubiorev.2016.05.009] [PMID: 27181909]

[191] Nation DA, Sweeney MD, Montagne A, *et al.* Blood-brain barrier breakdown is an early biomarker of human cognitive dysfunction. Nat Med 2019; 25(2): 270-6.
[http://dx.doi.org/10.1038/s41591-018-0297-y] [PMID: 30643288]

[192] Molinuevo JL, Ayton S, Batrla R, *et al.* Current state of Alzheimer's fluid biomarkers. Acta Neuropathol 2018 Nov; 28 Nov; 136(6): 821-53.
[http://dx.doi.org/10.1007/s00401-018-1932-x] [PMID: 30488277]

CHAPTER 11

DNA Sensors for Diagnosis of Infectious Diseases

Lærke Bay Marcussen[1,2,#], Kamilla Vandsø Petersen[2,#], Birgitta Ruth Knudsen[2] and Marianne Smedegaard Hede[3,*]

[1] *Department of Biomedicine, Aarhus University, Denmark*

[2] *Department of Molecular Biology and Genetics, Aarhus University, Denmark*

[3] *VPCIR.COM, Denmark*

Abstract: Infectious diseases are the cause of more than 5 million deaths annually, which corresponds to approximately 10% of all deaths worldwide. Rapid and reliable diagnosis is a key aspect in reducing the number of deaths associated with infectious diseases since fast commencement of the correct treatment will not only improve patient survival but also reduce the risk of spreading the disease. Moreover, fast and reliable diagnosis prevent the wrong medicine from being prescribed, something that otherwise may lead to hmedication overuse and increased drug resistance. DNA based sensors are a group of diagnostic sensors that have attracted much attention due to their potentials for specific, sensitive, and fast detection of disease associated target molecules. In the following chapter, we will go through examples of different DNA sensors and describe the wide variety of readout systems that have been applied for DNA-sensor mediated detection of infectious diseases.

Keywords: DNA-sensors, Diagnostics, Infectious diseases, Pathogen detection.

INTRODUCTION

Infectious diseases are caused by microorganisms, also called pathogens, which are infectious agents for particular diseases. These pathogens include bacteria, viruses, fungi and the unicellular and multicellular eukaryotic organisms collectively termed parasites. The infectious diseases are typically identified through a diagnostic test that allows the detection of presence or absence of a pathogen by recognizing specific variables, more precisely the molecular biomarkers which include proteins, small metabolites, nucleotide sequences, cytokines *etc.* Theoretically, all biomarkers which can distinguish pathogens from non-pathogens are potential indicators of infectious diseases and can be utilized

---

* **Corresponding author Marianne Smedegaard Hede:** VPCIR.COM, Denmark; E-mail: msh@vpcir.com[#] The authors contributed equally to the work

Han-Sheng Chuang & Yi-Ping Ho (Eds.)

for diagnostic examinations, besides being useful for monitoring response to therapy and potentially predicting therapeutic outcomes. The availability of a reliable, rapid, specific and sensitive diagnostic test is therefore crucial, because it gives the clinicians the ability to fast diagnose the disease onset, which may affect therapy effectiveness, and avoid long-term complications and pathogen transmissions, thereby limiting the risk of epidemics and pandemics. Furthermore, fast and precise diagnosis has the possibility to reduce cases of unnecessary usage of broad-spectrum antibiotics and hopefully decrease the pathogen resistance to antibiotics.

The ideal biomarker presents specific characteristics of the pathogen which offers the possibility to develop a biosensor for detection of these recognition elements in a specific and sensitive manner. Depending on the pathogen of interest, the discovery of suitable biomarkers can be achieved by several approaches including biomolecule screening techniques and bioinformatics analysis. Samples used for diagnostic examination can be body fluids, biopsies or swaps. Development of biosensors has been a challenging task due to the limited quantity of biomarkers in biological samples. To address the challenge, an array of amplification systems has been developed for the enhancement of detection sensitivity.

Numerous biosensors targeting different biomarkers have been developed for detection of pathogens and some have been approved by the Food and Drug Administration (FDA) in the United States as medical devices for point of care diagnostic tests. This chapter is aimed to review examples of technical approaches that have been used for developing DNA based biomolecular sensors able to detect biomarkers for specific disease-causing pathogens. Several amplification systems used for signal enhancement and selected readout strategies are also covered.

DNA BASED BIOMOLECULAR SENSORS

DNA used as biosensors can be categorized in multiple ways. In this section they are classified into two groups. The first group is based on catalytic activity inherent in the DNA itself *e.g.* DNAzymes [1]. When such sensors recognize specific biomarkers, the biomarkers are converted to detectable products, while the sensor itself is left unchanged. The second type of DNA based biosensors can react with one or more molecules resulting in detectable changes in the biosensors. Selected examples are presented in this section.

DNA Biomolecules with Inherent Activity for the Detection

DNAzymes

Deoxyribozymes, also named DNAzymes, are single-stranded DNA molecules identified to perform different chemical reactions often with catalytic activity. They can be designed to perform various functions, including oxidative or hydrolytic DNA cleavage, DNA/RNA ligation, DNA phosphorylation, and RNA cleavage [2].

RNA-cleaving DNAzymes are among the most studied groups. These are comprised of an inherent catalytic core of varying length and secondary-structure complexity with two flanked substrate-binding domains (Fig. **1**). They catalyze a site-specific cleavage of RNA molecules at a particular phosphodiester location between unpaired purine and a paired pyrimidine residues. The mechanism is dependent on cofactors but does not need activity from any other molecules. After cleaving the target RNA molecule, the DNAzyme-RNA-complex dissociates and the DNAzyme is able to subsequently bind and cleave additional RNA molecules allowing signal amplification [1, 3]. DNAzymes are not known to exist in nature but can be isolated by *in vitro* selection from random catalytic DNA sequence pools [3]. By changing the sequence of the substrate-recognition domains, the specificity of the DNA enzyme can be modified to target different RNA substrates. This can be utilized for the diagnosis of infectious diseases based on the detection of RNAs in pathogens [4].

The DNAzyme contains a catalytic core (depicted yellow in Fig. (**1**)) and two flanking substrate-recognition arms (black) which bind target mRNA. The DNAzyme catalyses the cleavage reaction on mRNA substrate which subsequently dissociates allowing the DNAzyme to perform an additional cleavage cycle.

To date, RNA-cleaving DNAzymes have been developed to recognize specific bacterial pathogens such as *Escherichia coli* and *Clostridium difficile* [5]. The method includes labeling of DNAzymes with a fluorophore and quencher adjacent to the RNA cleavage site, which makes the DNAzyme activity directly measurable [6]. A high recognition specificity is achieved by using a double selection approach in which a DNA library is negatively selected against the cellular mixture prepared from unintended (non-target) bacteria, followed by a positive selection against the same mixture derived from a specific bacterial pathogen that is the target for detection [7]. The DNAzymes have the disadvantage of possibly creating off-targets resulting in false positives or negatives. But they also present several advantages based on the thermal stability, ease of production, modification and the possibility of labeling for directly detection.

Many variations of DNAzyme design have been reported. For example the incorporation of aptamers to increase specificity or the use of urea hydrolization in order to ease detection [8]. In addition to the intrinsic properties of DNAzymes as enzymes they are also compatible with DNA amplification techniques which will make the technique even more sensitive [2, 3]. Systems for amplification and readout strategies will be described later in this chapter.

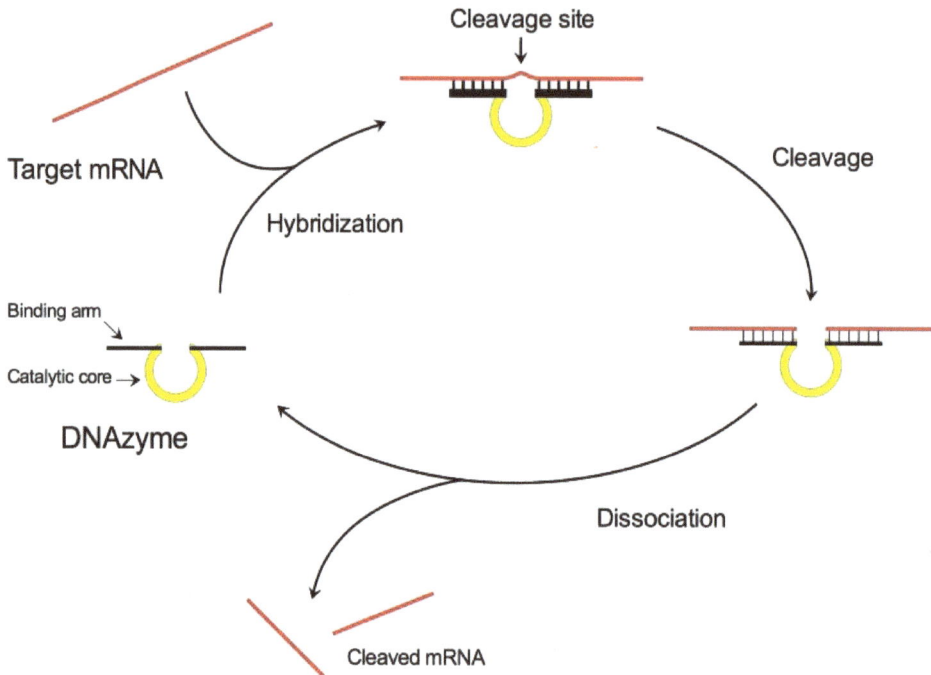

Fig. (1). Representative illustration of DNAzyme-based mRNA cleavage.

Sensors Based on DNA Conformational Changes

Aptamers

Aptamers find their applications in specific detection of a wide range of targets ranging from small molecules and proteins to whole cells and viruses. Biosensors based on aptamers are often called aptasensors. They consist of either a short single-stranded DNA sequence, RNA or peptide molecules which can be selected by *in vitro* techniques to bind the target molecule of interest [9, 10].

It is possible to construct or isolate nucleic aptamers through a variety of methods but most frequently by *in vitro* selection using a technique known as SELEX

(Systematic Evolution of Ligands using Exponential Enrichment), discovered by Gold and Szostak in the 1990s [11, 12] (Fig. **2**). The SELEX methodology comprises steps that are repeated in order to search for nucleotides that bind with the highest affinity to the target molecule. The steps are selection, elution and amplification. First, the target molecule of interest is incubated with a large library of random oligonucleotides. The bound target molecules are separated from the unbound library components. In the case of proteins, the aptamers can distinguish between closely related but non-identical proteins by molecular recognition binding mechanisms of structure compatibility, induced fit, hydrogen bridges and electrostatic interactions. This step is generally coupled with several other methods to increase the specificity to the target molecule. In the last step of the SELEX cycle, polymerase chain reaction (PCR) amplification is used to create a new library of the target-bound library components to be used in the next selection round [11].

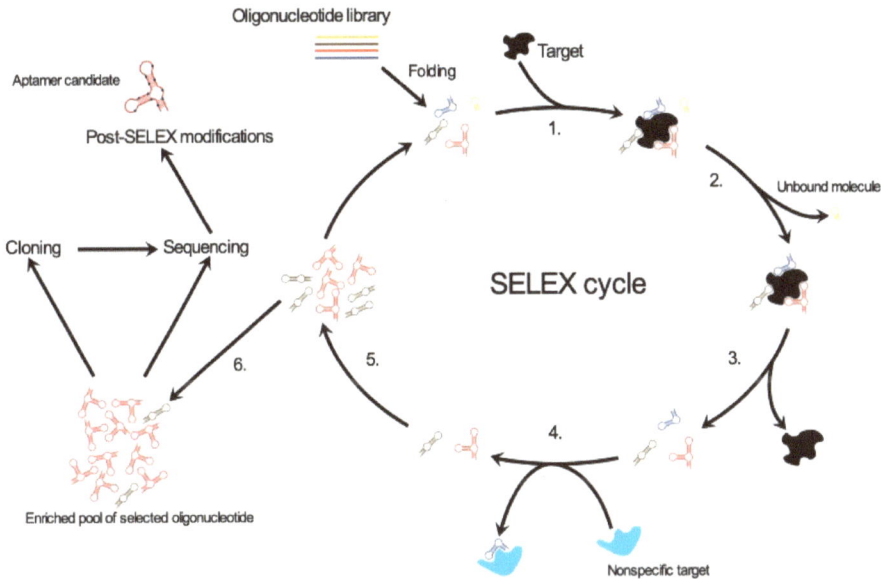

Fig. (2). Schematic representation of the basic principle of SELEX. **1.** The target molecule of interest is incubated with a large library of folded single stranded oligonucleotides. **2.** The three-dimensional structure of the oligonucleotide binds to specific regions on the target molecule while unbound molecules are removed by a washing step (positive selection). **3.** The target-bound oligonucleotides are eluted. **4.** Additional steps can be performed as the negative selection to exclude unspecific binding *e.g.* by incubation with nonspecific target molecules, as illustrated in this figure. **5.** The remaining nucleic acids are amplified by PCR and denatured into single strands to create a new library for the next selection round. **6.** After the last round of SELEX an enriched pool of the selected oligonucleotide is produced and can be cloned using plasmids and sequenced. At last affinity information can be obtained by further analysis and post-SELEX modifications can be performed. The number of screenings is determined by the type of library and the degree of enrichment of the specific sequence obtained from each cycle.

It is also possible to design a multiplexed scheme to detect a variety of aptamer-target reactions simultaneously [13]. Furthermore, negative selection is often executed to improve target specificity. In this process the oligonucleotide library is incubated with nonspecific target molecules, excluding those that bind unspecific to such off targets.

Selected aptamers are cloned and sequenced to identify sequences or secondary/tertiary structures that interact with target molecules. This step may be followed by larger scale productions with great accuracy [14]. A great advantage of aptamers is the ability of modification by various chemical reactions to increase stability, binding efficiency and nuclease resistance which extends the degradation time [15]. Also, it has the advantage of allowing direct detection as well as being compatible with amplification systems which makes the technique more sensitive [10].

Since the high affinity and specificity for some ligands cannot be recognized by antibodies such as ions or small molecules, these nucleic acids based aptasensors are often called "chemical antibodies". They are beneficial for POC tests for the detection of target pathogens causing various infectious diseases because of the benefits of great stability, selectivity and sensitivity [16].

The recognition components may be pathogen related toxins or proteins, whole cells or nucleic acids. Many aptamers have been applied to preclinical studies which indicates the great potential of oligonucleotide aptamers as a diagnostic tool. Some of the nucleic aptamers designed to detect human pathogens in specific ways are listed below in Table **1**.

Table 1. Overview of selected nucleic acid aptamers for detection of pathogenic organisms [17 - 20].

Nucleic Acid Aptamers				
Gram Positive Bacteria	**Gram Negative Bacteria**	**Viruses**	**Protozoa**	**Fungi**
Staphylococcus aureus	*Escherichia coli*	*Avian influenza virus*	*Plasmodium falciparum*	Several species of *Penicillium* genus
Campylobacter jejuni	*Vibrio parahemolyticus*	*Human immunodeficiency virus (HIV)*	*Schistosoma japonicum*	Several species of the *Aspergillus* genus
Listeria monocytoges	*Salmonella enterica*	*SARS coronavirus*	*Leishmania infantum*	*Fusarium* genus

(Table 1) cont.....

Nucleic Acid Aptamers				
Gram Positive Bacteria	Gram Negative Bacteria	Viruses	Protozoa	Fungi
Lactobacillus acidophilus	Francisella tularesis	Human papillomavirus (HPV)	Cryptosporidium parvum	
Streptococcus pyrogenes	Pseudomonas aeruginosa	Hepatitis B virus Hepatitis C virus	Trypanosoma spp.	
*Mycobacterium tuberculosis	*Mycobacterium tuberculosis	Ebola virus		
Bifidobacterium bifidum		Chikungunya		
Bacillus antracia				
Bacillus thuringiensis				

*are both Gram positive and Gram negative [21].

The sensing systems for the nucleic acid aptamer-based detection of pathogenic components can be done by incorporating different signal transducers which can be measured either directly or using signal amplifying tools *e.g.* isothermal nucleic amplification systems.

Enzymatic Biosensors

Concerning biochemistry, a substrate is a molecule upon which an enzyme catalyzes a reaction. Enzymes are capable of recognizing only a specific substrate or a class of substrates enabling specific reactions. Hence, pathogen derived nucleic acid modifying enzymes present in a sample can be detected by detecting their interaction with one or more specially designed nucleic acid substrates.

In the case of a single substrate, the enzyme binds the substrate and creates an enzyme-substrate-complex followed by the transformation of the substrate into products. The enzyme is released and able to react with another available substrate. Thus, a continuous transformation of substrates into products may be achieved, given that sufficient amount of substrates are available. To detect a specific pathogen, substrates can be created to match the activity of an enzyme biomarker specific for a pathogenic bacteria, fungi or protozoa [18].

Primers and Probes

Pathogens causing infectious diseases are frequently detectable by their unique nucleic acid sequences which can be identified by different techniques. The principle of the individual variants can be utilized to distinguish among various pathogens and non-pathogens which can be useful for diagnostic POC tests [22].

By knowing the unique target sequence, it is possible to design a probe, a short synthetic DNA or RNA sequence, which spontaneously hybridizes by Watson-Crick base pairing [23]. This can be performed in either solution or on solid support. The different techniques are often performed at different temperatures and in order to avoid unspecific hybridization, the annealing temperature must be taken into account. Various labeling techniques can be developed for measurements of the bound probe. However, sensitivity of this procedure may be challenging and amplification may be necessary [24]. This can be done by designing a primer, short oligonucleotide sequence, which functions as a starting point for DNA/RNA synthesis. This results in the generation of a copy of the target strand and can be utilized for amplification of the signal. Since, the primer is elongated from the 3' end it gives the opportunity to label the 5' end. The principle of using primers and DNA/RNA synthesis has been used in many different amplification systems [15].

AMPLIFICATION SYSTEMS

Biological samples often contain limited material for the measurement. Therefore, diagnostic tests usually require one or more amplification steps to make the detection possible or more distinguishable from the background noise. Sensitive diagnostic tests are desirable because early treatment at the disease onset will lower the risk of transmission and death. Increased sensitivity can be achieved by various amplification systems, such as (quantitative)polymerase chain reaction (q)PCR, rolling circle amplification (RCA) and loop-mediated isothermal amplification (LAMP) [25].

Polymerase Chain reaction (PCR)

PCR relies on an enzyme-driven process for amplifying short DNA sequences *in vitro*. It employs predesigned oligonucleotide primers complementary to a specific pathogenic nucleic sequence. It is well known that PCR enables exponential growth in the number of copies of the pathogenic target DNA through multiple reaction cycles. The process consists of three steps, DNA strand separation (denaturation), primer hybridization, and primer extension by DNA synthesis. One cycle is carried out by repetitively changing the temperature of the reaction mixture, resulting in two double-stranded DNA molecules identical to the target sequence [26].

First, the two strands of the parent DNA molecule are separated by heating. Second, two primers anneal - one at each end, thereby flanking the target DNA. In the last step, DNA synthesis is carried out by a thermostable DNA polymerase. This is done by catalyzing growth from the DNA primers which are extended toward each other. Each cycle creates two double-stranded DNA molecules identical to the target sequence and thereby the target DNA is exponentially amplified, even from one single copy. This makes the technique very sensitive and useful for diagnostics by using primers specific for the pathogens causing infectious diseases [22]. Subsequently, the amplified products can be detected and analyzed by different processing techniques.

An alternative approach to the traditional PCR is termed qPCR or real-time PCR. This approach allows real-time measurement of DNA synthesis by using labelling methods generating a signal recorded during each cycle [27]. The choice of labeling depends on the compatibility of the experimental design. With qPCR the number of starting templates can be quantified by comparing the exact cycle number at which amplified products formed significantly over baseline with a pre-derived standard. The practical advantages of qPCR compared to the conventional PCR include speed, simplicity, reproducibility and quantitative capacity. The drawbacks are the complexity of the reactions that requires skilled personnel and delicate equipment.

Numerous medical devices based on the principle of PCR are approved by FDA and have been implemented as routinely infectious disease diagnostic tests *e.g. Chlamydia trachomatis, Neisseria gonorrhoeae, Streptococcus pneumoniae, Clostridium difficile* and *Mycobacteria* [28].

Another variation of the PCR principle is a technique widely used for the amplification of specific RNA sequences, termed reverse transcription PCR, (RT-PCR). The enzyme reverse transcriptase uses RNA template rather than DNA. It elongates from DNA primers which are annealed to the RNA template producing a complementary single-stranded DNA strand in a process called reverse transcription. DNA polymerase converts the single stranded DNA into double-stranded DNA,which is used as a template for amplification by standard or real-time PCR reaction, as described above [29]. RT-PCR can be used for determination of the presence of RNA in a sample, thus, it is a potential diagnostic tool. An example of this is viral RNA, *e.g.* the Zika virus. DNA primers specific for the envelope region of the Zika virus genome can anneal and be used for RT-PCR followed by real-time PCR [30].

The PCR-based techniques, in general, have the disadvantage of the requirement of controlled heating and cooling cycles, thus specialized heat-stable DNA polymerases are needed, which limits its applicability. Yet, different isothermal amplification systems have been developed. Examples of these are rolling circle amplification (RCA) and loop-mediated isothermal amplification (LAMP) [31, 32].

Rolling Circle Amplification (RCA)

In diagnostic tools, RCA is typically used for isothermal rapid amplification of small synthetic oligonucleotide circles. Hybridization of a complementary primer to the circle allows oligonucleotide synthesis using the circle as a template to roll upon, resulting in a long single stranded DNA product with tandem repeats of a sequence complementary to the circle sequence. The RCA-based assay gives the possibility to concentrate many signals in a localized area, thus amplifying the detection sensitivity [33]. It is possible to design circular DNA templates of interest and, consequently, also create DNA products with functional sequences, including DNA aptamers, DNAzymes, or restriction sites [34]. Many different strategies, based on the RCA principle, have been developed. An example is the DNA circle template-mediated enzymatic ligation based on the different ligation approaches of substrate oligonucleotide sequences to create a DNA circle usable as a template for RCA. A common substrate for this process is padlock probes [35] (Fig. **3**). These are single stranded DNA molecules with sequences at both ends, which are complementary to the target region. They are designed in such a way that annealing to the target sequence brings the ends of the padlock probe together without leaving any gap. Hence, the target DNA is used as a ligation template allowing the ends of the padlock probe to be ligated. This creates a circle usable for RCA with either the same target as the primer or by adding an external short DNA primer. This method is very selective due to the necessity of the padlock probe to get circularized, which requires complete hybridization of the probe to the target DNA. Various pathogen-specific enzymes have also been used to convert linear DNA molecules to closed circles that could template RCA. Such systems have been used for the detection of the malaria-causing parasite [36 - 38], tuberculosis causing *Mycobacteria* [39, 40], and the AIDS causing HIV [41]. Moreover, the system has been used to measure the activity of cancer relevant drug targets in small biological samples [42 - 45].

A.

B.

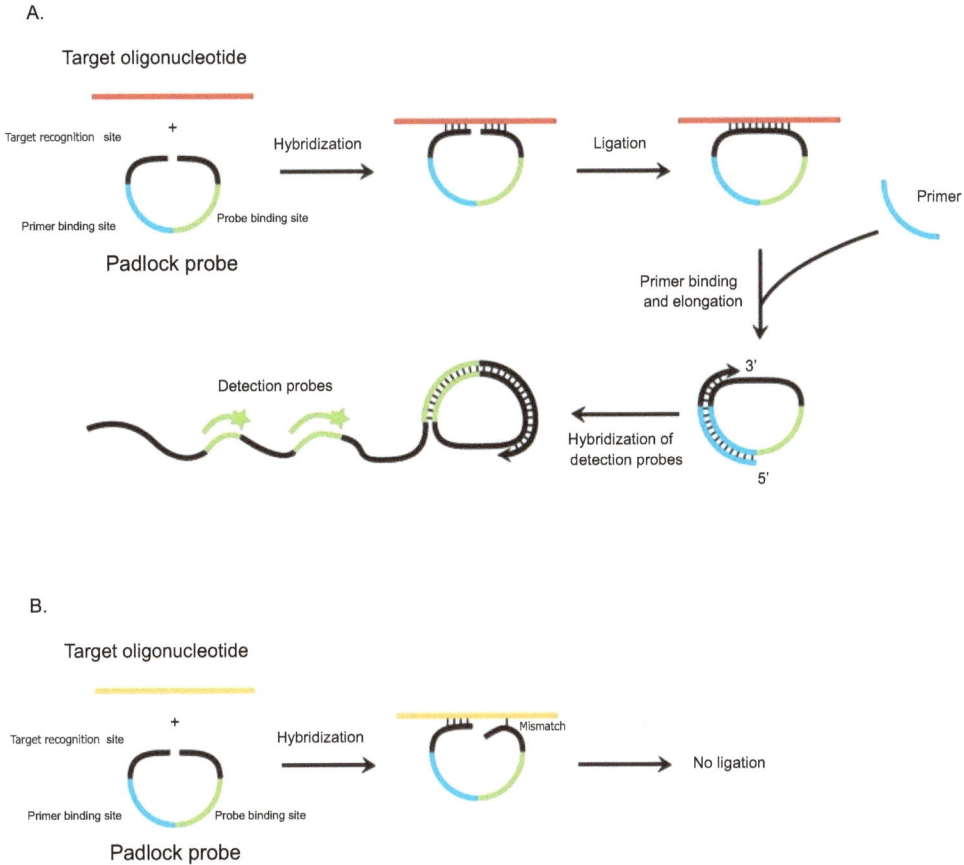

Fig. (3). Schematic representation of the rolling circle amplification (RCA) technology exemplified by padlock probes.

A. The padlock probe contains two terminal binding sites which are complementary to a target oligonucleotide strand (red). During a perfect match these two ends will hybridize to a target strand and form a closed circle by the addition of ligase. The target strand dissociates and binding of a DNA primer (blue) enables strand elongation performed by a DNA polymerase using the circularized probe as a template. The elongation step results in a long tandem single stranded RCA product containing several copies of the closed circle which can be detected through the hybridization of sequence specific fluorescently labeled probes (green) complementary to the sequence amplified. B. Mismatch between the target oligonucleotide to the padlock probe leads to no ligation, thus no circle is formed and no amplification will occur.

Loop-mediated Isothermal Amplification (LAMP)

LAMP is an isothermal amplification system which relies on an auto-cycling strand displacement of DNA synthesis [46]. Four primers are used as starting points for elongation. These consist of two inner and two outer primers which are designed to recognize six distinct regions on the target DNA sequence. At first, all four primers are used to produce two dumbbell structures, however only the inner primers are used in the elongation steps. The reaction is initiated by strand invasion by one of the inner primers (Fig. **4**). A DNA polymerase possesses strand displacement as it elongates from the primer, separating the target duplex DNA. As a result, this reaction proceeds at a constant temperature. When the strand is displaced, the 5' end product hybridizes to form a loop-structure which serves as a template for further DNA synthesis leading to a complementary strand and opening of the 5' end loop. An outer primer hybridizes to the target DNA and extends, displacing the complementary strand and releasing the first single stranded DNA products in the formation of a dumbbell. A DNA polymerase extends from the 3' end and opens up the loop at the 5' end converting the dumbbell to a stem loop structure. This serves as an initiator for LAMP cycling. In the subsequent LAMP cycling the second inner and outer primers hybridize to the other ends on the target sequence. One inner primer hybridizes to the loop on the products initiating displacement DNA synthesis, yielding the original stem-loop DNA and a new with a stem twice as long. By incubating the mixture of samples, primers, DNA polymerase with strand displacement activity and substrates, it is possible to both amplify and detect the reaction in a single step. The detection can be performed by a variety of methods. For larger volumes some can be observed by the eyes while others can be recorded using different strategies including real-time measurements [32, 47].

LAMP has been applied to detect a variety of pathogens including severe acute respiratory syndrome (SARS) coronavirus, Human immunodeficiency virus-1 (HIV-1), *Staphylococcus aureus* and *Streptococcus pneumoniae* [48].

READOUT STRATEGIES

Detection of the signal produced by the DNA biosensors is possible with several different readout strategies. This section will cover a selection of readout strategies and their applications in diagnosis of infectious diseases. The strategies will be divided into two groups: label-dependent and label-free.

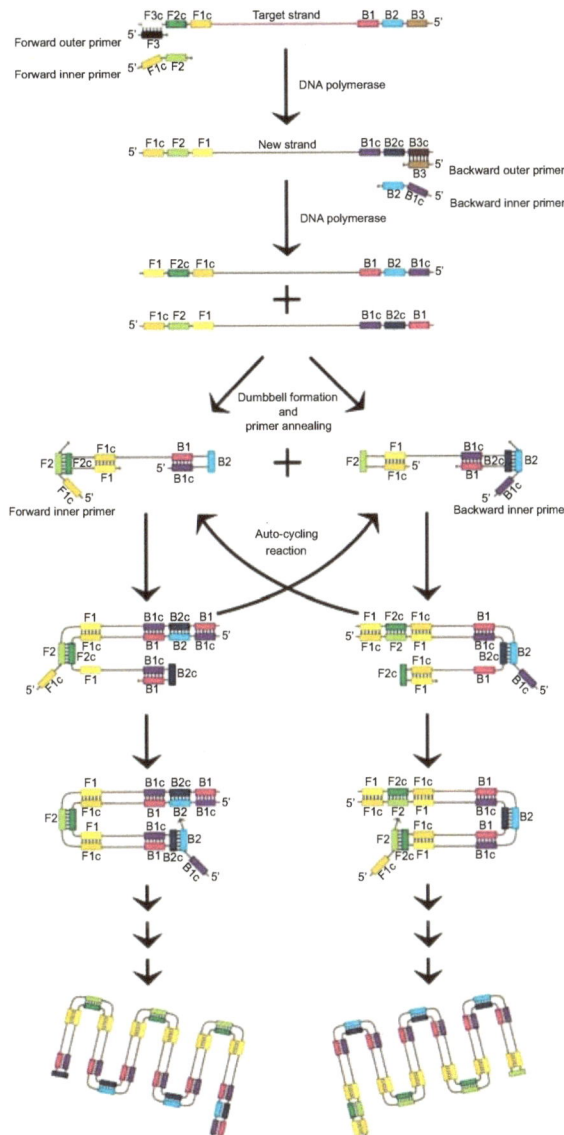

Fig. (4). Loop-mediated isothermal amplification (LAMP): Four different primers, two inner and two outer primers, are designed to recognize six distinct sequences on the target strands. The outer primers are complementary to the regions; F3c and B3c. The inner primers bind to the sequences F2c and B2c. They also contain flanking sequences complementary to the regions F1 and B1. The four primers anneal to the target sequences. A strand-displacement DNA polymerase synthesizes new DNA strands by elongating the primers from the 3' end. After this step the target DNA sequence and the outer primers F3 and B3 are no longer required, and are thus not used in the amplification steps. F1 and F1c are complementary, as are B1 and B1c. These hybridize to form loops resulting in two dumbbell-structures which contain annealing sites for both inner primers. The amplification is achieved by a strand-displacement DNA polymerase synthesizing from the 3' ends of both the open loops and inner primers producing long concatemers each with more sites for initiation.

Label-dependent Readouts for DNA Sensors

Label-dependent biosensing assays are most commonly used. In labeled assays a target or the product of a target analyte is usually sandwiched between the capture and detection agents. The capture agents can be immobilized on *i.e.* a solid surface, chips or nanoparticles, while detection agents are conjugated to tags such as fluorophores, enzymes or nanoparticles. Advantages of labeled biosensors are that they usually provide quantitative detection and high sensitivity. Moreover, capture and detection agents consists of different target binding sites, which increases specificity and reduces background [49].

Fluorescence

Fluorescence is a well-known detection technique known to be highly sensitive and to enable single-molecule detection. Fluorescence is commonly used as a readout strategy in many established assays and diagnostic methods. It is, however, facing challenges such as autofluorescence and photostability when employing biological samples [50]. A DNA structure can itself be directly labeled with fluorescence or indirectly with fluorescently labelled nucleotides, probes or antibodies. The use of nucleic acids in diagnostic settings usually require amplification before the detection is possible. Amplification is commonly performed by PCR with different DNA polymerases. PCR can for example amplify specific regions of pathogenic DNA or RNA. Fluorescent real-time detection of amplified products can be mediated by dyes intercalating in the DNA, by using probes or primers that changes conformation following target amplification, or by fluorescently labelled probes or primers that targets the amplification product [51]. Many methods based on PCR amplification are approved by the FDA for diagnosis of infectious diseases. One example is the COBAS AmpliScreen HIV-1 Test in which amplified HIV-1 RNA is detected with specific fluorescently labeled probes [52].

Amplification with common PCR requires thermocycling, which is not well suited for POC diagnostic methods. Instead isothermal amplification can be used. Isothermal amplification can amplify DNA at a single temperature. Different isothermal amplification reactions have been employed in the study of new diagnostic methods for infectious diseases. One such isothermal reaction is the previously described LAMP method, that uses strand displacement DNA polymerases to amplify from DNA or RNA templates. LAMP is highly efficient and produces large amount of DNA in short time [53].

A LAMP based method has been used for sequence-specific detection of HIV-1 from whole blood samples. HIV-1 specific primers were employed for LAMP amplification which was detected with sequence-specific visual detection mediated by a fluorescein labeled primer and a complementary quencher labelled oligonucleotide. The fluorescein labeled primer was present during LAMP amplification while the quencher labeled oligonucleotide was added in the end. If the specific HIV-1 target was present in the sample the fluorescein-primer binds to the amplicon and gives a fluorescent signal. If no HIV-1 target is present the fluorescein-primer is free to bind the quencher labeled oligonucleotide, and the fluorescence was quenched [54]. LAMP has also been used for similar assays with primers specific for other infectious agents *i.e. Salmonella* [55], *Listeria monocytogenes* [56] and *Plasmodium falciparum* [57].

Another isothermal amplification method used in the development of diagnostic tests is RCA in which a primer is elongated to a long single-stranded product containing several tandems repeats complementary to the circular template [34]. RCA and subsequent detection of RCA products with fluorescently labeled oligonucleotides has been used to detect the product of target-specific enzymatic reactions on specially designed DNA sensors. One such method, detecting the presence of tuberculosis-causing mycobacteria, relies on a mycobacterial enzyme called topoisomerase 1A (TOP1A) as a biomarker. Detection of mycobacteria was performed with an anchored DNA substrate able to capture TOP1A and being converted into a closed circle product in an isolated reaction with the enzyme. This circle was used as a template for RCA, and the RCA products were hybridized to fluorescently labeled probes, allowing detection of specific enzymatic activities at a single molecule level with fluorescence microscopy in an extremely sensitive manner [39]. Similar methods have been used to detect HIV via virus encoded integrases [41], and malaria by detecting the presence of the malaria causing parasite, *P. falciparum*, using *P. falciparum* encoded topoisomerase 1 as a biomarker [36, 37]. A similar system has also been employed to measure the activity of cancer relevant targets in small biological samples and even in single cells [42 - 45].

DNA probes are not only used to detect amplified products but also to detect, localize, and quantify specific nucleic acid sequences for diagnostic purposes. Fluorescently labeled probes can be used in methods such as fluorescent in situ hybridization (FISH). FISH can be used to localize specific DNA sequences in a patient's cell or tissue sample. FISH can use primary patient material and specifically identify pathogens. The method does, however, have low sensitivity in relation to PCR and requires targeted identification [58]. Many studies have investigated the potential of FISH in pathogen detection and have shown that FISH can be used for rapid detection of *Leishmania* [59], *Helicobacter pylori* [60], or *Staphylococcus aureus* [61] with probes targeting ribosomal RNA specific for the pathogen in formalin-fixed, paraffin-embedded biopsy samples.

Another way to detect specific products is with molecular beacons. Molecular beacons are oligonucleotides with hairpin shapes labeled with a fluorophore and a quencher at each end in close proximity. In the hairpin shape, the fluorophore is quenched. Upon hybridization to a target sequence, the beacon undergoes conformational changes, which restores the fluorescence of the fluorophores. Molecular beacons can be used alone or multiplexed to detect the presence of multiple target sequences [62]. Beacons are most often used to detect amplified products of the target sequence, as in the FDA approved NucliSENS EasyQ® MRSA Assay to detect the presence of methicillin-resistant *S. aureus* [63]. Molecular beacons have also been employed in the recently developed TB diagnostic method named Xpert MTB/RIF, a method recommended by the World Health Organization (WHO) [64]. This method used real-time PCR to amplify the mycobacterial RNA polymerase gene. The method enables simultaneous diagnosis of TB and detection of resistance towards treatment with the drug Rifampicin by using fluorescently labelled beacons specific for different mutations within the gene known to cause the resistance [65].

The before mentioned FISH technology can also be performed with molecular beacons as probes, which have been reported to provide higher discriminatory power over corresponding linear probes. The beacon targeted 16S ribosomal RNA specific to *Pseudomonas* and the bacteria was detected in solution with flow cytometry [66]. Several FISH kits have been approved by the FDA. One example is the hemoFISH Masterpanel [67] that detects a panel of bacterial species such as *S. aureus*, *E. coli* and *K. pneumoniae* with probes targeting the conserved 16S ribosomal RNA specific for each species [68].

Fluorescence resonance energy transfer (FRET) relies on the transfer of energy between a donor fluorophore and an acceptor fluorophore in close proximity. This allows the detection of molecular interactions by measuring conformational changes both *in vitro* or *in vivo* [69]. Fluorescently labeled FRET probes have been used to study the development of diagnostics methods. For instance, FRET have been combined with PCR to detect and differentiate *Salmonella* species. This method is based on the detection of a highly conserved gene among *Salmonella* species called tetrathionate reductase response regulator gene (ttrR), which is an ideal target for molecular probes. The ttrR gene is amplified by PCR and FRET probes, with a low level of polymorphism resulting in different melting point for the salmonella organisms, hybridized to the amplified region resulting in species specific detection of *Salmonella* [70]. FRET has also been combined with reverse-transcription PCR for the detection of influenza A virus in poultry [71]. A similar method has been used to study faster ways to genotype Human papillomavirus (HPV) types 6 and 11. In this case FRET real-time PCR was used to detect HPV and probe specific melting temperature analysis could differentiate between the two subtypes [72].

Although fluorescence is the most commonly used readout strategy, several other label-dependent methods exists, some of which will be described next.

Horseradish Peroxidase

Horseradish Peroxidase (HRP) is widely used for colorimetric or chemiluminescent detection via the ability of HRP to convert a substrate into a colored product or emission of light. HRP is often used as label in biosensing assays. The enzyme converts substrates into colored, fluorescent or redox active molecules [73]. HRP has been used in several diagnostic assays, *i.e.* in an FDA approved detection of a panel of stool bacterial pathogens such as *Campylobacter coli*, *Salmonella*, *Shigella*, and *E. coli*. For this purpose, pathogenic DNA was amplified in the presence of biotin, immobilized by hybridization to capture probes on a silica surface, and bound to anti-biotin HRP conjugated antibodies. The colorless colorimetric HRP substrate 3,3',5,5'-Tetramethylbenzidine (TMB) was added to the filter and converted to a blue color visual on the filters by HRP detected with an optical reader [74].

A HRP-based readout for a DNA sensor has been used to detect the malaria causing parasite *P. falciparum* in saliva. In this setup, HRP enables a colorimetric readout of DNA circles generated by a pathogen specific enzymatic reaction on the DNA sensor followed by RCA. In order to do this, biotin coupled deoxynucleotides were incorporated into the RCA product, which was bound to a silica filter and coupled to streptavidin conjugated HRP. TMB was added to the filter and converted to a blue color visual on the filters [37]. HRP has been used in similar colorimetric readout methods for the detection of TB. A patient sample was amplified with isothermal amplification with biotin and bound to HRP. The HRP substrate TMB was added and oxidized by HRP, again creating a visual color change on the silica filter visual by naked eye [75]. A similar method using a cellulose-paper-based colorimetric assay has been used to detect pathogen DNA of *M. tuberculosis*. The cellulose paper was functionalized with tysol groups in order to immobilize sulfhydryl-modified oligonucleotide probes complimentary to a segment of *M. tuberculosis*. DNA from *M. tuberculosis* was subjected to PCR in the presence of biotin. The amplified biotinylated target sequence was hybridized to the probes on the cellulose paper. Streptavidin-HRP was again added and able to oxidize TMB to create a detectable color change on the paper [76].

Another HRP-based colorimetric sensor system have been used to detect HPV16. This system utilizes a biotinylated capture probe immobilized on a streptavidin covered surface. The capture probe binds to the target DNA. The target was then bound by the ssDNA region of a hybrid ssDNA-dsDNA detection probe. The double-stranded DNA contained bindings sites for a DNA binding protein conjugated to HRP facilitating the binding of more than one HRP per target without amplification [77].

Metallic Nanoparticles

Another method to detect DNA sensors are via metallic nanoparticles. The colors displayed from nanoparticles (NPs) is dependent on several factors such as shape, size and state of aggregation [78]. One such NP is Au (gold), which holds several advantages over other NPs. AuNPs are highly suitable for in vitro diagnostics and are widely used for biosensor applications due to their optical and electronic properties. Irradiation of Au with light of one specific wavelength causes oscillation of electrons in the conduction band, which can lead to a color change of the AuNP. This color change is observable by eye. Other advantages of AuNPs are relatively simple synthesis in common chemical laboratories, possibilities within surface modifications which rely on highly stable Au-S bonds, and finally a biosafety better than that of other nanoparticles [79, 80].

AuNPs can be used for colorimetric readout strategies based on aggregation or dispersion of the particles. AuNPs have been used as a readout strategy for the lateral flow assay (LFA). LFA is commonly used for POC diagnosis *i.e.* the pregnancy test. LFA works on polymer paper strips usually composed of a nitrocellulose membrane divided in a sample pad, conjugate pad, absorbing pad, a test zone and a control zone. The test zone can be coupled to a capture probe specific for the target while the control zone is coupled to a probe that captures a control. A sample is applied to the sample pad and is absorbed by the absorbing pad creating a flow through the strip. The conjugate pad contains AuNP modified probes or antibodies that disperses and binds to the sample. The targets are sandwiched between the capture probe and the AuNP modified probe, which created a red color in the target and control zone if the target is present [79, 81].

The sensitivity of LFA is not as high as more technically complicated methods such as *e.g.* PCR. Therefore, various studies have been made to improve the sensitivity of LFA for POC diagnosis. By combining DNA probes with HRP-AuNP dual labels Mao *et al.* were able to detect DNA samples via the generation of the characteristic red band on the LFA membrane [82]. A similar DNA biosensor has been used for the detection of microRNAs in biological samples [83]. A preamplification step with PCR can increase the sensitivity of the method [84]. This has, for instance, been used for the detection of *Vibrio cholerae* with a LFA based DNA biosensor that captured the amplified DNA of *V. cholerae* as generated by PCR of a patient sample [85].

AgNPs are not used as much as AuNPs. Synthesis of AgNPs is more difficult and functionalization of the particles is less efficient [86]. Not many studies utilizing AgNPs for DNA sensor-based diagnostics of infectious diseases have been reported. One example is detection of dengue virus RNA with DNA-triangular silver nanoparticle (TAg) nanoprobes. Detection relies on aggregation of the DNA-TAg probes when no target RNA is present in the sample, which leads to a color change due to optical properties of the AgNPs [87]. Instead of being used for direct detection, AgNPs have been used to enhance other detection methods in metal-enhanced fluorescence (MEF). MEF occurs when fluorophores are within a short distance of metal nanostructures. MEF has been shown to enhance the fluorescence of Cy5 and Cy3 fluorophores markedly and can be used to increase sensitivity in many fluorescently based assays [88]. Detection of *Salmonella enterica* via its chromosomal oriC locus directly from blood has been performed with the help of the MEF technology. This method relies on a glass surface covered with AgNPs. An anchor probe coupled to the silver covered glass surfaces captures the oriC target sequence. A fluorescently labeled probe, binding to the target, enables detection, which is enhanced by the silver particles that hence increase the sensitivity of the method [89].

A method based on AuNP labeled detection probes combined with AgNP enhancement in a microarray format has been approved by the FDA for detection of Clostridium difficile. Capture oligonucleotides specific for *C. difficile* toxins DNA are bound to the microarray surface. Mediator oligonucleotides bind to the target and an AuNP probe. Ag enhancement of the Au probe results in Au-Ag aggregates that scatter detectable light [90].

Quantum Dots

Quantum dots (QD), are semiconductor nanocrystals with photophysical and electrical properties. Due to the small size of QDs, approximately 2-5 nm, the electrons within the dots are confined in small spaces, leading to the emission of light. The emitted fluorescence from QDs is determined by particle size with the smaller particles producing energy in the blue spectrum and the larger particles producing energy in the red spectrum [91]. QDs comprise optical properties over organic fluorophores such as higher fluorescent quantum yield, better resistance towards photo-bleaching, and longer fluorescent life-time [92]. QD can be functionalized with molecules such as biotin or avidins, which allow subsequent binding to oligonucleotides, aptamers or antibodies. In addition to this, QDs can itself replace fluorescent labels and can, for instance, be conjugated to oligonucleotides [93]. QDs can also be used instead of fluorescent dyes in techniques, such as *in situ* hybridization in which QDs are more suitable for long-term tracking and localization of genes or proteins. Sequence specific DNA probes labeled with QDs have *i.e.* been used to detect *E. coli* [94].

A QD-based DNA nanosensor has been able to detect the activity of mycobacterial topoisomerase 1 activity. This sensor consists of a single-stranded oligonucleotide with the recognition sequence specific for the mycobacterial enzyme. The oligonucleotide is dual-labeled with biotin and Cy5, and is assembled with streptavidin functionalized QDs. Detection of the sensor relies on the mechanism of FRET. In this case, the energy transfer from the QD to the Cy5 leads to quenching of the QD fluorescence. Upon cleavage of the DNA nanosensor by mycobacterial enzymes the Cy5 will be removed and the QD able to emit fluorescence. Viable mycobacteria was hence represented as increases in QD emission [40].

QDs have moreover been studied for multiplexed detection of bacteria and viruses. For this purpose, several QDs barcodes have been developed. The QD-based barcodes contain different ratios of fluorescent QDs, each with a unique color corresponding to a particular target. Positive detection of a target occurs when there is a simultaneous detection of the barcode signal and a secondary fluorophore. QDs barcodes can be conjugated with capture oligonucleotides specific for the target bacteria or virus, as is the secondary fluorophore. These components are mixed in a solution with the sample to be analyzed, and a sandwich structure is formed if the target is present A positive signal is the result of the fluorescence emitted from the QDs and the secondary fluorophore. A negative signal is identical to the initial emitted fluorescence from the QD barcode [95, 96]. In combination with DNA probes QD barcodes have been used for the detection of infectious diseases such as relevant HBV viral genomes in clinical samples [97] and for the rapid screening of genetics biomarkers of HIV, malaria, HBV, HCV and syphilis in a multiplexed assay [98].

Label-free Detection

WHO has described the ideal diagnostic test as affordable, sensitive, specific, user-friendly, rapid and robust, equipment-free and deliverable to end users (ASSURED) [99]. Although this is the goal in many studies worldwide, in reality, such perfects kits are still to be developed. The strengths and weaknesses of currently used label-free detection methods will be discussed below.

Different types of sensors have different capabilities. While label dependent DNA sensors where the target biomarker is detected using *e.g.* fluorescent labeled probes, display very high sensitivity, labeling takes time and money [100]. Much effort has therefore been put into development of label-free DNA sensors without sacrificing the benefits of label dependent sensors. A broad range of label-free sensors detecting pathogenic DNA have been described [101, 102]. Label-free detection of DNA may be achieved by taking advantage of the hybridization of the target DNA molecule to immobilized DNA. The sensor is then designed in such a way that the hybridization leads to a change in absorption spectra, electrochemical properties or other easily read parameters [101, 102, 111, 103 - 110]. In recent years, visualization techniques have reached a resolution that allows direct visualization of DNA without any labels.

In the following section, we will go through some of the most promising label-free DNA sensor systems and techniques that may be used for DNA sensing in the future.

Electrochemical

As mentioned previously, one way to detect the presence of pathogenic DNA is to exploit the inherent ability of DNA to bind (hybridize) efficiently to a specific (complementary) DNA sequence in a highly predictable and controllable manner. Immobilizing a DNA sequence that will hybridize to unlabeled DNA from the pathogen of interest and then recording the binding event is therefore a flexible and attractive method for detecting infectious diseases. It is thus not surprising that much work has focused on this class of sensors despite the need for preparative steps including DNA purification and potentially amplification.

A relatively simple method for detecting hybridization between immobilized DNA and DNA in a sample is the use of electrochemical sensors where a hybridization induced difference in voltage is registered and used to read out the hybridization event. Such sensors have been developed for a range of infectious agents including prokaryotes such as *Streptococcus pyogenes* and *Neisseria gonorrhoeae*, to mention just a few [111, 112], as well as viral DNA [113, 114] and DNA from eukaryotic parasites [107, 115].

Metal oxides frequently form the base of electrochemical sensors. An example is a sensor developed for the detection of *Leishmania donovani*, the causative agent of Visceral Leishmaniasis. This sensor consists of single stranded DNA immobilized on a nickel oxide film on an indium tin-coated glass plate. Hybridization of pathogen derived DNA to the sensor is detected using methylene blue, which generates an electrochemical signal for ssDNA as opposed to dsDNA. The signal was hence significantly reduced in the presence of leishmanial DNA complementary to the ssDNA on the sensor [107]. A similar biosensor was published by the same group in a paper presenting a sensor targeting *N. gonorrhoeae* using a zinc oxide based sensor [111].

Biosensors may also be produced to accurately detect pathogenic strains, such as Shiga toxin producing *E. coli*. Narang *et al.* recently published a quantitative sensor doing just this, which was based on a fluorine doped tin oxide (FTO), molybdenum diselenide nano-urchin [106] hereby demonstrating the flexibility and easily obtained adjustability of DNA biosensors in general, and electrochemical sensors, in particular.

In some cases, in order to improve sensitivity and specificity, electrochemical sensors have been coupled with preceding amplification of the target DNA with PCR. This strategy has been successfully used for development of a sensor detecting *Streptococcus pneumoniae* derived DNA [116, 117]. The drawback is an extra step and device requirement connected with PCR amplification. It is, therefore, interesting that integrated devices for both DNA amplification and detection using an electrochemical approach are emerging [118]. Specialized and expensive equipment is, however, still needed, which also reduces the deliverability and applicability sought by WHO.

Gold Nanoparticles

As previously described, aggregation of Au (gold) nanoparticles (AuNPs) leads to a significant alteration of the absorption spectra accompanied by a visible change of color of the gold suspension [119]. This easily detectable change has made gold aggregation an attractive point-of-care adaptable method for monitoring DNA hybridization. The sensor system may be designed in a way so that target DNA, present in a sample, hybridizes to complementary sequences immobilized on the AuNPs. The AuNPs are, hence, brought together by the DNA bridges leading to detectable changes in absorption spectra. This approach was used, for example, in the production of sensors for *Klebsiella pneumoniae* [120]. Interestingly, the sensitivity was only one order of magnitude lower than PCR, which is considered one of the most sensitive methods for DNA detection available.

Higher sensitivity to changes resulting from hybridization of DNA and accompanying aggregation of AuNPs can be obtained by exploiting gold nano rods as compared to spherical AuNPs [105]. Gold nano rods remain less studied than their spherical counterparts. They have, however, been used for generating a sensor DNA system for detection of Hepatitis B [103] and *Chlamydia trachomatis* derived DNA found in the urine of a patient [104]. In the latter case the aggregation was read using transmission electron microscopy, which will be discussed later.

Although detection of specific pathogens is often preferred, universal sensors detecting all bacteria are desired in some situations such as *e.g.* testing for bacteria in the urine. Such a sensor has been developed based on the aggregation of gold nano rods tricked by a highly conserved 16S rDNA region found in most bacteria [121]. This is a perfect example of how DNA sensors can be adapted to fit the many and highly varying needs in diagnosis.

Atomic Force Microscopy (AFM)

In AFM, a microprobe is used for scanning a surface (the sample). During scanning, the intermolecular and interatomic forces between an ultrafine needle/probe and the sample are registered and converted into a topographic image of the surface. There are two main strategies for scanning the surface. The probe may be kept in a constant height above the surface. Alternatively, scanning can be done by tapping the surface with the probe.

With a resolution of 0.1 nm, AFM is able to create an image of a DNA strand with sufficient resolution for detection of the DNA sequence, modifications [122], and topology [123 - 127]. DNA hybridization events may be detected with AFM with very high specificity allowing the detection of even a single nucleotide mismatch [125 - 128]. Furthermore, despite the need for extensive sample preparation in terms of DNA purification and sample drying, direct visualization of the pathogenic DNA itself is beneficial compared to the indirect measurement of a signal induced by the target DNA. On top of visualizing hybridization events, the high resolution of AFM enables it to detect binding to or structural modifications of the immobilized DNA [123, 124, 129]. AFM could hence be employed to detect nucleic acid modifications performed specifically by enzymes expressed by the target organism. AFM is therefore interesting for use in combination with DNA sensors, but unfortunately, portable, cheap, and point-of-care friendly AFM instruments with high resolution are, however, still currently not available

Transmission Electron Microscopy (TEM) and Scanning Electron Microscopy (SEM)

When a wave of electrons is sent through an ultrathin sample, the electrons interact with the atoms of that sample. This leads to the electrons being differentially transmitted through the sample based on variations in the material and thickness. This is the backbone of the TEM technology. The resolution obtained with TEM is so high that it is possible to use this technology for sequencing DNA at the single molecule level. Since the structure and sequence of DNA molecules can be determined using TEM, DNA sensors taking advantage of this imaging system can be envisioned. Biomolecules may be damaged by the electron dose normally applied during high resolution TEM. It is, therefore, among other things, important to choose proper conditions for imaging such as reduced voltage or cooling [130 - 132].

SEM is based on the scanning of a surface using a beam of electrons and the detection of the scattered electrons. SEM share many features of TEM in terms of benefits and drawbacks in reading DNA sensors. The maximal resolution and magnification are greater in TEM, but the sample preparation is simpler for SEM than TEM, giving it an advantage when it comes to speedy and user-friendly diagnosis [130].

Surface Plasmon Resonance (SPR)

When polarized light is shone unto a thin conducting layer positioned at the interface of two media with different refractive index, a phenomenon denoted SPRpolymer occurs, which leads to a drop in the intensity of the reflected light. A typical setup for SPR analysis is a glass prism and an aqueous liquid separated by a thin gold layer. SPR occurs at a certain wavelength and angle of the incoming light. This can be used to detect the binding of analytes to a potential binding partner. If binding occurs, the refractive index will change, leading to a change in the angle at which the intensity of the reflected light drops.

Diagnosis of infectious diseases can be achieved using the SPR technology for detecting DNA from pathogens by detecting the hybridization of pathogenic DNA to immobilized DNA complementary to a specific DNA sequence in the microbial genome. Such tests have been developed for quantitative detection of DNA from pathogenic bacteria such as *Salmonella enterica* serovars typhi [109], *Neisseria meningitidis* [110], and *Brucella melitensis* [108].

Nanopores

As implied by the name, the nanopore technology is based on nanometer sized pores which are positioned in an electrically resistant membrane. These pores may be solid-state nanopores made from *e.g.* silicon [133]. Alternatively, they can be formed by biological materials such as α-hemolysin [134] or the mycobacterial porin MspA [135] both of which are proteins forming pores of a few nanometers. DNA can be led through the pore using an ionic current. The change in current as the DNA passes through the pore enables for sequencing with very long reads [136].

The MinION nanopore sequencer is a small portable device for sequencing using the nanopore technology which has been used successfully *e.g.* for identification of pathogens from positive blood cultures [137]. On top of the portability, there are no capital costs, which opens a cost-efficient possibility for doing occasional diagnosis using nanopore technology.

Although the use of nanopore based technology in diagnosis recently has been focusing predominantly on sequencing, it can be used as a method for reading out some of the DNA sensor strategies discussed previously. One of these strategies is that pathogens can be detected via biomarkers that trigger the formation of covalently closed single stranded DNA circles and subsequent RCA. It has hence been demonstrated that RCA products attached to beads could be identified and quantified using a nanopore [138]. Moreover, specific DNA sequences in solution can be detected using nanopores by analyzing beads coated with complementary bait DNA [139].

CONCLUDING REMARKS

Great progress has been achieved with regards to specific and sensitive detection of infectious diseases. Much of this progress has involved DNA sensors. In this chapter, we have provided examples of how DNA sensors can be designed to allow detection of disease-associated target molecules. The detected target molecule may be DNA from pathogenic organisms, or other molecules found only in the case of infection with the disease causing organism. High sensitivity can be achieved through one or more rounds of signal amplification using techniques such as PCR or RCA. Novel visualization and measuring techniques are continuously emerging, exploiting developments within nanotechnology. Many of these techniques are already being implemented for DNA sensor read-out and the interdisciplinary partnership between medicine, physics, chemistry, and biology will no doubt continue to offer increasingly accurate and cheap diagnostic tests helping save millions of lives every year.

CONSENT FOR PUBLICATION

Not applicable.

CONFLICT OF INTEREST

The authors confirm that this chapter contents have no conflict of interest.

ACKNOWLEDGEMENT

The authors would like to acknowledge associate professor Magnus Stougaard for fruitful discussions about DNA sensors in general and their use in diagnostics in particular. We would also like to thank Michael Kire for his great contribution to the construction of illustrations. Last but not least, we would like to acknowledge the support from the Dagmar Marshalls Foundation, Fabrikant Einar Willumsens Mindelegat, and Familien Erichsens Mindefond.

REFERENCES

[1]   Joyce F, Torrey N, Road P, *et al.* A DNA enzyme with MgZ + -dependent phosphoesterase RNA activity. Chemistry (Easton) 1995; 655-60.

[2]   Zhang J. RNA-Cleaving DNAzymes : Old Catalysts with New Tricks for Intracellular and In Vivo Applications 2018; 1-20.

[3]   Santoro SW, Joyce GF. A general purpose RNA-cleaving DNA enzyme. Proc Natl Acad Sci USA 1997; 94(9): 4262-6.
[http://dx.doi.org/10.1073/pnas.94.9.4262] [PMID: 9113977]

[4]   Ali MM, Aguirre SD, Lazim H, Li Y. Fluorogenic DNAzyme probes as bacterial indicators. Angew Chem Int Ed Engl 2011; 50(16): 3751-4.
[http://dx.doi.org/10.1002/anie.201100477] [PMID: 21412961]

[5]   Zhang W, Feng Q, Chang D, Tram K, Li Y. In vitro selection of RNA-cleaving DNAzymes for bacterial detection. Methods 2016; 106: 66-75.
[http://dx.doi.org/10.1016/j.ymeth.2016.03.018] [PMID: 27017912]

[6]   Shen Z, Wu Z, Chang D, *et al.* A Catalytic DNA Activated by a Specific Strain of Bacterial Pathogen. Angew Chem Int Ed Engl 2016; 55(7): 2431-4.
[http://dx.doi.org/10.1002/anie.201510125] [PMID: 26676768]

[7]   Liu M, Chang D, Li Y. Discovery and Biosensing Applications of Diverse RNA-Cleaving DNAzymes. Acc Chem Res 2017; 50(9): 2273-83.
[http://dx.doi.org/10.1021/acs.accounts.7b00262] [PMID: 28805376]

[8]   Zhou W, Ding J, Liu J. Theranostic DNAzymes. Theranostics 2017; 7(4): 1010-25.
[http://dx.doi.org/10.7150/thno.17736] [PMID: 28382172]

[9]   Davis JJ, Tkac J, Humphreys R, Buxton AT, Lee TA, Ko Ferrigno P. Peptide aptamers in label-free protein detection: 2. Chemical optimization and detection of distinct protein isoforms. Anal Chem 2009; 81(9): 3314-20.
[http://dx.doi.org/10.1021/ac802513n] [PMID: 19320493]

[10]   Park KS. Nucleic acid aptamer-based methods for diagnosis of infections. Biosens Bioelectron 2018; 102: 179-88.
[http://dx.doi.org/10.1016/j.bios.2017.11.028] [PMID: 29136589]

[11]   Tuerk C, Gold L. Systematic evolution of ligands by exponential enrichment: Chemi-SELEX. Science (80-) 1990; 249: 505-10.

[12]   Ellington AD, Szostak JW. © 19 90 Nature Publishing Group. Lett To Nat 1990; 346: 818-22.
[http://dx.doi.org/10.1038/346818a0]

[13]   Ko Ferrigno P. Non-antibody protein-based biosensors. Essays Biochem 2016; 60(1): 19-25.
[http://dx.doi.org/10.1042/EBC20150003] [PMID: 27365032]

[14]   Pan Q, Luo F, Liu M, *et al.* Oligonucleotide aptamers : promising and powerful diagnostic and therapeutic tools for infectious diseases 2018; 77: 83-98.
[http://dx.doi.org/10.1016/j.jinf.2018.04.007]

[15]   Röthlisberger P, Hollenstein M. Aptamer chemistry 2018; 77: 83-98.
[http://dx.doi.org/10.1016/j.addr.2018.04.007]

[16]   Jayasena SD. Aptamers: an emerging class of molecules that rival antibodies in diagnostics. Clin Chem 1999; 45(9): 1628-50.
[http://dx.doi.org/10.1093/clinchem/45.9.1628] [PMID: 10471678]

[17]   Zhang Y, Lai SB, Juhas M. Recent Advances in Aptamer Discovery and Applications. Molecules 2019; 24.
[http://dx.doi.org/10.3390/molecules24050941]

[18]   Rocchitta G, Spanu A, Babudieri S, *et al.* Enzyme biosensors for biomedical applications: Strategies for safeguarding analytical performances in biological fluids. Sensors (Switzerland) 2016; 16.
[http://dx.doi.org/10.3390/s16060780]

[19]   Jayasena SD. Aptamers: an emerging class of molecules that rival antibodies in diagnostics. Clin Chem 1999; 45(9): 1628-50.
[http://dx.doi.org/10.1093/clinchem/45.9.1628] [PMID: 10471678]

[20]   Davydova A, Vorobjeva M, Pyshnyi D, Altman S, Vlassov V, Venyaminova A. Aptamers against pathogenic microorganisms. Crit Rev Microbiol 2016; 42(6): 847-65.
[http://dx.doi.org/10.3109/1040841X.2015.1070115] [PMID: 26258445]

[21]   Trifiro S, Bourgault AM, Lebel F, René P. Ghost mycobacteria on Gram stain. J Clin Microbiol 1990; 28(1): 146-7.
[http://dx.doi.org/10.1128/JCM.28.1.146-147.1990] [PMID: 1688872]

[22]   Valones MA, Guimarães RL, Brandão LA, de Souza PR, de Albuquerque Tavares Carvalho A, Crovela S. Principles and applications of polymerase chain reaction in medical diagnostic fields: a review. Braz J Microbiol 2009; 40(1): 1-11.
[http://dx.doi.org/10.1590/S1517-83822009000100001] [PMID: 24031310]

[23]   Crick F, Watson J. 1953.Nature Publishing Group

[24]   Lorenz TC. Polymerase chain reaction: basic protocol plus troubleshooting and optimization strategies. J Vis Exp 2012; 1-15.
[http://dx.doi.org/10.3791/3998] [PMID: 22664923]

[25]   Gill P, Ghaemi A. Nucleic acid isothermal amplification technologies: a review. Nucleosides Nucleotides Nucleic Acids 2008; 27(3): 224-43.
[http://dx.doi.org/10.1080/15257770701845204] [PMID: 18260008]

[26]   Mullis K, Faloona F, Scharf S, Saiki R, Horn G, Erlich H. Specific enzymatic amplification of DNA in vitro: the polymerase chain reaction. Cold Spring Harb Symp Quant Biol 1986; 51(Pt 1): 263-73.
[http://dx.doi.org/10.1101/SQB.1986.051.01.032] [PMID: 3472723]

[27]   Cottrez F, Auriault C, Capron A, Groux H. Quantitative PCR: validation of the use of a multispecific internal control. Nucleic Acids Res 1994; 22(13): 2712-3.
[http://dx.doi.org/10.1093/nar/22.13.2712] [PMID: 8041636]

[28]   Maurin M. Real-time PCR as a diagnostic tool for bacterial diseases. Expert Rev Mol Diagn 2012; 12(7): 731-54.
[http://dx.doi.org/10.1586/erm.12.53] [PMID: 23153240]

[29]   Shiao Y. A new reverse transcription-polymerase chain reaction method for accurate quantification 2003; 12: 1-12.

[30]   Burkhalter KL, Savage HM. Detection of Zika Virus in Desiccated Mosquitoes by Real-Time Reverse Transcription PCR and Plaque Assay 2017; 23: 2-3.

[31]   Fire A, Xu SQ. Rolling replication of short DNA circles. Proc Natl Acad Sci USA 1995; 92(10): 4641-5.
[http://dx.doi.org/10.1073/pnas.92.10.4641] [PMID: 7753856]

[32]   Wen Y-M, Wang Y-X. Loop Mediated isothermal amplification (LAMP). Rev Med Virol 2009; 19: 57-64.
[http://dx.doi.org/10.1002/rmv.600] [PMID: 19058172]

[33]   Stone C, Mahony J. Point-of-care (POC) Tests for Infectious Diseases– The Next Generation! Ann Infect Dis Epidemiol 2018; 3: 1-8.

[34]   Ali MM, Li F, Zhang Z, *et al.* Rolling circle amplification: a versatile tool for chemical biology, materials science and medicine. Chem Soc Rev 2014; 43(10): 3324-41.
[http://dx.doi.org/10.1039/c3cs60439j] [PMID: 24643375]

[35]   Nilsson M, Malmgren H, Samiotaki M, Kwiatkowski M, Chowdhary BP LU. Padlock probes: circularizing oligonucleotides for localized DNA detection. Science (80-) 1994; 2085-8.
[http://dx.doi.org/10.1126/science.7522346]

[36] Tesauro C, Juul S, Arno B, *et al.* Specific detection of topoisomerase I from the malaria causing P. falciparum parasite using isothermal rolling circle amplification. Conf Proc . Annu Int Conf IEEE Eng Med Biol Soc IEEE Eng Med Biol Soc Annu Conf 2012; 2012: 2416–2419.

[37] Hede MS, Fjelstrup S, Lötsch F, *et al.* Detection of the Malaria causing Plasmodium Parasite in Saliva from Infected Patients using Topoisomerase I Activity as a Biomarker. Sci Rep 2018; 8(1): 4122.
[http://dx.doi.org/10.1038/s41598-018-22378-7] [PMID: 29515150]

[38] Juul S, Nielsen CJF, Labouriau R, *et al.* Droplet microfluidics platform for highly sensitive and quantitative detection of malaria-causing Plasmodium parasites based on enzyme activity measurement. ACS Nano

[39] Franch O, Han X, Marcussen B, *et al.* A new DNA sensor system for specific and quantitative detection of mycobacteria 2019; 587-97.
[http://dx.doi.org/10.1039/C8NR07850E]

[40] Jepsen ML, Harmsen C, Godbole AA, *et al.* Specific detection of the cleavage activity of mycobacterial enzymes using a quantum dot based DNA nanosensor 2016; 358-64.
[http://dx.doi.org/10.1039/C5NR06326D]

[41] Wang J, Liu J, Thomsen J, *et al.* Novel DNA sensor system for highly sensitive and quantitative retrovirus detection using virus encoded integrase as a biomarker. Nanoscale 2017; 9.
[http://dx.doi.org/10.1039/C6NR07428F]

[42] Stougaard M, Lohmann JS, Mancino A, *et al.* Single-molecule detection of human topoisomerase I cleavage-ligation activity. ACS Nano 2009; 3(1): 223-33.
[http://dx.doi.org/10.1021/nn800509b] [PMID: 19206270]

[43] Kristoffersen EL, Givskov A, Jørgensen LA, *et al.* Interlinked DNA nano-circles for measuring topoisomerase II activity at the level of single decatenation events. Nucleic Acids Res 2017; 45(13): 7855-69.
[http://dx.doi.org/10.1093/nar/gkx480] [PMID: 28541438]

[44] Keller JG, Tesauro C, Coletta A, *et al.* On-slide detection of enzymatic activities in selected single cells. Nanoscale
[http://dx.doi.org/10.1039/C7NR05125E]

[45] Andersen FF, Stougaard M, Jørgensen HL, *et al.* Multiplexed detection of site specific recombinase and DNA topoisomerase activities at the single molecule level. ACS Nano 2009; 3(12): 4043-54.
[http://dx.doi.org/10.1021/nn9012912] [PMID: 19950974]

[46] Chang CC, Chen CC, Wei SC, Lu HH, Liang YH, Lin CW. Diagnostic devices for isothermal nucleic acid amplification. Sensors (Basel) 2012; 12(6): 8319-37.
[http://dx.doi.org/10.3390/s120608319] [PMID: 22969402]

[47] Yan L, Zhou J, Zheng Y, *et al.* Isothermal amplified detection of DNA and RNA. Mol Biosyst 2014; 10(5): 970-1003.
[http://dx.doi.org/10.1039/c3mb70304e] [PMID: 24643211]

[48] Drapała D, Kordalewska M. Loop-mediated Isothermal Amplification (LAMP) as a diagnostic tool in detection of infectious diseases. PhD Interdiscip J 2011; 12: 19-23.

[49] Mandy LY Sin, Kathleen E Mach, Pak Kin Wong and JCL. Advances and challenges in biosensor-based diagnosis of infectious diseases 2014; 14: 225-44.

[50] Aitken CE, Marshall RA, Puglisi JD. An oxygen scavenging system for improvement of dye stability in single-molecule fluorescence experiments. Biophys J 2008; 94(5): 1826-35.
[http://dx.doi.org/10.1529/biophysj.107.117689] [PMID: 17921203]

[51] Niemz A, Ferguson TM, Boyle DS. Point-of-care nucleic acid testing for infectious diseases 2013; 29: 240-50.

[52] COBAS Ampliscreen HIV-1 Test

[53] Article R. Loop-mediated isothermal amplifi cation (LAMP): a rapid , accurate , and cost-effective diagnostic method for infectious diseases 2009; 62-9.

[54] Curtis KA, Rudolph DL, Owen SM. Sequence-Specific Detection Method for Reverse Transcription , Loop-Mediated Isothermal Amplification of HIV-1 2009; 972: 966-72.

[55] Hara-kudo Y. Loop-mediated isothermal amplification for the rapid detection of Salmonella 2005; 253: 155-61.
[http://dx.doi.org/10.1016/j.femsle.2005.09.032]

[56] Sheng MT, Zhang ZX. Rapid and Sensitive Detection of Listeria monocytogenes by Loop-Mediated Isothermal Amplification 2011; 511-6.

[57] Sirichaisinthop J, Buates S, Watanabe R, *et al.* Short Report : Evaluation of Loop-Mediated Isothermal Amplification (LAMP) for Malaria Diagnosis in a Field Setting 2011; 85: 594-6.

[58] Frickmann H, Zautner AE, Moter A, *et al.* Critical Reviews in Microbiology Fluorescence in situ hybridization (FISH) in the microbiological diagnostic routine laboratory : a review 2017; 7828.
[http://dx.doi.org/10.3109/1040841X.2016.1169990]

[59] Frickmann H, Alnamar Y, Essig A, *et al.* Rapid identification of Leishmania spp. in formalin-fixed, paraffin-embedded tissue samples by fluorescence in situ hybridization. Trop Med Int Health 2012; 17(9): 1117-26.
[http://dx.doi.org/10.1111/j.1365-3156.2012.03024.x] [PMID: 22776353]

[60] Can F, Yilmaz Z, Demirbilek M, *et al.* Diagnosis of Helicobacter pylori infection and determination of clarithromycin resistance by fluorescence in situ hybridization from formalin-fixed, paraffin-embedded gastric biopsy specimens. Can J Microbiol 2005; 51(7): 569-73.
[http://dx.doi.org/10.1139/w05-035] [PMID: 16175205]

[61] Wang P. Simultaneous detection and differentiation of Staphylococcus species in blood cultures using fluorescence in situ hybridization. Med Princ Pract 2010; 19(3): 218-21.
[http://dx.doi.org/10.1159/000285294] [PMID: 20357507]

[62] Tyagi S, Kramer FR. Molecular Beacons in Diagnostics 2012; 6: 2-7.

[63] NucliSENS EasyQ® MRSA Assay

[64] Xpert MTB/RIF

[65] Boehme CC, Nabeta P, Hillemann D, *et al.* Rapid molecular detection of tuberculosis and rifampin resistance. N Engl J Med 2010; 363(11): 1005-15.
[http://dx.doi.org/10.1056/NEJMoa0907847] [PMID: 20825313]

[66] Lenaerts J, Lappin-scott HM, Porter J. Improved Fluorescent In Situ Hybridization Method for Detection of Bacteria from Activated Sludge and River Water by Using DNA Molecular Beacons and Flow Cytometry 2007; 73: 2020-3.

[67] HemoFISH masterpanel

[68] Davenport M, Mach KE, Shortliffe LMD, Banaei N, Wang TH, Liao JC. New and developing diagnostic technologies for urinary tract infections. Nat Rev Urol 2017; 14(5): 296-310.
[http://dx.doi.org/10.1038/nrurol.2017.20] [PMID: 28248946]

[69] Selvin PR. The renaissance of fluorescence resonance energy transfer 7

[70] Zhang J, Wei L, Kelly P, *et al.* Detection of Salmonella spp. using a generic and differential FRET-PCR. PLoS One 2013; 8(10)e76053
[http://dx.doi.org/10.1371/journal.pone.0076053] [PMID: 24146814]

[71] Luan L, Sun Z, Kaltenboeck B, *et al.* Detection of influenza A virus from live-bird market poultry swab samples in China by a pan-IAV, one- step reverse-transcription FRET. Nat Publ Gr 2016; pp. 1-9.

[72]   Combrinck CE, Seedat RY, Burt FJ. FRET-based detection and genotyping of HPV-6 and HPV-11 causing recurrent respiratory papillomatosis. J Virol Methods 2013; 189(2): 271-6.
[http://dx.doi.org/10.1016/j.jviromet.2013.01.025] [PMID: 23473839]

[73]   Veitch NC. Horseradish peroxidase : a modern view of a classic enzyme 2004; 65: 249-59.
[http://dx.doi.org/10.1016/j.phytochem.2003.10.022]

[74]   Great Basin Stool Bacterial Pathogens Panel

[75]   Ng BYC, Wee EJH, West NP, *et al.* Naked-Eye Colorimetric and Electrochemical Detection of Mycobacterium tuberculosis—toward Rapid Screening for Active Case Finding. ACS Sens 2016; 1: 173-8.
[http://dx.doi.org/10.1021/acssensors.5b00171]

[76]   Saikrishnan D, Goyal M, Rossiter S, Kukol A. A cellulose-based bioassay for the colorimetric detection of pathogen DNA. Anal Bioanal Chem 2014; 406(30): 7887-98.
[http://dx.doi.org/10.1007/s00216-014-8257-y] [PMID: 25354892]

[77]   Aktas GB, Skouridou V, Masip L. Novel signal amplification approach for HRP-based colorimetric genosensors using DNA binding protein tags. Biosens Bioelectron 2015; 74: 1005-10.
[http://dx.doi.org/10.1016/j.bios.2015.07.077] [PMID: 26264267]

[78]   Aldewachi H, Chalati T, Woodroofe MN, *et al.* Gold nanoparticle-based colorimetric biosensors 2018; 18-33.
[http://dx.doi.org/10.1039/C7NR06367A]

[79]   Zhou W, Gao X, Liu D, *et al.* Gold Nanoparticles for In Vitro Diagnostics 2017; 115: 10575-636.

[80]   Holzinger M, Goff A, Le , Cosnier S. Nanomaterials for biosensing applications : a review 2014; 2: 1-10.
[http://dx.doi.org/10.3389/fchem.2014.00063]

[81]   He Y, Zhang S, Zhang X, *et al.* Ultrasensitive nucleic acid biosensor based on enzyme-gold nanoparticle dual label and lateral flow strip biosensor. Biosens Bioelectron 2011; 26(5): 2018-24.
[http://dx.doi.org/10.1016/j.bios.2010.08.079] [PMID: 20875950]

[82]   Mao X, Ma Y, Zhang A, *et al.* Disposable Nucleic Acid Biosensors Based on Gold Nanoparticle Probes and Lateral Flow Strip 2009; 81: 1660-8.

[83]   Xuefei G, Xu H, Baloda M, *et al.* Visual Detection of microRNA with Lateral Flow Nucleic Acid Biosensor 2014; 578-84.

[84]   Lie P, Liu J, Fang Z, *et al.* ChemComm A lateral flow biosensor for detection of nucleic acids with high sensitivity and selectivity w 2012; 236-8.

[85]   Chua A, Yean CY, Ravichandran M, Lim B, Lalitha P. A rapid DNA biosensor for the molecular diagnosis of infectious disease. Biosens Bioelectron 2011; 26(9): 3825-31.
[http://dx.doi.org/10.1016/j.bios.2011.02.040] [PMID: 21458979]

[86]   Larguinho M, Baptista PV. Gold and silver nanoparticles for clinical diagnostics - From genomics to proteomics. J Proteomics 2012; 75(10): 2811-23.
[http://dx.doi.org/10.1016/j.jprot.2011.11.007] [PMID: 22119545]

[87]   Vinayagam S, Rajaiah P, Mukherjee A, Natarajan C. DNA-triangular silver nanoparticles nanoprobe for the detection of dengue virus distinguishing serotype. Spectrochim Acta A Mol Biomol Spectrosc 2018; 202: 346-51.
[http://dx.doi.org/10.1016/j.saa.2018.05.047] [PMID: 29800899]

[88]   Sabanayagam CR, Lakowicz JR. Increasing the sensitivity of DNA microarrays by metal-enhanced fluorescence using surface-bound silver nanoparticles 2007; 35: 1-9.

[89]   Tennant SM, Zhang Y, Galen JE, *et al.* Ultra-Fast and Sensitive Detection of Non-Typhoidal Salmonella Using Microwave-Accelerated Metal- Enhanced Fluorescence ("'MAMEF'") 2011; 6: 1-8.

[90] FDA. Clostridium Difficile Toxin Gene Amplification Assay

[91] Knudsen BR, Jepsen ML, Ho Y, *et al.* Quantum dot-based nanosensors for diagnosis via enzyme activity measurement 2014; 7159.
[http://dx.doi.org/10.1586/erm.13.17]

[92] Resch-genger U, Grabolle M, Cavaliere-jaricot S, *et al.* Quantum dots versus organic dyes as fluorescent labels 2008; 5: 763-75.
[http://dx.doi.org/10.1038/nmeth.1248]

[93] Zhang Y, Wang T. Quantum Dot Enabled Molecular Sensing and Diagnostics 2012; 2.
[http://dx.doi.org/10.7150/thno.4308]

[94] Wu SM, Zhao X, Zhang ZL, *et al.* Quantum-dot-labeled DNA probes for fluorescence in situ hybridization (FISH) in the microorganism Escherichia coli. ChemPhysChem 2006; 7(5): 1062-7.
[http://dx.doi.org/10.1002/cphc.200500608] [PMID: 16625674]

[95] Hauck TS, Giri S, Gao Y, Chan WC. Nanotechnology diagnostics for infectious diseases prevalent in developing countries. Adv Drug Deliv Rev 2010; 62(4-5): 438-48.
[http://dx.doi.org/10.1016/j.addr.2009.11.015] [PMID: 19931580]

[96] Wang Y, Yu L, Kong X, Sun L. Application of nanodiagnostics in point-of-care tests for infectious diseases. Int J Nanomedicine 2017; 12: 4789-803.
[http://dx.doi.org/10.2147/IJN.S137338] [PMID: 28740385]

[97] Kim J, Biondi MJ, Feld JJ, Chan WC. Clinical Validation of Quantum Dot Barcode Diagnostic Technology. ACS Nano 2016; 10(4): 4742-53.
[http://dx.doi.org/10.1021/acsnano.6b01254] [PMID: 27035744]

[98] Giri S, Sykes EA, Jennings TL, Chan WC. Rapid screening of genetic biomarkers of infectious agents using quantum dot barcodes. ACS Nano 2011; 5(3): 1580-7.
[http://dx.doi.org/10.1021/nn102873w] [PMID: 21355538]

[99] Kosack CS, Page A, Klatser PR. A guide to aid the selection of diagnostic tests 2017; 639-45.
[http://dx.doi.org/10.2471/BLT.16.187468]

[100] Daniels JS, Pourmand N. Label-free impedance biosensors: Opportunities and challenges. Electroanalysis 2007; 19(12): 1239-57.
[http://dx.doi.org/10.1002/elan.200603855] [PMID: 18176631]

[101] Abu-Salah KM, Zourob MM, Mouffouk F, Alrokayan SA, Alaamery MA, Ansari AA. DNA-Based Nanobiosensors as an Emerging Platform for Detection of Disease. Sensors (Basel) 2015; 15(6): 14539-68.
[http://dx.doi.org/10.3390/s150614539] [PMID: 26102488]

[102] Datta M, Desai D, Kumar A. Gene Specific DNA Sensors for Diagnosis of Pathogenic Infections. Indian J Microbiol 2017; 57(2): 139-47.
[http://dx.doi.org/10.1007/s12088-017-0650-8] [PMID: 28611490]

[103] Wang X, Li Y, Wang H, *et al.* Gold nanorod-based localized surface plasmon resonance biosensor for sensitive detection of hepatitis B virus in buffer, blood serum and plasma. Biosens Bioelectron 2010; 26(2): 404-10.
[http://dx.doi.org/10.1016/j.bios.2010.07.121] [PMID: 20729056]

[104] Parab HJ, Jung C, Lee JH, Park HG. A gold nanorod-based optical DNA biosensor for the diagnosis of pathogens. Biosens Bioelectron 2010; 26(2): 667-73.
[http://dx.doi.org/10.1016/j.bios.2010.06.067] [PMID: 20675117]

[105] Stone J, Jackson S, Wright D. Biological applications of gold nanorods. Wiley Interdiscip Rev Nanomed Nanobiotechnol 2011; 3(1): 100-9.
[http://dx.doi.org/10.1002/wnan.120] [PMID: 20967876]

[106] Narang J, Mishra A, Pilloton R, *et al.* Development of MoSe(2) Nano-Urchins as a Sensing Platform

for a Selective Bio-Capturing of Escherichia. coli Shiga Toxin DNA. Biosens 2018; 8.
[http://dx.doi.org/10.3390/bios8030077]

[107] Mohan S, Srivastava P, Maheshwari SN, Sundar S, Prakash R. Nano-structured nickel oxide based
       DNA biosensor for detection of visceral leishmaniasis (Kala-azar). Analyst (Lond) 2011; 136(13):
       2845-51.
       [http://dx.doi.org/10.1039/c1an15031f] [PMID: 21611668]

[108] Sikarwar B, Singh VV, Sharma PK, *et al*. DNA-probe-target interaction based detection of Brucella
       melitensis by using surface plasmon resonance. Biosens Bioelectron 2017; 87: 964-9.
       [http://dx.doi.org/10.1016/j.bios.2016.09.063] [PMID: 27665519]

[109] Singh A, Verma HN, Arora K. Surface plasmon resonance based label-free detection of Salmonella
       using DNA self assembly. Appl Biochem Biotechnol 2015; 175(3): 1330-43.
       [http://dx.doi.org/10.1007/s12010-014-1319-y] [PMID: 25391546]

[110] Kaur G, Paliwal A, Tomar M, Gupta V. Detection of Neisseria meningitidis using surface plasmon
       resonance based DNA biosensor. Biosens Bioelectron 2016; 78: 106-10.
       [http://dx.doi.org/10.1016/j.bios.2015.11.025] [PMID: 26599479]

[111] Ansari AA, Singh R, Sumana G, Malhotra BD. Sol-gel derived nano-structured zinc oxide film for
       sexually transmitted disease sensor. Analyst (Lond) 2009; 134(5): 997-1002.
       [http://dx.doi.org/10.1039/b817562d] [PMID: 19381396]

[112] Singh S, Kaushal A, Khare S, Kumar A. DNA chip based sensor for amperometric detection of
       infectious pathogens. Int J Biol Macromol 2017; 103: 355-9.
       [http://dx.doi.org/10.1016/j.ijbiomac.2017.05.041] [PMID: 28502856]

[113] Li X, Scida K, Crooks RM. Detection of hepatitis B virus DNA with a paper electrochemical sensor.
       Anal Chem 2015; 87(17): 9009-15.
       [http://dx.doi.org/10.1021/acs.analchem.5b02210] [PMID: 26258588]

[114] Rasouli E, Shahnavaz Z, Basirun WJ, *et al*. Advancements in electrochemical DNA sensor for
       detection of human papilloma virus - A review. Anal Biochem 2018; 556: 136-44.
       [http://dx.doi.org/10.1016/j.ab.2018.07.002] [PMID: 29981317]

[115] Gokce G, Erdem A, Ceylan C, Akgöz M. Voltammetric detection of sequence-selective DNA
       hybridization related to Toxoplasma gondii in PCR amplicons. Talanta 2016; 149: 244-9.
       [http://dx.doi.org/10.1016/j.talanta.2015.11.071] [PMID: 26717837]

[116] Campuzano S, Pedrero M, García JL, García E, García P, Pingarrón JM. Development of
       amperometric magnetogenosensors coupled to asymmetric PCR for the specific detection of
       Streptococcus pneumoniae. Anal Bioanal Chem 2011; 399(7): 2413-20.
       [http://dx.doi.org/10.1007/s00216-010-4645-0] [PMID: 21229236]

[117] Sotillo A, Pedrero M, de Pablos M, *et al*. Clinical evaluation of a disposable amperometric magneto-
       genosensor for the detection and identification of Streptococcus pneumoniae. J Microbiol Methods
       2014; 103: 25-8.
       [http://dx.doi.org/10.1016/j.mimet.2014.04.014] [PMID: 24858449]

[118] Park YM, Lim SY, Shin SJ, *et al*. A film-based integrated chip for gene amplification and
       electrochemical detection of pathogens causing foodborne illnesses. Anal Chim Acta 2018; 1027: 57-
       66.
       [http://dx.doi.org/10.1016/j.aca.2018.03.061] [PMID: 29866270]

[119] Aldewachi H, Chalati T, Woodroofe MN, Bricklebank N, Sharrack B, Gardiner P. Gold nanoparticle-
       based colorimetric biosensors. Nanoscale 2017; 10(1): 18-33.
       [http://dx.doi.org/10.1039/C7NR06367A] [PMID: 29211091]

[120] Ahmadi S, Kamaladini H, Haddadi F, Sharifmoghadam MR. Thiol-Capped Gold Nanoparticle
       Biosensors for Rapid and Sensitive Visual Colorimetric Detection of Klebsiella pneumoniae. J
       Fluoresc 2018; 28(4): 987-98.

[http://dx.doi.org/10.1007/s10895-018-2262-z] [PMID: 30022376]

[121] Wang X, Li Y, Wang J, *et al.* A broad-range method to detect genomic DNA of multiple pathogenic bacteria based on the aggregation strategy of gold nanorods. Analyst (Lond) 2012; 137(18): 4267-73.
[http://dx.doi.org/10.1039/c2an35680e] [PMID: 22836346]

[122] Oliveira SC, Oliveira-Brett AM. DNA-electrochemical biosensors: AFM surface characterisation and application to detection of in situ oxidative damage to DNA. Comb Chem High Throughput Screen 2010; 13(7): 628-40.
[http://dx.doi.org/10.2174/1386207311004070628] [PMID: 20402643]

[123] Pyne AL, Hoogenboom BW. Imaging DNA Structure by Atomic Force Microscopy. Methods Mol Biol 2016; 1431: 47-60.
[http://dx.doi.org/10.1007/978-1-4939-3631-1_5] [PMID: 27283301]

[124] Lyubchenko YL, Shlyakhtenko LS. Imaging of DNA and Protein-DNA Complexes with Atomic Force Microscopy. Crit Rev Eukaryot Gene Expr 2016; 26(1): 63-96.
[http://dx.doi.org/10.1615/CritRevEukaryotGeneExpr.v26.i1.70] [PMID: 27278886]

[125] Ngavouka MDN, Capaldo P, Ambrosetti E, Scoles G, Casalis L, Parisse P. Mismatch detection in DNA monolayers by atomic force microscopy and electrochemical impedance spectroscopy. Beilstein J Nanotechnol 2016; 7: 220-7.
[http://dx.doi.org/10.3762/bjnano.7.20] [PMID: 26977379]

[126] Gilmore JL, Yoshida A, Takahashi H, *et al.* Analyses of nuclear proteins and nucleic acid structures using atomic force microscopy. Methods Mol Biol 2015; 1262: 119-53.
[http://dx.doi.org/10.1007/978-1-4939-2253-6_8] [PMID: 25555579]

[127] Dubrovin EV, Presnova GV, Rubtsova MY, Egorov AM, Grigorenko VG, Yaminsky IV. The Use of Atomic Force Microscopy for 3D Analysis of Nucleic Acid Hybridization on Microarrays. Acta Naturae 2015; 7(2): 108-14.
[http://dx.doi.org/10.32607/20758251-2015-7-2-108-114] [PMID: 26085952]

[128] Wang J, Bard AJ. Monitoring DNA immobilization and hybridization on surfaces by atomic force microscopy force measurements. Anal Chem 2001; 73(10): 2207-12.
[http://dx.doi.org/10.1021/ac001344a] [PMID: 11393842]

[129] Liu J, Wang X, Zhang W. Atomic Force Microscopy Imaging Study of Aligning DNA by Dumbbell-like $Au-Fe_3O_4$ Magnetic Nanoparticles. Langmuir 2018; 34(49): 14875-81.
[http://dx.doi.org/10.1021/acs.langmuir.8b01784] [PMID: 30011364]

[130] Marini M, Falqui A, Moretti M, *et al.* The structure of DNA by direct imaging. Sci Adv 2015; 1(7)e1500734
[http://dx.doi.org/10.1126/sciadv.1500734] [PMID: 26601243]

[131] Egerton RF. Radiation damage to organic and inorganic specimens in the TEM. Micron 2019; 119: 72-87.
[http://dx.doi.org/10.1016/j.micron.2019.01.005] [PMID: 30684768]

[132] Egerton RF, Li P, Malac M. Radiation damage in the TEM and SEM. Micron 2004; 35(6): 399-409.
[http://dx.doi.org/10.1016/j.micron.2004.02.003] [PMID: 15120123]

[133] Lee K, Park KB, Kim HJ, *et al.* Recent Progress in Solid-State Nanopores. Adv Mater 2018; 30(42)e1704680
[http://dx.doi.org/10.1002/adma.201704680] [PMID: 30260506]

[134] Kasianowicz JJ, Brandin E, Branton D, Deamer DW. Characterization of individual polynucleotide molecules using a membrane channel. Proc Natl Acad Sci USA 1996; 93(24): 13770-3.
[http://dx.doi.org/10.1073/pnas.93.24.13770] [PMID: 8943010]

[135] Faller M, Niederweis M, Schulz GE. The Structure of a Mycobacterial Outer-Membrane Channel. Science (80-) 2004.
[http://dx.doi.org/10.1126/science.1094114]

[136] Leggett RM, Clark MD. A world of opportunities with nanopore sequencing. J Exp Bot 2017; 68(20): 5419-29.
[http://dx.doi.org/10.1093/jxb/erx289] [PMID: 28992056]

[137] Ashikawa S, Tarumoto N, Imai K, *et al.* Rapid identification of pathogens from positive blood culture bottles with the MinION nanopore sequencer. J Med Microbiol 2018; 67(11): 1589-95.
[http://dx.doi.org/10.1099/jmm.0.000855] [PMID: 30311873]

[138] Kühnemund M, Nilsson M. Digital quantification of rolling circle amplified single DNA molecules in a resistive pulse sensing nanopore. Biosens Bioelectron 2015; 67: 11-7.
[http://dx.doi.org/10.1016/j.bios.2014.06.040] [PMID: 25000851]

[139] Adela Booth M, Vogel R, Curran JM, *et al.* Detection of target-probe oligonucleotide hybridization using synthetic nanopore resistive pulse sensing. Biosens Bioelectron
[http://dx.doi.org/10.1016/j.bios.2013.01.044]

CHAPTER 12

Unconventional Microfluidics for Biosensing

Yi Zhang[*]

School of Mechanical and Aerospace Engineering, Nanyang Technological University, Singapore

Abstract: Conventional microfluidics handles liquids in a continuous fashion in microchannels. It has been widely adopted in bioanalysis for its many advantages including the ability to manipulate single cells. The footprint of the conventional microfluidic chip is small. However, it requires sophisticated external control and sensing systems to function, which limits the applications of conventional microfluidics to the laboratory environment. For point-of-care applications in the resource-limited environment, standalone diagnostic platforms, such as digital microfluidics-based platforms, are more desirable. Digital microfluidics manipulates fluids in discrete volumes in the form of droplets. In this chapter, we introduce the principle of digital microfluidics and focus on the two main forms of digital microfluidics that are actuated by the magnetic force and the electrowetting on dielectrics. We will discuss the actuation mechanisms in details and compare the pros and cons of the two most popular digital microfluidic platforms. We will also look into the applications of the digital microfluidics in biosensing and diagnostics. Example of digital microfluidics-based nucleic acids, proteins and cells analysis will be deliberated with a focus on the suitability of those assays on digital microfluidic platforms for point-of-care applications.

Keywords: Biosensing, Digital Microfluidics, Diagnostics, DNA/RNA, EWOD, ELISA, Magnetic Digital Microfluidics, Sample-To-Answer.

INTRODUCTION

About three decades ago, microfluidics was proposed as a new way of manipulating a minute amount of fluids in a controlled manner [1, 2]. Earlier research in the field of microfluidics focused on the microdevice fabrication and the fundamentals of the fluidic behavior at microscale [1, 3, 4]. Later on, a wide range of microfluidic applications in biology, chemistry and clinical research had been developed [5, 8]. These innovations led to the invention of valuable assays, such as the single cell analysis, sample-to-answer analysis and point-of-care (POC) diagnostics, which were previously impossible due to the lack of proper

---

[*] **Corresponding author Yi Zhang:** School of Mechanical and Aerospace Engineering, Nanyang Technological University, Singapore; E-mail: yi_zhang@ntu.edu.sg

tools. Nowadays, microfluidics manifests in many forms including the continuous flow microfluidics, droplet microfluidics,(9) digital microfluidics [10, 11], and paper-based microfluidics [12, 13]. among others.

In the course of its development, many varieties of microfluidic systems have been proposed. These systems can be broadly categorized into the closed microfluidics in which the fluids are confined in a closed space, and the open microfluidics in which the fluids are exposed to the ambient environment. Because the closed microfluidics is the earliest and most widely recognized form of microfluidic system, it is referred to as the conventional microfluidics. Hence, the open microfluidic system is considered the unconventional form of microfluidics in this chapter.

The conventional microfluidics downscales the fluidic components such as pipes, containers, chambers, valves and pumps to microns and utilizes these microfluidic components to control the fluids. The conventional microfluidic platform manipulates the fluids in a closed fluidic network consisting of micro channels and chambers. The fluid flows within these microfluidic components and follows a path defined by them. Other than at the inlet and outlet, the fluid is not in direct contact with the ambient environment.

Because their scale matches that of biological entities, the conventional microfluidic systems have many advantageous features that are highly coveted in biomedical applications. For example, microfluidics systems reduce reagent consumption hence the cost of bioassays. They also reduce the required sample volume per assay, which allows users to acquire more information with limited sample availability. The Reynolds number (Re), which describes the relative effect of the inertial flow and the viscous flow (**Equation 1**), is small in microfluidic systems. As a result, the flow is usually laminar in the microchannel. When multiple streams enter the same microchannel, they flow in parallel layers and do not mix, and the mass exchange between these streams is accomplished only by diffusion. Although the laminar flow would be problematic during fluidic mixing, it enables several applications unique to microfluidics. One application that exploits the laminar flow is an H-sensor or T-sensor [14]. These diffusion-based devices are commonly used to sort micro/nano particles [14]. and generate the concentration gradient [15]. The microfluidic systems are also able to provide a precise spatio-temporal control of the fluidic environment for controlled delivery of bioagents and controlled stimulation of biological entities. Moreover, the small scale of microfluidic components enables a high degree of integration and parallelization. These unique features make the microfluidic systems well-suited for high-throughput screening.

$$Re = \frac{\rho v D}{\mu} \qquad \qquad (1)$$

In spite of the aforementioned benefits, the conventional microfluidics has several limitations that hinder its applications to biosensing and clinical diagnostics, particularly in the field of POC diagnostics. Because the conventional microfluidic system could integrate and streamline multiple processes, it has been acclaimed as the go-to solution for the sample-in-answer-out analysis, which is a key feature of a POC diagnostic platform. Nevertheless, this claim is true only to a certain extent. The conventional microfluidics is the foundation of many micro total analysis systems (μTAS) a.k.a. Lab on a Chip (LOC) systems that are capable of automated sample-in-answer-out analysis [7]. For example, an LOC for the molecular diagnostics could streamline the upstream sample preparation, the assay reaction, and the downstream or real time detection. It is able to extract the DNA from the sample input, amplify the DNA using Polymerase Chain Reaction (PCR) or isothermal reactions, and detect the DNA using real time readout or gel electrophoresis post-amplification. This sample-in-answer-out analysis has greatly simplified the assay procedures and eliminated the error due to human interference.

However, the sample-in-answer-out ability alone is not sufficient for a fully functional POC diagnostic platform. POC diagnostic platforms are most sought after by users in resource-constrained environments or homecare environments where the infrastructure support and the intellectual support are lacking. Consumables and supplies that are readily available in the laboratories and hospitals are scarce in these resource-limited settings. To operate a conventional microfluidic device, the microfluidic chip needs to be coupled to the pressure source and the control system through tubing and interface connectors. Additional optical or electrochemical sensors are often required for signal readout. These peripherals for the conventional microfluidic system are usually bulky and expensive. As a result, the μTAS based on the conventional microfluidic system is often a "chip in the lab" rather than a "lab on a chip". Therefore, the conventional microfluidic system is not appropriate for the POC diagnostics due to the complexity of its fluidic operation, the high cost associated with the control system, and the large footprint of the required peripherals that renders the microfluidic device unportable.

While the conventional microfluidics provides an excellent tool to study fundamental biological and clinical problems in the laboratory setting, alternative microfluidic technologies that offer a simple equipment-free fluidic operation are much better suited for POC applications.

The conventional microfluidics is a closed system that uses microstructures, such as microchannels and microchambers, to define a closed flow path. The fluids are usually driven through the microfluidic network by the pressure difference supplied by a pump. In comparison, the open microfluidics usually does not have any confinement structures. It may occasionally have structures that provide partial confinement. Examples of open microfluidics include the digital microfluidics [10, 11], the paper-based microfluidics [13]. and the open-channel microfluidics [16, 18]. Because of the open design, the fluids cannot be driven by the conventional pumping mechanisms. Instead, various other mechanisms, such as magnetic force, capillary force, electrowetting, acoustic force, have been employed to actuate the fluids on the open microfluidic platform. Some of these actuation mechanisms exploit the intrinsic properties of the fluids and the substrate materials to operate in an equipment-free manner. Compared to the closed microfluidic system, the open microfluidic system is more versatile and more well-suited for POC applications.

This chapter is aimed to elaborate the digital microfluidics including both the magnetic digital microfluidics and the electrowetting-on-dielectrics (EWOD)-based microfluidics. For each of these systems, we will introduce its working principle, fabrication methods as well as its key characteristics, and discuss the suitability in POC applications.

DIGITAL MICROFLUIDICS

Digital microfluidics is so named because the fluids are digitized into discrete volumes that form droplets spontaneously on an open surface that is chemically rendered low in surface energy (Fig. **1**). The fluidic operation on the digital microfluidic platform is realized by controlling the motion of these droplets. For example, liquid addition and mixing are realized by merging multiple droplets; liquid aliquoting is realized by splitting big droplets into small ones; waste liquid disposal and particle washing are realized by separating the particles from one droplet and merging them with another droplet. No microstructure is needed to contain the fluid as each droplet is self-contained. The droplet serves as a virtual fluidic container in which reagents are stored and reactions take place.

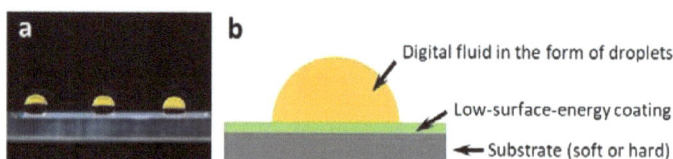

Fig. (1). Digital microfluidics. a) Discrete droplets on a digital microfluidic platform. b) Schematics of droplets on a substrate with a low-surface-energy coating.

Digital microfluidics is categorized based on its actuation mechanisms. Commonly used actuation methods include magnetic force [10, 19 - 22], electrowetting-on-dielectrics (EWOD) [11, 23, 24], surface acoustic wave [25 - 28], and optowetting [29, 30]. Among these actuation methods, magnetic force and EWOD are the most popular and well-established actuation methods for digital microfluidics. In this chapter, we will focus on these two methods, provide a comprehensive review of their current development status, and discuss their suitability for POC applications.

MAGNETIC DIGITAL MICROFLUIDICS

To actuate droplets on an open surface with magnetic force, a magnetic medium is required to make the droplets responsive to magnetic stimulus. Here, the term "magnetic" is used as a generic term that broadly refers to materials with ferromagnetic, paramagnetic, and superparamagnetic properties. The magnetic medium that serves as the actuator could manifest in the form of magnetic particles [19, 21, 31 - 33], a magnetic solution [34, 35], or a flexible magnetic surface substrate (Fig. **2**) [36 - 38].

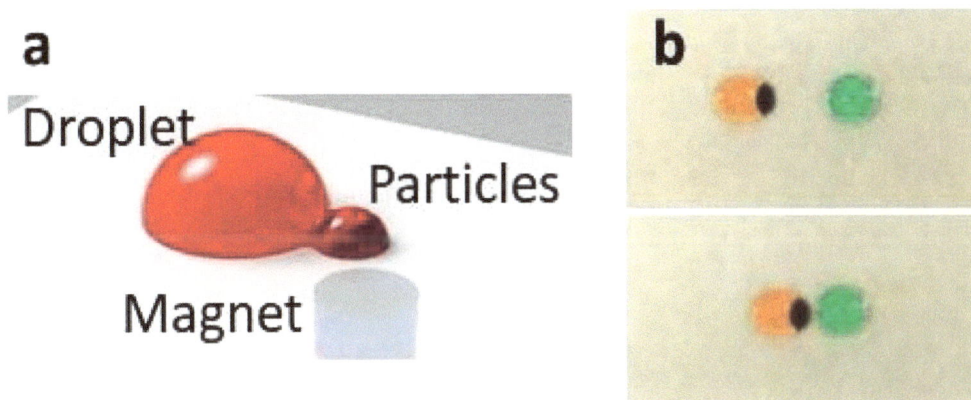

Fig. (**2**). **a**) Schematics of the droplet manipulation on the magnetic digital microfluidic platform. **b**) Droplet transport with magnetic particles added to the droplet. Fig. (**2b**) is reproduced from Ref. [21]. with permission from Wiley.

The most commonly used magnetic medium is the magnetic particles. Occasionally, magnetic salt is added to the droplet to create a magnetic ionic solution that responds to the external magnetic field. But magnetic particles are more desirable than the magnetic ionic solution because the high ionic strength in the solution would have a negative impact on the biosensing assays.

The surface of magnetic particles could be either hydrophilic or hydrophobic. When hydrophilic magnetic particles are added to the droplets, they form a cluster inside the droplets. A permanent magnet is placed below the substrate to control the movement of the magnetic particle cluster. Due to the surface tension of the droplet, the droplet tends to hold the magnetic particles within. As a result, the droplet would travel together with the magnetic particle cluster. Under certain circumstances, the surface tension of the droplet might not be sufficient to withhold the magnetic particle cluster inside the droplet. In such scenarios, the magnetic particle cluster would extract itself from the droplet.

The fundamental mechanism of magnetically actuated droplets on a plain hydrophobic surface has been comprehensively studied [39]. Three factors have been determined to affect the droplet operations: the droplet volume, the magnetic force and the moving speed. Given the same external magnetic field and the same type of particles, the magnetic force F_m is proportional to the particle mass loading M.

$$F_m = K_m \left(\frac{M}{\rho}\right) \tag{2}$$

where ρ is the particle density and K_m is the proportional factor related to the gradient of the external magnetic field and the magnetic susceptibility of the particles.

As the droplet moves with the magnetic particle cluster, it experiences a frictional force that is proportional to the velocity U and the diameter D of the droplet contact area.

$$F_f \propto UD = K_f U V^{1/3} \tag{3}$$

where K_f is the proportional factor related to the friction coefficient. The radius R of the droplet contact area is approximately proportional droplet volume V to the 1/3 power.

Another factor that is crucial in determining the droplet operation is the capillary force F_c surrounding the magnetic particle cluster, which is proportional to the diameter d of the magnetic particle plug. Assuming the magnetic particle plug is a hemisphere in shape, the radius r is proportional to the 1/3 power of the particle mass loading M.

$$F_c \propto d = K_c M^{1/3} \qquad (4)$$

where K_c is the proportional factor related to the surface tension of the fluid.

Depending on the relative strength of the magnetic force F_m, the frictional force F_f and the capillary force F_c, the droplet operation may be divided into 3 phases (21) (Fig. 3). If the capillary force F_c is smaller than the magnetic force F_m as well as the frictional force F_f, the magnetic particle cluster would extract itself from the droplet. This particle extraction process usually occurs with a low particle loading, a large droplet volume and a high moving speed. If the capillary force F_c is greater that the magnetic force F_m, the droplet would move together with the magnetic particle plug. This steady droplet transport process occurs with a large particle mass loading, a small droplet volume and a relatively low moving speed. Because the droplet moves steadily at a constant velocity, the frictional force F_f is equal to the magnetic force F_m. Another undesired operation occurs when the particle loading becomes too small. In this scenario, the magnetic force F_m is smaller than the capillary force F_c as well as the frictional force F_f, which means that the magnetic particle cluster could not break the surface tension but the magnetic force is too small to pull the droplet. As a result, the magnet would disengage from the magnetic particles and the droplet.

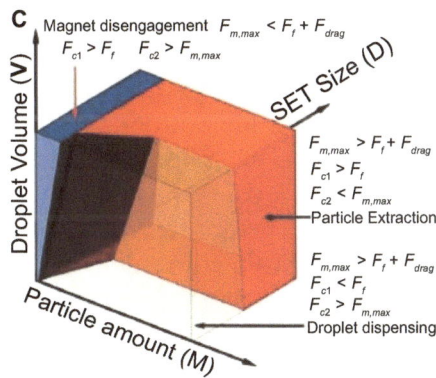

Fig. (3). Phase diagram of droplet manipulation on the surface energy trap-assisted magnetic digital microfluidic platform. Reproduced from Ref. [21]. with permission from Wiley.

The external magnetic field can also be applied through electromagnets. Several magnetic digital microfluidic platforms implement a micro coil-based electromagnet array fabricated on a thin film printed circuit board. By changing the polarity of the current, the resulted alternating magnetic field generates a magnetic field gradient to control the movement of the magnetic particles and the droplets.

If the particles are hydrophobic, they do not form a cluster inside the droplet. Instead, the magnetic particles spread over the droplet surface. The droplet encapsulated by the confluent layer of hydrophobic particles is called a liquid marble [22, 40 - 43]. The magnetic medium can be added in two ways. One may use hydrophobic magnetic particles that consist of magnetic core and a hydrophobic coating, to encapsulate the liquid marble [42]. Alternatively, soluble magnetic salt or hydrophilic magnetic particles may be added into the droplet as the magnetic medium while non-magnetic hydrophobic particles are used to encapsulate the liquid marble [44 - 45]. In both cases, the liquid marble would respond to the stimulus of external magnetic field. Compared to the droplets used in regular magnetic digital microfluidics, the major advantage of the liquid marble is its high stability on any surface. Unlike the "naked" droplet which would spread and wet the hydrophilic surface, the hydrophobic particles on the surface of the liquid marble creates a solid-solid interface and prevents the liquid from wetting the hydrophilic substrate, thereby maintaining the shape of the liquid marble. Moreover, the particle layer is able to reduce the evaporation [46 - 47]. which is a serious concern in digital microfluidics.

Another type of magnetic medium is the magnetically responsive flexible substrate. Such a substrate is usually fabricated by adding magnetic particles or permanent magnets to the silicone rubber. Micro/nanostructures are often introduced on the substrate during the rubber casting to increase the surface roughness thus the apparent contact angle [48]. When a magnet is brought to the vicinity of the flexible substrate from the bottom, the magnet pulls the substrate down and creates a potential well. The droplet has the tendency to roll to the bottom of the well where the energy level is the lowest. As the magnet moves, the potential well changes its location. The droplet rolls with the potential well, and the droplet transport is realized. This method does not require the addition of extraneous substances, such as the magnetic particles and ionic salts, to the droplet for the magnetic actuation. However, the size of the potential well is relatively big, and the number of droplets can be manipulated concurrently on a single flexible substrate is limited. On a rigid substrate, the closely placed droplets do not influence each other. In contrast, the closely placed droplets would fall into the same potential well hence cannot be manipulated independently.

Assisted Magnetic Digital Microfluidics

The simplest magnetic digital microfluidic system manipulates droplets on a Teflon-coated plain surface without any additional features. The required volume of the droplet and the mass of magnetic particles are dictated by the assay requirements. These two parameters are usually fixed for a particular assay. As a result, the only parameter that can be adjusted for droplet manipulation is the magnet moving speed. A low moving speed is used for droplet transport, and a high moving speed is required to extract magnetic particles from the droplet. However, under certain assay conditions, the mass of the magnetic particles required would be too high, and it would be impossible to extract the particles from the droplet under any feasible moving speed. One solution to this problem is to add assistive features to facilitate the droplet manipulation in combination with magnetic particles. The assistive features may manifest in the form of physical microstructures or chemical modifications that would interact with the droplets.

Microstructure-Assisted Magnetic Digital Microfluidics

The physical microstructures are introduced to the magnetic digital microfluidic platform mainly to facilitate the particle extraction process. Microscale constrictions are placed along the droplet moving path (Fig. **4**). These micro constrictions provide a narrow passage which only allows the magnetic particle cluster to squeeze through, but not the droplets. The constriction is usually imposed laterally by a microchannel or paired micro pillars (Fig. **4a**) [31, 32, 50 - 52]. Alternatively, the constriction is imposed vertically with an overhanging microstructure that prevents the droplet from moving further by holding the top part of the droplet (Fig. **4b**) [49]. As a droplet moves towards a constricted region, the magnetic particle cluster is able to squeeze through the micro constrictor but the liquid droplet is stopped from advancing further along the path. As a result, the magnetic particle cluster is extracted from the droplet.

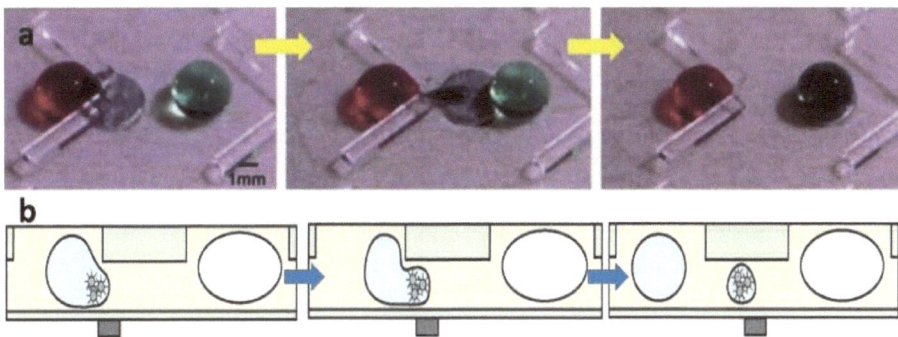

Fig. (4). Physical microstructure-assisted magnetic digital microfluidic platform. a) Constrictions from the side. b) Constrictions from the top. Fig. (**4a**) is reproduced from Ref. [32]. with permission from the Royal Chemistry Society. Fig. (**4b**) is reproduced from Ref. [49]. with permission from Elsevier.

As discussed above, the droplet moving on a plain surface experiences only one force in the opposite direction of the movement (*i.e.,* the frictional force). As the moving speed increases, the frictional force increases proportionally. Once the frictional force exceeds the capillary force surrounding the magnetic particle cluster, the particle extraction takes place. However, under certain circumstances, a large quantity of magnetic particles is required to perform an assay, which imposes a large capillary force surrounding the magnetic particle cluster. Under such a condition, the frictional force alone is insufficient to overcome the capillary force at any feasible moving speed. The micro constrictor provides a mechanism to anchor the droplet for easy particle extraction. Once the droplet comes in contact with the micro constrictor, an additional resistance force F_s acts on the droplet. The additional resistance force works together with the frictional force to hold the droplet while the magnetic particle cluster is pulled away from the droplet by the magnet. The combined resistance force and the frictional force are sufficient to overcome the capillary force surrounding the large magnetic particle cluster, thereby facilitating the particle extraction.

The microstructure-assisted magnetic digital microfluidics has simplified the particle extraction, an important fluidic operation required for heterogeneous assays. Because the droplet volume and the magnetic particle loading are determined by the assay requirements, the users are unable to realize the particle extraction by adjusting these two parameters. By incorporating micro constrictions to facilitate the particle extraction process, it becomes easier to translate various diagnostic assays on the magnetic digital microfluidic platform without having to worry about the fluidic operations.

Chemical Modification-Assisted Magnetic Digital Microfluidics

Although the physical microstructures greatly ease the particle extraction process, the complexity added to the device fabrication makes the microstructure-assisted magnetic digital microfluidic platform less attractive. An improved approach uses surface chemical modifications to facilitate the droplet manipulation.

The substrate on which the droplets sit in a magnetic digital microfluidic platform has a low surface energy. The low surface energy is achieved by a thin film coating with Teflon or other fluorosurfactants and fluoroalkalines. The low surface energy renders the substrate omniphobic to ensure smooth movement of the droplet. As the droplet moves on the substrate, it experiences a frictional force which provides the resistance to hold back the droplet during the particle extraction. The microstructure-assisted device avails the additional resistance force provided by the microstructure for droplet manipulation. The additional resistance force can also be provided by the chemical surface modification.

Certain regions on the low-surface-energy substrate are chemically rendered hydrophilic with high surface energy [21, 33]. When a droplet moves over these high-energy regions, the surface tension pins down the contact line and traps the droplet. We therefore refer to these high-surface-energy regions as the surface energy trap (SET). The SET provides the additional resistance force needed to facilitate the droplet manipulation.

When a droplet is pulled over a SET by the magnetic particle cluster at a constant speed, the droplet experiences several forces (Fig. 5). The magnetic force F_m, which is proportional to the particle mass loading M, pulls the droplet forward. Two forces are exerted on the droplet in the opposite direction of the droplet movement. The drag force F_{drag} is approximately proportional to the length scale of the droplet or $V^{1/3}$. The surface tension F_i is proportional to the diameter of the SET D. Once the droplet moves over a SET, the contact line of the droplet is pinned down due to the high surface tension, forming one necking point (NP1) around the SET with a capillary force F_{c1} that is proportional to the diameter of the SET D. Meanwhile, the magnetic particle cluster keeps pulling the droplet, forming another necking point (NP2) around the magnetic particle cluster with a capillary force F_{c2} that is proportional to the length scale of the magnetic particle mass loading or $M^{1/3}$. Depending on the relative magnitude of these forces, one of the following three scenarios would occur given a constant moving speed of the magnet. First, if the magnetic force F_m is smaller than the combined resistance force (*i.e.,* $F_i + F_{drag}$), the capillary force F_{c1} is greater than the surface tension F_i around the SET, and the capillary force F_{c2} is greater than the magnetic force F_m, the magnet would disengage from the magnetic particle cluster, which is an undesired scenario. This scenario often occurs when the magnetic particle loading is too small. The desired droplet operations are the particle extraction and the fluidic dispensing. The particle extraction occurs when the magnetic force F_m is greater than the combined resistance force F_i+F_{drag}, the capillary force F_{c1} is greater than the surface tension F_i, but the capillary force F_{c2} is less than the magnetic force F_m. Under these conditions, the necking point NP2 around the magnetic particle cluster would break. In contrast, when the magnetic force F_m is greater than the combined resistance force F_i+F_{drag}, the capillary force F_{c1} is less than the surface tension F_i, but the capillary force F_{c2} is greater than the magnetic force F_m, the necking point NP1 would break, resulting in the liquid dispensing. With the assistance of these chemical surface modifications, a full range of droplet operations, including the droplet transport, droplet mixing, particle extraction, liquid dispensing and cross-platform transport, have been demonstrated on the magnetic digital microfluidic platform [21]. (Figs. **5, 6**).

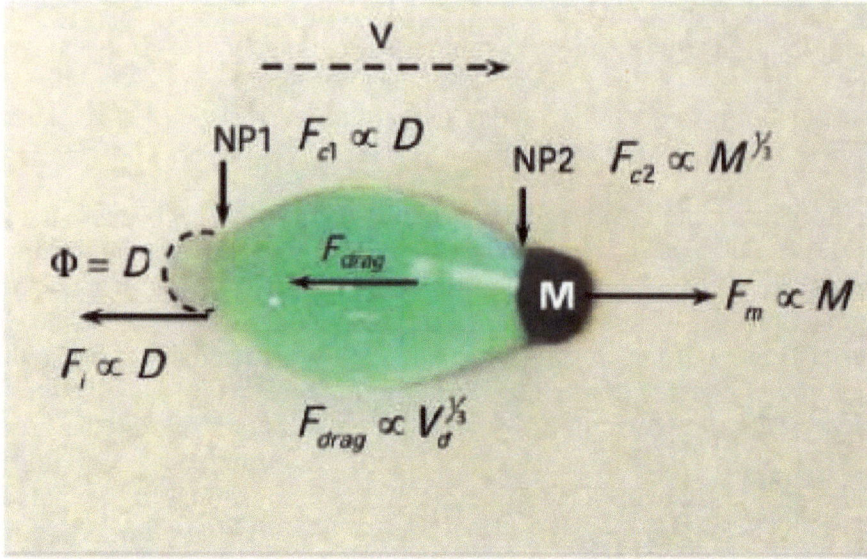

Fig. (5). Force diagram a droplet experiences when moving over a surface energy trap. Reproduced from Ref. [21]. with permission from Wiley.

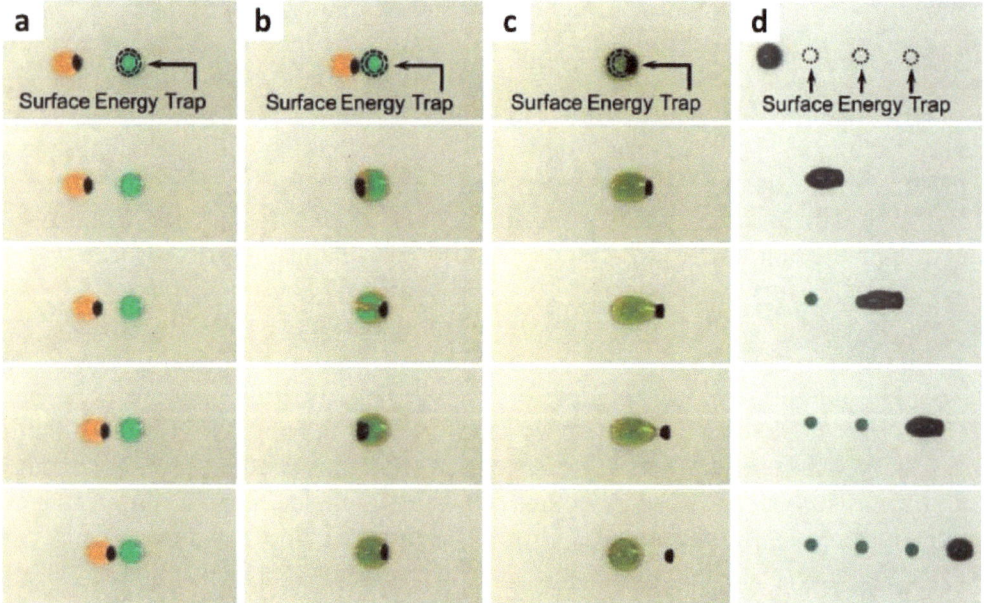

Fig. (6). Droplet manipulations with the assistance of the surface energy traps on the magnetic digital microfluidic platform. a) Droplet moving, b) droplet coalesce and mixing, c) magnetic particle extraction, and d) passive liquid dispensing. Reproduced from Ref. [21]. with permission from Wiley.

EWOD-BASED DIGITAL MICROFLUIDICS

The droplet actuation on the EWOD-based digital microfluidic platform relies on the pressure gradient induced by the electrical potential exerted on one side of the droplet, which causes asymmetric droplet deformation and droplet movement [23, 53]. Although both single-plate and two-plate configurations have been demonstrated for EWOD-based digital microfluidics, the two-plate configuration is more common. In the two-plate configuration, the droplet is sandwiched between the two flat substrates (Fig. **7**). The top plate is usually made of indium-tin-oxide (ITO) glass which serves as a conductive electrode as the ground and provides a transparent window for easy visualization. The metal actuation electrode is fabricated on the bottom plate using microfabrication techniques. An insulating material is deposited on top of the actuation electrode as the dielectric layer. A Teflon thin film is then coated on both plates to ensure smooth droplet movement.

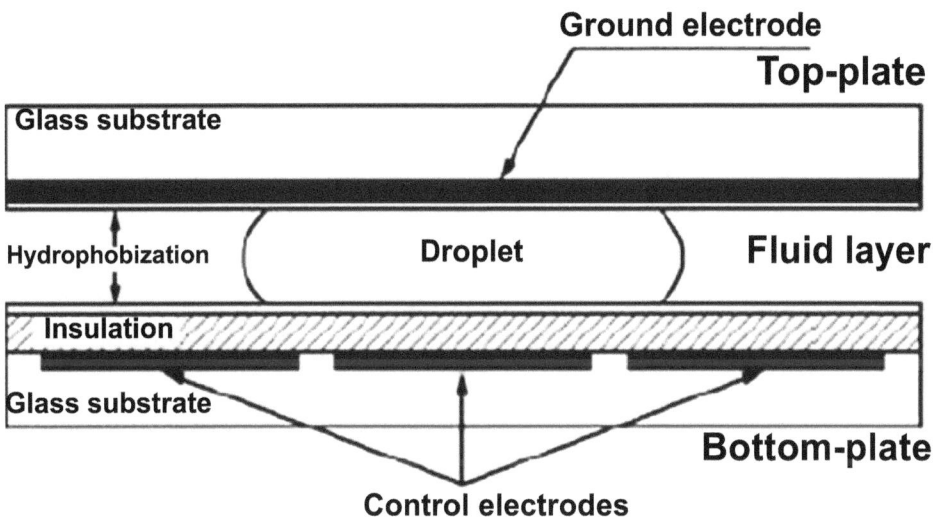

Fig. (7). Schematics of EWOD-based digital microfluidic platform. Reproduced from Ref. [23]. with permission from Springer Nature.

To actuate a droplet using EWOD, the size of the electrode must be smaller than the contact size of the droplet so that the droplet would occupy more than one electrode when sandwiched between the two plates. Initially, the contact angle on the two sides of the droplet are identical. Once the electrical potential is applied to one side of the droplet through an activation electrode, the contact angle changes according to the Young-Lippmann relationship [53]:

$$cos\theta = cos\theta_0 + \frac{\varepsilon_0 \varepsilon_r V^2}{2\gamma d} \quad\quad (5)$$

where θ_0 is the initial contact angle without the applied voltage, θ is the contact angle as a result of the electrowetting effect under the applied voltage. ε_0 and ε_r are the vacuum permittivity and the relative permittivity of the dielectric layer, respectively. γ is the surface tension of the filling media, which is usually air but occasionally silicone oil or organic solvent. V is the applied voltage, and d is the thickness of the dielectric layer.

When the droplet occupies more than one electrode, and only one of the electrodes is activated, the contact angles on the two sides of the droplet become different. This asymmetry in the contact angle results in a pressure gradient across the droplet, which drives the droplet from the side with a larger contact angle to the side with a smaller contact angle (*i.e.,* from the zero-potential electrode to the high potential electrode). The driving force is approximated according to the following equation [54]:

$$L\gamma(cos\theta - cos\theta_0) = \frac{\varepsilon_0 \varepsilon_r V^2}{2d} \quad\quad (6)$$

Continuous droplet actuation on the EWOD-based digital microfluidic platform is realized by activating the electrodes along the droplet moving path in sequence. Once the droplet reaches the designated location, all electrodes are deactivated, the droplet restores its symmetry, and the droplet movement stops.

One unique and advantageous feature of the EWOD-based digital microfluidic system is its ability to actively split the droplet to accomplish liquid dispensing [53, 55]. The active droplet splitting is accomplished by activating both electrodes on the two ends of the droplet. Consequently, the liquid flows from the center of the droplet to the ends. As the fluid leaves the original droplet center, the center gradually narrows until the Laplacian pressure is large enough to break the surface tension, resulting in two daughter droplets. This mechanism is usually used for symmetric droplet splitting. For liquid dispensing, an asymmetric droplet splitting mechanism is derived by imposing a physical restriction on the parent droplet. Usually, a reservoir with a small opening is used to hold the parent droplet in position [55]. A linear array of actuation electrodes is connected to the opening of the reservoir. As the actuation electrodes are activated in sequence, it draws a liquid column from the reservoir. The liquid column would break at certain point as its length increases, resulting in a daughter droplet of smaller volume compared to the parent droplet. The daughter droplets dispensed using this approach are reasonably uniform and can be prepared on demand.

EWOD-based digital microfluidics is also capable of passive liquid dispensing by patterning the Teflon thin film coating with hydrophilic features, similar to that of the magnetic digital microfluidic.

MAGNETIC DIGITAL MICROFLUIDICS *VS* EWOD-BASED DIGITAL MICROFLUIDICS

Magnetic digital microfluidics and EWOD-based digital microfluidics have their respective advantages or disadvantages. Magnetic digital microfluidics can be manipulated either manually or automatically with a motorized translational stage, whereas the EWOD-based digital microfluidics must be operated using an automated control system. On one hand, the automation of the EWOD system is more accurate and efficient. On the other hand, the manual operation of magnetic digital microfluidics allows it to be deployed in the resource-constrained environment for POC applications. The major advantage of the EWOD-based digital microfluidics over magnetic digital microfluidics is its ability to actively dispense daughter droplets of desired volumes Magnetic digital microfluidics can only passively dispense fluids through the SETs.

The most unique feature of magnetic digital microfluidics is the multiple functions of the magnetic particles added to the droplets. The particles are used both as the droplet actuator and the solid substrate for biochemical reactions. Both the droplet motion and the biochemical reaction can be controlled by a permanent magnet. As a result, magnetic digital microfluidics is well-suited for heterogeneous solid phase reactions. EWOD could incorporate microparticles as the solid substrate for heterogeneous bioreactions. Nonetheless, additional mechanisms, such as magnetic force or acoustic wave, are required to manipulate these particles in addition to the electrowetting mechanisms used for the droplet actuation.

In terms of the device fabrication, the magnetic digital microfluidics is significantly simpler than the EWOD-based device. Magnetic digital microfluidics only requires a hydrophobic coating on a plain surface, and an optional layer with assistive features. In contrast, the EWOD-based device demands a more complex fabrication process for multiple layers consisting of a dielectric layer, an electrode layer and a transparent conductive layer in addition to the hydrophobic coating.

In terms of the droplet manipulation, magnetic digital microfluidics is more tolerant of the fluid properties, capable of manipulating various types of fluids with vastly different surface tension, conductivity and permittivity. In contrast, EWOD is very sensitive to the fluidic properties. The surface tension, conductivity and permittivity of the fluid have a strong influence on the electrowetting property of the fluid, hence the droplet actuation.

APPLICATIONS OF DIGITAL MICROFLUIDICS IN BIOSENSING AND POC DIAGNOSTICS

Digital microfluidics has been demonstrated in a number of preparative and analytical bioassays including the DNA/RNA extraction, small molecule detection by enzymatic assays, targeted gene analysis by PCR, and targeted protein analysis by enzyme-linked immunosorbent assay (ELISA) among others. In digital microfluidics, the droplets function as the virtual reaction chambers in which all the reactions are contained. Therefore, no physical microchamber or other microstructure is required to contain the fluids.

Nucleic Acids-Based Assay

One of the most common applications of digital microfluidics is the DNA extraction. The DNA extraction is accomplished based on the reversible binding/desorption mechanism of the DNA molecules on the surface of magnetic particles that function as the solid substrate. The surface of the magnetic particle is coated with a layer of silica. First, the biosample is incubated with the silica magnetic particles in an aqueous binding buffer containing chaotropic salts with a high ionic strength and a low pH. In this buffer, only the DNA molecules in the biosample have the tendency to bind to the silica surface. Once the DNA molecules bind to the particle surface, buffers containing a high concentration of organic solvent are used to wash away the salt from the binding buffer and other unwanted cellular components from the biosample. After washing, an aqueous elution buffer with a low ionic strength and a high pH is incubated with the particles to elute the DNA molecules from the solid phase into the liquid phase for the subsequent analysis. On the magnetic digital microfluidic platform, the magnetic particles are moved through droplets containing the required buffers. Assistive features are sometimes used to help particles split from one droplet and merge with another. On the EWOD-based digital microfluidic platform, this liquid exchange process is realized by immobilizing the particles with a magnet and driving the buffer droplets over the immobilized particles in sequence. This droplet-based DNA extraction process is often coupled with the downstream DNA detection assays for the sample-to-answer analysis of clinical samples on the digital microfluidic platform. To do so, the droplet containing the eluted DNA is moved to merge with a PCR reaction buffer droplet containing the primer set that recognizes the target DNA sequence. Alternatively, the magnetic particles with the DNA bound to the surface may be directly merged with the PCR buffer droplet. The low-ionic-strength and high-pH buffer used in PCR favors the desorption of the DNA from the particle surface, eluting the DNA molecules into the PCR reaction buffer for the amplification. Subsequently, the PCR could be performed with or without the presence of the magnetic particles because the particles do not affect the PCR reaction. Nevertheless, it is a good practice to remove the particles because the particles would interfere the fluorescent signals during real-time PCR.

Several works have demonstrated the sample-to-answer DNA/RNA sensing on the digital microfluidic platform, particularly on the magnetic digital microfluidic platform. During the H5N1 avian flu outbreak in 2007, Pipper and colleagues used their magnetic digital microfluidic platform for point-of-care avian flu diagnostics by extracting the viral RNA with magnetic particles and detecting the isolated RNA using the real time reverse-transcriptase PCR (RT-PCR) on the magnetic digital microfluidic platform [19]. The same group used a similar device to analyze a biomarker of transfected white blood cell. On this platform, the PCR was performed not by changing the temperature of the heating unit, but by moving the droplet between four heating units held at constant temperatures required for the DNA denaturation, primer annealing and amplicon elongation [20]. The magnetic droplet actuation was accomplished by placing the permanent magnet on a rotational motor. Zhang and colleagues used a surface modification-assisted magnetic digital microfluidic platform to analyze cancer genetic biomarkers [21]. In this work, the SETs were implemented to facilitate the particle extraction during the sample preparation and the liquid dispensing during the DNA aliquoting. With the assistance of these SETs, authors demonstrated the sample-to-answer analysis of multiple cancer genetic markers with a single sample preparation by splitting the isolate DNA into multiple aliquots.

Several POC molecular diagnostic platforms have been developed based on the magnetic digital microfluidics. Zhang and colleagues developed a POC cancer biomarker analysis system based on the physical structure-assisted magnetic digital microfluidics. Micropillars were used to form a narrow slit to facilitate the particle extraction [32]. The authors demonstrated the sample-to-answer analysis of the cancer biomarker using the whole blood sample. They also demonstrated the detection of bacterial pathogens using an isothermal DNA amplification method in addition to PCR. Chiou and colleagues developed a similar sample-to-answer cancer biomarker molecular analysis system using the physical structure-assisted magnetic digital microfluidics [31]. Instead of using a permanent magnet to control the motion of the magnetic particles, an array of micro-coil electromagnets is activated in sequence to actuate the droplet. Shih and colleagues demonstrated a two-plate magnetic digital microfluidic cartridge for the sample-to-answer diagnostics of infectious diseases [56]. The sealed cartridge contained all the reagents and magnetic particles required to analyze the target DNA/RNA in the form of droplets. The cartridge was filled with oil to separate the droplets and prevent the evaporation. This platform used an automated droplet manipulation system by placing the magnet on a rotational motor. In addition to the movement in the planar direction, the magnet also moved in the vertical direction to pull the magnetic particles to the top plate. The magnetic particle cluster was able to move on the top plate until it reached the designated location where it was lowered to bottom plate and merged with another droplet. With an integrated fluorescent detection system, successful POC diagnostics of Chlamydia trachomatis and hepatitis C had been demonstrated using a real time isothermal amplification technique as well as PCR.

Molecular diagnostics has also been demonstrated on the EWOD-based digital microfluidic platform. Sista and colleagues developed a cartridge-based POC diagnostic platform for automated droplet manipulation through EWOD [57]. The authors used Chargeswitch® magnetic particles as the solid substrate for DNA/RNA extraction. The surface charge of these particles switched from negative to positive in the binding buffer, and switched from positive to negative in the elution buffer. This mechanism was used for the reversible DNA binding/desorption in the DNA extraction process. In this process, the buffer droplets were driven over the magnetic particle cluster in sequence while a permanent magnet was placed below the EWOD actuation electrode to immobilize the magnetic particles during the liquid exchange. The on-chip thermal cycling was carried out in the space domain by moving the PCR droplet between zones held at 60°C and 95°C, respectively. Using this platform, the authors demonstrated the sample-to-answer detection of the methicillin-resistant *Staphylococcus aureus* and the *Candida albicans*. This platform was successfully commercialized by the Advanced Liquid Logic Inc [58]. The company also demonstrated multiplexed PCR on this platform for the diagnostics of methicillin-resistant *Staphylococcus aureus* (MRSA), *Mycoplasma pneumoniae*, and *Candida albicans*. In this application, the sample preparation was performed off-chip and introduced onto the EWOD-based magnetic digital microfluidic platform for the subsequent PCR analysis which was carried out by driving multiple reaction droplets in parallel between different temperature zones.

Protein-Based Assay

Immunoassays are often used to detect the presence as well as the quantity of the protein of interest in the biological sample. Sandwich ELISA is one of the most common forms of immunoassays widely used in clinical diagnostics. In the sandwich ELISA, a pair of antibodies or other binding agents (*e.g.* peptide or aptamers) are used to recognize the target of interest. The capture antibody is immobilized on the solid substrate, usually the surface of a microwell plate, via passive adsorption or covalent linking. After adding the sample to the microwell, the target protein is captured by the capture antibody via the ligand-receptor recognition. The detector antibody that recognizes a different epitope of the target protein may be added separately or together with the sample. After washing away the excess sample and reagents, the capture antibody, detector antibody and the target protein form a sandwich structure. The detector antibody is either directly conjugated to an enzyme or indirectly tagged with an enzyme through a secondary antibody. This enzyme, which is immobilized to the solid substrate with the detector antibody, develops the chemical substrate and generates a colorimetric, fluorescent or chemiluminescent signal that correlates to the amount of the protein target.

In digital microfluidics, the ELISA is established by conjugating the capture antibody to the surface of the magnetic particles that serve as the solid substrate (Fig. **8**). After the addition of the sample and the detector antibody, the sandwich structure together with the enzyme is immobilized on the particle surface. The washing process in this particle-based ELISA process is carried out by moving the magnetic particles through a series of washing buffer droplets or by holding the magnetic particles in place while driving the washing buffer droplets over the particles in sequence.

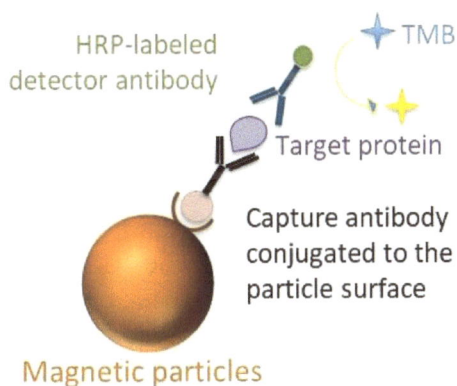

Fig. (8). Schematic illustration of magnetic particle-based ELISA. Reproduced from Ref [74] with permission from Wiley.

Particle-based protein detection has been demonstrated on several physical structure-assisted magnetic digital microfluidic platforms. Shikida and colleagues fabricated a device with a series of open chambers separated by a partially open gate [49]. The gate closed from the top and left a narrowing opening at the bottom. As it moved towards the gate, the droplet was stopped by the partially closed gate whereas the magnetic particles squeezed through the narrow opening at the bottom and continued moving forward. Instead of ELISA, the authors demonstrated a single-step enzymatic reaction with enzymes being immobilized on the particle surface. The same group presented a similar device with narrow microchannels that connect micro chambers as the restriction to assist the particle extraction [52]. Kim and colleague designed a micropillar array to facilitate the particle extraction for particle-based ELISA on a magnetic digital microfluidic platform [50]. The aqueous phase and the oil phase were separated by the micropillar array. When the magnetic particles moved from the aqueous phase to the oil phase, the micropillar array stopped the aqueous solution but allowed the magnetic particles to pass through the array via the spacing between the micropillars.

Wheeler's group has demonstrated several EWOD digital microfluidics-based immunodiagnostic platforms. Ng and colleagues performed both competitive and noncompetitive ELISA on the EWOD-based digital microfluidic platform by conjugating the capture antibody to magnetic particles [59]. A permanent magnet was used to hold the magnetic particles in position during the washing process. The reagents in the form of droplets were driven over the particle cluster one at a time. Using this platform, the authors detected the thyroid stimulating hormone (TSH) and 17β-estradiol (E2). The authors applied a similar platform for the detection of the rubella immunity [60]. The operation procedure was similar to the previous case. But the target of interest was the antibody instead of the antigen. The antigen was conjugated to the magnetic particles as the capture agent instead. Shamsi and colleagues incorporated the electrochemistry sensing modality in the EWOD-based digital microfluidics [61]. In addition to the actuation electrodes, the working electrode, the reference electrode and the counter electrodes were also fabricated on the top plate. The ELISA was performed by conjugating the capture antibody to the magnetic particles that served as the solid substrate. The horseradish peroxidase (HRP)-conjugated detector antibody converted the substrate 3,3',5,5'-tetramethylbenzidine (TMB) into an oxidized molecule that were detected amperometrically through the electrochemistry sensing electrodes on the top plate. Rackus and colleagues improved the sensitivity of the electrochemical immunoassay by introducing nanostructured electrodes to the EWOD-based digital microfluidic platform [62]. The nanostructured working electrode was fabricated by the electrodeposition of gold on to the top plate. The signal obtained using the nanostructured electrode was significantly enhanced with an enhancement factor over 600 folds compared to the regular planar electrode. The rubella virus was conjugated to the magnetic particles as the capture agent to detect the immunoglobin against the virus. A secondary antibody conjugated with the alkaline phosphatase converted the pAPP substrate molecule to the pAP which was an electroactive reporter. Ng and colleagues brought the EWOD digital microfluidics-based immunodiagnostic platform to the field to detect the immunity against measles and rubella viruses in the resource-limited settings in Kenya [63]. Using an automated EWOD system, the authors achieved a sensitivity of 86% and a specificity of 80% for the measles virus, and a sensitivity of 81% and a specificity of 91% for the rubella virus.

The EWOD-based digital microfluidic platform was also used for the protein sample preparation. Seale and his colleagues performed the immunoprecipitation on the digital microfluidic platform to purify the human serum albumin (HSA) spiked in the fetal bovine serum and recovered 80% of HSA [64]. Mei and colleagues attempted to deplete proteins from the human serum on the EWOD-based digital microfluidic platform [65]. In this case, magnetic particles were conjugated with anti-HSA and protein A/G to deplete the HSA the immunoglobins, respectively. The authors managed to deplete over 95% of the total proteins in 10 minutes on the digital microfluidic platform.

Cell Assay

Droplets are excellent micro bioreactors. Each droplet is a virtual cell culture chamber with a large surface-to-volume ratio for effective gas exchange. The essential gases, such as oxygen and carbon dioxide, could diffuse through the droplet efficiently. The potential issue associated EWOD-based cell culture is the damages to cells caused by the electricity and the joule heating [66]. It has been shown that the DNA integrity and the gene expression are significantly altered when a high-frequency actuation signal is applied through a large electrode for a long period of time [67]. The joule heating could raise the temperature in the droplet to as high as 56°C and cause cell death [68]. This issue could be solved by carefully evaluating the cell viability under various actuation conditions and select the condition that does not damage the cells.

Compared to the liquid buffers used in the nucleic acid and protein assays, the cell culture medium is a more complex matrix containing buffers, proteins, ions and other additives that are essential for the cell growth. The relatively high concentrations of proteins and ions significantly interfere with the electrowetting property and hinder the droplet transport on the digital microfluidic platform. One main issue associated with the high concentration of proteins in the cell culture medium is caused by the protein adsorption on the hydrophobic Teflon surface of the digital microfluidic platform [67]. The protein adsorption causes the droplets to stick to the surface and impedes the droplet movement. One common solution to this problem is by using an immiscible carrier solution to encapsulate the cell culture medium droplet. As a result, only the carrier fluid is in contact with the actuation electrodes. On the EWOD-based digital microfluidic platform, the carrier fluid is selected with a good electrowetting property for easy actuation. The culture medium droplet would move together with the carrier fluid droplet upon the application of the electrical potential. An alternative approach was to introduce additives, such as graphene oxide and Pluronic, to the cell culture medium to prevent the protein adsorption on the Teflon-coated surface. With these additives, the droplet could be transported freely by EWOD in spite of high protein concentration.

Using these approaches, a number of cell-based assays have been successfully demonstrated on the EWOD-based digital microfluidic platform. Barbulovic-Nad and colleagues performed a cytotoxicity assay by culturing the Jurkat T-cells in suspension [69]. The authors used the Pluronic as the additive to prevent the protein adsorption. The actuation conditions were optimized to minimize the adverse effect on the cells. It was shown that the sensitivity of the cytotoxicity assay was 20 times higher on the EWOD-based digital microfluidic platform than that on the conventional microwell plate. The same group also developed a digital microfluidics-based adherent cell culture system [70]. This system used a hydrophilic patch to passively dispense a fibronectin-based extracellular matrix (ECM) as the cell culture substrate. The adherent cells were cultivated on the passively dispensed ECM in droplets. The waste liquid was removed, and new reagents for the cell passage were subsequently added to the ECM by driving the droplets over the hydrophilic zone. Authors successfully demonstrated the seeding, cultivation and passage of several cell lines in 150-nL droplets on this platform for several weeks. In addition to the cell culture, functional cell assays were also demonstrated on the EWOD-based digital microfluidic platform. For example, Srigunapalan and colleagues patterned the top plate of EWOD-based digital microfluidic platform with hydrophilic patches and used these patches as the solid substrate for the "upside-down" culture of the adherent primary endothelial cells [71]. After the cell culture, a monocyte adhesion assay was performed by adding a droplet containing monocytes to the primary endothelial cell culture. The primary endothelial cells activated by the TNFα showed significantly stronger adhesion to the monocytes. Using the silicone oil as the carrier fluid, Zhou and colleagues actuated the alginate hydrogels embedded with cells and arranged them in 2D arrays as a way of printing tissue engineering models [72]. The cultivation of small animal embryo was also successfully demonstrated by Son and colleagues [73]. The droplet containing the zebra fish embryo was transported on the EWOD-based digital microfluidic platform with an actuation voltage around 100 V_{rms} at 8 kHz. Subsequently, the zebra fish embryos were evaluated by allowing them to hatch in the fresh water. Embryos that were subjected to EWOD manipulation under the aforementioned conditions were able to hatch normally.

Compared to the EWOD-based system, the magnetic digital microfluidic platform is less severely affected by the buffer conditions of the cell culture medium. The magnetic actuation is insensitive to the protein content and the ionic strength of the buffer. However, the cell culture on the magnetic digital microfluidic platform has not been systematically studied. Very few works have demonstrated cell culture on the magnetic digital microfluidic work. Zhang and colleagues cultivated bacteria in the droplets containing a serial dilution of antibiotics and performed the antimicrobial susceptibility testing (AST) on the magnetic digital microfluidic platform [33]. In this work, the authors used the SETs to passively dispense antibiotics from the stock solution droplet for the generation of the serial dilution. An array of surface energy traps of different sizes was used to dispense liquid of desired volumes. The size of the surface energy traps determined the volume of the daughter droplets. A serial dilution of antibiotics was created after merging the daughter droplets with the dilution buffer droplets which contained the bacterial cells and the culture broth. The bacteria were cultured in droplets over night to determine the minimal inhibitory concentration of the antibiotics.

CONCLUDING REMARKS

Since its emergence, microfluidics has been closely associated with bioanalysis. The conventional microfluidic platform has greatly advanced the fundamental research in the field of biology, but its highly complexity and sophisticated peripherals have limited its applications to the laboratory settings. In POC applications, a standalone microfluidic platform with minimal peripherals is highly coveted. Unconventional microfluidics, particularly the digital microfluidics, meets this requirement. Due to its simple fluidic operation and unique virtual reaction chamber concept, digital microfluidics has been developed into true POC diagnostic platforms capable of sample-to-answer analysis. In spite these advantages, digital microfluidics still has several limitations that remain to be addressed. For example, the open design is prone to evaporation. Although carrier oil is often added to prevent the evaporation, the additional thermal mass complicates the biochemical reactions such as PCR. The future work on digital microfluidics should focus on the system integration that combine several modules for droplet motion control, environment (*e.g.* temperature, pressure) control and chip-to-world interface. Although digital microfluidic systems are still not as popular as the conventional microfluidic systems, we believe digital microfluidics could find niche applications in medical diagnosis.

CONSENT FOR PUBLICATION

Not applicable.

CONFLICT OF INTEREST

The authors confirm that this chapter contents have no conflict of interest.

ACKNOWLEDGEMENT

The author would like to thank the funding support from Singapore Ministry of Education (Tier 1 RG49/17) and Nanyang Technological University (Start-Up Grant).

REFERENCES

[1]   Gravesen P, Branebjerg J, Jensen OS. Microfluidics-a review. J Micromech Microeng 1993; 3(4): 168.
        [http://dx.doi.org/10.1088/0960-1317/3/4/002]

[2]   Whitesides GM. The origins and the future of microfluidics. Nature 2006; 442(7101): 368-73.
        [http://dx.doi.org/10.1038/nature05058] [PMID: 16871203]

[3]   de Jong J, Lammertink RG, Wessling M. Membranes and microfluidics: a review. Lab Chip 2006; 6(9): 1125-39.
        [http://dx.doi.org/10.1039/b603275c] [PMID: 16929391]

[4]   Suh YK, Kang S. A review on mixing in microfluidics. Micromachines (Basel) 2010; 1(3): 82-111.
        [http://dx.doi.org/10.3390/mi1030082]

[5]   Daw R, Finkelstein J. Lab on a chip. Nature 2006; 442: 367.
        [http://dx.doi.org/10.1038/442367a]

[6]   Dittrich PS, Manz A. Lab-on-a-chip: microfluidics in drug discovery. Nat Rev Drug Discov 2006; 5(3): 210-8.
        [http://dx.doi.org/10.1038/nrd1985] [PMID: 16518374]

[7]   Haeberle S, Zengerle R. Microfluidic platforms for lab-on-a-chip applications. Lab Chip 2007; 7(9): 1094-110.
        [http://dx.doi.org/10.1039/b706364b] [PMID: 17713606]

[8]   Mark D, Haeberle S, Roth G, Von Stetten F, Zengerle R. Microfluidic lab-on-a-chip platforms: requirements, characteristics and applications Microfluidics Based Microsystems. Springer 2010; pp. 305-76.

[9]   Teh S-Y, Lin R, Hung L-H, Lee AP. Droplet microfluidics. Lab Chip 2008; 8(2): 198-220.
        [http://dx.doi.org/10.1039/b715524g] [PMID: 18231657]

[10]   Zhang Y, Nguyen N-T. Magnetic digital microfluidics - a review. Lab Chip 2017; 17(6): 994-1008.
        [http://dx.doi.org/10.1039/C7LC00025A] [PMID: 28220916]

[11]   Choi K, Ng AH, Fobel R, Wheeler AR. Digital microfluidics. Annu Rev Anal Chem (Palo Alto, Calif) 2012; 5: 413-40.
        [http://dx.doi.org/10.1146/annurev-anchem-062011-143028] [PMID: 22524226]

[12]   Martinez AW, Phillips ST, Whitesides GM, Carrilho E. Diagnostics for the developing world: microfluidic paper-based analytical devices. ACS Publications 2009.

[13]   Li X, Ballerini DR, Shen W. A perspective on paper-based microfluidics: Current status and future trends. Biomicrofluidics 2012; 6(1): 11301-1130113.

[http://dx.doi.org/10.1063/1.3687398] [PMID: 22662067]

[14] Weigl BH, Yager P. Microfluidic diffusion-based separation and detection. Science 1999; 283(5400): 346-7.
[http://dx.doi.org/10.1126/science.283.5400.346]

[15] Lin B, Levchenko A. Spatial manipulation with microfluidics. Front Bioeng Biotechnol 2015; 3: 39.
[http://dx.doi.org/10.3389/fbioe.2015.00039] [PMID: 25905100]

[16] Lazar IM, Karger BL. Multiple open-channel electroosmotic pumping system for microfluidic sample handling. Anal Chem 2002; 74(24): 6259-68.
[http://dx.doi.org/10.1021/ac0203950] [PMID: 12510747]

[17] Khare K, Zhou J, Yang S. Tunable open-channel microfluidics on soft poly(dimethylsiloxane) (PDMS) substrates with sinusoidal grooves. Langmuir 2009; 25(21): 12794-9.
[http://dx.doi.org/10.1021/la901736n] [PMID: 19572521]

[18] Hamedi MM, Ünal B, Kerr E, Glavan AC, Fernandez-Abedul MT, Whitesides GM. Coated and uncoated cellophane as materials for microplates and open-channel microfluidics devices. Lab Chip 2016; 16(20): 3885-97.
[http://dx.doi.org/10.1039/C6LC00975A] [PMID: 27714038]

[19] Pipper J, Inoue M, Ng LFP, Neuzil P, Zhang Y, Novak L. Catching bird flu in a droplet. Nat Med 2007; 13(10): 1259-63.
[http://dx.doi.org/10.1038/nm1634] [PMID: 17891145]

[20] Pipper J, Zhang Y, Neuzil P, Hsieh TM. Clockwork PCR including sample preparation. Angew Chem Int Ed Engl 2008; 47(21): 3900-4.
[http://dx.doi.org/10.1002/anie.200705016] [PMID: 18412211]

[21] Zhang Y, Wang TH. Full-range magnetic manipulation of droplets via surface energy traps enables complex bioassays. Adv Mater 2013; 25(21): 2903-8.
[http://dx.doi.org/10.1002/adma.201300383] [PMID: 23529938]

[22] Zhao Y, Xu Z, Niu H, Wang X, Lin T. Magnetic liquid marbles: Toward "lab in a droplet". Adv Funct Mater 2015; 25(3): 437-44.
[http://dx.doi.org/10.1002/adfm.201403051]

[23] Fair RB. Digital microfluidics: is a true lab-on-a-chip possible? Microfluid Nanofluidics 2007; 3(3): 245-81.
[http://dx.doi.org/10.1007/s10404-007-0161-8]

[24] Jebrail MJ, Bartsch MS, Patel KD. Digital microfluidics: a versatile tool for applications in chemistry, biology and medicine. Lab Chip 2012; 12(14): 2452-63.
[http://dx.doi.org/10.1039/c2lc40318h] [PMID: 22699371]

[25] Ding X, Li P, Lin S-CS, *et al.* Surface acoustic wave microfluidics. Lab Chip 2013; 13(18): 3626-49.
[http://dx.doi.org/10.1039/c3lc50361e] [PMID: 23900527]

[26] Guttenberg Z, Müller H, Habermüller H, *et al.* Planar chip device for PCR and hybridization with surface acoustic wave pump. Lab Chip 2005; 5(3): 308-17.
[http://dx.doi.org/10.1039/B412712A] [PMID: 15726207]

[27] Wang Z, Zhe J. Recent advances in particle and droplet manipulation for lab-on-a-chip devices based on surface acoustic waves. Lab Chip 2011; 11(7): 1280-5.
[http://dx.doi.org/10.1039/c0lc00527d] [PMID: 21301739]

[28] Yeo LY, Friend JR. Surface acoustic wave microfluidics. Annu Rev Fluid Mech 2014; 46: 379-406.
[http://dx.doi.org/10.1146/annurev-fluid-010313-141418]

[29] Chiou PY, Moon H, Toshiyoshi H, Kim C-J, Wu MC. Light actuation of liquid by optoelectrowetting. Sens Actuators A Phys 2003; 104(3): 222-8.
[http://dx.doi.org/10.1016/S0924-4247(03)00024-4]

[30]   Park S-Y, Teitell MA, Chiou EPY. Single-sided continuous optoelectrowetting (SCOEW) for droplet manipulation with light patterns. Lab Chip 2010; 10(13): 1655-61.
[http://dx.doi.org/10.1039/c001324b] [PMID: 20448870]

[31]   Chiou C-H, Shin DJ, Zhang Y, Wang T-H. Topography-assisted electromagnetic platform for blood-to-PCR in a droplet. Biosens Bioelectron 2013; 50: 91-9.
[http://dx.doi.org/10.1016/j.bios.2013.06.011] [PMID: 23835223]

[32]   Zhang Y, Park S, Liu K, Tsuan J, Yang S, Wang T-H. A surface topography assisted droplet manipulation platform for biomarker detection and pathogen identification. Lab Chip 2011; 11(3): 398-406.
[http://dx.doi.org/10.1039/C0LC00296H] [PMID: 21046055]

[33]   Zhang Y, Shin DJ, Wang T-H. Serial dilution via surface energy trap-assisted magnetic droplet manipulation. Lab Chip 2013; 13(24): 4827-31.
[http://dx.doi.org/10.1039/c3lc50915j] [PMID: 24162777]

[34]   Guo Z-G, Zhou F, Hao J-C, Liang Y-M, Liu W-M, Huck WTS. "Stick and slide" ferrofluidic droplets on superhydrophobic surfaces. Appl Phys Lett 2006; 89(8)081911
[http://dx.doi.org/10.1063/1.2336729]

[35]   Misuk V, Mai A, Giannopoulos K, Alobaid F, Epple B, Loewe H. Micro magnetofluidics: droplet manipulation of double emulsions based on paramagnetic ionic liquids. Lab Chip 2013; 13(23): 4542-8.
[http://dx.doi.org/10.1039/c3lc50897h] [PMID: 24108233]

[36]   Biswas S, Pomeau Y, Chaudhury MK. New Drop Fluidics Enabled by Magnetic-Field-Mediated Elastocapillary Transduction. Langmuir 2016; 32(27): 6860-70.
[http://dx.doi.org/10.1021/acs.langmuir.6b01782] [PMID: 27300489]

[37]   Seo KS, Wi R, Im SG. Kim DH. A superhydrophobic magnetic elastomer actuator for droplet motion control. Polym Adv Technol 2013; 24(12): 1075-80.
[http://dx.doi.org/10.1002/pat.3190]

[38]   Wenzel RN. Surface Roughness and Contact Angle. J Phys Chem 1949; 53(9): 1466-7.
[http://dx.doi.org/10.1021/j150474a015]

[39]   Long Z, Shetty AM, Solomon MJ, Larson RG. Fundamentals of magnet-actuated droplet manipulation on an open hydrophobic surface. Lab Chip 2009; 9(11): 1567-75.
[http://dx.doi.org/10.1039/b819818g] [PMID: 19458864]

[40]   Aussillous P, Quéré D. Liquid marbles. Nature 2001; 411(6840): 924-7.
[http://dx.doi.org/10.1038/35082026] [PMID: 11418851]

[41]   Zhao Y, Xu Z, Parhizkar M, Fang J, Wang X, Lin T. Magnetic liquid marbles, their manipulation and application in optical probing. Microfluid Nanofluidics 2012; 13(4): 555-64.
[http://dx.doi.org/10.1007/s10404-012-0976-9]

[42]   Zhao Y, Fang J, Wang H, Wang X, Lin T. Magnetic liquid marbles: manipulation of liquid droplets using highly hydrophobic Fe3O4 nanoparticles. Adv Mater 2010; 22(6): 707-10.
[http://dx.doi.org/10.1002/adma.200902512] [PMID: 20217774]

[43]   Ooi CH, Nguyen N-T. Manipulation of liquid marbles. Microfluid Nanofluidics 2015; 19(3): 483-95.
[http://dx.doi.org/10.1007/s10404-015-1595-z]

[44]   Khaw MK, Ooi CH, Mohd-Yasin F, Nguyen AV, Evans GM, Nguyen N-T. Dynamic behaviour of a magnetically actuated floating liquid marble. Microfluid Nanofluidics 2017; 21(6): 110.
[http://dx.doi.org/10.1007/s10404-017-1945-0]

[45]   Khaw MK, Ooi CH, Mohd-Yasin F, Vadivelu R, John JS, Nguyen N-T. Digital microfluidics with a magnetically actuated floating liquid marble. Lab Chip 2016; 16(12): 2211-8.
[http://dx.doi.org/10.1039/C6LC00378H] [PMID: 27191398]

[46] Tosun A, Erbil H. Evaporation rate of PTFE liquid marbles. Appl Surf Sci 2009; 256(5): 1278-83.
[http://dx.doi.org/10.1016/j.apsusc.2009.10.035]

[47] Dandan M, Erbil HY. Evaporation rate of graphite liquid marbles: comparison with water droplets. Langmuir 2009; 25(14): 8362-7.
[http://dx.doi.org/10.1021/la900729d] [PMID: 19499944]

[48] Chen G, Gao Y, Li M, Ji B, Tong R, Law M-K, *et al.* Rapid and flexible actuation of droplets via a low-adhesive and deformable magnetically functionalized membrane. J Mater Sci 2018; 53(18): 13253-63.
[http://dx.doi.org/10.1007/s10853-018-2563-2]

[49] Shikida M, Takayanagi K, Inouchi K, Honda H, Sato K. Using wettability and interfacial tension to handle droplets of magnetic beads in a micro-chemical-analysis system. Sens Actuators B Chem 2006; 113(1): 563-9.
[http://dx.doi.org/10.1016/j.snb.2005.01.029]

[50] Kim JA, Kim M, Kang SM, Lim KT, Kim TS, Kang JY. Magnetic bead droplet immunoassay of oligomer amyloid β for the diagnosis of Alzheimer's disease using micro-pillars to enhance the stability of the oil-water interface. Biosens Bioelectron 2015; 67: 724-32.
[http://dx.doi.org/10.1016/j.bios.2014.10.042] [PMID: 25459055]

[51] Shikida M, Nagao N, Imai R, Honda H, Okochi M, Ito H, *et al.* A palmtop-sized rotary-drive-type biochemical analysis system by magnetic bead handling. J Micromech Microeng 2008; 18(3)035034
[http://dx.doi.org/10.1088/0960-1317/18/3/035034]

[52] Shikida M, Takayanagi K, Honda H, Ito H, Sato K. Development of an enzymatic reaction device using magnetic bead-cluster handling. J Micromech Microeng 2006; 16(9): 1875.
[http://dx.doi.org/10.1088/0960-1317/16/9/017]

[53] Cho SK, Moon H, Kim C-J. Creating, transporting, cutting, and merging liquid droplets by electrowetting-based actuation for digital microfluidic circuits. J Microelectromech Syst 2003; 12(1): 70-80.
[http://dx.doi.org/10.1109/JMEMS.2002.807467]

[54] Berthier J, Dubois P, Clementz P, Claustre P, Peponnet C, Fouillet Y. Actuation potentials and capillary forces in electrowetting based microsystems. Sens Actuators A Phys 2007; 134(2): 471-9.
[http://dx.doi.org/10.1016/j.sna.2006.04.050]

[55] Ren H, Fair RB, Pollack MG. Automated on-chip droplet dispensing with volume control by electro-wetting actuation and capacitance metering. Sens Actuators B Chem 2004; 98(2-3): 319-27.
[http://dx.doi.org/10.1016/j.snb.2003.09.030]

[56] Shin DJ, Trick AY, Hsieh Y-H, Thomas DL, Wang T-H. Sample-to-answer droplet magnetofluidic platform for point-of-care hepatitis C viral load quantitation. Sci Rep 2018; 8(1): 9793.
[http://dx.doi.org/10.1038/s41598-018-28124-3] [PMID: 29955160]

[57] Sista R, Hua Z, Thwar P, *et al.* Development of a digital microfluidic platform for point of care testing. Lab Chip 2008; 8(12): 2091-104.
[http://dx.doi.org/10.1039/b814922d] [PMID: 19023472]

[58] Hua Z, Rouse JL, Eckhardt AE, *et al.* Multiplexed real-time polymerase chain reaction on a digital microfluidic platform. Anal Chem 2010; 82(6): 2310-6.
[http://dx.doi.org/10.1021/ac902510u] [PMID: 20151681]

[59] Ng AH, Choi K, Luoma RP, Robinson JM, Wheeler AR. Digital microfluidic magnetic separation for particle-based immunoassays. Anal Chem 2012; 84(20): 8805-12.
[http://dx.doi.org/10.1021/ac3020627] [PMID: 23013543]

[60] Ng AH, Lee M, Choi K, Fischer AT, Robinson JM, Wheeler AR. Digital microfluidic platform for the detection of rubella infection and immunity: a proof of concept. Clin Chem 2015; 61(2): 420-9.
[http://dx.doi.org/10.1373/clinchem.2014.232181] [PMID: 25512641]

[61]   Shamsi MH, Choi K, Ng AH, Wheeler AR. A digital microfluidic electrochemical immunoassay. Lab Chip 2014; 14(3): 547-54.
[http://dx.doi.org/10.1039/C3LC51063H] [PMID: 24292705]

[62]   Rackus DG, Dryden MD, Lamanna J, *et al.* A digital microfluidic device with integrated nanostructured microelectrodes for electrochemical immunoassays. Lab Chip 2015; 15(18): 3776-84.
[http://dx.doi.org/10.1039/C5LC00660K] [PMID: 26247922]

[63]   Ng AHC, Fobel R, Fobel C, *et al.* A digital microfluidic system for serological immunoassays in remote settings. Sci Transl Med 2018; 10(438)eaar6076
[http://dx.doi.org/10.1126/scitranslmed.aar6076] [PMID: 29695457]

[64]   Seale B, Lam C, Rackus DG, Chamberlain MD, Liu C, Wheeler AR. Digital Microfluidics for Immunoprecipitation. Anal Chem 2016; 88(20): 10223-30.
[http://dx.doi.org/10.1021/acs.analchem.6b02915] [PMID: 27700039]

[65]   Mei N, Seale B, Ng AH, Wheeler AR, Oleschuk R. Digital microfluidic platform for human plasma protein depletion. Anal Chem 2014; 86(16): 8466-72.
[http://dx.doi.org/10.1021/ac5022198] [PMID: 25058398]

[66]   Jones TB, Fowler JD, Chang YS, Kim C-J. Frequency-based relationship of electrowetting and dielectrophoretic liquid microactuation. Langmuir 2003; 19(18): 7646-51.
[http://dx.doi.org/10.1021/la0347511]

[67]   Ng AH, Li BB, Chamberlain MD, Wheeler AR. Digital microfluidic cell culture. Annu Rev Biomed Eng 2015; 17: 91-112.
[http://dx.doi.org/10.1146/annurev-bioeng-071114-040808] [PMID: 26643019]

[68]   Au SH, Fobel R, Desai SP, Voldman J, Wheeler AR. Cellular bias on the microscale: probing the effects of digital microfluidic actuation on mammalian cell health, fitness and phenotype. Integr Biol 2013; 5(8): 1014-25.
[http://dx.doi.org/10.1039/c3ib40104a] [PMID: 23770992]

[69]   Barbulovic-Nad I, Yang H, Park PS, Wheeler AR. Digital microfluidics for cell-based assays. Lab Chip 2008; 8(4): 519-26.
[http://dx.doi.org/10.1039/b717759c] [PMID: 18369505]

[70]   Barbulovic-Nad I, Au SH, Wheeler AR. A microfluidic platform for complete mammalian cell culture. Lab Chip 2010; 10(12): 1536-42.
[http://dx.doi.org/10.1039/c002147d] [PMID: 20393662]

[71]   Srigunapalan S, Eydelnant IA, Simmons CA, Wheeler AR. A digital microfluidic platform for primary cell culture and analysis. Lab Chip 2012; 12(2): 369-75.
[http://dx.doi.org/10.1039/C1LC20844F] [PMID: 22094822]

[72]   Zhou J, Lu L, Byrapogu K, Wootton DM, Lelkes PI, Fair R. Electrowetting-based multi-microfluidics array printing of high resolution tissue construct with embedded cells and growth factors. Virtual Phys Prototyp 2007; 2(4): 217-23.
[http://dx.doi.org/10.1080/17452750701747278]

[73]   Son SU, Garrell RL. Transport of live yeast and zebrafish embryo on a droplet digital microfluidic platform. Lab Chip 2009; 9(16): 2398-401.
[http://dx.doi.org/10.1039/b906257b] [PMID: 19636473]

[74]   Kanitthamniyom P, Zhang Y, Magnetic digital microfluidics on a bioinspired surface for point-of-care diagnostics of infectious disease. Electrophoresis 2019; 40: 1178–1185.
[http://dx.doi.org/10.1002/elps.201900074] [PMID: 30770588]

SUBJECT INDEX

A

Abnormal 350, 396, 401
  microtubule-associated tau proteins 350
  mitochondrial transport machinery 396
  neural transmissions 401
  protein aggregation processes 350
Acousto-optic modulators (AOMs) 232
Actin cytoskeleton 273
Activity 14, 15, 79, 141 177, 180, 185, 262,
      357, 361, 389, 390, 397, 396, 401, 403,
      437, 438, 442, 445, 450, 455
  catalytic 437, 438
  cellular 262
  conjugated enzyme 361
  cortical network 403
  cytochrome oxidase 397
  decreased bilateral inferior frontal 403
  electrical 262
  excessive left frontoparietal 403
  exonuclease 177
  fast spiking 401
  inhibited proteasome 396
  instrumental 390
  metabolic signaling pathway 397
  microglia 357
  neural 185
  protease 180
  small GTPases 180
  urease enzyme 141
Acute 107, 271 134
  myocardial infarction 107
  respiratory distress syndrome 271
  respiratory syndrome 134
Adsorption 7, 78, 79, 80, 124, 142, 171, 274
  electrostatic 78
  hydrogen 79, 80
Agents 68, 307, 312, 357, 366, 406, 416, 436,
      449, 450, 456, 489, 490
  bioterror 307
  first amyloid imaging PET 357
  infectious 436, 450, 456
  interfering 68, 366
  therapeutic 406

Aggregates 187, 393, 394, 397
  toxic cytoplasmic 393
Alkaline-phosphatase enzyme probe 89
Alternating current voltammetry (ACV) 90
Alumina membrane 414
  nanoporous 414
Alzheimer's 351, 354, 355, 366, 389
  CSF profile 354
  disease and related disorders association
      (ADRDA) 389
  disease brain tissue 351
  disease models 366
  disease neuroimaging initiative (ADNI)
      355
Amplicons 179, 324, 450
  self-probing 179
Amplification 6, 13, 213, 214, 228, 230, 311,
      312, 322, 439, 440, 443, 444, 446, 448,
      449, 456, 457
  downstream EXPAR 6
  enzymatic 322
  platinum nanocatalyst 13
Amplification process 5, 84
  downstream signal 5
Amyloidosis 350, 391
Amyloid precursor protein (APP) 349, 351,
      352, 396, 408
Amyotrophic Lateral Sclerosis 392, 403, 408,
      409, 410
Analyzers 233, 234 329, 399, 418, 419
  high-throughput exosome 418
  microfluidic biofluid 329
  rotating 234
  voltage-based nanoparticle 419
Android 320 414
  smartphone 320
  oxidation technique 414
Anti-avian influenza virus antibody 107
Antibiotics 319, 437, 492
  broad-spectrum 437
Antibodies 2, 7, 8, 82, 83, 106, 107, 108, 130,
      133, 138, 142, 146, 228, 319, 361, 362,
      365, 488, 489
  biotin-tagged 133

Nucleic acid 2, 3, 5, 10, 308, 312, 314, 321, 333, 336, 441, 442, 458
  amplification tests (NAATs) 308, 312, 314, 321, 333, 336
  Aptamers 441, 442
  hybridization 171
  modifications 458
  molecule 10
  probes 2, 3, 5
NW 121, 144
  gate bias configurations 121
  sensor 121, 144

O

Oligomers, detecting small nucleic acid 49
Oligonucleotide library 441
Oligonucleotides 83, 84, 87, 88, 89, 133, 177, 196, 228, 393, 440, 450, 451, 454, 455
  antisense 393
  folded single stranded 440
  hybridized 196
  labeled 450
  labelled 450
  random 440
  single-stranded 133, 455
  small sequence of 87, 88
  target-bound 440
Optical 37, 230
  heterodyne technique 230
  lithography techniques 37
Outer mitochondrial membrane (OMM) 394, 397
Ovarian cancer 108, 142
  epithelial 142
Oxidation 12, 29, 65, 66, 67, 69, 76, 78 79, 80, 81, 106, 107, 118, 119, 124, 394, 413
  electrochemical 79
  electrochemical-reduced graphene 413
  enzymatic 78
  lipid 394
  photo-induced 12
Oxidation reaction 67, 310
  water-activated 310
Oxidative stress 108, 388, 395, 397, 407, 420
  excessive 395
  increased 388
Oxygen plasma treatment 129

P

Paired helical filament (PHF) 400
Parkinson's disease (PD) 71, 108, 110, 391, 392, 394, 395, 397, 398, 400, 403, 406, 407, 408, 409
Pathogens 9, 49, 82, 230, 311, 312, 436, 437, 438, 441, 442, 444, 447, 450, 452, 456, 457, 459, 460, 486
  bacterial 9, 230, 438, 452, 486
  detecting food 49
  disease-causing 437
  urinary 82
Pathology 71, 348, 349, 350, 360, 367, 391, 419, 420
  amyloid 350
  histological 332
  vascular 349
  white matter 360
Peptide nucleic acid (PNA) 7, 106, 109, 118, 188
Photo-elastic modulation (PEM) 234, 235
Photoinduced electron transfer (PET) 172, 176, 182, 183, 311, 347, 357, 388, 390, 400, 409
Photonic crystal-enhanced microscopy (PCEM) 41
Photoresists, conventional 46
Physical deposition methods 30
Pittsburgh compound B (PiB) 357, 399, 400, 409
Plasma 355, 409
  tau proteins 355
  uric acid 409
Plasmodium falciparum 441, 450
Plasmonic nanostructures 218, 219, 222, 238, 248, 249
  subwavelength 219
Plasmonic nanotechnology 218
Polymerase chain reaction (PCR) 84, 177, 178, 196, 197, 310, 311, 440, 443, 444, 449, 453, 457, 472, 486
Presynaptic 356
  plasma membrane protein 356
  vesicle protein 356
Principal component analysis (PCA) 326, 329, 400
Printed circuit board (PCB) 116, 414, 476
Probe protein-protein interactions 184

Chuang & Ho

Prognosis 100, 261, 347, 351, 369, 392, 403,
    407, 422
Progression 261, 288 354, 355, 357, 359, 360,
    368, 390, 397, 401, 402, 403, 410
  of Alzheimer's disease 390
  retrogenesis 360
  shear-mediated 288
  topographical neurodegeneration 359
Properties 116, 147, 261, 263, 276, 417, 454,
    456
  electrical 116, 147, 276, 454
  electrochemical 456
  haemorheological 292
  magnetic oscillation 417
  mechanical 263
  non-Newtonian 261
Prostate-specific antigen (PSA) 108, 109, 117,
    118, 135, 136, 138, 142
Protein(s) 51, 134, 141, 142, 146, 173, 184,
    185, 187, 189, 196, 197, 262, 308, 318,
    319, 351, 353, 356, 357, 388, 393, 394,
    395, 396, 397, 405, 406, 487, 490
  bacterial 308
  Based Assay 487
  dysfunctional 397
  enzyme 184
  fusion 186
  induced fluorescence enhancement (PIFE)
    173
  keratin 146
  misfolded 388, 406
  nucleocapsid 134
  phosphorylated 353
  synaptic 356, 357
  tetracysteine-tagged 189
  toxic 351, 406
  transmembrane 262
Proteostasis 393
Proton motive force (PMF) 394
Pseudomonas aeruginosa 442
PVC 71
  based composite membranes 71
  Membrane-Containing Sensors 71

Q

Quantum dot (QDs) 15, 49, 50, 172, 173, 174,
    181, 324, 326, 414, 416, 454, 455
Quartz crystal microbalances (QCM) 44, 45,
    148

R

Radio frequency (RF) 31
Radioimmunoassay 2, 8
Raman spectroscopy 250
Rationalized fabrication procedure 126
RBC 264, 265, 266, 267, 269, 274, 275, 276
  aggregation, measurement of 274, 276
  deformability reduced 269
  deformation 264, 265, 266, 267
  depleted plasma 275
  in passing funnel constriction 265
RCA 140, 141, 445
  amplified detection process 140
  based assay 445
  reaction 140
  technique 141
Reactions 32, 37, 38, 39, 45, 65, 66, 72, 79,
    80, 81, 82, 86, 110, 140, 171, 290, 311,
    438, 441, 442, 444, 447
  antibody-antigen 311
  aptamer-target 441
  assay 472
  biocatalytic 89
  chemical 32, 65, 171, 290, 438, 441
  electrochemical 66, 82
  enzyme-catalyzed 72
  photochemical 37, 38
  urease enzyme 140
Real-time 10, 332
    machine learning analysis 332
    multiple targets tracking 10
Red blood cell (RBCs) 12, 261, 262, 263, 265,
    266, 267, 268, 269, 270, 273, 274, 276,
    277, 291
Redox reaction 3, 65, 67, 68, 413
Reduction 66, 118, 129, 388, 391, 417
  immunomagnetic 388, 391, 417
  nanowire width 118
  reaction 66, 129
Regulation 87, 334, 397
  mitochondrial dynamics 397
  post-transcriptional 87
Relative angle shift (RAS) 226, 227
Remote image analysis 321
Resistance 67, 71, 264, 272, 274, 418, 436,
    441
  charge transfer 67
  fluidic 418

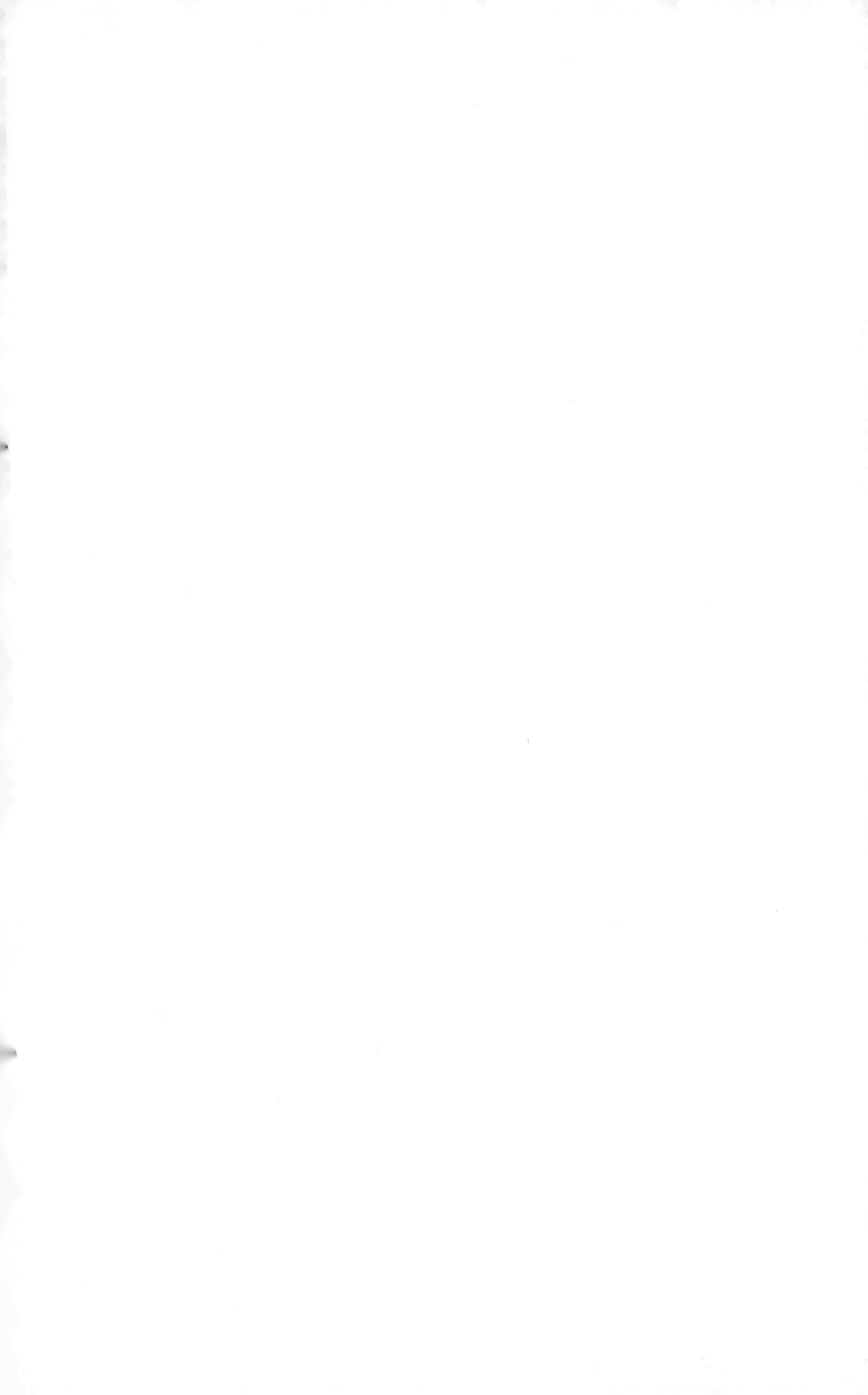

*9 789811 464782 *